I0044322

Hematology: Blood Cells Research

Hematology: Blood Cells Research

Editor: Martha Roper

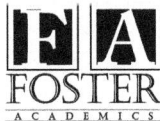

FA
FOSTER
ACADEMICS

www.fosteracademics.com

www.fosteracademics.com

FA
FOSTER
ACADEMICS

Cataloging-in-Publication Data

Hematology : blood cells research / edited by Martha Roper.
    p. cm.
Includes bibliographical references and index.
ISBN 978-1-63242-481-5
1. Hematology. 2. Blood cells. 3. Blood--Diseases. I. Roper, Martha.
RC636 .H46 2017
616.15--dc23

© Foster Academics, 2017

Foster Academics,
118-35 Queens Blvd., Suite 400,
Forest Hills, NY 11375, USA

ISBN 978-1-63242-481-5 (Hardback)

This book contains information obtained from authentic and highly regarded sources. Copyright for all individual chapters remain with the respective authors as indicated. All chapters are published with permission under the Creative Commons Attribution License or equivalent. A wide variety of references are listed. Permission and sources are indicated; for detailed attributions, please refer to the permissions page and list of contributors. Reasonable efforts have been made to publish reliable data and information, but the authors, editors and publisher cannot assume any responsibility for the validity of all materials or the consequences of their use.

Trademark Notice: Registered trademark of products or corporate names are used only for explanation and identification without intent to infringe.

Printed and bound in the United States of America.

Contents

Preface

Blood cells refer to the cells formed by hematopoiesis in the blood. They are also referred to as haematopoietic cells, hematocyte, etc. Hematology comprises the study of blood and blood cells along with the diseases related to it. The aim of this text is to familiarize the readers with all the important topics of hematology and its research. While understanding the long-term perspectives of the topics, the book makes an effort in highlighting their impact as a modern tool for the growth of the discipline. The various studies that are constantly contributing towards advancing technologies and evolution of this field are examined in detail in the text. It is an essential guide for both academicians and those who wish to pursue this discipline further.

All of the data presented henceforth, was collaborated in the wake of recent advancements in the field. The aim of this book is to present the diversified developments from across the globe in a comprehensible manner. The opinions expressed in each chapter belong solely to the contributing authors. Their interpretations of the topics are the integral part of this book, which I have carefully compiled for a better understanding of the readers.

At the end, I would like to thank all those who dedicated their time and efforts for the successful completion of this book. I also wish to convey my gratitude towards my friends and family who supported me at every step.

Editor

Effects of Danshensu on Platelet Aggregation and Thrombosis: *In Vivo* Arteriovenous Shunt and Venous Thrombosis Models in Rats

Chen Yu[1*◊], **Dong Qi**[2◊], **Wei Lian**[3], **Qing-Zhong Li**[1], **Hong-Juan Li**[1], **Hua-Ying Fan**[4*]

1 School of Pharmacy, Binzhou Medical University, Yantai, Shandong, China, 2 Department of Nephrology, Yantai Yu-Huang-Ding/Qingdao University Hospital, Yantai, Shandong, China, 3 Yantai Yan-Tai-Shan Hospital, Yantai, Shandong, China, 4 School of Pharmacy, Yantai University, Yantai, Shandong, China

Abstract

Danshensu, a type of dihydroxyphenyl lactic acid, is one of the most abundant active phenolic acids in the dried root of *Salvia miltiorrhizae* (Lamiaceae)—widely used traditional Chinese medicine. The effects of danshensu on platelet aggregation and thrombus formation in rats were examined using various methods. It was found that danshensu significantly reduced thrombus weight in 2 experimental thrombosis models; dose-dependent inhibition of adenosine diphosphate (ADP) and arachidonic acid (AA)-induced platelet aggregation occurred in normal and blood stasis-induced rats; Danshensu also significantly mitigated blood viscosity, plasma viscosity and hematocrit levels. Moreover, danshensu significantly inhibited venous thrombosis-induced expression of cyclooxygenases-2 (COX-2) rather than cyclooxygenases-1(COX-1) in the venous walls, down regulated thromboxane B_2 (TXB$_2$) and up regulated 6-keto prostaglandin $F_{1\alpha}$ (6-keto-PGF$_{1\alpha}$), normalizing the TXB$_2$/6-keto-PGF$_{1\alpha}$ ratio. In addition, danshensu did not induce gastric lesions and even had protective effects on aspirin-induced ulcer formation at doses as high as 60 mg/kg. These findings suggest that the antithrombotic and antiplatelet aggregation effects of danshensu are attributed to its highly selective inhibition of COX-2 and ability to normalize the thromboxane A$_2$(TXA$_2$)/prostacyclin(PGI$_2$) balance. These findings suggest that danshensu have great prospects in antithrombotic and antiplatelet therapy.

Editor: Pablo Garcia de Frutos, IIBB-CSIC-IDIBAPS, Spain

Funding: This study was supported by the Project of National Natural Science Foundation of China (Grant No. 81303259), URL: http://www.nsfc.gov.cn/, Shandong Province Natural Science Foundation (No. ZR2010HL065), URL: http://www.sdnsf.gov.cn/portal/, Research Award Fund for Outstanding Young and Middle-aged Scientists of Shandong Province of China (project No. BS2013YY046), URL: http://www.sdstc.gov.cn/, and the Programs for Science and Technology Development and Plan of Yanta (No. 2013WS262), URL: http://www.ytstc.gov.cn/. The funders had no role in study design, data collection and analysis, decision to publish, or preparation of the manuscript.

Competing Interests: The authors have declared that no competing interests exist.

* Email: yuchen810624@163.com (CY); katiefhydong@sina.com (HYF)

◊ These authors contributed equally to this work.

Introduction

Thrombus formation accelerates the progression of various cardiovascular and cerebrovascular disorders. Thromboembolic complications of arteriosclerosis, heart attack, stroke and peripheral vascular disease are the principal causes of death in developed countries. Arterial and venous thrombi comprises primarily platelet aggregates.

Platelets mediate the initiation of thrombosis through platelet adhesion, activation and aggregation [1]. A collaborative meta-analysis of randomized trials has demonstrated that antiplatelet therapy is beneficial in treating thromboembolic diseases and preventing serious vascular events, arterial occlusion and venous thromboembolism in a wide range of patients who are at high risk for occlusive vascular events [2]. Thus, the inhibition of platelet function has the potential to treat circulatory diseases, spurring the development of many antiplatelet and antithrombotic agents and prompting an examination of their effects in preventing thrombosis.

Danshen, the dried root of *Salvia miltiorrhizae* (Lamiaceae), is one of the most widely used traditional herbal medicines against various cardiovascular and cerebrovascular diseases, including coronary heart disease, myocardial infarction, stroke and hypertension. Danshen contains hydrophilic phenolics and lipophilic quinones, which have many pharmacological and therapeutic properties [3].

Increasing data have demonstrated that danshensu is an abundant and representative phenolic acid in danshen [4]. Danshensu (chemical structure shown in Fig. 1) known as β 3,4-dihydroxyphenyl-lactic acid—has several mechanisms by which it elicits its therapeutic effects. Danshensu can mitigate cardiovascular and cerebrovascular disturbances [5] by improving microcirculation, increasing blood flow, relaxing the coronary arteries and promoting anticoagulation [6].

However, the antithrombotic and antiplatelet effects and mechanisms of danshensu are unknown. The purpose of this study was to determine the effects and mechanisms of danshensu with regard to platelet aggregation, thrombus formation and blood circulation so as to provide pharmacological evidence that supports its clinical application.

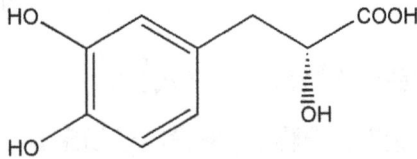

Figure 1. Chemical structure of danshensu ($C_9H_{10}O_5$, molecular weight = 198.17).

Results

Effects on platelet aggregation *in vivo*

To assess the effect of danshensu on platelet aggregation, we measured the inhibition of platelet aggregation on danshensu induced by ADP and AA in normal rats. As shown in Fig. 2, compared with the control group, ADP and AA-induced platelet aggregation was altered by pretreatment with danshensu and aspirin. Danshensu dose-dependently inhibited AA-induced platelet aggregation by approximately 13.9% at 15 mg/kg, 17.9% at 30 mg/kg and 21.5% at 60 mg/kg, respectively. This result showed that similar inhibition in the ADP-induced platelet aggregation. The inhibition of platelet aggregation induced by ADP was 10.5%, 14.6% and 23.5% at doses of 15, 30, and 60 mg/kg, respectively.

Further, we determined effect of danshensu on platelet aggregation in blood stasis rats induced by AA. Blood stasis increased platelet aggregation compared with the control group as shown in Fig. 3, which was also modified by pretreatment with danshensu in a dose-dependent manner. This inhibitory effect of danshensu at dose of 60 mg/kg was comparable with that of aspirin at 20 mg/kg in blood stasis rats.

Effect on thrombus formation

Two rat models of thrombosis were developed by installing an arteriovenous shunt and ligating the inferior vena cava to study the antithrombotic activity and mechanism of danshensu *in vivo*. Pretreatment with danshensu (15 to 60 mg/kg) decreased throm-

bus formation dose-dependently in the arteriovenous shunt model. The inhibition of thrombus formation was about 12.6%, 18.2% and 29.6% respectively (Fig. 4).

As shown in Fig. 5, this result was confirmed by inferior vena cava model. Residual thrombi from the occlusive vessels of all rats were measured. Compared with the thrombotic control group, aspirin at 20 mg/kg decreased the thrombus weight from 35.37 ± 3.03 mg to 24.14 ± 4.23 mg versus 29.65 ± 5.62 mg with 15 mg/kg, 25.78 ± 3.95 mg with 30 mg/kg and 23.84 ± 2.26 mg with 60 mg/kg of danshensu, respectively. Antithrombotic activity of danshensu at dose of 60 mg/kg is comparable with that of aspirin at 20 mg/kg.

Effects on COX and possible mechanisms

Inhibitory effects of danshensu and aspirin against 2 cyclooxygenases (COX) isoforms were first examined *in vitro* using enzymatic assays. While danshensu had little inhibitory effect on COX-1, danshensu decreased COX-2 activity at 20 to 200 μM even at 200 μM yielding an IC_{50} value of approximately 44 μM (Fig. 6 A vs B).

In contrast, aspirin inhibited COX-1 and COX-2, with geometric mean IC_{50} values of 39.8 and 60.7 μM, respectively. The IC_{50} ratios of COX-1 to COX-2 for danshensu and aspirin exceeded 10 and 0.67 respectively, it is demonstrated that danshensu selectively inhibits COX-2 over COX-1 by approximately 20-fold.

The effects of danshensu on COX-1 and COX-2 levels were examined using western blot technique. As shown in Fig. 7, the expression of COX-1 and COX-2 induced by inferior vena cava ligation was significantly elevated when compared with control group. It is clear that aspirin significantly inhibited both COX-1 and COX-2 expression while danshenu only significantly inhibited COX-2 but not COX-1 expression (Fig. 7B vs D). This observation indicates that danshensu exerts its antiplatelet effect by selectively targeting on COX-2.

Next, we measured the serum concentrations of TXB_2 and 6-keto-PGF1α in the rats. TXB_2 and 6-keto-PGF$_{1\alpha}$ levels increased significantly, accompanying a rise in the TXB_2/6-keto-PGF$_{1\alpha}$

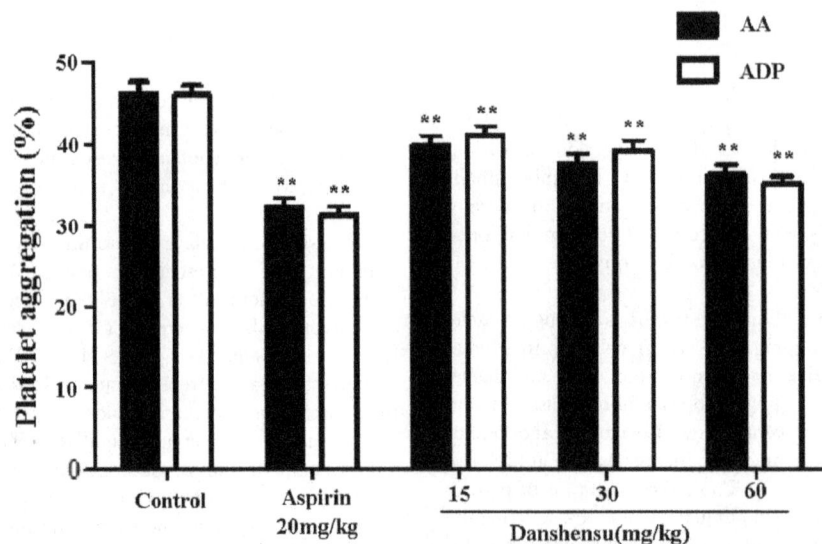

Figure 2. Effect of danshensu on platelet aggregation in normal rats. Blood was drawn 60 min after intragastric danshensu administration. Platelet aggregation was induced by diphosphate (ADP) and arachidonic acid (AA). Data are expressed as mean ± SEM (each group, n = 10). **$P < 0.01$ with control group.

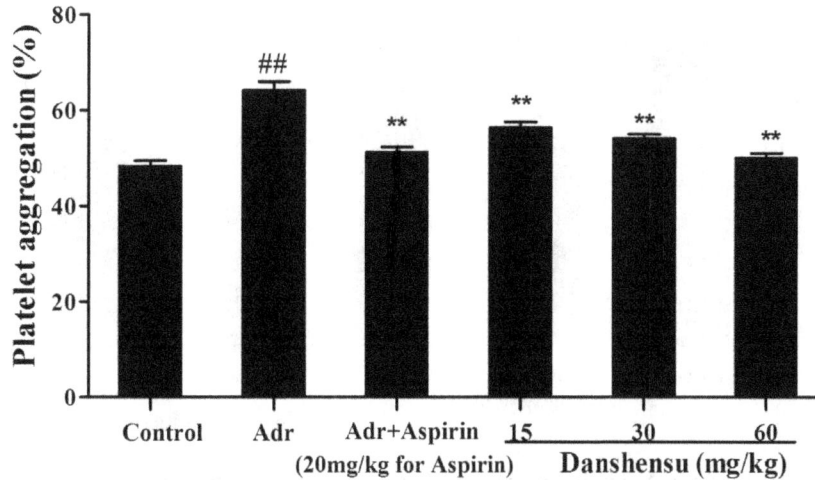

Figure 3. Effect of danshensu on platelet aggregation in blood stasis rats. Blood was drawn 60 min after intragastric danshensu administration. Platelet aggregation was induced by arachidonic acid (AA). Data are expressed as mean ± SEM (each group, n = 10). The blood stasis model was built during the interval between when 2 injections of adrenaline hydrochloride (Adr) were given to rats placed in ice-cold water. ##$P <$ 0.01 compared with normal control. *$P <$0.05 **$P <$0.01 compared with Adr control.

ratio in the 2 thrombosis models. Aspirin significantly reduced TXB_2 and 6-keto-$PGF_{1\alpha}$ levels, decreasing the TXB_2/6-keto-$PGF_{1\alpha}$ ratio. Danshensu downregulated TXB_2 and increased 6-keto-$PGF_{1\alpha}$ levels, especially at 30 and 60 mg/kg, normalizing the TXB_2/6-keto-$PGF_{1\alpha}$ ratio better than aspirin (Tables 1 and 2).

Effect on hemorheology

whole blood viscosity (WBV) at all shear rates, plasma viscosity (PV) and hematocrit values (Hct) significantly rose in blood stasis rats, but danshensu significantly reduced blood viscosity, plasma viscosity and hematocrit, particularly at 30 and 60 mg/kg (Table 3).

Protective effects of danshensu on gastric mucosa

We examined the gastrointestinal (GI) effects of oral administration of danshensu and aspirin in rats for 7 days. The ulcer index for all groups is summarized in Fig. 8. Aspirin resulted in gastric lesions and the ulcer index was significantly higher than the

control group. In contrast, danshensu did not induce gastric lesions, even at as high as 60 mg/kg.

We also investigated the effect of danshensu on aspirin-induced gastric lesions. The macroscopic findings of open stomachs are shown in Fig. 9A, we found that oral administration of aspirin (200 mg/kg body weight) induced severe mucosal damage in the gastric corpus of mice. Danshensu had no damaging effects on the stomach. In addition co-administration of danshensu with aspirin could inhibit aspirin-induced ulcer formation. Fig. 9B shows the ulcer score of gastric hemorrhagic ulcers in each group. These data suggest that danshensu has gastroprotective activities and it also prevents aspirin-induced gastric ulcer formation.

Discussion

Many life-threatening diseases, such as atherosclerosis, cerebrovascular thrombosis, coronary artery disease, stroke and tumor metastasis are related with platelet dysfunctions [7]. Many

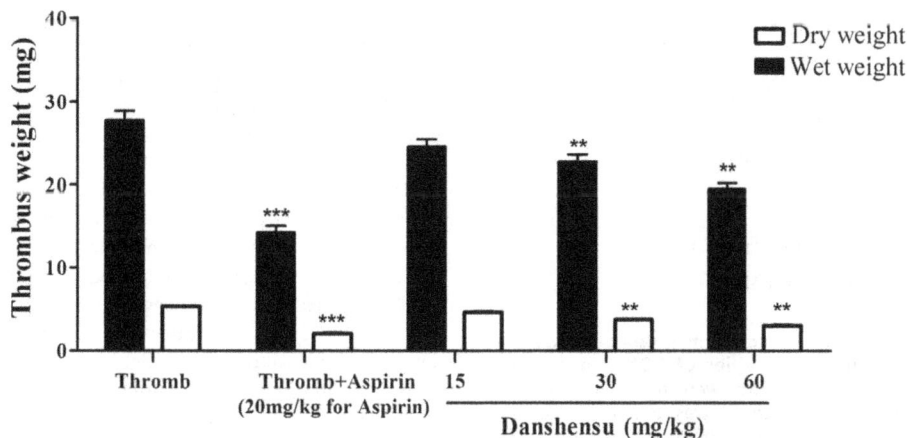

Figure 4. Antithrombotic activity of danshensu in the rat model of arteriovenous shunt. The drug or solvent was administered orally 60 min before thrombogenic challenge. Data are expressed as mean ± SEM (each group, n = 10). Thromb: thrombosis. *$P <$0.05, **$P <$0.01, ***$P <$ 0.001 compared with thrombotic control group.

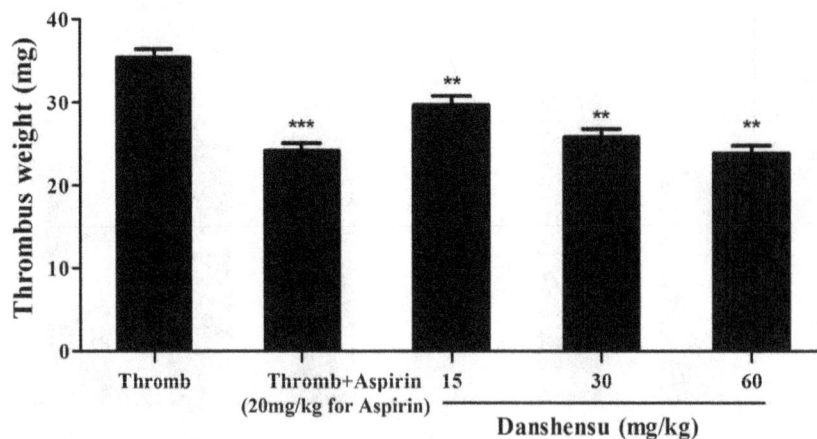

Figure 5. Antithrombotic activity of danshensu in the rat model of ligating inferior vena cava. The drug or solvent was administered orally 60 min before the thrombogenic challenge. Data are expressed as mean ± SEM (each group, n = 10). Thromb: thrombosis. *$P<0.05$, **$P<0.01$, ***$P<0.001$ compared with thrombotic control group.

available antiplatelet agents interfere with platelet function at various levels of activation, which results in several clinical disadvantages, including gastrointestinal side effects and hemorrhage. For this reason, a search for safer and more effective

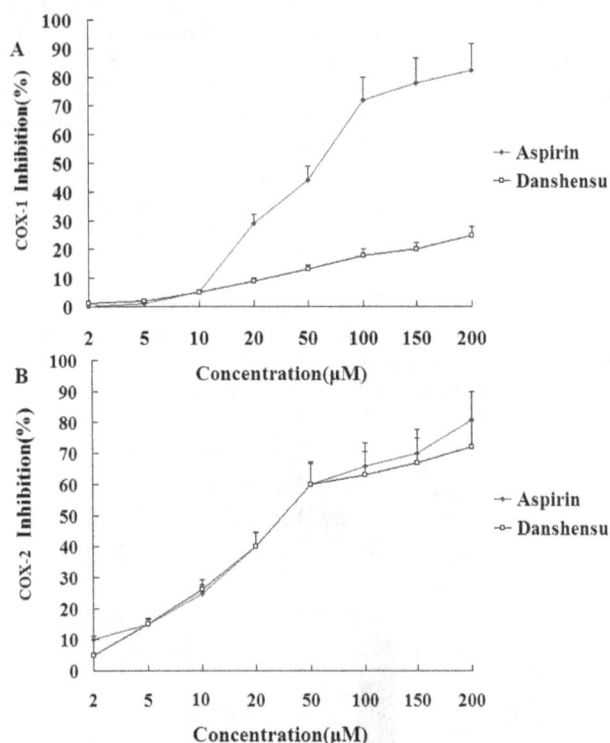

Figure 6. Direct effect of various concentrations of danshensu and aspirin on the enzymatic activities of COX-1 and COX-2. Danshensu and aspirin (water, as a control) were incubated with COX-1 (A) or COX-2 (B) for 10 min and then AA was added. COX enzyme activities are reflected by the amount of PGE_2 produced. PGE_2 production was measured by ELISA. Enzyme activity in the sample without treatment (water alone) served as control and results are expressed as inhibitory rate of COX-1 and COX-2 activity compared with solvent control.

antiplatelet agents without these adverse effects would be highly desirable. In recent years, new therapeutic agents have been derived from Chinese herbs and there is growing interest in this area.

In this study, we examined the antiplatelet and antithrombotic effects of danshensu and the pharmacological mechanisms. We determined effects of danshensu on platelet function by measuring ADP and AA-induced platelet aggregation. Our results showed that danshensu produced marked antiplatelet effect on ADP and AA platelet agonists ex vivo aggregation. This inhibitory effect of danshensu at dose of 60 mg/kg was comparable with aspirin at 20 mg/kg in blood stasis-induced rats.

The effects of danshensu on thrombus formation were studied in arteriovenous shunt model and inferior vena cava model; these models simulate arterial and venous thrombosis observed in humans [8]. Our results demonstrated that danshensu has potent antithrombotic effects against arterial and venous thrombosis.

To assess the effect of danshensu on microcirculation, we evaluated hemorheologic parameters in blood stasis model. Blood stasis can result in platelet aggregation and hemorheological abnormalities. Hemorheological disorders mediate the pathogenesis and development of many cardiovascular and cerebrovascular diseases [9]. In this study, rats were injected subcutaneously with adrenaline hydrochloride (Adr) and treated with cold stress. As a result, blood viscosity, plasma viscosity and hematocrit increased significantly compared with the control group. Our results suggest that Adr combined with exposure to ice-cold water induces blood stasis resulting in hemorheological abnormalities. Platelet aggregation is believed to be a factor that determines blood viscosity [10], consistent with our results that danshensu improves hemorheologic parameters, ameliorates blood stasis and promotes circulation by decreasing whole blood viscosity, secondary to the inhibitory effect on platelet aggregation.

In our study, Danshensu exhibited apparent antiplatelet and antithrombotic activity. In order to explore the further mechanisms of antiplatelet and anti-thrombosis, the activity and expression of COXs were measured. We also evaluated the levels of TXB_2 and 6-keto-$PGF_{1\alpha}$ in both arterial and venous thrombosis models. Our results indicated that danshensu could selectively inhibit COX-2 rather than COX-1 to regulate the balance of TXA_2/PGI_2. Therefore, danshensu exhibited superior antiplatelet and antithrombotic effects compared with aspirin.

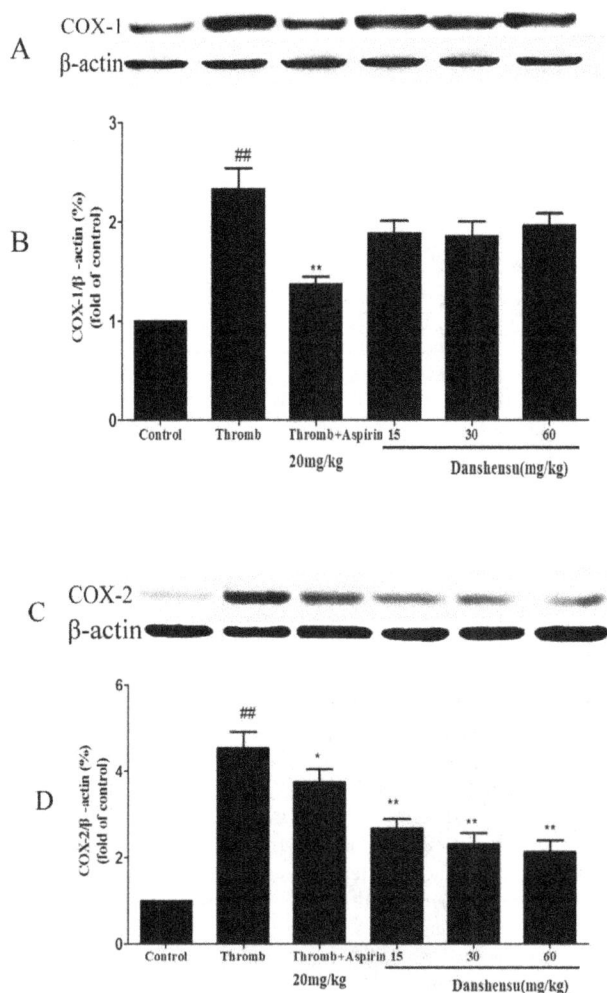

Figure 7. The effects of danshensu on COX expression. Rats were given 15, 30 and 60 mg/kg danshensu intragastrically and 20 mg/kg aspirin for 7 days. Venous thrombus formation was induced by inferior vena cava (IVC) ligation to produce thrombus after last administration.Vein walls were harvested from venous thrombosis and the expression of COX-1 and COX-2 was assessed by western analysis (A and C). β-actin was measured to confirm equal loading of proteins. Densitometric analysis of COX-1 (B) and COX-2 (D) expression is represented by the mean from 3 separate experiments. Data were normalized to β-actin levels. Thromb: thrombosis. ##$P<0.01$ compared with normal control. *$P<0.05$, **$P<0.01$ compared with thrombotic control group.

Disruption of the TXA_2-PGI_2 balance increases the risk of thrombosis [11]. TXA_2 and PGI_2 are metabolites of arachidonic acid, which is hydrolyzed by COXs and transformed into endoperoxides, prostaglandins (PGs) and TXA_2 [12]. COXs exist as 2 distinct isoforms: COX-1 and COX-2. COX-1 which is constitutively expressed in most tissues and has high levels of activity in the the gastrointestinal tract, is thought to exert homeostatic properties that are crucial for gastric physiologic function, including mucosal protectionwhereas COX-2 is absent from most healthy tissues but is induced by proinflammatory and proliferative stimuli after exposure to cytokines, immunological stimuli and growth factors [13,14]. TXA_2 is a potent inducer of platelet aggregation and vasoconstriction and its levels rise in thrombus models. In contrast, PGI_2 is a potent platelet inhibitor.

An increase in TXA_2 results in the adhesion, aggregation and release of platelets. However, PGI_2 inhibits platelet aggregation [15,16]. In our study, aspirin significantly decreased both TXB_2 and 6-keto-$PGF_{1\alpha}$ levels due to its non-selective and irreversible COX inhibition. Aspirin exerts its antiplatelet activity through inhibition of both COX-1 and COX-2, therefore inhibits not only the production of TXA_2 in platelets, but also the production of anti-aggregatory PGI_2 in vessel walls. This phenomenon is referred to as the "aspirin dilemma"[17] and is considered to be a reason underlying the insufficient efficacy and unclear dose–response effects of aspirin [18,19]. Compared with aspirin, danshensu with higher selectivity for COX-2 is able to normalize the TXA_2/PGI_2 balance better, by upregulating 6-keto-$PGF_{1\alpha}$ and downregulating TXB_2 simultaneously.

Finally, we evaluated the protective effects of danshensu on gastric mucosa. We compared the ulcerogenic effects of danshensu and aspirin on gastric mucosa and demonstrated that danshensu did not cause any apparent ulceration of the gastric mucosa in rats, even at a dose of 60 mg/kg. In contrast, aspirin had a potent ulcerogenic effect at the antithrombotic dose(20 mg/kg) and produced severe hemorrhagic necrotic lesions in the gastric mucosa even at a dose of 200 mg/kg Aspirin-induced gastric lesion was completely inhibited by the coadministration of danshensu. The observed differences in gastric ulcerogenic properties between danshensu and aspirin may be related with the difference in COX-1 selectivity. COX-1-derived PGs are thought to play a dominant role in gastric mucosal defense and cytoprotection and it has been confirmed that selective inhibition of COX-1 alone may not cause ulcers, but inhibition of both COX-1 and COX-2 is required for the development of gastric lesions [20,21]. Thus, danshensu by selectively inhibit COX-2 only, is considered to be potentially less damaging to the gastrointestinal tract than aspirin that also block COX-1.

In conclusion, our findings suggest that danshensu has potent antithrombotic effects and antiplatelet aggregation activity without inducing GI adverse events. This might be attributed to danshensu's mechanism of its functions as a highly selective COX-2 inhibitor with an ability to normalize TXA_2/PGI_2 balance superior to aspirin. Thus, Danshensu may have good prospects in antithrombotic and antiplatelet therapy.

Materials and Methods

Chemicals and reagents

Danshensu (purity 98%) was provided by Nanjing Zelang Medical Biological Technology Co. Ltd (Nanjing, China). Aspirin (purity 98%) was produced by Anhui Fengyuan Pharmaceutical Co. Ltd (Anhui, China). Arachidonic acid (AA) was purchased from Sigma-Aldrich Chemical Co. (USA). Heparin sodium was purchased from Jiangsu Wanbang Biochemical Medicine Co. Ltd. (Jiangsu, China). Adrenaline hydrochloride was purchased from Tianjin Jinyao Amino Acids Co. Ltd. (Tianjin, China). COX inhibitor screening assay kits were purchased from Cayman Chemical Company (Ann Arbor, MI, USA). Primary antibodies against COX-1, COX-2, β-actin and horseradish peroxidase (HRP)-conjugated secondary antibody were purchased from Santa Cruz Biotechnology, Inc. The thromboxane B_2 (TXB_2) and 6-keto prostaglandin $F_{1\alpha}$ (6-keto-$PGF_{1\alpha}$) radioimmunoassay kits were produced by Tianjin Jiuding Engineering of Medicine and Biology Co. Ltd. (Tianjin, China).

Animals and treatments

Male Sprague-Dawley rats (weight approximately 300 g, 3–4 months each) were purchased from Shandong Lvye Pharmaceu-

Table 1. Effects of danshensu on plasma TXB_2 and 6-keto-$PGF_{1\alpha}$ levels and TXB_2-6-keto-$PGF_{1\alpha}$ ratio in rats in the arteriovenous shunt model.

Group	Dose(mg/kg)	TXB_2 (pg/mL)	6-keto-$PGF_{1\alpha}$ (pg/mL)	TXB_2/6-keto-$PGF_{1\alpha}$
Normal		180.0±8.3	487.3±16.6	0.38±0.01
Thromb		552.2±18.9##	602.5±20.4##	0.93±0.03##
Thromb+Aspirin	20	56.5±1.9***	190.5±7.5***	0.30±0.01***
Thromb +Danshensu	15	258.1±10.2**	621.7±19.8*	0.40±0.01**
	30	228.7±11.5**	638.3±22.1**	0.37±0.02**
	60	206.4±8.9**	649.2±15.8**	0.35±0.02**

Blood was drawn from the abdominal aorta at the end of arteriovenous shunt test period and anticoagulated with indomethacin-EDTA-Na_2. Plasma samples were prepared by centrifugation and analyzed by radioimmunoassay. Data are expressed as mean±SEM (each group, n=10). #$P<0.05$, ##$P<0.01$ compared with normal group, *$P<0.05$, **$P<0.01$, ***$P<0.001$ compared with thrombotic control group.

tical Co. Ltd., China (certificate No. SCXK (Lu) 20030008). Male ICR mice (weight approximately 25 g, 8–9 weeks each) were purchased from the Animal Department of the College of Medicine, Beijing University (certificate no. SCXK (Jing) 2006–0008).

Animals were acclimated for at least 1 week to a temperature of 24±1°C and humidity of 55±5%. The animals were maintained with free access to standard diet and tap water. The experimental procedures were approved by the Office of Experimental Animal Management.

Committee of Shandong Province, China (certificate No. SYXK (Lu) 20090015). Rats were given 15, 30 and 60 mg/kg danshensu and 20 mg/kg aspirin intragastrically (i.g.). All drugs were dissolved in 0.9% normal saline as vehicle. The control rats were given 0.9% normal saline. All drugs and saline were administered orally to rats once daily at 9 AM for 7 days. All *in vivo* experiments were conducted 60 min after the treatment.

Assay of *ex vivo* Platelet Aggregation in Rats

Blood was collected after the last administration of danshensu and saline. All rats were anesthetized with 10% chloral hydrate and blood was collected from the abdominal aorta and anticoagulated with citrate (3.8%; 1 vol anticoagulant: 9 vol blood). Platelet-rich plasma (PRP) was prepared by centrifuging the blood at 1000 rpm for 8 min and at 3000 rpm for 15 min to prepare platelet-poor plasma (PPP). The platelet concentration was adjusted to $1.8-2\times10^9$/mL with PPP. Then, 0.3 mL of PRP was placed in a cuvette and stirred with a rotor at 37°C for 5 min,

after which 6 μM ADP and 100 μM AA was added. Aggregation was measured with a platelet aggregometer (LBY-NJ4, Pulisheng Instrument Co. Ltd. China). Results were recorded as light transmission at maximal aggregation after the addition of an aggregating agent. Data are expressed as percentage of maximal aggregation.

In vivo arteriovenous shunt thrombosis

Rat arterial-venous shunts (silk thread model) were prepared with 2 2-cm-long polyethylene tubes (1 mm i.d.), linked by a central section (8 cm long; 2 mm i.d.) that contained a 5-cm piece of silk thread and was filled with saline solution that contained heparin 50 U/kg. Rats were anesthetized with chloral hydrate (350 mg/kg, i.p.) and an arterial-venous shunt was placed between the right carotid artery and left jugular vein [22,23]. After blood was circulated through the shunt for 15 minutes, both ends of the tube were pinched, the silk thread was removed from the shunt tube and the wet and dry weights were measured by subtracting the pre-experiment weight of the 5-cm silk thread. The rate of inhibition of thrombosis formation was calculated as inhibition (%) = (A-A_1)/A×100%, where A is the thrombus weight of the thrombosis control group and A_1 is the weight after treatment with the agents. The sham group did not undergo the surgery. All rats fasted overnight before the operation.

Venous thrombosis model

Venous thrombus formation was induced by inferior vena cava (IVC) ligation to produce a stasis thrombus as described [24,25].

Table 2. Effects of danshensu on plasma TXB_2 and 6-keto-$PGF_{1\alpha}$ levels and TXB_2-6-keto-$PGF_{1\alpha}$ ratio in rats the venous thrombosis model.

Group	Dose(mg/kg)	TXB_2 (pg/mL)	6-keto-$PGF_{1\alpha}$ (pg/mL)	TXB_2/6-keto-$PGF_{1\alpha}$
Normal		197.0±8.2	528.3±16.8	0.37±0.03
Thromb		605.2±21.9##	652.5±24.6##	0.95±0.03##
Thromb+Aspirin	20	106.5±4.2***	395.0±14.5***	0.29±0.01***
Thromb +Danshensu	15	358.1±12.8**	663.7±24.2*	0.50±0.02**
	30	328.7±10.6**	684.3±25.1**	0.45±0.02**
	60	306.4±8.2***	719.2±20.9**	0.40±0.02**

Blood was drawn from the abdominal aorta at the end of venous thrombus formation period and anticoagulated with indomethacin-EDTA-Na_2. Plasma samples were prepared by centrifugation and analzyed by radioimmunoassay. Data are expressed as mean±SEM (each group, n=10). #$P<0.05$, ##$P<0.01$ compared with normal group, *$P<0.05$, **$P<0.01$, ***$P<0.001$ compared with thrombotic control group.

Table 3. The effect of danshensu on the hemorheological parameters in rats.

Group	WBV(mPa.s)			PV(mPa.s)	Hct(%)
	Low shear rate	Medium shear rate	High shear rate		
Normal Control	22.72±1.21	5.88±0.25	4.44±0.11	1.41±0.08	0.41±0.02
Adr Control	39.55±1.35##	9.01±0.32##	6.52±0.23##	2.06±0.06##	0.45±0.02##
Adr Aspirin 20 mg/kg	26.59±0.87**	6.82±0.21**	5.02±0.19**	1.66±0.06*	0.44±0.04
Adr Danshensu 15 mg/kg	35.36±2.25*	8.64±0.51*	6.28±0.31*	1.89±0.08*	0.45±0.02*
Adr Danshensu 30 mg/kg	31.24±1.08**	7.74±0.23**	5.65±0.18**	1.67±0.09*	0.44±0.02*
Adr Danshensu 60 mg/kg	27.12±1.05**	6.65±0.19**	4.78±0.12**	1.45±0.42**	0.43±0.02*

Rats were treated by subcutaneous injection of adrenaline hydrochloride and cold stress. The normal control rats received only saline. Next, blood was collected 30 min after drug administration. Hemorheologic parameters were analyzed by routine laboratory assays. Data are expressed as mean±SEM (each group, n = 10). #$P<0.05$, ##$P<0.01$ compared with normal control. *$P<0.05$ **$P<0.01$ compared with Adr control. Adr: adrenaline hydrochloride, WBV: whole blood viscosity, PV: plasma viscosity, Hct: hematocrit.

Rats were anesthetized with chloral hydrate (350 mg/kg, i.p.). After the rats were fixed on a temperature-controlled heating pad (38°C) to maintain body temperature, the abdomen was opened surgically. The intestines were moved gently to one side and covered with saline-moistened gauze and the vena cava was exposed by blunt dissection. One millimeter above the bifurcation of the vena iliaca and vena cava, the free vein was ligated by tightening the proximal and distal segments using 4-0 suture (Shinva Medical, China) to induce blood stasis. The abdominal cavity was closed provisionally and blood stasis was maintained for 4 h. After the abdomen was reopened, the ligated venous segment was excised and opened longitudinally to remove the thrombus. The vein wall and thrombus were divided by blunt or sharp dissection. The isolated thrombus was blotted of excess blood and weighed immediately. Harvested vein samples were homogenized for subsequent biochemical analysis. Sham operation was performed in the control group.

Measurement of plasma TXB$_2$ and 6-keto-PGF$_{1\alpha}$

Blood was drawn from the abdominal aorta at the end of the arteriovenous shunt test period or venous thrombosis model.

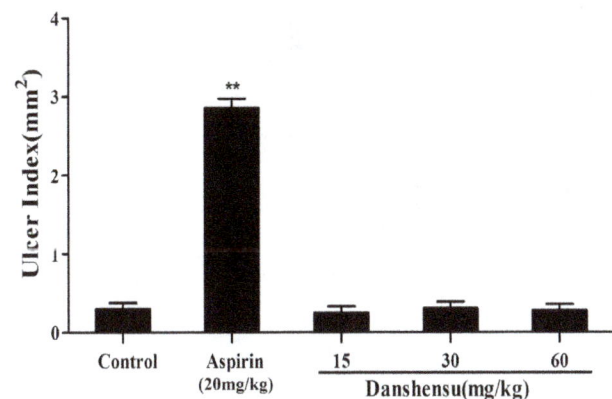

Plasma was prepared by centrifuging blood at 4000 rpm for 5 min. TXA$_2$ and PGI$_2$ levels were estimated by measuring their stable hydrolysis products—TXB$_2$ and 6-keto-PGF$_{1\alpha}$, respectively—per standard procedures using EIA kits (Cayman Chemical) and expressed as pg/mL.

Figure 8. Gastric ulcerogenic response induced by danshensu and aspirin in rats. The test compounds were administered orally at the indicated dose (mg/kg) to rats for 7 days. The animals were sacrificed after the last drug administration and the total length of mucosal lesions in each stomach was used to create an ulcer index. Data are presented as the mean ± SEM (each group, n = 10). **$P<0.01$ versus the control group.

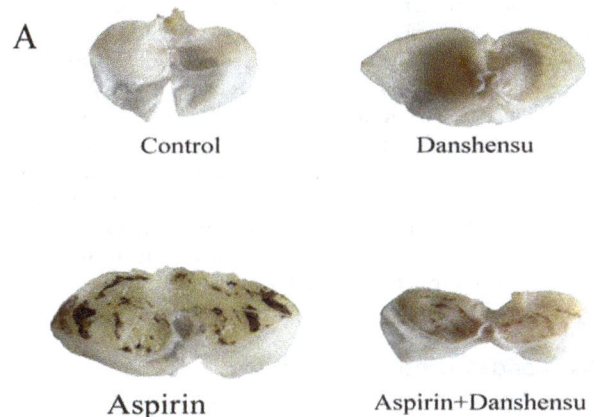

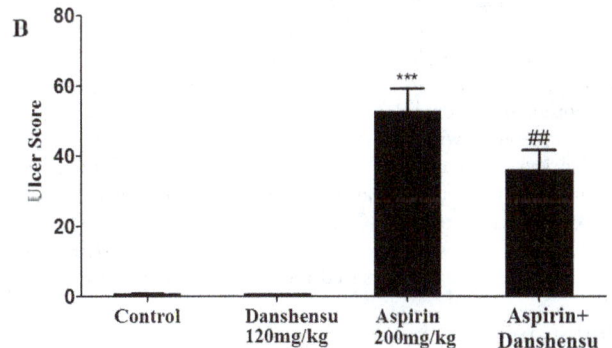

Figure 9. Effects of danshensu on aspirin-induced gastric lesions in mice. A: Photographs of gastric mucosa in the control group and danshensu, aspirin and aspirin + danshensu treatment groups are shown. B: The hemorrhagic ulcer index (mm^2) for each condition. Values are shown as the mean ± SEM(each group, n = 10). **$P<0.01$ compared with the control rats. ##$P<0.01$ compared with the aspirin-treated rats.

Effects of Danshensu on COX activity and expression

The inhibition of COX-1 and COX-2 by danshensu and aspirin was determined using COX inhibitor screening assay kits per the manufacturer's instructions. Danshensu and aspirin (with the same volume of water serving as control) were incubated directly with COX-1 or COX-2 in reaction buffer for 10 min. Then, AA was added as substrate and the reaction continued for another 2 min. Then, 0.1 N HCl and saturated stannous fluoride solution were added immediately to stop the enzymatic reaction. The amount of prostaglandin E_2 (PGE_2) that was generated by COX was measured using Cayman ELISA kits. The effects of danshensu and aspirin on COX activity were evaluated by comparing the amounts of PGE_2 production between reactions with and without the drugs. Inhibitory rates were calculated, based on PGE_2 production, as follows: Inhibitory rate (%) = (PGE_2 in Control groups-PGE_2 in drug-treated groups) ×100/PGE_2 in Control groups.

To measure COX-1 and COX-2 expression, venous walls from the venous thrombosis were analyzed by western blot. Venous samples were homogenized mechanically on ice and centrifuged at 4500 g for 10 minutes at 4°C; total proteins were then collected from the supernatants and the protein content was measured using a BCA protein assay kit.

Samples were separated by SDS-PAGE for immunoblot analysis. After the electrophoresis running for 60 min, proteins were transferred onto polyvinylidenedifluoride (PVDF) membranes. The membranes were blocked with 3% skim milk and saturated in Tris-buffered saline with 1% Tween 20 for 1 h at room temperature. Then, the membrane was incubated with primary anti-COX-1 and anti-COX-2 (1:300; Cayman Chemical) overnight at 4°C. The membranes were washed 3 times for 5 min each and incubated in horseradish peroxidase (HRP)-conjugated secondary antibody solution for 1 h at room temperature. The blots were washed again and visualized by using an enhanced chemiluminescence (ECL) detection kit (Beyotime Institute of Biotechnology) and exposure to photographic film. Images were collected and the respective bands were quantitated by densitometric analysis using the DigDoc100 program.

Effects of danshensu on blood stasis

The blood stasis model was established per previous reports [26]. The rats were divided randomly into 6 groups of 10 rats each: normal control, model group given 0.9% normal saline, aspirin (20 mg/kg) and Danshensu (15, 30 and 60 mg/kg). All drugs and saline were administered orally to the rats once per day at 9 AM for 7 days. After the sixth administration, blood stasis was induced by placing the rats in ice-cold water between 2 injections of adrenaline hydrochloride (Adr). All other rats were injected subcutaneously with Adr (0.8 mg/kg), except the control rats, which were injected with 0.9% (w/v) NaCl saline solution. Two hours after the first injection, all rats except the control group were soaked in ice water (0–2°C) for 5 min and reinjected with Adr (0.8 mg/kg) subcutaneously 2 h later to effect blood stasis. Afterward, the rats were placed into cages and fed freely.

Blood samples were collected and anticoagulated with heparin 30 min after the last administration of drugs or saline on the following day. Hemorheologic parameters, including WBV at various shear rates, PV and Hct, were measured by routine laboratory assays. Another aliquot of blood was collected into plastic tubes that contained 3.8% citrate and prepared PRP and PPP as described in *Assay of ex Vivo Platelet Aggregation in Rats*. Platelet aggregation was measured by arachidonic acid-induced.

Ulcerogenic Effects of Danshensu on Gastric Mucosa

Rats were sacrificed by cervical dislocation and the stomachs were removed immediately to determine the gastric ulcer index after the platelet aggregation assayas described with modifications [27,28]. The stomach tissues were split longitudinally and opened along the greater curvature. The total length (mm) of visible mucosal lesions in each stomach sample was measured and used to establish an ulcer index. An independent observer scored the macroscopic appearance of the gastric mucosa. The ulcer area was calculated as $\pi/4 \times a \times b$ mm^2, where a is the long axis and b is the short axis. The ulcer area was expressed as an ulcer index.

Effects of danshensu on aspirin-induced gastric lesion in mice

To investigate the effect of danshensu on aspirin-induced gastric lesions, male ICR mice were randomly divided into 4 groups. Group 1 received 1% carboxymethylcellulose in water as vehicle, Group 2 received danshensu treatment (120 mg/kg body weight), Group 3 received aspirin treatment (200 mg/kg body weight, suspended in 1% carboxymethylcellulose in water) and Group 4 received treatment of aspirin and danshensu. All drugs were administered orally once per day at 9 AM for 7 days. The mice were anesthetized with ether and sacrificed. One hour after the last administration, the isolated stomach was ligated at pylorus and cardia ends, filled with 1.5 mL of 2% formalin and immersed in 2% formalin for 15 min. Then, the stomach was cut along the greater curvature and the lengths of lesions on the stomach wall were measured as described [29].

Statistical analysis

Data were analyzed using SigmaStat 3.1 (SPSS Inc.; Chicago, IL) and expressed as mean±standerd error of means (SEM). P< 0.05 was considered to be statistically significant.

Acknowledgments

Chen Yu and Dong Qi contributed equally to this work.

Author Contributions

Conceived and designed the experiments: CY DQ. Performed the experiments: CY DQ. Analyzed the data: WL QZL HJL. Contributed reagents/materials/analysis tools: HJL HYF. Wrote the paper: CY DQ.

References

1. Ruggeri ZM, Loredana Mendolicchio G (2007) Adhesion Mechanisms in Platelet Function Circulation Research. 100: 1673–1685.
2. Antithrombotic Trialists' Collaboration. (2002) Collaborative meta-analysis of randomisedtrials of antiplatelet therapy for prevention of death, myocardial infarction and stroke in high risk patients. BMJ; 324: 71–86.
3. Kang DG, Oh H, Sohn EJ, Hur TY, Lee KC, et al. (2004) Lithospermic acid B isolated from Salviae miltiorrhiza ameliorates ischaemia/reperfusion-induced renal injury in rats. Life Sci. 75: 1801–1816.
4. Chan K, Chui SH, Wong DY, Ha WY, Chan CL, et al (2004) Protective effects of Danshensu from the aqueous extract of Salvia miltiorrhiza (danshen) against homocysteine-induced endothelial dysfunction, Life Sci. 75: 3157–3171.
5. Zhao GR, Zhang HM, Ye TX, Xiang ZJ, Yuan YJ, et al (2008) Characterization of the radical scavenging and antioxidant activities of Danshensu and salvianolic acid B. Food and Chemical Toxicology. 46: 73–81.
6. Chan K, Chui SH, Wong DY, Ha WY, Chan CL, et al (2004) Protective effects of Danshensu from the aqueous extract of Salvia miltiorrhiza (Danshen) against homocysteine-induced endothelial dysfunction. Life Sciences; 75: 3157–3171.

7. Tran H, Anand SS (2004) Oral antiplatelet therapy in cerebrovascular disease, coronary artery disease and peripheral arterial disease. J Am Med Assoc. 292: 1867–1874.

8. Damiano BP, Mitchell JA, Giardino E, Corcoran T, Haertlein BJ, et al (2001) Antiplatelet and Antithrombotic Activity of RWJ-53308, A Novel Orally Active Glycoprotein IIb/IIIa Antagonist. Thromb Res. 104: 113–126.

9. Nosal' R, Jancinova V (2002) Cationic amphiphilic drugs and platelet phospholipase A2 (cPLA2). Thromb Res. 105: 339–345.

10. Ryu KH, Han HY, Lee SY, Jeon SD, Im GJ, et al (2009) Ginkgo biloba extract enhances antiplatelet and antithrombotic effects of cilostazol without prolongation of bleeding time. Thrombosis Research. 124: 328–334.

11. Baskurt OK, Meiselman HJ (2003) Blood Rheology and Hemodynamics. Semin Thromb Hemost. 29: 435–450.

12. Takeuchi K (2012) Pathogenesis of NSAID-induced gastric damage: importance of cyclooxygenase inhibition and gastric hypermotility. World J Gastroenterol18(18).: 2147–2160.

13. Halter F, Tarnawski AS, Schmassmann A (2001) Cyclooxygenase 2-implications on maintenance of gastric mucosal integrity and ulcer healing: controversial issues and perspectives. Gut. 49: 443–453.

14. Masferrer JL, Zweifel BS, Seibert K (1990) Selective regulation of cellular cyclooxygenase by dexamethasone and endotoxin in mice. J Clin Invest. 86: 1375–1379

15. Lechi C, Andrioli G, Gaino S, Tommasoli R, Zuliani V, et al (1996). The antiplatelet effects of a new nitroderivative of acetylsalicylic acid–an in vitro study of inhibition on the early phase of platelet activation and on TXA2 production. Thrombosis and Haemostasis. 76(5): 791–798.

16. Weiss HJ, Turitto VT (1979) Prostacyclin (prostaglandin I2, PGI2) inhibits platelet adhesion and thrombus formation on subendothelium. Blood. 53(2): 244–250

17. Patrono C, Garcia Rodriguez LA, Landolfi R, Baigent C (1979) Low-dose aspirin for the prevention of atherothrombosis. N Engl J Med. 353(22): 2373–83.

18. Collaboration AT (2002). Collaborative meta-analysis of randomised trials of antiplatelet therapy for prevention of death, myocardial infarction and stroke in high risk patients. BMJ. 324 (7329): 71–86.

19. Sakata C, Kawasaki T, Kato Y, Abe M, Suzuki K, et al (2013) ASP6537, a novel highlcy selective cyclooxygenase-1 inhibitor, exerts potent antithrombotic effect without "aspirin dilemma". Thrombosis Research 132: 56–62.

20. Wooten JG, Blikslager AT, Ryan KA, Marks SL, Law JM, et al (2008) Cyclooxygenase expression and prostanoid production in pyloric and duodenal mucosae in dogs after administration of nonsteroidal anti-inflammatory drugs. Am J Vet Res. 69(4): 457–64.

21. Wallace JL, McKnight W, Reuter BK, Vergnolle N (2000) NSAID-induced gastric damage in rats: Requirement for inhibition of bothe cyclooxygenase 1 and 2. Gastroenterology. 119: 706–14.

22. Umar A, Boisseau M, Yusup Az, Upur H, Bégaud B, et al (2004). Interactions between aspirin and COX-2 inhibitors or NSAIDs in a rat thrombosis model. Fundam Clin Pharmacol. 18(5): 559–563.

23. Umoisseau M, Garreau C, Begaud B, Molimard M, Moore N (2003) Effects of armagnac extracts on human platelet function in vitro and on rat arteriovenous shunt thrombosis in vivo. Thromb Res. 110, 135–140.

24. Henke PK, Varga A, De S, Deatrick CB, Eliason J, et al (2004). Deep vein thrombosis resolution is modulated by monocyte CXCR2-mediated activity in a mouse model. Arterioscler Thromb Vasc Biol. 24: 1130–1137.

25. Henke PK Varma MR, Deatrick KB, Dewyer NA, Lynch EM, et al (2006) Neutrophils modulate post-thrombotic vein wall remodeling but not thrombus neovascularization. Thromb Haemost 2006; 95: 272–281.

26. Chen XP, Wang XW, Zhang YY, Xu XF, Ke WB, et al (2007) Effect of ethanol extract of terminalia chebula on microrheological characteristics in acute blood stasis model rat. Chin J Hemorh. 17(4): 525–528.

27. Sakata C, Kawasaki T, Kato Y, Abe M, Suzuki K, et al (2013) ASP6537, a novel highly selective cyclooxygenase-1 inhibitor, exerts potent antithrombotic effect without"aspirin dilemma" Thrombosis Research. 132: 56–62

28. Mei XT, Xu DH, Xu SK, Zheng YP, Xu SB (2013) Zinc(II)-curcumin accelerates the healing of acetic acid-induced chronicgastric ulcers in rats by decreasing oxidative stress and downregulationof matrix metalloproteinase-9, Food and Chemical Toxicology. 60: 448–454

29. Guth PH, Aures D, Paulsen G (1989) Topical aspirin plus HCl gastric lesion in the rat. Gastroen-terology. 76–88.

2

A New Flow-Regulating Cell Type in the Demosponge *Tethya wilhelma* – Functional Cellular Anatomy of a Leuconoid Canal System

Jörg U. Hammel*[¤a], **Michael Nickel**[¤b]

Institut für Spezielle Zoologie und Evolutionsbiologie mit Phyletischem Museum, Friedrich-Schiller-Universität Jena, Erbertstr. 1, 07743, Jena, Germany

Abstract

Demosponges possess a leucon-type canal system which is characterized by a highly complex network of canal segments and choanocyte chambers. As sponges are sessile filter feeders, their aquiferous system plays an essential role in various fundamental physiological processes. Due to the morphological and architectural complexity of the canal system and the strong interdependence between flow conditions and anatomy, our understanding of fluid dynamics throughout leuconoid systems is patchy. This paper provides comprehensive morphometric data on the general architecture of the canal system, flow measurements and detailed cellular anatomical information to help fill in the gaps. We focus on the functional cellular anatomy of the aquiferous system and discuss all relevant cell types in the context of hydrodynamic and evolutionary constraints. Our analysis is based on the canal system of the tropical demosponge *Tethya wilhelma*, which we studied using scanning electron microscopy. We found a hitherto undescribed cell type, the reticuloapopylocyte, which is involved in flow regulation in the choanocyte chambers. It has a highly fenestrated, grid-like morphology and covers the apopylar opening. The minute opening of the reticuloapopylocyte occurs in an opened, intermediate and closed state. These states permit a gradual regulation of the total apopylar opening area. In this paper the three states are included in a theoretical study into flow conditions which aims to draw a link between functional cellular anatomy, the hydrodynamic situation and the regular body contractions seen in *T. wilhelma*. This provides a basis for new hypotheses regarding the function of bypass elements and the role of hydrostatic pressure in body contractions. Our study provides insights into the local and global flow in the sponge canal system and thus enhances current understanding of related physiological processes.

Editor: David J. Schulz, University of Missouri, United States of America

Funding: Funding for this research came from Deutsche Forschungs Gemeinschaft (www.dfg.de) research grant HA 6405/1-1 to JUH. The funder had no role in study design, data collection and analysis, decision to publish, or preparation of the manuscript.

Competing Interests: The authors have declared that no competing interests exist.

* Email: joerg.hammel@uni-jena.de

¤a Current address: Center for Materials and Coastal Research, Helmholtz-Zentrum Geesthacht, Max-Planck-Straße 1, 21502, Geesthacht, Germany
¤b Current address: Bionic consulting, Bruckenäcker 4, 70565, Stuttgart, Germany

Introduction

Sponges are sessile filter-feeding animals. Accordingly, the canal or aquiferous system is their most distinct anatomical feature. Functionally speaking it can be considered the most important organizational unit besides the skeletal elements which give the sponge its structure. In accordance with their feeding habits, all physiological processes in sponges rely on the ability to process high volumes of water through the body. Only in this way are they able to obtain the required nutrients and oxygen and get rid of metabolic waste products.

Research into the biomechanics and fluid dynamics of filter-feeding and into biological fluid transport systems in general has revealed a close interdependence between hydrodynamic constraints, the micro- and macro-morphology of the cellular elements involved and, indeed, the structure of the anatomy in its entirety [1–6]. A number of hydrodynamic constraints and optimality principles have been suggested to play a role in shaping the general architecture of the canal system [3], but the key features appear to be flow resistance and pressure drop [2]. Pressure drop can be

understood as the resistance which fluid encounters when it passes through a filter. In the incurrent canal system in sponges, small apertures in the form of ostia and prosopyles contribute significantly to the pressure drop within the system (Figure 1). Further on, the apopylar apertures and the microvilli collar of the choanocyte chambers are also thought to play a significant role (Figure 1). While the effect of pressure drop in sponges has been considered to varying extents in general models of flow on an organismal scale, almost nothing is known about the influence of cell morphologies on local flow conditions or their implication for hydrodynamics on an organismal scale. Local flow regimes are of the utmost importance, however, especially when it comes to functional considerations such as nutrient uptake and gas exchange.

From a biological perspective resistance has a significant influence on two central aspects of filter feeding. On the one hand it determines the power required to move the fluid through the system. On the other hand it determines, in the context of morphological constraints and anatomy, the flow velocity of the

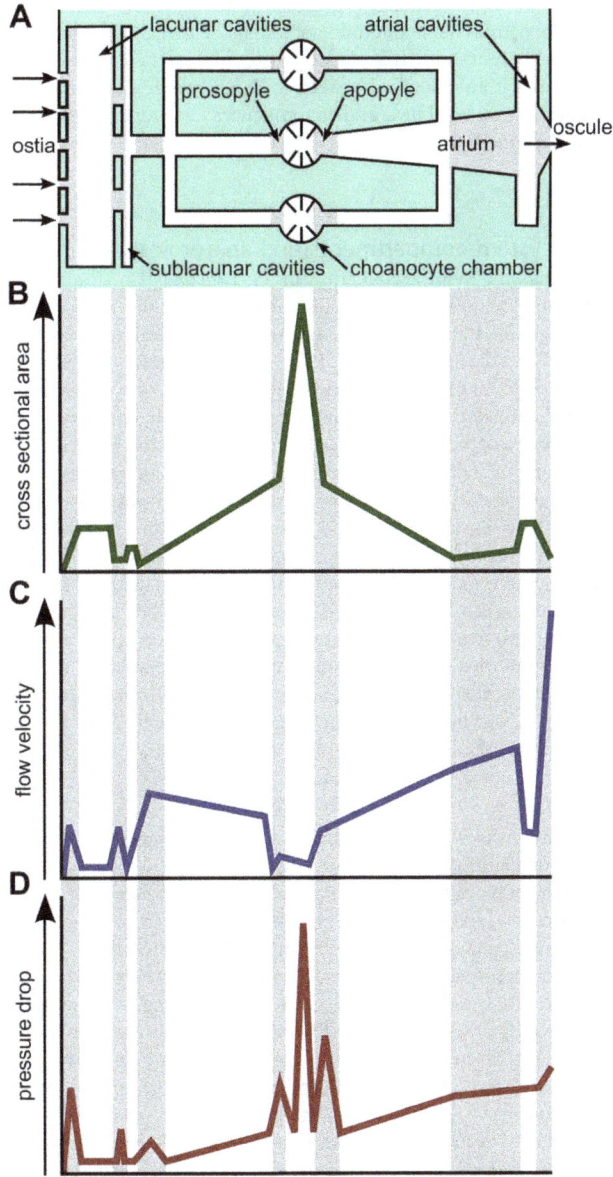

Figure 1. Scheme of hydrodynamic conditions in different sections of the leuconoid canal system based on morphometric and anatomical data on the sponge canal system as well as on fundamental physical laws in hydrodynamics [3,4,6,9–11,46]. (A) Structural representation of the main canal system elements in the direction of flow. (B) Schematic diagram of the change of available total cross sectional area along the flow path. (C) Schematic diagram of flow velocities in the canal system. (D) Schematic diagram of the change of pressure drop along the flow path.

cellular entities involved in the canal system. The morphometric and anatomical data pertaining to the architecture of the canal system and the cell types involved then needs to be integrated into basic fluid dynamic theory in order to gain a deeper and more detailed understanding of the hydrodynamic situation as a whole in sponge canal systems. Current understanding is based on general information regarding leucon-type canal systems [3,4,9,10] and recent specific morphometric and hierarchical data pertaining to the aquiferous system [6]. Flow velocity within the canal system is affected most prominently by the total available cross-sectional area of every functional unit in it (Figure 1A–C) [3,4,11]. Slower flow velocities are caused by an increase in total available cross-sectional area on any given hierarchical level [4,9]. However, the cross-sectional area of single segments on a hierarchical level is usually small. Overall increases in cross-sectional area are related to increases in the number of small sized segments on the respective level [6,12]. As the lower cross-sectional area of small sized canals is a consequence of their smaller diameter we can draw from the following two equations a direct relationship between pressure drop and resistance:

$$R = \frac{8 \cdot \eta \cdot l}{\pi \cdot r^4} \qquad (1)$$

$$\Delta P = Q \cdot R \qquad (2)$$

Where R is resistance, η the viscosity of the fluid, l the length of a canal segment, r the canal diameter, ΔP is pressure drop and Q is flow. According to equation (1), radius has the greatest influence on resistance, which allows us to conclude that numerous small sized canals will lead to high resistance and therefore necessitate a high level of pumping power. Equation (2) describes the relationship between pressure drop within the system and flow, viz. resistance. Sites with high local resistance in the system contribute significantly to pressure drop, especially when small sized elements are involved (Figure 1D). All considerations so far have remained on a local scale, however, focusing on single canal system elements. In order to come up with a comprehensive functional morphological interpretation, the complete architecture of the canal system and the specific sub-elements defined in the context of hydrodynamics as functional units need to be taken into account on both the local and the organismal scale. In order to do this, two fundamental principles of resistance theory have to be considered. (1) Total resistance for serial segments is the sum of all the segments included. (2) For segments arranged in parallel, total resistance is given by the following equation.

$$R_{tot} = \frac{1}{\sum_{k=1}^{n} \frac{1}{R_k}} \qquad (3)$$

As a consequence, the high resistance of numerous small sized canal segments - on any hierarchical level - turns out to make a much smaller contribution to total resistance on the organismal scale than indicated by the high individual values.

At present, the model for flow regimes in sponges [9] considers some of the physical and hydrodynamic constraints mentioned above [3,4,11], but with regard to morphological and architectural information is restricted to statistical morphometric data [3]. Modern imaging and analysis techniques have made detailed and even complete morphometric data available for biophysical considerations of general canal system anatomy [6,12–14]. The

fluid in the canal system. Particle capture rates are greatly influenced by the prevailing Reynolds number and are therefore related to flow velocity and anatomy [7,8]. We are consequently faced with complex interdependencies between cellular morphology and anatomy, energy expenditure and filter-feeding. In order to understand these complex relationships in sponges we need detailed information regarding the hierarchy and three-dimensional architecture of the canal system, quantitative morphometric data pertaining to individual canal segments, flow velocity measurements and detailed morphological data regarding the studies in question have revealed that the architectural complexity of the canal system anatomy in leucon-type sponges is much higher than previously thought, featuring phenomena such as bypass elements or highly asymmetric branching which need to be included in an updated flow model in order to explain canal system hydrodynamics on a local scale as well as an organismal one. However, in order to obtain a sufficiently detailed picture of the hydrodynamics of the canal system to put together a new biophysical model of flow, data from a single species needs to be available for all the prerequisites mentioned above. Flow inside the canal system of sponges is influenced not only by the system's gross morphological architecture but subject too to constraints imposed by cellular elements. Most studies into sponge aquiferous systems have focused either on the architecture and morphology of the canal system in general or on the way in which choanocytes work. The present study aims to provide an overview, from a functional morphological and hydrodynamic perspective, of all relevant cellular structures within the leucon-type poriferan aquiferous system of one exemplary species.

The tropical demosponge *Tethya wilhelma* SARÀ, SARÀ, NICKEL & BRÜMMER 2001 was chosen as a model on which to assess the way in which the morphology of cellular elements of the canal system relates to functional morphological aspects derived from hydrodynamic constraints. The general architecture of the canal system had already been examined for this species on an organismic scale [6,15]. Being one of the rare sponge species continuously cultivable under laboratory conditions [16–19] and even exhibiting regular asexual reproduction by budding [20], *T. wilhelma* is an emerging model demosponge for various types of functional investigation including physiological, genetic and morphological studies.

Morphologically speaking, the following series of elements are considered the functional modules of the aquiferous system [21]: Ostia>(sub dermal lacunae)>incurrent canals>prosopyls>choanocyte chambers>apopyles>excurrent canals>oscule(s). Ostia are the microscopic incurrent openings into the system, while the oscule or oscules are the excurrent openings. The choanocyte chambers act as displacement pumps and generate the pressure differential which drives the water through the system [10]. Their in- and excurrent openings are called the proso- and apopyle.

There are large discrepancies in our current morphological understanding of the various elements of and cell types involved in the aquiferous system. Although some cell types (e.g. endopinacocytes and choanocytes in particular) have been studied in detail, thorough comparative cytological studies based on broad taxon sampling are scarce. The most comprehensive review is to be found in Simpson's compendium of sponge biology [21], though the information in it is unfortunately fairly general. A more recent and detailed study into cell types in demosponges focuses on systematic and evolutionary aspects of aquiferous system characters [22]. Detailed morphological studies of cell types which contribute to functionally important elements of the aquiferous system help us, when they consider the hydrodynamic environment in which such cells are found, to assess their functional role [23,24]. This applies to apopylar cells (cone cells), central cells and any other cell type located in hydrodynamically pivotal sites in choanocyte chambers.

Theoretical and experimental investigations into choanocyte chambers have shown on the basis of choanocyte arrangement and orientation that the chambers can be understood as positive displacement pumps or, in technical terms, as peristaltic pumps [10,11]. Experimentally and theoretically consistent models for filter feeding in sponges do exist, though definitive experimental evidence is still lacking since science currently lacks the technical

observation methodologies for *in vivo* studies [1,25]. However, in order to complement our understanding of functional morphology, the present study is intended to provide a detailed analysis of cell types within the canal system of *T. wilhelma* with respect to their impact on local flow and consequences for hydrodynamics on an organismic level.

Results

Canal system compartments and anatomical details

The canal system architecture in *T. wilhelma* is of the leucon type with some striking manifestations of specific canal system elements. The incurrent canal system features voluminous cortical lacunar sub-dermal cavities. This cortical lacunar network is connected to an underlying network of sub-lacunar cavities located at the choanosome/cortex boundary. Both lacunar systems consist of an extensive network of anastomosing oval-shaped/flat canals. Branching off from the lacunar- and sub-lacunar cavities, high numbers of ramifying canals lead into the choanosome. Due to the roughly globular shape of the body, the canals of the incurrent and excurrent canal systems are significantly intertwined in the choanosome region. Within the excurrent canal system the atrium region stands out by virtue of its volume and can be characterized as a larger sized canal resembling a vestibule which opens directly into the outflow opening (oscule) (Figure 2). Depending on the state of morphological (re-)organization and environmental flow conditions, varying numbers of oscules are present, from one in the majority of cases to several in more rare cases.

Ostia

Specimens of *T. wilhelma* exhibit ostia of varying sizes, with no direct correlation with body size discernible - at least not in the specimens investigated here (Figure 3). The diameters of single ostia in all the specimens studied (N = 10) ranged from fully closed to a typical maximum of <15 μm. Ostia greater than this in diameter were present only in very low numbers. Depending on environmental flow conditions, ostia appear as single openings, in small groups or as ostia fields (Figure 3A). Smaller sized ostia are formed by intracellular pores (Figure 3B, Figure S1), whereas larger ones are made up like intercellular ostia by groups of several cells (Figure 3C). In both cases the exopinocytes involved in the formation of ostia are in direct contact with adjacent exopinocytes and endopinacocytes. Where specimens of *T. wilhelma* had been cultured under steady flow conditions over a long period of time, ostia fields covering the topmost portion of the surface of the sponge were observable. In this case, ostia were generally larger (up to 43 μm). Tissue bridges between the ostia usually varied in length between 5 μm and 20 μm.

Choanocyte chambers

Choanocyte chambers are almost globular in *T. wilhelma* and possess one apopylar and one to several prosopylar openings (Figure 4A). The number of choanocytes within a choanocyte chamber is dependent on chamber size and body size (~50–90 choanocytes/chamber, 70±13 choanocytes/chamber (N = 15 taken from 4 specimens)). The choanocytic prosopyle is formed by an interstice between adjacent choanocytes which lack filopodial extensions, which means that the prosopyle itself lacks any kind of specialized choanocytic prosopylar structure (Figure 4A).

Prosopyles

Prosendopinacocytes form internal, single-cell pores known as pinacocytic prosopyles (Figure 4F). The mean diameter of these

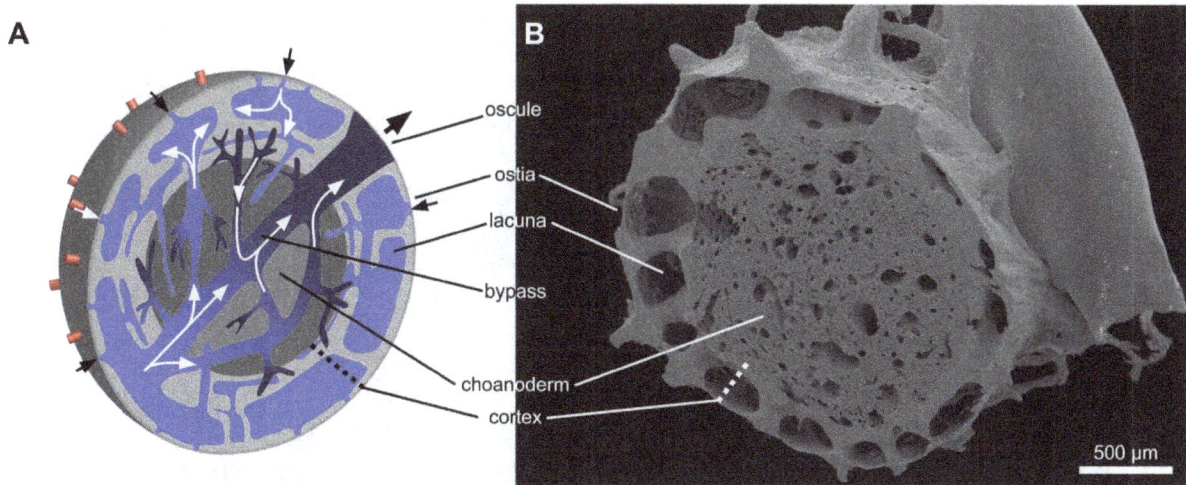

Figure 2. Schematic organization (A) and habitus (B) of *T. wilhelma* **aquiferous system.** (A) Potential flow directions in the canal system are indicated with arrows (after [15]). A color gradient from light to dark blue in the canals indicates the allocation of the corresponding elements to the incurrent and excurrent system. Due to the presence of bypasses in the canal system flow directions cannot be assigned with certainty to all sections. This might even cause backflows from the excurrent to the incurrent system. Main features/structures of the canal system are labeled in the scanning electron micrograph (B) as well as in the schematic drawing (A).

pore-based openings into the choanocyte chambers is about 7.4 µm. The prosendopinacocytes which form the pinacocytic prosopyle come into direct contact with the basal part of choanocyte cell bodies (Figure 4G).

Apopyles

The choanocytic apopyle is formed by apopylar cells (Figure 4B–D), two to three of which (depending on the size of the choanocyte chamber) form a ring-like structure (Figure 4B). Each apopylar cell bears a single cilium 3.9 µm in length (Figure 4D). In a cross-sectional view the ring formed by apopylar cells around the apopylar opening displays a characteristic double cone shape [26] (Figure 4C). On the choanocytic face the apopylar cells come into contact with choanocytes by way of a thin velum which forms the edge of the inner part of the ring/pore structure. This velum comes into direct contact with the choanocyte microvilli collar. The single cilium of the apopylar cells projects into the apopylar opening (Figure 4B–D). Facing the apopyle the cells connect to an apopylar pore-forming apendopinacocyte, which in turn touches a hitherto undescribed cell type spanning the apopylar opening (Figure 4B, Figure 5).

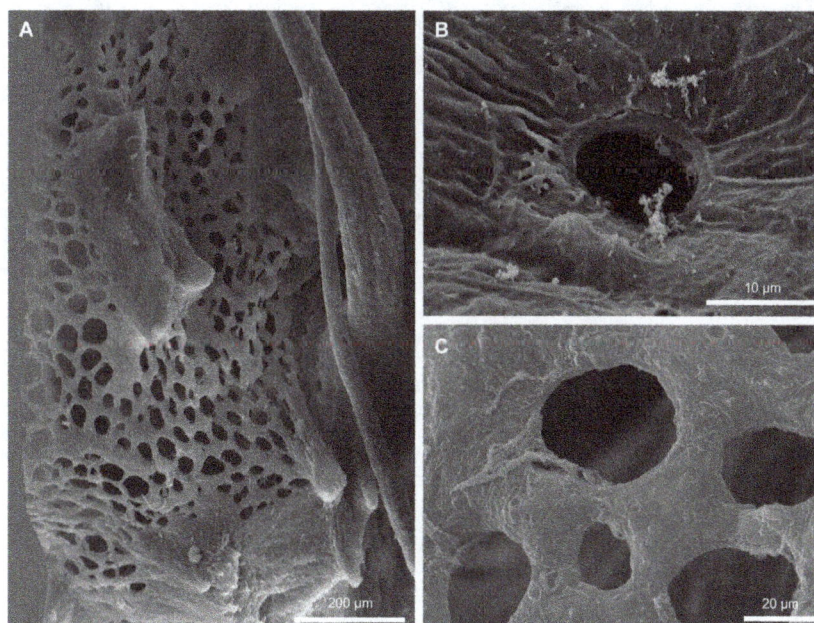

Figure 3. Scanning electron micrograph of an ostia pore field (A), a single ostium (B) and details of ostia in an ostia pore field (C).

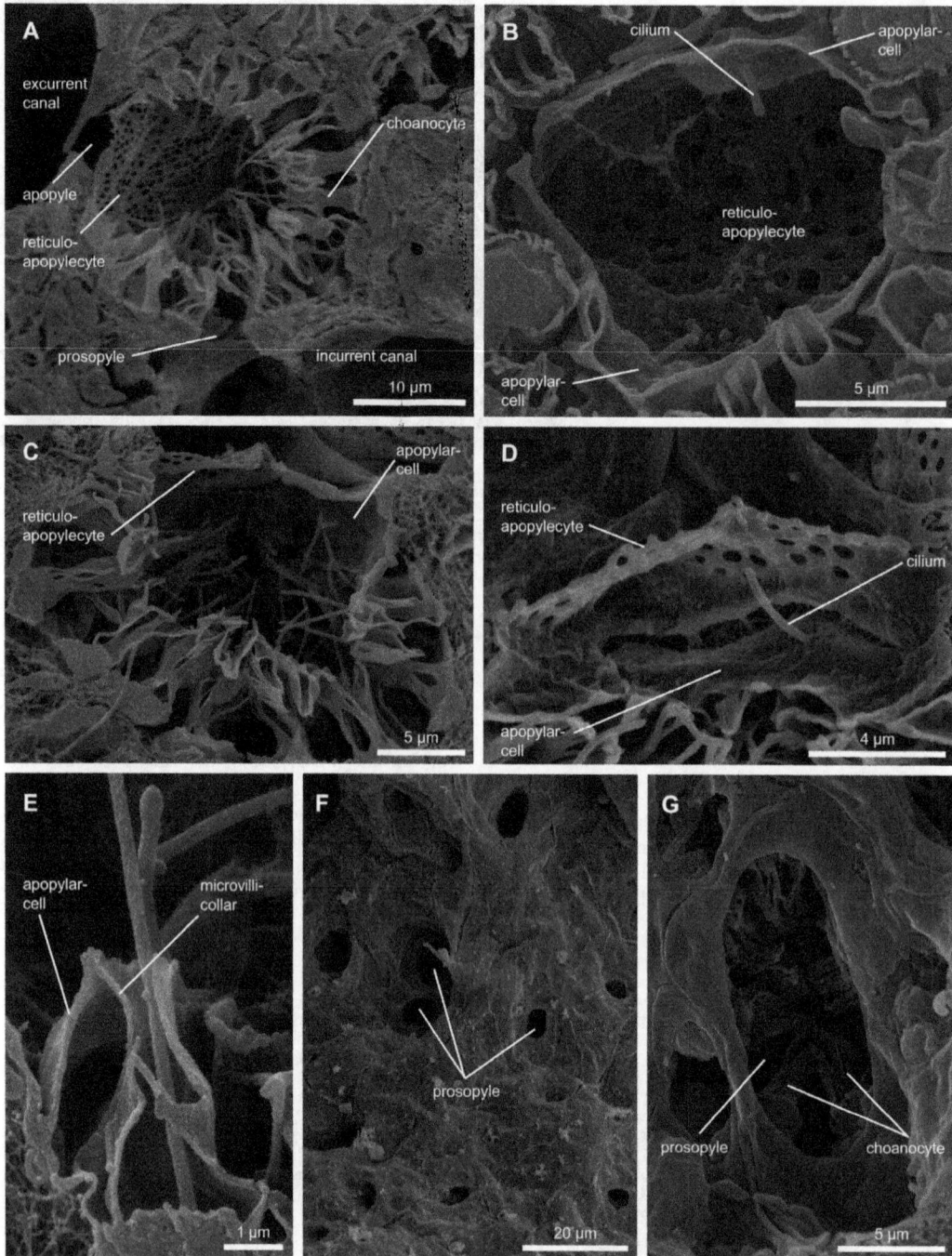

Figure 4. Scanning electron micrograph of cellular structures in the choanocyte chamber. (A) Overview of a choanocyte chamber connected to an incurrent- and excurrent canal with the relevant cellular prosopylar and apopylar elements and the location of the new cell type: reticuloapopylocyte. (B) Circular arrangement of apopylar cells and the position adjacent to reticuloapopylocyte. Hydrodynamic sealing of apopylar velum and microvilli collar. (C) Arrangement of cilium bearing apopylar cells, choanocytes and reticuloapopylocytes in the choanocytic apopyle. (D) Detailed view of an apopylar cell with its cilium directing into the flow at the apopyle. (E) Detailed view of the apopylar velum and microvilli collar contact side which results in a hydrodynamic sealing. (F) Overview of prosopylar openings in the incurrent canal system. (G) Pore cell forming a prosopylar opening. In the background microvilli collars of choanocytes are visible.

A new mesh-forming cell type within the apopyle - Reticuloapopylocyte

Reticuloapopylocytes – a previously unknown type of cell - have a high number of small intracellular pores which give them a mesh or grid-like morphology (Figure 5). These pores have openings of about 0.53 µm±0.07 µm (N = 82, taken from 1 specimen) (Figure 5E–F) and are found in an opened and closed state (Figure 5D). Reticuloapopylocytes, then, are able to adopt a gradient of opening states from totally open and highly fenestrated to partially or almost completely closed. When all reticuloapopylocyte pores are open, the functional cross-sectional area of the

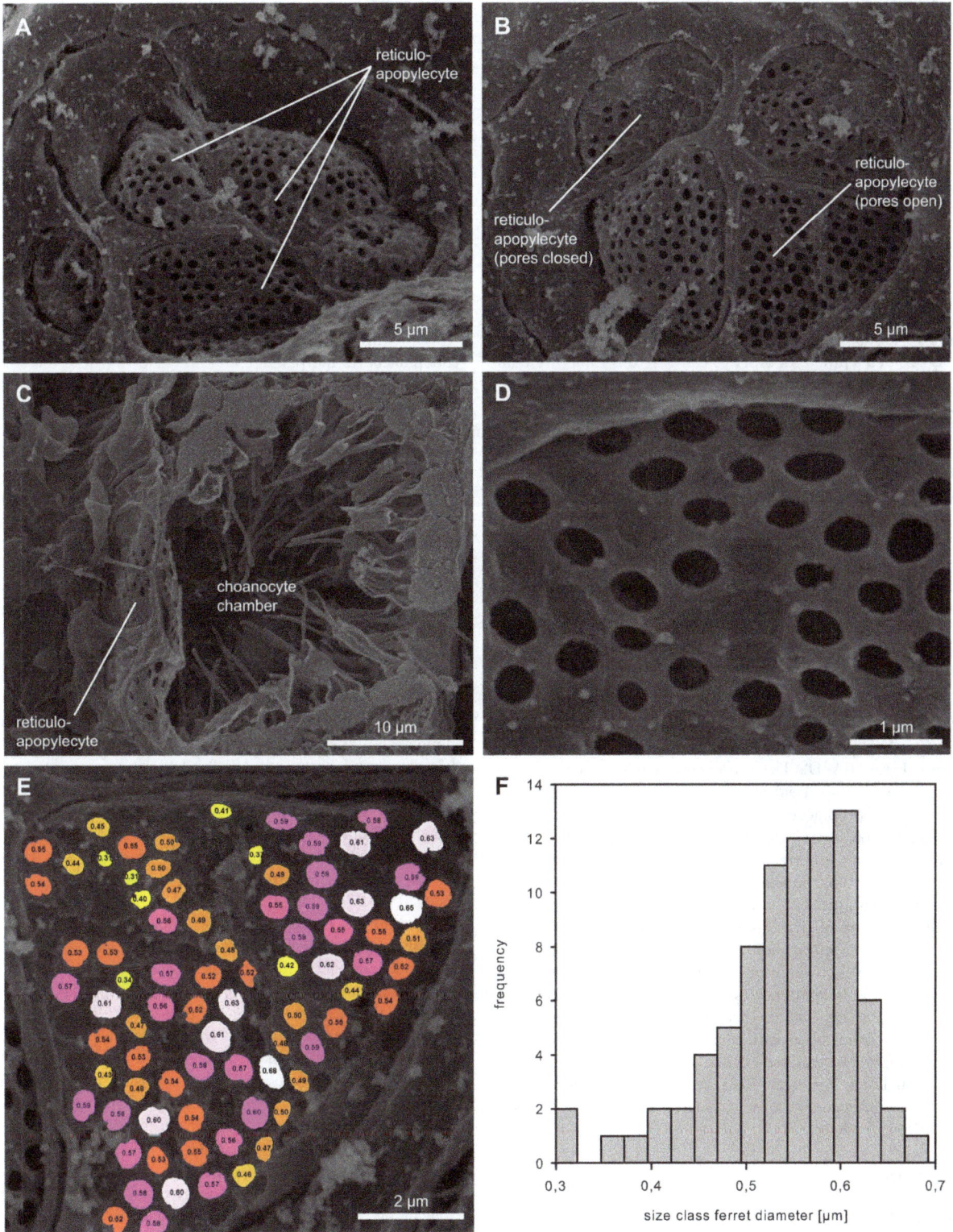

Figure 5. Scanning electron micrographs of reticuloapopylocytes. (A) View on reticuloapopylocytes from the excurrent canal with adjacent endopinacocytes and most of the pores open. (B) View on reticuloapopylocytes from the excurrent canal with one cell having most of the pores closed. (c) Overview of the position of reticuloapopylocytes in the apopyle (cross section through a choanocyte chamber). (D) Detailed view on pores of reticuloapopylocytes in an open and closed state. (E) Color coded and labeled ferret pore diameter of reticuloapopylocyte. (F) Distribution of ferret pore diameters in reticuloapopylocytes.

apopyle equals approximately 50% of the total area which would be present if the reticuloapopylocyte was absent. Typically, the cross-sectional area available to flow is much lower. The cell itself is very thin, usually below 0.5 μm, which is why the high level of fenestration leads to a grid-like morphology. Where a single reticuloapopylocyte spans the apopylar opening, it is almost circular in shape. In the case of larger apopylar openings, two or more reticuloapopylocytes form a mesh-like covering (Figure 5A–C).

Using the pore measurements presented in figure 5E–F, we calculated how reticuloapopylocytes contribute to the resistance of flow. Taking as a basis the cross-sectional area of pores and entire cells, we calculated the radius of pores and the radius of the apopylar opening. For the sake of simplification, we assumed that both were circular. By putting the measurements presented into equations 1 and 3, we calculated reticuloapopylocyte resistance to be $4.12 \cdot 10^{-3}$ Pa s μm^{-3}. In order to compare this value, we then calculated the resistance of the same apopyle opening without the reticuloapopylocyte and found it to be $3.13 \cdot 10^{-3}$ Pa s μm^{-3}. An apopylar opening with the same available cross-sectional area as the reticuloapopylocyte (12.87 μm^2) would give rise to a single apopyle with a radius of 2.03 μm and a resistance of $5.45 \cdot 10^{-3}$ Pa s μm^{-3}. The resistance of an apopyle with a reticuloapopylocyte is therefore 1316 times greater than that of the same apopylar opening unaltered. A smaller apopyle with the same available cross-sectional area as observed in the reticuloapopylocyte would lead to a 17-fold increase in resistance compared to the reference apopyle.

Pinacocytes

The prosendopinacocytes lining the walls of the lacunar and sublacunar cavities and the incurrent canal walls are less than 0.5 μm thick except for a small swelling incorporating the nucleus. Their overall shape is irregular and adopted to the local canal geometry (Figure 6A–D). The prosendopinacocytes in our study never displayed the T-shaped or umbrella-like morphology characteristic of exopincocytes (Figure 6F).

T. wilhelma possesses two types of apendopinacocytes which line the walls of excurrent canals and the atrium region, respectively. The type present in and around the atrium region bears a single 5.5 μm±0.79 μm (N = 16, taken from 4 specimens) long cilium (Figure 6C,E). Monociliated apendopinacocytes exhibit a fusiform cell morphology and appear to be arranged in a highly ordered fashion within the atrium region (Figure 6A,C). As in the case of prosendopinacocytes, the main cell body is very thin, usually below 0.5 μm, with the exception of the part holding the nucleus. Away from the atrium, monociliated apendopinacocytes become less frequent and non-ciliated apendopinacocytes start to dominate in lining the canal walls. Non-ciliated apendopinacocytes are no different on the micro morphological level to non-ciliated prosendopinacocytes.

Discussion

1. Morphology

Ostia. The diameters displayed by ostia in *T. wilhelma* were highly variable, ranging from total closure to more than 40 μm when open. The ability to open and close ostia within a relatively short period of time for flow-regulating purposes has been documented in a number of different sponge species (e.g. [27,28]). For this reason ostia diameters and numbers within specimens appear highly variable at any given time.

Pinacocytes. Biophysically, pinacocytes encounter a number of mechanical forces including shear stress and drag which are generated by flow along the canal system. Some of these forces result from direct interactions between the fluid and the pinacocyte surface which in turn contribute to general flow resistance and the resulting velocity profile. The boundary layer of the flow profile is particularly important in the context of particle feeding as it is involved in the slowdown and sedimentation of particles for phagocytosis along the canal walls [29].

The morphologies of apendopinacocytes, and most likely endopinacocytes in general, might reflect local hydrodynamics [30]. For the purposes of comparison, arterial endothelial cells have been shown under pulsatile but unidirectional laminar flow to align in the direction of flow [5]. In areas of flow separation and/or flow reversal (e.g. branching), they adopt an unaligned polygonal-shaped organization [5]. However, since our knowledge of local flow regimes in canals is very limited, it cannot yet be claimed with certainty that there is a direct correlation between endopinacocyte morphology and flow. Nevertheless, the fact that apendopinacocytes in *T. wilhelma* are aligned in an ordered way in the atrium region in particular is of great interest, for it is theoretically possible, taking fluid dynamics and morphometric data into account [6], that flow there might develop a pronounced unidirectional laminar profile.

T. wilhelma apendopinacocytes in and around the atrium region are monociliated. A morphologically similar cell type is characteristic of all Homoscleromorpha [22,31,32]. However, the monociliated endopinacocytes of Homoscleromorpha bear a much longer cilium and have been proposed to be actively involved in flow generation, something which is highly unlikely in *T. wilhelma* where the short cilium would make flow generation by apendopinacocytes relatively inefficient compared to that by choanocytes [10]. We propose as an alternative that the short apendopinacocyte cilium in *T. wilhelma* functions as a stereocilium and is involved in local flow sensing. The fact that the monociliated apendopinacocytes of the freshwater sponge *Ephydatia muelleri* (LIEBERKÜHN, 1856), which are located in exactly the same position as in *T. wilhelma*, have recently been demonstrated to have a sensory function backs up this claim [30]. The nonmotile primary cilium in *Ephydatia muelleri* consists of 9 circularly arranged microtubule doublets ("9+0" fashion), but lacks the central ones ("9+1" fashion) characteristic of motile cilia and flagellae [30,33].

Choanocyte chambers. The choanocyte chambers in *T. wilhelma* exhibit two specializations which are presumed to have a substantial impact on local and global fluid dynamics: (1) monociliated apopylar cells and (2) reticuloapopylocytes. In *T. wilhelma* apopylar cells form a ring-shaped reduction of the choanocytic apopylar opening which is double cone-shaped in cross-section. A functional morphological interpretation of the location of this cell type in a hydrodynamically pivotal site is discussed below. Apart from their role in preventing back flow, the function of apopylar cells is currently unclear, especially with regard to the cilium. However, since the cilium projects freely into the apopylar opening we propose that it is involved in flow sensing. Verifying this experimentally, however, will be technically challenging. As in the case of monociliated apendopinacocytes, ultrastructural data pertaining to microtubule arrangement might help to answer this question.

2. Functional Anatomy

Hydrodynamic situation in sections of the canal system and implications for the function of cell types. The development of ostia pore fields (see Figure 3), as observed in T. wilhelma under steady state flow conditions, can be explained as a result of fundamental fluid dynamic principles. As explained by

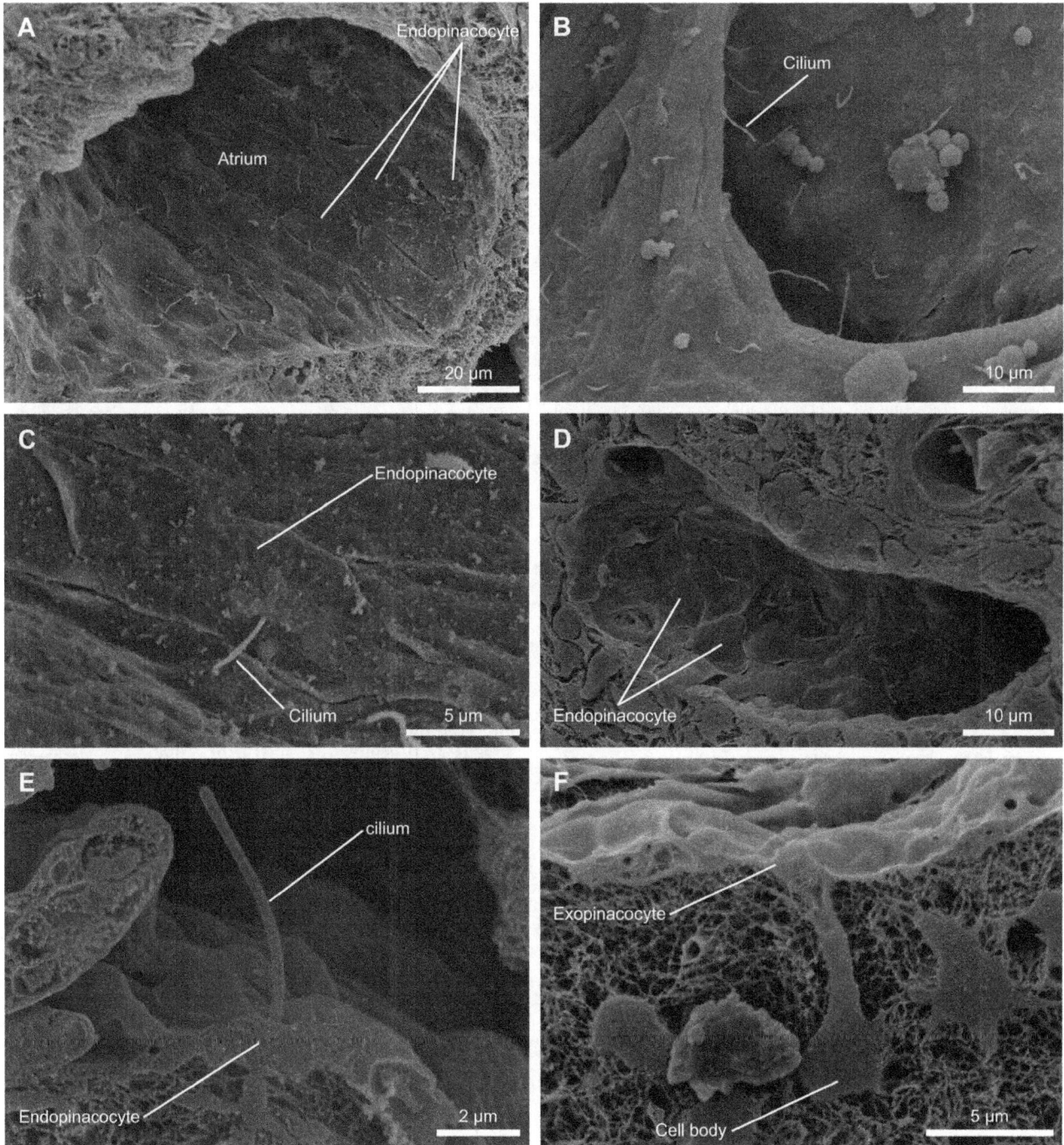

Figure 6. Scanning electron micrographs of pinacocytes. (A) Highly ordered apendopinacocytes in the atrium region. (B) Monociliated apendopinacocytes in the excurrent canal system. (C) Detailed view of a monociliated apendopinacocyte. (D) Prosendopinacocytes lining the walls of the incurrent canal system. (E) Detail of the cilium of an apendopinacocyte. (F) Cross section of an exopinacocyte lining the outer surface of *T. wilhelma*. Note the T-shaped umbrella like cross sectional morphology with the cell body of the pinacocyte sunk into the extra cellular matrix.

equations 1 and 3 in the introduction, pore fields drastically reduce the total resistance of the global influx and therefore reduce global pumping energy costs. Even though the parallel arrangement of small sized elements in the canal system reduces resistance on an organismic scale, resistance in each single element remains high. Therefore, the systemic resistance of individual canal segments influences the amount of water passing through certain areas of the sponge body. This can be quantified by the term perfusion, the amount of water passing through a defined volume of the sponge body over a given time interval. Consequently, resistance is a factor which can be used directly to control the perfusion of certain areas of the sponge body and to adjust local flow. No studies to our knowledge have yet addressed this aspect of local flow regulation from a detailed theoretical and experimental perspective. However, it seems on the basis of all the available data and fluid dynamics models that a local regulation of perfusion is possible within specific areas of the sponge, and that this is most efficient in regions which (1) have a significant impact on flow resistance and (2) can be mechanically modified by the sponge. Both requirements are fulfilled when it comes to ostia and the oscule, and in principle in the case of small sized canal segments too. As T. wilhelma normally only possesses one oscule, flow theory and the continuity of flow would suggest that oscule contraction would only cause very slight variation in local flow. This is supported by studies into ostia contraction in T. wilhelma (unpublished data) and other species, which have demonstrated that single ostia can be contracted individually [34]. Unless new methodologies become available, however, it will only be possible to demonstrate this quantitatively and experimentally in a transparent sponge species which permits in situ high resolution flow measurements to be taken within the canal system. The question of whether and how small sized canal segments influence perfusion is closely related to the pronounced regular body contractions observed in T. wilhelma. Predicting the effects of canal contractions on local flow during a contraction and expansion cycle is difficult, as information on the exact dynamics of canal contractions can only be obtained indirectly from the overall kinetics inferable from time-lapse sequences [13,35]. However, local body contractions and contraction waves across the body have been reported both for T. wilhelma and other sponges [36] and are presumed to be related to local changes in canal diameter and to result in changes in perfusion (see equation 1).

In terms of local hydrodynamics, the most complex functional unit within the canal system is the choanocyte chamber. From experimental and theoretical studies into sponges and choanoflagellates, we know a good deal about particle filtering at the level of choanocytes (e.g. [2,10,25,37]). However, we still lack detailed knowledge of flow fields in choanocyte chambers. A schematic drawing of simulated flow fields is given in figure 7. Hydrodynamically pivotal sites within the choanocyte chamber are marked with stars (Figure 7) and refer to structures with a significant impact on flow resistance. These include the prosopylar openings (Figure 1D), where resistance is determined by the diameter of the opening. It is presumed that the small size of these openings causes flow to accelerate compared to its velocity in adjacent canal segments. Predicting the situation for choanocytes is difficult as we lack information on how flow in the near field surrounding the choanocytes is affected by neighboring cells. In choanoflagellates, which are morphologically and functionally very similar to choanocytes microvilli collar height, density, spacing, angle and flagella length have been demonstrated to be interdependent [2]. The choanocytes in T. wilhelma have a smaller number of almost erect microvilli which are oriented parallel to each other and can be expected to reduce resistance to flow. This in turn can be expected to reduce pressure drop at the level of choanocyte chambers, if velocity is the fixed parameter or a slower flow an pumping capacity compared to choanoflagellates if pressure drop is the reference constant determining flow. Downstream in the direction of flow apopylar openings form the next anatomical structure crucial to pressure drop. In T. wilhelma, as in some other sponges [23,26,28,31,38–43], apopylar cells directly adjacent to the apopylar opening form a cone-shaped ring structure which makes contact with the neighboring choanocytes. The exact function of this structure is hard to pinpoint. Comparative experimental studies into flow fields around sessile and free swimming choanoflagellates might serve as a starting point. The studies in question have demonstrated that the boundary layer (e.g. the height above the substratum in a sessile choanoflagellate) has a significant influence on far and near field flow in terms of the development of eddies [16]. Applying these observations to

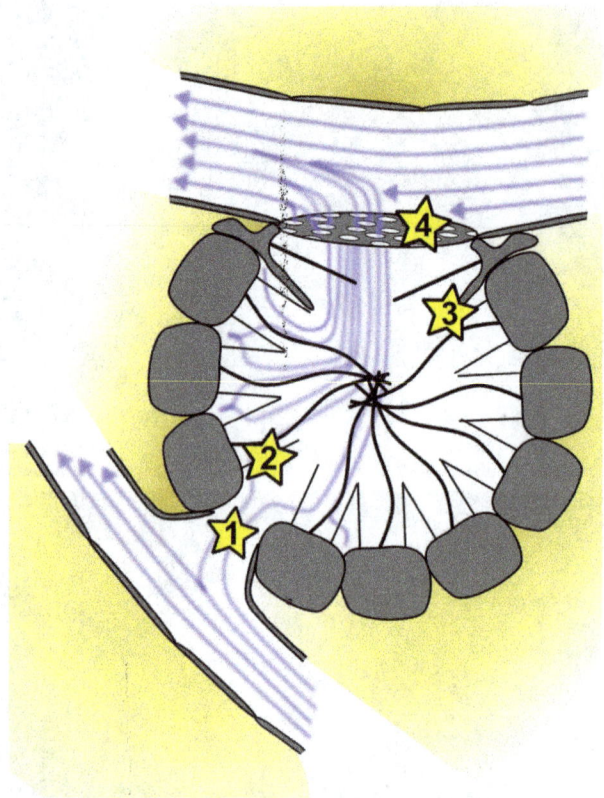

Figure 7. Schematic drawing of a choanocyte chamber with indicated flow directions and hydrodynamically pivotal sites (stars): 1. prosopyle, 2. microvilli collar, 3. contact side between apopylar velum of monociliated apopylar cells and microvilli collar of choanocytes at the apopylar opening, 4. reticuloapopylocyte.

choanocyte chambers may suggest that if no additional structures were present, eddies would develop between choanocytes and the apopylar opening. The direction of flow of eddies in this location would be opposite to the direction of outflow and would result in a significant disturbance of flow at the apopylar opening. In order to prevent the development of eddies in this location an additional boundary structure is needed. In T. wilhelma, the cone-shaped ring of apopylar cells around the opening fulfils this requirement by forming a ceiling seal with the microvilli collar tips of adjacent choanocytes, thus seeming to prevent backflow through eddies, which would significantly reduce local and global pumping efficiencies.

3. Functional aspects of the new cell type

From a hydrodynamic point of view, reticuloapopylocytes are the second functional morphological extravagance to be found in connection with T. wilhelma choanocyte chambers. Their location in the canal system and their morphology give rise to a number of hypotheses regarding their function. Reticuloapopylocytes might (1) serve as filtering devices, (2) be related to passive flow, and (3) serve as local flow-regulating devices.

A role in particle filtration, suggested by their sieve-like nature, can very likely be ruled out. We have never observed particles stuck on reticuloapopylocytes, nor witnessed any phagocytosic events. Considering the size of the pore(s) (~0.5 μm) and the size of a typical food particle (2 μm–5 μm), we would expect the pores to be clogged by retained particles within a very short period of time. From particle feeding experiments and our understanding of hydrodynamic constraints, we know that the majority of particles are restrained with great efficiency by the microvilli collar of choanocytes at the latest [25,44]. In other words, in terms of efficiency, an additional downstream filtering element in the form of reticuloapopylocytes is simply not necessary, which renders this potential function obsolete under parsimonious evolutionary principles.

Experimental and theoretical studies into filter feeding animals, including several sponge species, have demonstrated using a Venturi tube principle how even actively pumping species benefit from and make use of ambient flow-induced passive ventilation [11,45,46]. A recent work on hexactinellids provides detailed calculations of the dimensions of canal system elements (especially canal segments, choanocyte chambers and their openings) in relation to their role in fostering passive flows [46]. In this context the presence of large bypass elements [15] and the highly asymmetric nature of branching in *T. wilhelma* [6] could be interpreted as factors which promote passive flows. However, this hypothesis is speculative as the impact of bypass elements on flow patterns inside sponges is not yet well understood on either the local or the organismic scale. It is therefore currently impossible to prove or reject this hypothesis for *T. wilhelma*. What is more, a closer look at the morphology and dimensions of apopylar openings in *T. wilhelma* in the context of resistance theory does not support the hypothesis of passive ventilation by ambient flow. This is underlined by the resistance values we calculated for reticuloapopylocyte-bearing apopyles, which are about 1300 time greater than in unchanged apopyles and 8000 times greater than in the hexactinellid *Aphrocallistes vastus* [46], where ambient current-induced passive flow has been demonstrated. We would expect the much greater pressure drop/resistance generated at fenestrated apopyles in comparison to non-specialized apopylar openings to prevent the induction of passive flow through choanocyte chambers in *T. wilhelma*.

The third hypothesis regarding local flow regulation is related to the fact that individual reticuloapopylocyte intracellular pores have been observed in both an open and a closed state, and to the detection of a specific myosin-heavy chain expression pattern in this new cell type [47] which indicates its ability to actively modify its state of opening. In this it is strikingly reminiscent of intracellular ostia, which possess the ability to open and close relatively rapidly in order to regulate flow [48–50]. Altering the available cross-sectional area of the apopyle by entirely or partially closing individual pores changes the resistance of the apopyle. Closing pores leads to (has the capacity to lead to?) a reduction in the volume of flow and possibly even to a complete shutdown of individual choanocyte chambers in distinct areas of the sponge body. A reduction in the volume of flow at an apopyle will result in a change in the perfusion of the portion of the sponge body in question. The ability to alter flow rates on a local scale with consequences on the regional and even organismal levels qualifies the reticuloapopylocyte as a simple and highly precise fine-tuning device. Theoretically, reticuloapopylocytes permit a gradual adjustment of resistance at the apopyle by closing increasing numbers of pores to create an almost continuous decrease in flow. However, as these cells are to be found deep in the sponge body and are thus not accessible to *in vivo* light microscopy, direct experimental evidence to back up or refute this hypothesis will be difficult to obtain.

4. Functional constraints in the evolution of apopylar elements

Body contraction-expansion cycles have been demonstrated in representatives of all four major lineages of sponges ([36] and Nickel unpublished data). Of all the species studied so far, the amplitude and frequency of body contractions have been highest in *T. wilhelma* [13,36]. The primary effectors of body contraction are endopinacocytes [35]. In the course of a body contraction cycle the canal lumen disappears almost entirely. The change in canal diameter leads to an increase in resistance in the canal system. This change in the hydrodynamic situation in the canal system during a body contraction cycle gives rise to three different functional constraints with regard to the evolution of apopylar elements: (1) Risk of damage to canal system elements caused by increasing pressure in the contraction phase. (2) A need to modify the perfusion of body parts, something which can be influenced by contraction and expansion phases (3) A need to generate increased Gauge pressure during the inflation of the canal system in the second kinetic phase (see [13,35]) of the expansion cycle.

An increase in Gauge pressure within the canal system during the relatively rapid contraction phase is the result of cumulative resistance caused by the reduction in canal diameter and the presence of just a single oscule through which all residual water has to be expelled. The increased Gauge pressure leads to constraint (1), which primarily affects all delicate structures in the canal system (e.g. choanocytes). From a technical point of view the solution would be a pressure regulator. In a very simple way in *T. wilhelma*, the reticuloapopylocytes constitute just such pressure regulators. A comparable role has been demonstrated for the morphologically highly similar sieve plates in the phloem of plants [51].

The exact role of body contractions in sponges is unclear. One hypothesis proposes a physiological need to flush the canal system by exchanging all the water in the aquiferous system in the course of a body contraction cycle. Experimental studies into body contraction cycles in different sponge species have demonstrated the presence of contraction waves which travel over the sponge body ([35] and own unpublished data) Over the course of a body contraction cycle, canal diameters undergo alterations which result in changes in resistance. These changes affect perfusion rates, as formulated by constraint (2) on the principle described in section 2 above.

An analysis of body contraction kinetics in sponges has revealed four different sub-phases [35]. The contraction and expansion stages exhibit two distinct kinetic phases each. Endopinacocytes have been identified as effectors of contraction [35]. The two different kinetic phases of the *T. wilhelma* expansion cycle are thought to have two effectors. In the early and more rapid expansion phase elastic energy loaded into a distinct higher ordered sub-volume of the extracellular matrix is released [52]. This results in a partial inflation of the aquiferous system which enables the choanocyte chambers to start working again. In the second, much slower kinetic phase, we propose that Gauge pressure plays a role in fully inflating the canal system. Fulfilling this functional constraint (3) basically requires the presence of two specific components of the sponge aquiferous system - reticuloapopylocytes and bypass elements. Reticuloapopylocytes increase Gauge pressure by increasing resistance, while bypass elements form direct connections between the incurrent and excurrent canal system [6,12,14,15]. Their function and impact on flow in sponges is still under debate, but hydrodynamics and resistance theory might shed light on their functional role in the context of body contraction cycles in *T. wilhelma*. The increased back pressure in the incurrent canal system generated by the presence of reticuloapopylocytes in pumping choanocyte chambers is coupled to the excurrent canal system via bypass elements. This increases Gauge pressure throughout the system, helping it to inflate.

A large number of the hypotheses and interpretations discussed above are based on theoretical considerations and fundamental physical rules, the morphology of specific cell types and the morphometric information available on the canal system. Again, experimental verification *in vivo* is not currently possible due to the lack of optical live imaging techniques for structures deep inside the sponge body. Non-destructive approaches, e.g. x-ray videography and tomography or magnetic resonance imaging, do not provide the required spatial and/or temporal resolution needed to simultaneously analyze morphology, flow and the kinetics of contraction. Furthermore, we are faced with highly complex interdependencies between the phenomena in question - e.g. pressure drop and gauge pressure being caused by bypasses and reticuloapopylocytes. A solution to this dilemma might be computational fluid dynamic modelling approaches based on exact canal system geometries obtained from biological entities. Depending on the effect to be studied, modeling approaches might enable us to reject and formulate new hypotheses, or even test the influence of specific structural elements by modifying the geometries used (e.g. including/excluding bypass elements). However, this would require detailed information on the morphology of the canal system, volume flow and temporal analysis data pertaining to the kinetics of body contractions.

Conclusions

Reticuloapopylocytes, described here in *Tethya wilhelma*, represent a new and functionally distinct type of cell. On the basis of related functional morphological and hydrodynamic constraints, we evaluated a range of hypotheses pertaining to the function of this new cell and its effect on local and organismic flow conditions. Compared to our understanding of the functional morphology and influence on fluid dynamics of the other cell types discussed in the present study, our knowledge of the apopyle in leuconoid canal systems is patchy, especially when it comes to understanding its role in flow conditions on a local and organismic scale and its relationship to particle filtration in general. All the studies concerned with flow in sponges so far have focused mainly on the relationship between flow conditions and the architecture of the canal system in general, or concentrated on ecological aspects. However, if we break groups of cells in the aquiferous system down into functional units, the most interesting one is constituted by choanocytes and apopyle-related cells. The fact that a putative flow-regulating cell type is able to cut off every single choanocyte chamber and connected canal system elements from a highly parallelized canal system configuration raises the question of whether the apopyle is in fact a general regulative element in all sponges. Further research needs to focus on morphological changes in apopyles which reflect functional plasticity, e.g. during contraction events or pumping arrests. This will require a highly differentiated fixation scheme for functional states which will have to be characterized, analysed and understood in detail.

Materials and Methods

Sponge material

Individuals of *T. wilhelma* were sampled from the type location in the aquarium of the zoological-botanical garden 'Wilhelma' (Stuttgart). As *T. wilhelma* is not considered an endangered or protected species, no special sampling permits were required to retrieve material for scientific experiments from the aquarium section of the zoological-botanical garden. A continuous culture of sponges was maintained in a 180 l aquarium at 26°C using artificial seawater under a light/dark cycle of 12:12 h. The sponges were fed regularly with commercial invertebrate food (Artifical Plancton, Aquakultur Genzel) [13].

Scanning electron microscopy

Specimens of *T. wilhelma* were fixed overnight in a precooled iso-osmolar solution of 1.25% glutaraldehyde, followed by a contrasting step in iso-osmolar 1% OsO_4 solution for 1.5 h. They were desilified in 5% hydrofluoric acid for 1 h and then embedded in styrenemethacrylate [53]. After semi-thin sectioning, we dissolved the plastic around the remaining sponge using xylene-treatment and dehydrated the samples in increasing concentrations of acetone. Specimens were critically point dried in an Emitech K850 CPD system and sputter coated in an Emitech K500 SC system. SEM images were taken on a Philips XL30ESEM instrument.

Morphometric measurements

Morphometric measurements of reticuloapopylocytes and other cells were performed using ImageJ [54]. For the analysis of reticuloapopylocyte pore sizes pores were semi-automatically segmented using the level sets algorithm in Fiji [55]. The ferret diameters (min and max) and area of reticuloapopylocytes and all segmented pores were measured using functions in ImageJ.

Acknowledgments

We are grateful to Martin S. Fischer (Jena) for infrastructure and financial support, Katja Felbel and Benjamin Weiss (Jena) for excellent technical assistance, Isabel Koch and Alex Mendosa (Wilhelma Stuttgart) for additional supply of sponges complementing our own cultures, Isabel Heim (Neubulach) for aquaristic knowledge, Christopher Arnold, Florian Wolf, Henry Jahn and Josefine Gaede for aquarium maintenance. David J. Schulz (Missouri) and an anonymous reviewer provided valuable comments to this manuscript.

Author Contributions

Conceived and designed the experiments: JUH MN. Performed the experiments: JUH MN. Analyzed the data: JUH MN. Contributed reagents/materials/analysis tools: JUH MN. Wrote the paper: JUH MN.

References

1. Riisgård HU, Larsen PS (2010) Particle capture mechanisms in suspension-feeding invertebrates. Marine Ecology Progress Series 418: 255–293.
2. Pettitt ME, Orme BAA, Blake JR, Leadbeater BSC (2002) The hydrodynamics of filter feeding in choanoflagellates. European Journal of Protistology 38: 313–332.
3. Murray CD (1926) The physiological principle of minimum work. I. The vascular system and the cost of flood volume. Proceedings of the National Academy of Sciences 12: 207–214.
4. LaBarbera M (1990) Principles of Design of Fluid Transport Systems in Zoology. Science 249: 992–1000.

5. Waters SL, Alastruey J, Beard DA, Bovendeerd PH, Davies PF, et al. (2011) Theoretical models for coronary vascular biomechanics: progress & challenges. Prog Biophys Mol Biol 104: 49–76.

6. Hammel JU, Filatov MV, Herzen J, Beckmann F, Kaandorp JA, et al. (2012) The non-hierarchical, non-uniformly branching topology of a leuconoid sponge aquiferous system revealed by 3D reconstruction and morphometrics using corrosion casting and X-ray microtomography. Acta Zoologica 93: 160–170.

7. Humphries S (2009) Filter feeders and plankton increase particle encounter rates through flow regime control. Proceedings of the National Academy of Sciences of the United States of America 106: 7882–7887.

8. Jorgensen CB (1983) Fluid Mechanical Aspects of Suspension Feeding. Marine Ecology Progress Series 11: 89–103.

9. Reiswig HM (1975) The aquiferous systems of three marine demospongiae. Journal of Morphology 145: 493–502.

10. Larsen PS, Riisgard HU (1994) The Sponge Pump. Journal of Theoretical Biology 168: 53–63.

11. Vogel S (1983) Life in moving fluids. The physical biology of flow. Princeton: Princeton University Press.

12. Bavestrello G, Burlando B, Sarà M (1988) The architecture of the canal systems of Petrosia ficiformis and Chondrosia reniformis studied by corrosion casts (Porifera, Demospongiae). Zoomorphology 108: 161–166.

13. Nickel M (2004) Kinetics and rhythm of body contractions in the sponge Tethya wilhelma (Porifera: Demospongiae). Journal of Experimental Biology 207: 4515–4524.

14. Burlando B, Bavestrello G, Sarà M (1990) The aquiferous systems of Spongia officinalis and Cliona viridis (Porifera) based on corrosion cast analysis. Bollettino di Zoologia 57: 233–239.

15. Nickel M, Donath T, Schweikert M, Beckmann F (2006) Functional morphology of Tethya species (Porifera): 1. Quantitative 3D-analysis of Tethya wilhelma by synchrotron radiation based X-ray microtomography. Zoomorphology 125: 209–223.

16. Schippers KJ, Sipkema D, Osinga R, Smidt H, Pomponi SA, et al. (2012) Cultivation of Sponges, Sponge Cells and Symbionts: Achievements and Future Prospects. Advances in Sponge Science: Physiology, Chemical and Microbial Diversity, Biotechnology 62: 273–337.

17. Fosså SA, Nilsen AJ (1996) Kapitel 3: Schwämme. Korallenriff-Aquarium, Band 5 Einzellige Organismen, Schwämme, marine Würmer und Weichtiere im Korallenriff und für das Korallenriff-Aquarium. Bornheim: Birgit Schmettkamp Verlag. pp. 35–65.

18. Arndt W (1933) Haltung und Aufzucht von Meeresschwämmen. In: Abderhalden, E, editor. Handbuch der Biologischen Arbeitsmethoden, Vol I: Methoden der Meeeresbiologie. Berlin: Urban & Schwarzenberg. pp. 443–464.

19. Kinne O (1977) Cultivation of animals - research cultivation, 3: Porifera. In: Kinne O, editor. Marine Ecology, Vol III (Cultivation). London: Wiley Interscience. pp. 627–664.

20. Hammel JU, Herzen J, Beckmann F, Nickel M (2009) Sponge budding is a spatiotemporal morphological patterning process: Insights from synchrotron radiation-based x-ray microtomography into the asexual reproduction of Tethya wilhelma. Frontiers in Zoology 6: 19.

21. Simpson TL (1984) The cell biology of sponges. Berlin Heidelberg New York: Springer.

22. Boury-Esnault N (2006) Systematics and evolution of Demospongiae. Canadian Journal of Zoology 84: 205–224.

23. De Vos C, Boury-Esnault N. (1990) The apopylar cell of sponges. In: Rützler K, editor; Woods Hole, MA. Smithsonian Institution Press, Washington, D.C. pp. 153–158.

24. Reiswig HM, Brown MJ (1977) The central cells of sponges. Zoomorphology 88: 81–94.

25. Leys SP, Eerkes-Medrano DI (2006) Feeding in a Calcareous Sponge: Particle Uptake by Pseudopodia. The Biological Bulletin 211: 157–171.

26. Langenbruch PF (1988) Body Structure of Marine Sponges: V. Structure of Choanocyte Chambers in Some Mediterranean and Caribbean Haplosclerid Sponges Porifera. Zoomorphology 108: 13–22.

27. Harrison FW (1972) Phase Contrast Photo Micrography of Cellular Behavior in Spongillid Porocytes Porifera Spongillidae. Hydrobiologia 40: 513–517.

28. Weissenfels N (1980) Structure and Function of the Fresh Water Sponge Ephydatia fluviatilis Porifera: 7. The Porocytes. Zoomorphologie 95: 27–40.

29. Shimeta J, Jumars PA (1991) Physical Mechanisms and rates of particle capture by suspensionfeeders. Oceanography and Marine Biology - An Annual Review 29: 191–257.

30. Ludeman D, Farrar N, Riesgo A, Paps J, Leys S (2014) Evolutionary origins of sensation in metazoans: functional evidence for a new sensory organ in sponges. BMC Evolutionary Biology 14: 3.

31. Vacelet J, Boury-Esnault N, De Vos C, Donadey C (1989) Comparative study of the choanosome of Porifera: II The Keratose sponges. Journal of Morphology 201: 119–129.

32. Boury-Esnault N, De Vos C, Donadey C, Vacelet J (1984) Comparative study of the choanosome of Porifera: I The Homoscleromorpha. Journal of Morphology 180: 3–17.

33. Sorokin S (1962) Centrioles and the formation of rudimentary cilia by fibroblasts and smooth muscle cells. The Journal of Cell Biology 15: 363–377.

34. Leys SP, Meech RW (2006) Physiology of coordination in sponges. Canadian Journal of Zoology 84: 288–306.

35. Nickel M, Scheer C, Hammel JU, Herzen J, Beckmann F (2011) The contractile sponge epithelium sensu lato–body contraction of the demosponge Tethya wilhelma is mediated by the pinacoderm. Journal of Experimental Biology 214: 1692–1698.

36. Nickel M (2010) Evolutionary emergence of synaptic nervous systems: what can we learn from the non-synaptic, nerveless Porifera? Invertebrate Biology 129: 1–16.

37. Leys SP, Hill A (2012) The physiology and molecular biology of sponge tissues. Adv Mar Biol 62: 1–56.

38. Weissenfels N (1982) Structure and Function of the Fresh Water Sponge Ephydatia fluviatilis Porifera: 9. Scanning Electron Microscope Histology and Cytology. Zoomorphology 100: 75–88.

39. Weissenfels N (1981) Structure and Function of the Fresh Water Sponge Ephydatia fluviatilis Porifera: 8. The Origin and Development of the Flagellated Chambers and Their Junction with the Excurrent Canal System. Zoomorphology 98: 35–46.

40. Langenbruch PF, Simpson TL, Scalera Liaci L (1985) Body structure of marine sponges: III The structure of choanocyte chambers in Petrosia ficiformis (Porifera, Demospongiae). Zoomorphology 105: 383–387.

41. Langenbruch PF, Jones WC (1990) Body structure of marine sponges: VI. Choanocyte chamber structure in the Haplosclerida (Porifera, Demospongiae) and its relevance to the phylogenesis of the group. Journal of Morphology 204: 1–8.

42. Langenbruch PF, Scalera Liaci L (1990) Structure of choanocyte chambers in Haplosclerid sponges. In: Rützler K, editor; Woods Hole, MA. Smithsonian Institution Press, Washington, D.C. pp. 245–251.

43. Saller U (1990) Formation and construction of asexual buds of the freshwater sponge Radiospongilla cerebellata (Porifera, Spongillidae). Zoomorphology 109: 295–301.

44. Riisgard HU, Larsen PS (2001) Minireview: Ciliary Filter Feeding and Bio-Fluid Mechanics – Present Understanding and Unsolved Problems. Limnology and Oceanography 46: 882–891.

45. Vogel S (1977) Current-induced flow through living sponges in nature. Proc Natl Acad Sci U S A 74: 2069–2071.

46. Leys SP, Yahel G, Reidenbach MA, Tunnicliffe V, Shavit U, et al. (2011) The sponge pump: the role of current induced flow in the design of the sponge body plan. PLoS One 6: e27787.

47. Steinmetz PRH, Kraus JEM, Larroux C, Hammel JU, Amon-Hassenzahl A, et al. (2012) Independent evolution of striated muscles in cnidarians and bilaterians. Nature 487: 231–U1508.

48. Jones WC (1962) Is there a nervous system in sponges? Biological Reviews 37: 1–50.

49. Emson RH (1966) The reactions of the sponge Cliona celata to applied stimuli. Comparative Biochemistry and Physiology 18: 805–827.

50. Elliott GR, Leys SP (2007) Coordinated contractions effectively expel water from the aquiferous system of a freshwater sponge. Journal of Experimental Biology 210: 3736–3748.

51. Jensen KH, Mullendore DL, Holbrook NM, Bohr T, Knoblauch M, et al. (2012) Modeling the hydrodynamics of Phloem sieve plates. Front Plant Sci 3: 151.

52. Nickel M, Bullinger E, Beckmann F (2006) Functional morphology of Tethya species (Porifera): 2. Three-dimensional morphometrics on spicules and skeleton superstructures of T. minuta. Zoomorphology 125: 225–239.

53. Weissenfels N (1982) Scanning electron microscope histology of spongy Ephydatia fluviatilis material. Microscopica Acta 85: 345–350.

54. Rasband WS (1997–2014) ImageJ. Bethesda, Maryland, USA; Available: http://rsb.info.nih.gov/ij/: National Institutes of Health.

55. Schindelin J, Arganda-Carreras I, Frise E, Kaynig V, Longair M, et al. (2012) Fiji: an open-source platform for biological-image analysis. Nat Meth 9: 676–682.

3

Differential Regulation of Human Aortic Smooth Muscle Cell Proliferation by Monocyte-Derived Macrophages from Diabetic Patients

Te-Chuan Chen[1], Mao-Ling Sung[2], Hsing-Chun Kuo[3,4], Shao-Ju Chien[5], Chia-Kuang Yen[2], Cheng-Nan Chen[6]*

1 Division of Nephrology, Kaohsiung Chang Gung Memorial Hospital and Chang Gung University College of Medicine, Kaohsiung, Taiwan, 2 Department of Cardiology, St. Martin De Porres Hospital, Chiayi, Taiwan, 3 Institute of Nursing and Department of Nursing, Chang Gung University of Science and Technology, Chronic Diseases and Health Promotion Research Center, CGUST, Taoyuan, Taiwan, 4 Research Center for Industry of Human Ecology, Chang Gung University of Science and Technology, Taoyuan, Taiwan, 5 Division of Pediatric Cardiology, Department of Pediatrics, Kaohsiung Chang Gung Memorial Hospital, Chang Gung University College of Medicine, Kaohsiung, Taiwan, 6 Department of Biochemical Science and Technology, National Chiayi University, Chiayi, Taiwan

Abstract

Macrophage accumulation in the arterial wall and smooth muscle cell (SMC) proliferation are features of type 2 diabetes mellitus (DM) and its vascular complications. However, the effects of diabetic monocyte-derived macrophages on vascular SMC proliferation are not clearly understood. In the present study, we investigated the pro-proliferative effect of macrophages isolated from DM patients on vascular SMCs. Macrophage-conditioned media (MCM) were prepared from macrophages isolated from DM patients. DM-MCM treatment induced HASMC proliferation, decreased $p21^{Cip1}$ and $p27^{Kip1}$ expressions, and increased microRNA (miR)-17-5p and miR-221 expressions. Inhibition of either miR-17-5p or miR-221 inhibited DM-MCM-induced cell proliferation. Inhibition of miR-17-5p abolished DM-MCM-induced $p21^{Cip1}$ down-regulation; and inhibition of miR-221 attenuated the DM-MCM-induced $p27^{Kip1}$ down-regulation. Furthermore, blocking assays demonstrated that PDGF-CC in DM-MCM is the major mediators of cell proliferation in SMCs. In conclusion, our present data support the hypothesis that SMC proliferation stimulated by macrophages may play critical roles in vascular complications in DM patients and suggest a new mechanism by which arterial disease is accelerated in diabetes.

Editor: Jozef Dulak, Faculty of Biochemistry, Poland

Funding: Grants CZRPG880253, CMRPF6A0073, CMRPG891581, CMRPG6C0071, CMRPG6C0011 and EZRPF6C0011 from Chang Gung Memorial Hospital-Kaohsiung Medical Center, Chang Gung Memorial Hospital, and Chang Gung University of Science and Technology, Chia-Yi Campus, Taiwan, and by the National Science Council, Taiwan (NSC101-2320-B-415-003-MY3, NSC102-2314-B-750-001, NSC101-2622-B-255-001-CC3, NSC102-2313-B-255-002). The funders had no role in study design, data collection and analysis, decision to publish, or preparation of the manuscript.

Competing Interests: The authors have declared that no competing interests exist.

* Email: cnchen@mail.ncyu.edu.tw

Introduction

Diabetes mellitus (DM) is associated with an increased risk for atherothrombotic complications such as peripheral artery disease, coronary artery disease, and myocardial infarction [1,2]. It is well documented that macrophage accumulation is a common feature of type 2 diabetes and its complications [3,4]. Recruitment of monocytes from the peripheral blood to the intima of the vessel wall and the monocytes' subsequent differentiation into macrophages are critical events in atherogenesis. In addition, pathological environments, such as hyperglycemia, may promote macrophage activation and secretion within DM tissues. It has been demonstrated that high-glucose (HG) treatments of human monocytes lead to the increased expression of inflammatory cytokine and chemokine genes [5]. Our previous study also reported that the macrophage inflammatory protein (MIP)-1α and 1β released by HG-treated monocyte-derived macrophages are major mediators for the induction of E-selectin expression in vascular endothelial cells (ECs) [6]. However, the effect of monocyte-derived macrophages isolated from diabetic patients on vascular smooth-muscle-cell (SMC) activation has not been completely understood.

The proliferation and phenotypic changes of vascular SMCs are key events in the development of atherosclerosis and its complications [7]. During the development of atherosclerotic plaque, SMCs migrate from the media into the intimal layer of the arterial wall, where they proliferate and produce an extracellular matrix (ECM), resulting in the formation of intimal hyperplasia [8]. Growth factors, inflammatory cytokines, and chemokines have been implicated as factors that mediate such SMC proliferation [9]. Among these factors, the platelet-derived growth factor (PDGF) family possesses the most potent mitogenic effects for SMC [10]. The G1-to-S phase transit of the cell cycle requires activation of the cyclin-cyclin-dependent kinase (CDK) complex. The cyclin-dependent kinase inhibitors (CKI) such as $p21^{Cip1}$ and $p27^{Kip1}$ have been shown to regulate the activity of these complexes in the G1 phase [11]. $p21^{Cip1}$ and $p27^{Kip1}$ are expressed in quiescent SMCs and are down-regulated following mitogen stimulation [12]. It has been shown that a hyperglycemic environment can activate vascular SMCs and cause vascular dysfunction [13]. In addition, it has also been found that hyperglycemic conditions have mitogenic effects on vascular SMCs [14]. Therefore, examining the proliferative response of vascular SMCs to hyperglycemia may potentially extend our understanding of the pathogenic mechanisms of vascular complications in diabetes.

The functions of SMCs may be modulated by their interaction with other vascular cells such as monocyte-derived macrophages. It has been reported that interactions between monocytes and vascular SMCs may contribute to monocyte retention within the vasculature [15]. Moreover, macrophages can release a wide range of regulatory factors that are growth mediators to affect cell proliferation. Previous studies have indicated that human monocyte-derived macrophages have an inhibitory effect on SMC growth [16,17]. Evidence also shows that palmitate-stimulated macrophages promote SMC proliferation via the secretion of bone morphogenetic protein (BMP) 2 and BMP4 [18]. Although there is considerable research on the role of macrophages in the development of atherosclerotic lesions, the contribution of macrophages under hyperglycemic conditions to SMC proliferation remains unclear.

SMCs in the media of the artery are encompassed by a network of ECM such as fibrillar collagen. Culturing SMCs on fibrillar collagen promotes the maintenance of the SMC contractile phenotype and exerts an anti-proliferative effect [19]. Since proliferation and accumulation of SMCs are believed to play important roles in the progression of macrophage-rich lesions to fibroatheromas [4], it was hypothesized that monocyte-derived macrophages differentiated from diabetic patients may alter gene expression and affect SMC proliferation. We found that the SMC proliferation induced by macrophages in hyperglycemia is mediated through the up-regulation of microRNA (miR)-17-5p and miR-221. This study presents evidence for a novel mechanism in which miRNAs act synergistically to induce SMC proliferation.

Methods

Materials

All culture materials were purchased from Gibco (Grand Island, NY, USA). Rat tail type I collagen was purchased from BD Biosciences (San Diego, CA). Mouse monoclonal antibodies (mAbs) against p21^{Cip1} and rabbit polyclonal antibodies (pAbs) against p27^{Kip1} were purchased from Cell Signaling Technology (Beverly, MA). mAbs against osteopontin (OPN) matrix gla protein (MGP) were purchased from Santa Cruz Biotech (*Santa Cruz*, CA, USA). Other chemicals of reagent grade were obtained from Sigma (St Louis, MO).

Subjects

The Ethics Committees of St. Martin De Porres Hospital (Chiayi City, Taiwan) approved the study protocol, and written informed consents were obtained from all patients before enrollment. The study group consisted of 13 patients with type 2 diabetes and 9 healthy control subjects. The patients had a mean ($\pm$SEM) age of 53.4$\pm$8.5 years, body mass index of 31.4$\pm$2.5 kg/m^2, fasting glucose of 185$\pm$12.4 mg/dL, triglyceride level of 182.9$\pm$16.1 mg/dL, LDL cholesterol level of 94.3$\pm$7.8 mg/dL, and hemoglobin A1$_C$ of 7.6$\pm$1.1%. All patients were treated with glyburide and metformin. None of the patients was primarily insulin dependent. In addition, we recruited 9 volunteers, who were admitted to the St. Martin De Porres Hospital for the purpose of routine physical examinations, as the control subject group. They had a mean ($\pm$SEM) age of 49.2$\pm$7.9 years, body

mass index of 22.7$\pm$1.3 kg/m^2, fasting glucose of 84.6$\pm$1.7 mg/dL, triglyceride level of 147.1$\pm$8.7 mg/dL, LDL cholesterol level of 95.2$\pm$3.8 mg/dL, and hemoglobin A1$_C$ of 4.7$\pm$0.4%. None of the normal subjects had infectious or inflammatory conditions, or cardiac, renal, or pulmonary decompensated diseases. Volunteers who smoked cigarettes, used alcohol or were under medications (hormonal replacement therapy, nonsteroidal anti-inflammatory drugs, corticosteroids, and anticoagulant drugs) were excluded from this normal subject group.

Human monocyte isolation

Human monocytes were isolated as previously described [6]. Peripheral blood mononuclear cells (PBMCs) were isolated by Histopaque 1077 density-gradient centrifugation. Monocytes were purified from PBMCs by negative selection using the magnetic-activated cell sorting (MACS) monocyte isolation kit (Miltenyi Biotech, Auburn, CA); PBMCs were first treated with FcγR blocking reagent (human IgG), followed by a hapten/antibody mixture (mixture of hapten-conjugated monoclonal anti-CD3, anti-CD7, anti-CD19, anti-CD45RA, anti-CD56, and anti-IgE antibodies). After treatment with MACS antihapten magnetic microbeads conjugated to monoclonal antihapten antibody, the labeled cells were passed over a MACS column, and the effluent was collected as the negative fraction representing enriched monocytes (>95% purity).

Preparation of macrophage-conditioned medium (MCM)

Differentiation of monocyte-derived macrophages from diabetes patients or normal control subjects was achieved by culturing the freshly isolated monocytes (5$\times$10^5 cells/mL) in RPMI-1640 medium supplemented with 10% autologous serum. After 4 days in culture, monocyte-derived macrophages were incubated for another 48 h in fresh serum-free RPMI medium. The conditioned medium was collected, centrifuged, filtered, and defined as diabetic (DM)-MCM and normal control (NC)-MCM.

Cell culture

Human aortic SMCs (HASMCs) were obtained commercially (Clonetics, Palo Alto, CA) and maintained in F12K medium supplemented with 10% FBS. Cells at passages 3 to 6 were used. Growth of the cells was arrested by incubating in F12K medium with 0.5% FBS for 48 hours before use.

Collagen matrices

Fibrillar collagen (0.1%) was prepared by mixing 4 mg/ml rat tail type I collagen (25%), 0.1 M NaOH (5%), 2$\times$ F12K medium (40%), FBS (10%), and complete medium (F12K with 10% FBS; 20%). The mixture (0.15 ml/cm^2) was allowed to form fibrillar collagen matrices for at least 1 h at 37°C. SMCs were cultured on the surface of fibrillar collagen as described [19].

MTT assay and flow cytometric analysis for cell proliferation

Cells were cultured on type I fibrillar collagen in 96-well plates. Cell proliferation was determined by 3-(4,5-dimethylthiazol-2-yl)-2,5-diphenyltetrazolium bromide (MTT) assay. After the incubation period, MTT solution was added to each well to a final concentration of 0.5 mg/mL, and the mixture was incubated at 37°C for 3 hours to allow MTT reduction. The formazan crystals were dissolved by adding dimethylsulfoxide (DMSO) and absorbance was measured at 570 nm with a spectrophotometer.

Cell-cycle distribution was determined by flow cytometry. Cells stained with propidium iodide were analyzed with a FACScalibur

(Becton Dickinson), and the data were analyzed by using a mod-fit cell cycle analysis program [19].

Real-time quantitative PCR

Total RNA preparation and the RT reaction were carried out as described previously [6]. Regular real-time quantitative PCR was performed to confirm PCR array results. PCRs were performed using an ABI Prism 7900HT according to the manufacturer's instructions. Amplification of specific PCR products was detected using the SYBR Green PCR Master Mix (Applied Biosystems). In addition, the designed primers in this study were: $p21^{Cip1}$ forward primer, 5'-CTGAA AGATG GACGC TCAAT-3'; $p21^{Cip1}$ reverse primer, 5'-CGTTT CA-GAA GCCAG AAGAG-3'; $p27^{Kip1}$ forward primer, 5'-CTGAA AGATG GACGC TCAAT-3'; $p27^{Kip1}$ reverse primer, 5'-CGTTT CAGAA GCCAG AAGAG-3'; OPN forward primer, 5'- TTGCA GCCTT CTCAG CCAA-3'; OPN reverse primer, .5'- GGAGG CAAAA GCAAA TCACT G-3'; MGP forward primer, 5'- GCTCA ATAGG GAAGC CTGTG AT-3'; MGP reverse primer, 5'- TTTCT TCCCT CAGTC TCATT TGG-3'; 18S rRNA forward primer, 5'-CGGCG ACGAC CCATT CGAAC-3', 18S rRNA reverse primer, 5'-GAATC GAACC CTGAT TCCCC GTC-3'. Quantification was performed using the $2^{-\Delta\Delta Ct}$ method [6].

Western blot analysis

SMCs were lysed with a buffer containing 1% NP-40, 0.5% sodium deoxycholate, 0.1% SDS, and a protease inhibitor mixture (PMSF, aprotinin, and sodium orthovanadate). The total cell lysate (50 μg of protein) was separated by SDS-polyacrylamide gel electrophoresis (PAGE) (12% running, 4% stacking) and analyzed by using the designated antibodies and the Western-Light chemiluminescent detection system (Bio-Rad, Hercules, CA), as previously described [19].

Inhibition of miR-17-5p and miR-221

Anti-miR inhibitors for miR-17-5p, miR-221, and corresponding negative controls were purchased from Ambion, Life Technologies (Austin, TX, USA). The SMCs were then transfected with the miRNA inhibitors or miRNA inhibitor negative control by Oligofectamine Transfection Reagent from Invitrogen, Life Technologies, in accordance with the manufacturer's procedure. The final concentration for miRNA inhibitor was 200 nmol/L. The transfection efficiency of miRNA inhibitors was further verified by Real-time quantitative PCR assay. After transfection with the miR-17-5p and miR-221 inhibitors, the expression levels of miR-17-5p and miR-221 were decreased by 75.3% and 78.7%, respectively.

ELISA for PDGF-BB and PDGF-CC

The levels of PDGF-BB and PDGF-CC in the MCM were determined by using sandwich ELISA (sensitivity 18 pg/mL; R&D) according to manufacturer's protocols, as previously described [19].

Statistical analysis

The results are expressed as mean ± standard error of the mean (SEM). Statistical analysis was performed by using an independent Student t-test for two groups of data and analysis of variance (ANOVA) followed by Scheffe's test for multiple comparisons. P values less than 0.05 were considered significant.

Results

The effect of DM-MCM on SMC proliferation

The effects of monocyte-derived macrophages from DM patients on cell proliferation were studied by treating SMCs cultured on fibrillar collagen with DM-MCM (vs. NC-MCM). SMCs were stimulated with the two types of MCM at different concentrations for 24 h, or $1 \times$ DM-MCM for the times indicated. Cell proliferation was analyzed by MTT assays. As shown in Figure 1A, proliferation of SMC was significantly increased (38%, 56% and 89% after cultivation for 24, 48 and 72 h, respectively) when cultivated with DM-MCM. SMCs cultured with NC-MCM had limited proliferation capacities (Figure 1A). SMCs treated with DM-MCM at different concentrations for 24 h showed a significantly higher growth rate when compared to the control cells (Figure 1B). Table 1 summarizes the flow cytometry analysis of cell distribution in the cell cycle phases. SMCs stimulated with DM-MCM for 24 and 48 h had marked decreases of cells in the G_0/G_1 phases and increases in the S-phase (Table 1).

DM-MCM decreased $p21^{Cip1}$ and $p27^{Kip1}$ and increased synthetic differentiation marker expression in SMCs

We examined the effects of DM-MCM on the expression of cell-cycle regulatory proteins $p21^{Cip1}$ and $p27^{Kip1}$. As shown in Figure 2B, SMCs with DM-MCM stimulation decreased the expressions of $p21^{Cip1}$ and $p27^{Kip1}$. However, there was no effect on $p21^{Cip1}$ and $p27^{Kip1}$ expression in SMCs cultured with NC-MCM (Figure 2A). Figure 2C shows that DM-MCM induced decreases in the mRNA expression of $p21^{Cip1}$ and $p27^{Kip1}$ after 12 h of DM-MCM stimulation.

We also examined the effect of DM-MCM on the expression of synthetic differentiation markers in SMCs. SMCs were cultured on fibrillar collagen, and the mRNA and protein expression of OPN and MGP was analyzed at various time points after cultivation. Real-time PCR analysis indicated the time-dependent increase in the levels of mRNA expression for OPN (Figure 3A) and MGP (Figure 3B) in SMCs on fibrillar collagen. The cultivation of SMCs by DM-MCM also caused significant increases in the OPN and MGP expression at 72 h on fibrillar collagen (Figure 3C).

miR-17-5p and miR-221 are involved in the regulation of HASMC proliferation

Recent studies have demonstrated that miRNAs are involved in regulating SMC gene expression and proliferation [20]. We therefore examined the effects of DM-MCM on the expression of miRNAs. Stimulation of SMCs with DM-MCM increased the expression of the miR-17-5p (Figure 4A) and miR-221 (Figure 4B), in a time-dependent manner.

To determine whether DM-MCM-induced cell proliferation was mediated by the up-regulation of miR-17-5p and miR-221, SMCs were pretreated with miR-17-5p and miR-221 inhibitors and subsequently stimulated with DM-MCM. The DM-MCM-induced SMC proliferation was significantly inhibited by pretreatments with miR-17-5p and miR-221 inhibitors (Figure 4C). The DM-MCM-induced decrease in the percentage of cells in the G_0/G_1 phases and the increase in the percentage of cells in the S-phase were also significantly inhibited by miR-17-5p and miR-221 inhibitors (Figure 4D).

In addition, SMCs were incubated with specific inhibitors of miR-17-5p and miR-221 for 1 h before and during stimulation with DM-MCM, and the expressions of $p21^{Cip1}$ and $p27^{Kip1}$ were analyzed. As shown in Figure 4E, miR-17-5p inhibitor significantly inhibited the DM-MCM-induced expression of $p21^{Cip1}$,

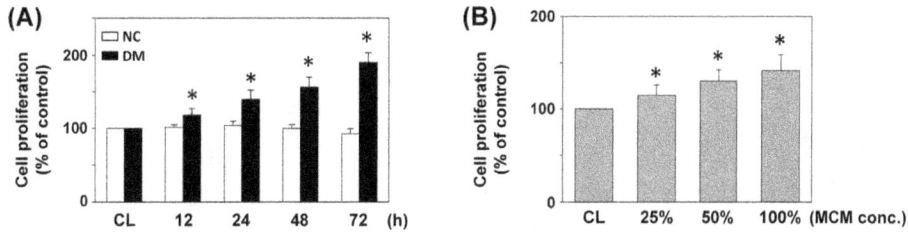

Figure 1. Effect of DM-MCM on cell viability of HASMCs. Bar graphs represent folds of controls (CL) SMCs, mean ± standard error of the mean (SEM) of 5 independent experiments. *P<0.05 versus CL SMCs. (A) SMCs were kept as CL or stimulated with NC-MCM or DM-MCM at the indicated time periods, or (B) stimulated with different concentrations of DM-MCM for 24 h. Cell proliferation was assayed by the MTT test.

whereas miR-221 inhibitor inhibited the DM-MCM-induced expression of p27^{Kip1}.

DM-MCM induced SMC proliferation was mediated by PDGF-CC

The effect of DM-MCM on SMC proliferation suggests that macrophages under a DM environment may release soluble mediators and exert paracrine effects on SMCs to induce cell proliferation. PDGF was identified in a search for serum factors that stimulate SMC proliferation [10]. As shown in Figure 5A, the incubation of SMCs with PDGF-CC neutralizing antibody, but not PDGF-BB, significantly inhibited DM-MCM-induced SMC proliferation. To confirm these results, the protein levels of PDGF-BB and PDGF-CC in NC- and DM-MCM were analyzed by ELISA. As shown in Figure 5B, culturing of monocyte-derive macrophages caused significant increases of PDGF-BB and PDGF-CC protein secretion in macrophages isolated from diabetic patients.

To further characterize the effect of the PDGF-BB or PDGF-CC in MCM on SMC proliferation and to determine the optimal PDGF concentrations, we examined the responses of SMC to 50% DM-MCM with different concentrations of the PDGF-BB and PDGF-CC (0–100 ng/mL) and their neutralizing antibodies. The results shown in Figure 5D indicated that PDGF-CC promoted SMC proliferation, and the effect was significantly inhibited by neutralizing antibody against PDGF-CC, while PDGF-BB had no significant effect on SMC proliferation (Figure 5C). Figure 5D also indicated that the optimal concentration of PDGF-CC was 50 ng/mL.

Discussion

Diabetic patients have an increased susceptibility to the development of atherosclerosis [21]. Atherosclerotic lesions in patients with diabetes are characterized by excessive macrophage infiltration, suggesting that the accumulation of monocyte-derived macrophages into the vasculature may be augmented under hyperglycemic conditions [3]. In addition, the migration and proliferation of SMCs are believed to play important roles in the progression of macrophage-rich lesions to fibroatheromas, and diabetic conditions have been shown to enhance this process [22]. It has been suggested that the macrophage-SMC coexistence as neighbors within the vessel walls induces regulatory signals involved in atherogenesis [23]. There is also evidence that hyperglycemia may enhance the interaction of macrophages and SMCs [24]. However, the pathophysiological mechanism of macrophage-SMC interaction remains poorly understood. The present study characterized the roles of two major monocyte-derived macrophage-induced mediators from diabetic patients in the regulation of p21^{Cip1} and p27^{Kip1} expressions by HASMCs. Several lines of evidence from the current study indicate that the effect of macrophages from DM patients on SMC proliferation was mediated by the down-regulation of expressions of p21^{Cip1} and p27^{Kip1} and that this down-regulation was mediated through the differential regulation of the miR-17-5p and miR-221. First, stimulation by DM-MCM induced decreased expression of p21^{Cip1} and p27^{Kip1}, as well as increased cell proliferation. Second, stimulation of SMCs by DM-MCM induced expression of miR-17-5p. Pretreatment of the cells with miR-17-5p inhibitor suppressed the DM-MCM-induced down-regulation of p21^{Cip1}

Table 1. Cell cycle analysis of SMCs stimulated with NC- and DM-MCM.

		% cells (mean ± SEM)		
	Duration (h)	G$_0$/G$_1$	S-phase	G$_2$/M
Control	0	87.4±2.1	6.5±0.8	6.1±1.2
NC-MCM	24	92.3±2.7	5.1±0.6	2.6±1.0
	48	92.9±1.9	3.9±0.4	3.2±0.8
	72	90.3±2.6	5.6±0.6	4.1±1.1
DM-MCM	24	72.1±4.8*	19.2±2.4*	8.7±1.4
	48	70.6±4.3*	22.3±2.7*	7.1±1.3
	72	65.7±6.6*	27.9±4.2*	6.4±0.9

SMCs were kept as controls or on fibrillar collagen with NG- or HG-MCM treatment. Cells were analyzed for DNA content by flow cytometry to show percentages in G$_0$/G$_1$, synthetic, or G$_2$/M phases of cell cycle. Data are mean ± SEM from three independent experiments.
*P<0.05 vs. control cells.

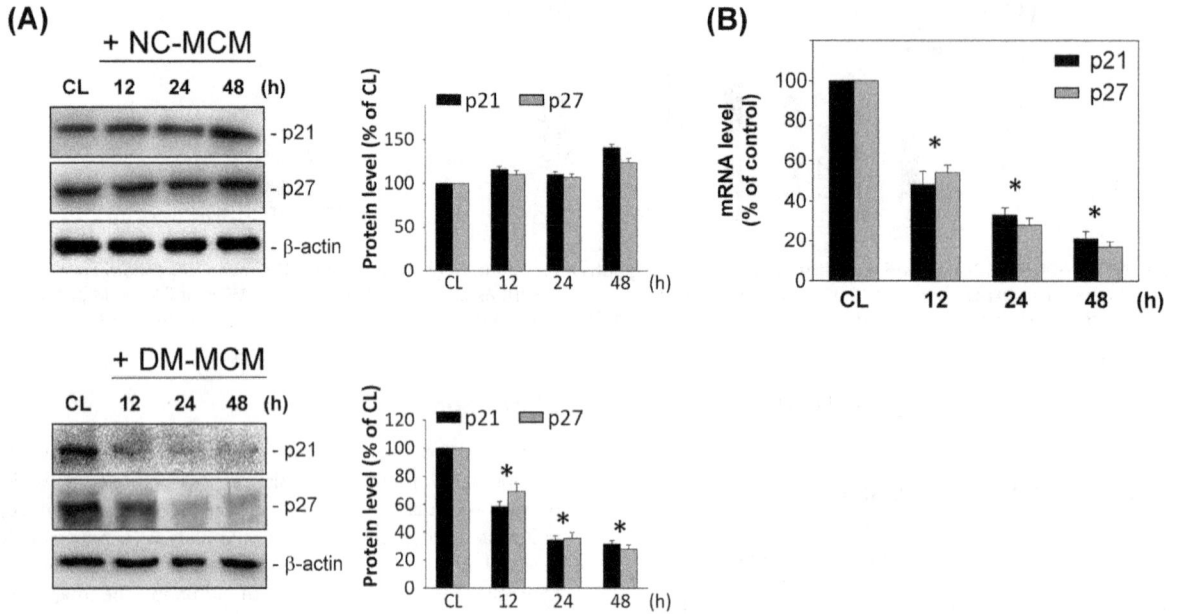

Figure 2. Effects of DM-MCM on p21^{Cip1} and p27^{Kip1} expression. Bar graphs represent folds of CL SMCs, mean $\pm$ SEM from 3 independent experiments. *$P<0.05$ versus CL SMCs. (A) SMCs were kept as CL or stimulated with NC-MCM or DM-MCM for the times indicated. Protein expressions were determined by Western blot analysis. Expression levels of p21^{Cip1} and p27^{Kip1} are presented as band densities (normalized to β-actin) relative to CL. (B) mRNA expressions were determined by real-time PCR analysis and normalized to 18S rRNA.

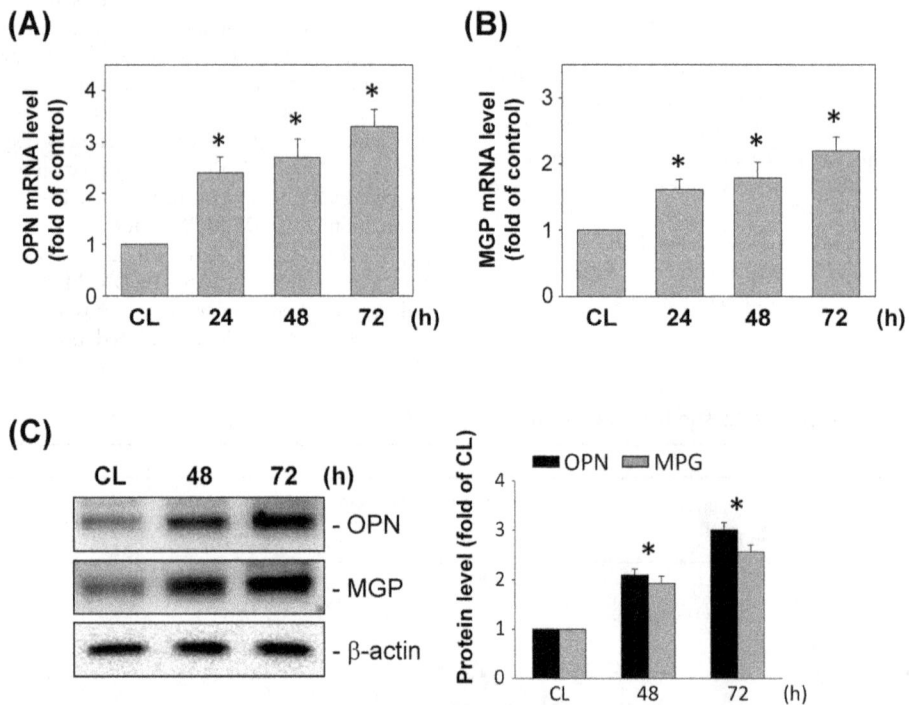

Figure 3. Effects of DM-MCM on synthetic differentiation marker expression in SMCs. Bar graphs represent folds of CL SMCs, mean $\pm$ SEM from 3 independent experiments. *$P<0.05$ versus CL SMCs. (A, B) DM-MCM induced mRNA expressions of osteopontin (OPN) and matrix gla protein (MGP) in SMCs. SMCs were kept as controls (CL) or stimulated with DM-MCM for the times indicated, and the mRNA expressions of OPN (A) and MGP (B) were determined using real-time PCR analysis and normalized to 18S rRNA. (C) SMCs were kept as CL or stimulated with DM-MCM for the times indicated. Protein expressions of OPN and MGP were determined by Western blot analysis. Expression levels of OPN and MGP are presented as band densities (normalized to β-actin) relative to CL.

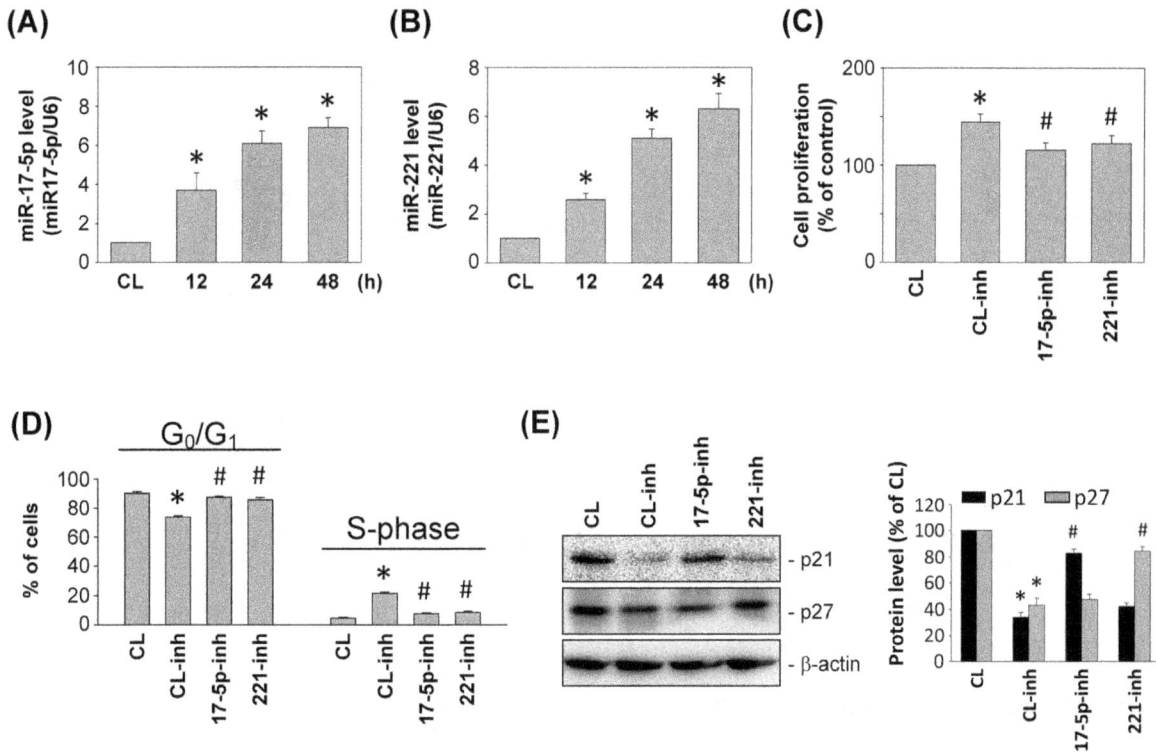

Figure 4. miR-17-5p and miR-221 are involved in the regulation of HASMC proliferation. (A, B) HASMCs were kept as controls (CL) or stimulated with DM-MCM for the times indicated. Relative miR-17-5p (A) and miR-221 (B) levels were determined through real-time PCR in HASMCs and normalized to U6 snRNA from 3 independent experiments. *$P<0.05$ versus CL SMCs. (C–E) SMCs were kept as CL or pretreated with miR-17-5p inhibitor (17-5p inh), miR-221 inhibitor (221 inh), or miRNA control inhibitor (CL inh) for 24 h, and then stimulated with DM-MCM for 24 h. The results are mean $\pm$ SEM from 3 independent experiments. *$P<0.05$ versus CL. #$P<0.05$ versus CL inhibitor (CL inh)-treated SMCs with DM-MCM stimulation. Cell proliferation was assayed by the MTT test (C). The distribution of the cell cycle was analyzed by flow cytometry (D). Protein expressions were determined by Western blot analysis. Expression levels of p21^{Cip1} and p27^{Kip1} are presented as band densities (normalized to β-actin) relative to CL (E).

and proliferation of the SMCs. Third, stimulation of SMCs with DM-MCM also induced expression of miR-221. Pretreatment of the cells with miR-221 inhibitor decreased the DM-MCM-induced down-regulation of p27^{Kip1} and SMC proliferation.

It is believed that extravasation of macrophages in the arterial wall promotes formation of atherosclerotic lesions. It has also been suggested that diabetes-elicited SMC proliferation occurs secondary to the increased macrophage infiltration into the arterial wall [22]. The effects of HG levels on the proliferative capacity of arterial SMCs are controversial. While several studies have demonstrated that HG levels can stimulate SMC proliferation [14,25], others have found no stimulatory effect [26,27]; yet another study has shown an inhibitory effect of HG levels on SMC proliferation [28]. By culturing HASMCs on fibrillar collagen that promotes the maintenance of SMC in a non-proliferative phenotype [19], we have been able to elucidate the factors that signal and control the modulation of HASMC proliferation. The present findings in HASMC cultures showed that treatment with DM-MCM had a stimulatory effect on the proliferation of HASMCs. During cell cycle progression, p21^{Cip1} and p27^{Kip1} have been shown to mediate cell cycle arrest by inhibiting Cdk activities [29]. In this study, mRNA and protein expressions of p21^{Cip1} and p27^{Kip1} were down-regulated in DM-MCM-stimulated HASMCs. Our data also demonstrated that treatment of SMCs with DM-MCM increased the percentage of cells in the S-phase, while the percentage of cells in the G$_0$/G$_1$ phases decreased.

Several studies have revealed the effects of miRNAs on the modulation of functions of SMCs [20,30,31], but the mechanism underlying the DM-MCM-induced proliferation of SMC remains largely unclear. Different miRNAs have been implicated in the regulation of the mitogenic response in SMCs [31,32]. miR-17-5p is one of the critical miRNAs for cell proliferation [33], and its up-regulation has been shown to modulate p21^{Cip1} expression in cancer cells [34]. miR-221 has also been implicated in the regulation of SMC proliferation and neointimal hyperplasia [35], and it has been reported to play an important role in the regulation of p27^{Kip1} down-regulation in SMCs [36]. The present study demonstrated that DM-MCM stimulates SMC proliferation through at least two miRNAs, as indicated by the DM-MCM-induction of increases in miR 17 5p and miR-221, which may be involved in the mitogenic action. We further showed that the inhibition of miR-17-5p inhibited the DM-MCM-induced down-regulation of p21^{Cip1} but had no effect on p27^{Kip1}, while the inhibition of miR-221 affected the down-regulation of p27^{Kip1} but had no effect on p21^{Cip1}. It has previously been shown that the differential regulation of cell-cycle regulatory proteins occurs by different mechanisms [37]. On the basis of these studies and our findings, it is reasonable to propose that DM-MCM may stimulate SMC proliferation through the differential regulation of p21^{Cip1} and p27^{Kip1} expressions regulated by different miRNAs.

It has been reported that a variety of regulatory molecules with the ability to regulate SMC or stem cell function in a paracrine fashion are released from macrophages [18,38]. It is thus

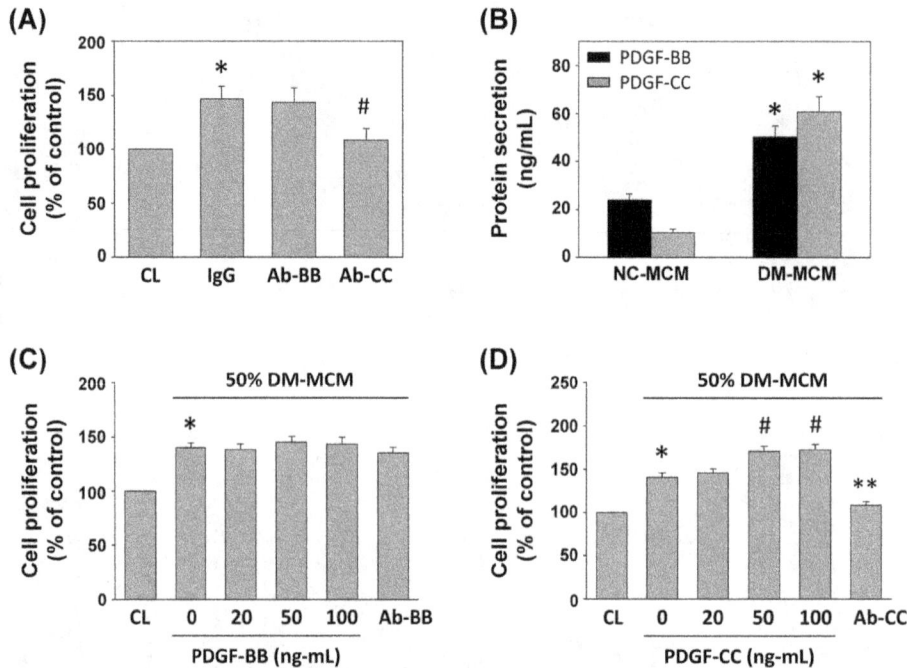

Figure 5. PDGF-CC is the major factor underlying DM-MCM-induced SMC proliferation. (A) Prior to culturing under control conditions (CL) or stimulation with DM-MCM, the DM-MCM and SMCs were pre-incubated with isotype-matched IgG or neutralizing antibodies against PDGF-BB (Ab-BB) or PDGF-CC (Ab-CC) individually for 2 h, and then stimulated with DM-MCM for 24 h. Cell proliferation was assayed by the MTT test from 3 independent experiments. *$P<0.05$ versus CL. #$P<0.05$ versus IgG-treated SMCs under DM-MCM stimulation. (B) The expression levels of PDGF-BB and PDGF-CC in MCM were determined by sandwich ELISA from 3 independent experiments. *$P<0.05$ versus NC-MCM. (C, D) SMCs were kept as CL or stimulated with 50% DM-MCM for 48 h. The proliferation of SMCs was obviously promoted by PDGF-CC at 50 and 100 ng/mL, and the promoting effect was inhibited by the neutralizing antibody against PDGF-CC (Ab-CC) (D). PDGF-BB has no significant effect on promoting SMC proliferation (C). Cell proliferation was assayed by the MTT assay from 3 independent experiments. *$P<0.05$ versus CL. #$P<0.05$ versus 50% DM-MCM-treated SMCs. **$P<0.05$ versus 50% DM-MCM-treated SMCs.

postulated that the elicited SMC growth in atherosclerotic lesions in diabetic conditions is due to the secretion of mediators from macrophages, and that macrophages may be directly affected by the diabetic environments. In our previous study, we observed that MIP-1α and 1β are significantly increased only in macrophages after differentiation under an HG environment [6]. In addition, it has been shown that levels of IGF-I in macrophage-rich regions in lesions of atherosclerosis from diabetic pigs were increased compared to non-diabetic controls [39]. Our present data demonstrated that MCM from DM patients significantly enhanced SMC proliferation, and this induction of cell proliferation by DM-MCM was inhibited following the neutralization of the PDGF-CC in DM-MCM. Hence, we suggest that the accumulation of macrophages in the arterial wall thereby increases the PDGF-CC level and contributes to SMC proliferation.

Taken together, our findings contribute new information about the mechanisms by which DM macrophages induce SMC proliferation. Treatment of SMCs with DM-MCM resulted in differential regulation of SMC–proliferation-mediated miRNAs. Activation of the miR-17-5p led to down-regulation of p21^{Cip1},

whereas activation of the miR-221 led to decreased expression of p27^{Kip1}. These findings provide insights into the mechanisms underlying the interplay between hyperglycemic macrophages with SMCs in modulating SMC function and gene expression, which may well be involved in the development of vascular complications in patients with diabetes.

Study limitations

There are some inherent limitations to this study. Although this study demonstrated that monocyte-derived macrophages differentiated from diabetic patients may affect SMC proliferation, the overall number of controls and patients was small. This association may therefore be correspondingly under- or over-estimated.

Author Contributions

Conceived and designed the experiments: TCC CNC. Performed the experiments: TCC MLS HCK SJC CKY. Analyzed the data: TCC MLS CNC. Contributed reagents/materials/analysis tools: MLS HCK. Wrote the paper: CNC.

References

1. Giacco F, Brownlee M (2010) Oxidative stress and diabetic complications. Circ Res 107: 1058–1070.
2. Rask-Madsen C, King GL (2013) Vascular complications of diabetes: mechanisms of injury and protective factors. Cell Metab 17: 20–33
3. Liang CP, Han S, Senokuchi T, Tall AR (2007) The macrophage at the crossroads of insulin resistance and atherosclerosis. Circ Res 100: 1546–1555.
4. Kanter JE, Johansson F, LeBoeuf RC, Bornfeldt KE (2007) Do glucose and lipids exert independent effects on atherosclerotic lesion initiation or progression to advanced plaques? Circ Res 100: 769–781.
5. Shanmugam N, Reddy MA, Guha M, Natarajan R (2003) High glucose-induced expression of proinflammatory cytokine and chemokine genes in monocytic cells. Diabetes 52: 1256–1264.

6. Chen TC, Chien SJ, Kuo HC, Huang WS, Sheen JM, et al. (2011) High glucose-treated macrophages augment E-selectin expression in endothelial cells. J Biol Chem 286: 25564–25573.

7. Lacolley P, Regnault V, Nicoletti A, Li Z, Michel JB (2012) The vascular smooth muscle cell in arterial pathology: a cell that can take on multiple roles. Cardiovasc Res 95: 194–204.

8. Owens GK, Kumar MS, Wamhoff BR (2004) Molecular regulation of vascular smooth muscle cell differentiation in development and disease. Physiol Rev 84: 767–801.

9. Tedgui A, Mallat Z (2006) Cytokines in atherosclerosis: pathogenic and regulatory pathways. Physiol Rev 86: 515–581.

10. Raines EW (2004) PDGF and cardiovascular disease. Cytokine Growth Factor Rev 15: 237–254.

11. Ahuja P, Sdek P, MacLellan WR (2007) Cardiac myocyte cell cycle control in development, disease, and regeneration. Physiol Rev 87: 521–544.

12. Findeisen HM, Gizard F, Zhao Y, Qing H, Heywood EB, et al. (2011) Epigenetic regulation of vascular smooth muscle cell proliferation and neointima formation by histone deacetylase inhibition. Arterioscler Thromb Vasc Biol 31: 851–860.

13. Bornfeldt KE, Tabas I (2011) Insulin resistance, hyperglycemia, and atherosclerosis. Cell Metab 14: 575–585.

14. Jeong IK, Oh da H, Park SJ, Kang JH, Kim S, et al. (2011) Inhibition of NF-κB prevents high glucose-induced proliferation and plasminogen activator inhibitor-1 expression in vascular smooth muscle cells. Exp Mol Med 43: 684–692.

15. Cai Q, Lanting L, Natarajan R (2004) Growth factors induce monocyte binding to vascular smooth muscle cells: implications for monocyte retention in atherosclerosis. Am J Physiol Cell Physiol 287: C707–714.

16. Proudfoot D, Fitzsimmons C, Torzewski J, Bowyer DE (1999) Inhibition of human arterial smooth muscle cell growth by human monocyte/macrophages: a co-culture study. Atherosclerosis 145: 157–165.

17. Schubert SY, Benarroch A, Ostvang J, Edelman ER (2008) Regulation of endothelial cell proliferation by primary monocytes. Arterioscler Thromb Vasc Biol 28: 97–104.

18. Chung JH, Jeon HJ, Hong SY, Lee da L, Lee KH, et al. (2012) Palmitate promotes the paracrine effects of macrophages on vascular smooth muscle cells: the role of bone morphogenetic proteins. PLoS One 7: e29100.

19. Chen CN, Li YS, Yeh YT, Lee PL, Usami S, et al. (2006) Synergistic roles of platelet-derived growth factor-BB and interleukin-1β in phenotypic modulation of human aortic smooth muscle cells. Proc Natl Acad Sci U S A 103: 2665–2670.

20. Robinson HC, Baker AH (2012) How do microRNAs affect vascular smooth muscle cell biology? Curr Opin Lipidol 23: 405–411.

21. Osório J (2010) Diabetes: Severe hypoglycemia associated with risk of vascular events and death. Nat Rev Cardiol 7: 666.

22. Askari B, Renard CB, Bornfeldt KE (2002) Regulation of smooth muscle cell accumulation in diabetes-accelerated atherosclerosis. Histol Histopathol 17: 1317–1328.

23. Matsumoto T, Kobayashi T, Kamata K (2010) Diabetic conditions act as matchmaker for monocytes and vascular smooth muscle cells. Am J Physiol Heart Circ Physiol 298: H731–733.

24. Febbraio M, Hajjar DP, Silverstein RL (2001) CD36: a class B scavenger receptor involved in angiogenesis, atherosclerosis, inflammation, and lipid metabolism. J Clin Invest 108: 785–791.

25. Yu S, Xi Z, Hai-Yan C, Ya-Li C, Shao-Hu X, et al. (2012) Interferon regulatory factor-1 as a positive regulator for high glucose-induced proliferation of vascular smooth muscle cells. J Cell Biochem 113: 2671–2678.

26. Suzuki LA, Poot M, Gerrity RG, Bornfeldt KE (2001) Diabetes accelerates smooth muscle accumulation in lesions of atherosclerosis: lack of direct growth-promoting effects of high glucose levels. Diabetes 50: 851–860.;

27. Indolfi C, Torella D, Cavuto L, Davalli AM, Coppola C, et al. (2001) Effects of balloon injury on neointimal hyperplasia in streptozotocin-induced diabetes and in hyperinsulinemic nondiabetic pancreatic islet-transplanted rats. Circulation 103: 2980–2986.

28. Peiró C, Lafuente N, Matesanz N, Cercas E, Llergo JL, et al. (2001) High glucose induces cell death of cultured human aortic smooth muscle cells through the formation of hydrogen peroxide. Br J Pharmacol 133: 967–974.

29. Tanner FC, Boehm M, Akyürek LM, San H, Yang ZY, et al. (2000) Differential effects of the cyclin-dependent kinase inhibitors p27^{Kip1}, p21^{Cip1}, and p16^{Ink4} on vascular smooth muscle cell proliferation. Circulation 101: 2022–2025

30. Li P, Zhu N, Yi B, Wang N, Chen M, et al. (2013) MicroRNA-663 Regulates Human Vascular Smooth Muscle Cell Phenotypic Switch and Vascular Neointimal Formation. Circ Res 113: 1117–1127.

31. Sun Y, Chen D, Cao L, Zhang R, Zhou J, et al. (2013) MiR-490-3p modulates the proliferation of vascular smooth muscle cells induced by ox-LDL through targeting PAPP-α. Cardiovasc Res 100: 272–279.

32. Liu X, Cheng Y, Chen X, Yang J, Xu L, et al. (2011) MicroRNA-31 regulated by the extracellular regulated kinase is involved in vascular smooth muscle cell growth via large tumor suppressor homolog 2. J Biol Chem 286: 42371–42380.

33. Cloonan N, Brown MK, Steptoe AL, Wani S, Chan WL, et al. (2008) The miR-17-5p microRNA is a key regulator of the G1/S phase cell cycle transition. Genome Biol 9: R127.

34. Ballarino M, Jobert L, Dembélé D, de la Grange P, Auboeuf D, et al. (2013) TAF15 is important for cellular proliferation and regulates the expression of a subset of cell cycle genes through miRNAs. Oncogene 32: 4646–4655.

35. Liu X, Cheng Y, Zhang S, Lin Y, Yang J, et al. (2009) A necessary role of miR-221 and miR-222 in vascular smooth muscle cell proliferation and neointimal hyperplasia. Circ Res 104: 476–487.

36. Davis BN, Hilyard AC, Nguyen PH, Lagna G, Hata A (2009) Induction of microRNA-221 by platelet-derived growth factor signaling is critical for modulation of vascular smooth muscle phenotype. J Biol Chem 284: 3728–3738.

37. Chiang JK, Sung ML, Yu HR, Chang HI, Kuo HC, et al. (2011) Homocysteine induces smooth muscle cell proliferation through differential regulation of cyclins A and D1 expression. J Cell Physiol 226: 1017–1026.

38. Lee MJ, Kim MY, Heo SC, Kwon YW, Kim YM, et al. (2012) Macrophages regulate smooth muscle differentiation of mesenchymal stem cells via a prostaglandin F$_{2α}$-mediated paracrine mechanism. Arterioscler Thromb Vasc Biol 32: 2733–2740.

39. Askari B, Carroll MA, Capparelli M, Kramer F, Gerrity RG, et al. (2002) Oleate and linoleate enhance the growth-promoting effects of insulin-like growth factor-I through a phospholipase D-dependent pathway in arterial smooth muscle cells. J Biol Chem 277: 36338–36344.

4

Inflammation-Induced Reactivation of the Ranavirus Frog Virus 3 in Asymptomatic *Xenopus laevis*

Jacques Robert*, Leon Grayfer, Eva-Stina Edholm, Brian Ward, Francisco De Jesús Andino

Department of Microbiology and Immunology, University of Rochester Medical Center, Rochester, United States of America

Abstract

Natural infections of ectothermic vertebrates by ranaviruses (RV, family *Iridoviridae*) are rapidly increasing, with an alarming expansion of RV tropism and resulting die-offs of numerous animal populations. Notably, infection studies of the amphibian *Xenopus laevis* with the ranavirus *Frog Virus 3* (*FV3*) have revealed that although the adult frog immune system is efficient at controlling RV infections, residual quiescent virus can be detected in mononuclear phagocytes of otherwise asymptomatic animals following the resolution of RV infections. It is noteworthy that macrophage-lineage cells are now believed to be a critical element in the RV infection strategy. In the present work, we report that inflammation induced by peritoneal injection of heat-killed bacteria in asymptomatic frogs one month after infection with *FV3* resulted in viral reactivation including detectable viral DNA and viral gene expression in otherwise asymptomatic frogs. *FV3* reactivation was most prominently detected in kidneys and in peritoneal HAM56+ mononuclear phagocytes. Notably, unlike adult frogs that typically clear primary *FV3* infections, a proportion of the animals succumbed to the reactivated *FV3* infection, indicating that previous exposure does not provide protection against subsequent reactivation in these animals.

Editor: Michael Klymkowsky, University of Colorado, Boulder, United States of America

Funding: This research was supported by the National Institutes of Health Grant (R24-AI-059830); LG was supported by a Life Sciences Research Fellowship from the Howard Hughes Medical Institute. The funders had no role in study design, data collection and analysis, decision to publish, or preparation of the manuscript.

Competing Interests: The authors have declared that no competing interests exist.

* Email: Jacques_Robert@urmc.rochester.edu

Introduction

Infections and die-offs caused by ranaviruses (RVs, family *Iridoviridae*) are increasing in prevalence concomitant with an unprecedented and alarming rise in the numbers of susceptible host species (including amphibians, bony fishes and reptiles) [1,2]. Notably, the remarkable ability of RVs to cross species barriers of numerous ectothermic vertebrates, suggests that these pathogens possess potent immune evasion mechanisms [3]. Furthermore, although some ectothermic vertebrate species are highly susceptible to RVs, others are more resistant and may serve as asymptomatic carriers that disseminate infectious virus. While RV infections and host pathogen interactions are increasingly documented for a variety of amphibian species, there is still very little known about mechanisms of ranaviral pathogenicity and host immune defenses to these large complex DNA viruses, whose genomes encode some 100 genes [4–6]. Using *X. laevis* and the RV *Frog Virus 3* (*FV3*), we have established a reliable experimental system to elucidate at the cellular and molecular levels interactions between RV pathogens and their amphibian hosts [7,8]. While our studies have shown the critical roles of CD8 T cells and antibody responses in controlling *FV3* infections, our findings also underscore a prominent role for macrophage-lineage cells both in the defense against RVs and as contributors to their immune evasion and possibly persistence [9].

In mammals, macrophage cell populations consist of long-lived, terminally differentiated and extensively heterogeneous immune cell populations, indispensable to host immunity and homeostasis.

As sentinels of the immune system, macrophages recognize viral infections through a repertoire of pattern recognition receptors, and facilitate viral clearance by producing an array of bioactive molecules, as well as by serving as antigen presenting cells able to activate T cells [10]. Conversely, distinct macrophage subsets may become productively infected by certain viruses (e.g., human immunodeficiency virus [HIV], measles, etc.), and serve as long-term viral reservoirs and agents of pathogen dissemination [11–13]. However, the viral strategy for utilizing macrophage lineages for immune escape, persistence and spread within their hosts has thus far been documented primarily for RNA viruses [13]. Notably, during the early stages of *FV3* infections, there is an accumulation of activated macrophages in the peritoneal cavity, exhibiting increased pro-inflammatory cytokine gene expression (IL-1β and TNFα) [14,15]. Intriguingly, subsequent to the resolution of the infection, peritoneal macrophages isolated from some, but not all asymptomatic animals harbor transcriptionally inactive *FV3* [14,15]. Based on these findings we have hypothesized that although adult frog macrophages are integral to anti-*FV3* immune responses, some of these cells are permissive to this pathogen and harbor quiescent, non-replicating virus. Similar to mammals, *Xenopus* peritoneal leukocytes (PLs) are a heterogeneous group of cells that, based on morphology and Giemsa staining patterns, include polymorphonuclear (PMN) granulocytes as well as monocytes and macrophage-like cells, and smaller lymphocytes [16,17]. We previously demonstrated that peritoneal injections of *X. laevis* with heat-killed *Escherichia coli* results in the accumulation of large numbers of PLs primarily composed (70 to 80%) of macrophages [18]. The present study examines the capacity to reactivate quiescent *FV3* in previously infected, asymptomatic *X. laevis* by inflammatory stimulation of these animals through intra-peritoneal administration of heat-killed *E. coli*.

Material and Methods

Animals

Outbred adult frogs were obtained from our *X. laevis* research resource for immunology at the University of Rochester (http://www.urmc.rochester.edu/smd/mbi/xenopus/index.htm). For all experiments outbred 2 year-old (~6 cm length) adult frogs were infected by intraperitoneal (i.p.) injection of 1×10^6 pfu of *FV3* in 0.2 ml of PBS modified to amphibian osmolarity (APBS) using a 1 ml sterile syringe with a 22 gauge, 1 ½ inch needle. Animals were maintained individually in 1 L container and reared by standard husbandry (feeding, cleaning). Virally infected animals were euthanized to minimize suffering as soon as abnormal behavior (listlessness, altered swimming and feeding, etc.) or signs of acute systemic infection (edema, floating a the surface) was detected or they displayed. Euthanasia was done by immersion in a 0.5% aqueous solution of tricaine methane sulfonate (MS-222), buffered with sodium bicarbonate.

Ethics Statement

Experiments involving frogs were carried out according to the Animal Welfare Act from the United States Department of Agriculture (USDA), the Public Health Service Policy (A-3292-01) and the Public Health Act of New York State. Any discomfort was minimized at all times. Animal care and all the protocols has been reviewed and approved by the University of Rochester Committee on Animal Resources (Approval number 100577/2003-151).

Frog Virus 3 Stocks and Animal Infections

Fathead minnow cells (FHM; American Type Culture Collection, ATCC No. CCL-42) were maintained in Dulbecco's modified Eagle's medium (DMEM; Invitrogen) supplemented with 10% fetal bovine serum (FBS; Invitrogen), penicillin (100 U/mL) and streptomycin (100 µg/mL) with 5% CO_2 at 30°C. *FV3* was grown by a single passage on FMH cells, purified by ultracentrifugation on a 30% sucrose cushion and quantified by plaque assay on FMH monolayer under an overlay of growth media containing 1% methylcellulose [14]. A6 kidney cells (ATCC No. CCL-102) were maintained in the same DMEM culture medium diluted to amphibian osmolarity (addition of 30% water).

Bacterial Stimulation

E. coli (XL1-blue, Stratagene, La Jolla, Ca.) cultured overnight at 37°C, were boiled for 1 hour, pelleted by centrifugation and resuspended in 1/10 of the initial volume (approximately 1×10^8 bacteria/ml) of APBS [19]. Infected frogs were injected i.p. with 300 µl of the heat-killed bacteria mixture (3×10^7 bacteria; corresponding to 3 mg of protein).

Plaque Forming Assays

FV3-infected kidneys, PLs or A6 cells were lysed in hypotonic buffer (Tris-HCL 50 mM; pH 7.5) by 3 freezing/thawing cycles and serially diluted in DMEM supplemented with 2.5% FBS. Five hundred µl of each dilution was plated in duplicate onto confluent monolayers of FHM cells in 6-well plates, and incubated at 30°C for 1 h with gentle agitation of volumes of viral particles every 20 min. Remaining volumes of viral particles were removed by

aspiration and 3 ml of overlay medium (DMEM supplemented with 2.5% FBS and 1% methyl-cellulose (Sigma) was added. Cells were incubated for 7 days at 30°C in 5% CO_2. Overlay media was aspirated and the cells stained for 10 min with 1% crystal violet in 20% ethanol.

PCR, RT-PCR and Quantitative Real-time PCR (qPCR)

RNA and DNA were extracted from cells and tissues using Trizol reagent following the manufacturer's protocol (Invitrogen). Total RNA (0.5 µg in in 20 µl) was used to synthesize cDNA with the iScript cDNA synthesis kit (Bio-Rad, Hercules, CA). One µl of cDNA template was used in all RT-PCRs and 50 ng DNA for PCR. Minus reverse transcriptase (RT) controls were included for every reaction, and all primers spanned at least one intron (Table 1). A water-only control was included in each reaction. PCR products were separated on 1.0% agarose gels and stained with ethidium bromide. Sizes of the products were determined using standardized markers of 1 kb plus from Invitrogen (Carlsbad, CA).

Cytospins and Cell Staining

Peritoneal leukocytes (PLs; 2×10^5 cells in 200 µl volume) were cytocentrifuged using a Shandon Southern cytospin centrifuge (600 rpm, 5 min.), fixed with 3.7% formalin for 1 min, permeabilized with 100% cold methanol (-20°C) and briefly washed with APBS. After blocking with 1% BSA in APBS for 1 hr, the PLs were incubated overnight with rabbit anti-*FV3* 53R serum [20] and mouse anti-HAM56 mAbs [21]. After washing, cells were incubated with DyLight 488-conjugated F(ab')2 Donkey Anti-Rabbit IgG (H+L) (Jackson ImmunoReaserch, PA) or DyLight 594-conjugated F(ab')2 Donkey Anti-Mouse IgG (H+L) (Jackson ImmunoResearch, PA), respectively. Cells then were stained with the fluorescent DNA intercalator (Hoechst-33258). Preparations were mounted in anti-fade medium (Molecular Probes, Oregon) and visualized with a Leica DMIRB inverted fluorescence microscope with a cooled charge-couple device (Cooke) controlled by Image-Pro software (Media Cybernetics).

Statistics

One-way ANOVA and Long-rank (Mantel Cox) comparisons tests were performed using GraphPad Prism version 6.00 for Windows, GraphPad Software, La Jolla California USA, (URL: www.graphpad.com).

Results

1. Detection of *FV3* DNA and transcripts in peritoneal leukocytes upon bacterial stimulation of previously challenged, asymptomatic adults

Intraperitoneal injection of heat killed (HK) bacteria (*E. coli*) into *X. laevis* adults results in a robust recruitment and accumulation of leukocytes in the peritoneal cavity within 3 days [14]. Based on Giemsa staining and morphological analysis, these elicited peritoneal leukocytes (PLs) were primarily composed of mononuclear phagocytes (>80%). To confirm these observations, we assessed the changes in the gene expression of macrophage and granulocyte growth factor receptors (M-CSFR and G-CSFR, respectively) during HK *E. coli*-elicited PL accumulation. Whereas the G-CSFR transcript levels showed an early transitory increase at 6 hrs following bacterial stimulation and declined to baseline levels by 24 hrs, the M-CSFR gene expression markedly increased from 24 hrs to 72 hrs post-stimulation (Fig. 1; corresponding to experiment 3 in Table 2). These data are in good concordance to

Table 1. Primer sequences used in this study.

Primers	Sequences
GAPDH	F: 5' - ACCCCTTCATCGACTTGGAC - 3'
	R: 5' - GGAGCCAGACAGTTTGTAGTG - 3'
EF-1α	F: 5' - CCTGAATCACCCAGGCCAGATTGGTG - 3'
	R: 5' - GAGGGTAGTGTGAGAAGCTCTCCACG - 3'
FV3 DNA Poly II	F: 5' - ACGAGCCCGACGAAGACTACATAG - 3'
	R: 5' - TGGTGGTCCTCAGCATCCTTTG - 3'
MCP	F: 5' - GACTTGGCCACTTATGAC - 3'
	R: 5' - GTCTCTGGAGAAGAAGAAGAA - 3'
MCSF-R	F: 5' - TGTATTCTTTGG ACT TGC CGT ATCTGG - 3'
	R: 5' - TTGTTTAGCTTCAAATTCTGGGTAATA - 3'

ªF, forward; R, reverse.

a predominant accumulation of mononuclear phagocytes 3 days after bacterial stimulation and further support our previous observations [14].

We next assessed whether HK *E. coli* stimulation of adult frogs with asymptomatic *FV3* infection (i.e., usually exhibiting undetectable levels of *FV3* DNA after immune clearance) may result in recruitment of macrophages harboring quiescent *FV3* from the periphery into the peritoneum and the reactivation of this quiescent virus. To this end, two-year old adult frogs were infected with a sub-lethal dose (10^6 PFU) of *FV3* and maintained for 30 days to ensure viral clearance, which usually occurs within 2 weeks [9]. At 30 days post-infection (dpi), the efficacy of viral clearance was evaluated by PCR and RT-PCR analysis of PLs. Subsequently (at 32 dpi), animals were injected with HK *E. coli* and PLs were again isolated 3 days later (35 dpi; Fig. 2A). Following these procedures, frogs were maintained under observation for further 60 more days (until 90 dpi total).

Initially, we examined whether viral DNA could be detected by PCR in PLs prior to bacterial stimulation, using *FV3* major capsid protein (MCP) and the viral DNA polymerase II-specific primers (vDNA pol II; *FV3* ORF 60R [22]). Before the inflammatory stimulus, detectable levels of *FV3* DNA were seen in 3 out of 15 frogs (1 prominently, and 2 at the limit of detection with this assay), indicating effective viral clearance at 30 dpi (Fig. 2B). In stark contrast, *FV3* DNA was detected in the PLs of 12 out 15 individuals 3 days after bacterial stimulation (35 dpi; Fig. 2C). Furthermore, the high intensity of some of the detected PCR products was suggestive of extensive viral loads (Fig. 1C; lane 3 and 6). As summarized in Table 2, comparable findings were obtained from 4 independent experiments. On average, 62% (28/45) of bacterially-stimulated frogs exhibited *FV3* reactivation (35 dpi), compared to only 6% seen in these animals just before the administration of the inflammatory stimulus (30 dpi). *FV3* was not detected in animal whole blood or purified blood leukocyte fractions (Fig. S1). This is consistent with previous observations indicating that *FV3* is only detected in blood circulation during early systemic infections [8,23].

To confirm that the inflammatory stimuli resulted in active infections, we examined *FV3* gene expression at 35 dpi (3 days post bacterial stimulation) of two integral viral genes: the early-expressed vDNA Pol II critical for RV replication and the late-expressed major capsid protein (MCP) that encodes the RV capsid subunits. RT-PCR analysis of cDNA synthesized from DNAse-treated RNA sample (Fig. 3) revealed that the expression of these

FV3 genes closely reflected the presence or absence of the *FV3* DNA (Fig. 2; Table 2). PLs from 8 of 15 HK *E. coli*-stimulated individuals showed significant FV3 gene expression (Fig. 3). Notably, similar results were obtained in the 3 additional experiments, whereas there was no detectable viral gene expression in cDNA samples mock-synthesized in absence of the reverse transcriptase (-RT), ruling out possible viral genomic DNA contamination of the RNA/cDNA samples (Fig. 3).

We conclude that the residual persisting *FV3* in a fraction of asymptomatic *X. laevis* adults may reestablish infections following bacterial stimulation. In addition, *FV3* gene expression suggests that FV3 detected in PLs after bacterial stimulation is transcriptionally active.

2. Reactivation of quiescent *FV3* by bacterial stimulation results in increased frog host mortality

To determine whether the inflammatory stimuli-induced *FV3* reactivation results in productive viral infections, we monitored animal survival over a period of 2 months. Strikingly, a significant fraction of these animals exhibited symptoms of acute ranaviral infection (Table 2) and ultimately succumbed from systemic viral infection (Fig. 4). It is noteworthy that *X. laevis* adult frogs are typically resistant to primary *FV3* infections [8]. Indeed, initial *FV3* inoculation of a control group from the same animal cohort resulted in a 10% mortality rate (see below and Table 2), which is consistent with our previous published observations [8,23]. In addition, only two animals died from bacterial stimulation alone (6%), likely reflecting complications from anesthesia. In contrast, the induction of systemic lethal infections was consistently obtained in several independent experiments and reached 36% animal mortality within a period of 60 days following bacterial stimulation (90 dpi total).

We additionally scored these animals for hallmark symptoms of RV disease including lethargy, skin redness (hemorrhage), shedding and edema [23]. Hemorrhage and tissue damages in the kidney and liver were also confirmed during necropsy of animals that died or were euthanized because of severe signs of sickness. We verified the occurrence of systemic *FV3* infection by PCR assays, and substantial viral DNA was detected in most tissues including spleens, livers and kidneys (Fig. 5).

Whereas *FV3* DNA was detected by PCR in most of the frogs that subsequently succumbed from FV3 infections, a few animals with undetectable viral loads in PLs following bacterial stimulation developed subsequent systemic *FV3* infections. It is possible that in

M-CSFR

G-CSFR

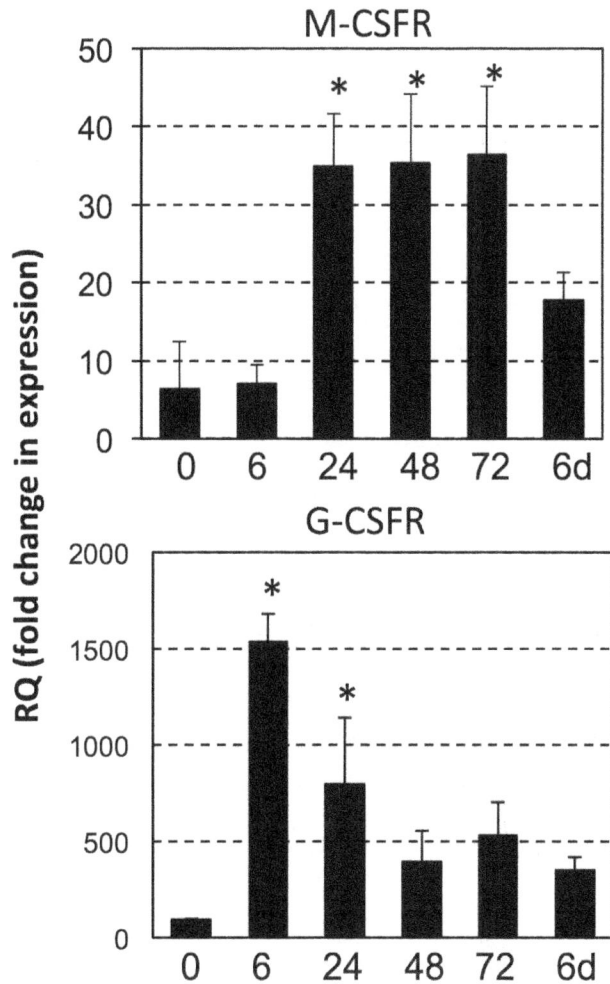

Figure 1. Change in gene expression of the macrophage marker M-CSFR and the granulocyte marker G-CSFR following injection of heat-killed bacteria. At different time points (6, 24, 48, 72 hrs and 6 days) following injection of heat killed *E. coli*, peritoneal phagocytes were isolated and assessed by qRT-PCR for genes expression of M-CFSR and G-CSFR. Gene expression was normalized relative to the GAPDH control. Results are means ± SEM; (*) over bars indicates significant differences between untreated control and experimental animals (3 individual per group).

these cases *FV3*-harboring macrophages (and/or other cells) were not recruited into the peritoneum or alternatively that the kinetics of reactivation in these animals were slower (than 33 dpi). Conversely, several frogs with detectable *FV3* DNA and viral gene transcripts did not develop systemic infection, suggesting that in these instances the host immune systems were effectively controlling the RV reactivated infections.

3. Detection of *FV3*-infected peritoneal macrophages after reactivation by bacterial stimulation

We have previously demonstrated that *X. laevis* peritoneal phagocytes harbor apparently quiescent *FV3* subsequent to general immune clearance of the viral infections [14,15]. We hypothesize that *FV3* could then persists in these macrophages, and serve as reservoir for viral dissemination upon appropriate re-

stimulation. We were therefore interested to determine whether *FV3* infected cells can be detected within mononuclear or polymorphonuclear peritoneal phagocyte populations. Accordingly, we examined PLs by fluorescence microscopy using the anti-53R Ab to detect *FV3* infected cells [20] and the macrophage marker HAM56 [21]. As we previously observed [14,18], PLs harvested from non-*FV3*-infected *X. laevis* 3 days after bacterial stimulation were mainly composed of macrophages, staining positive for HAM56 (Fig. 6A). More importantly, the anti-53R Ab positively stained a substantial fraction (from 20% to as much as 60% for the heavily infected animals) of peritoneal macrophages from animals with reactivated *FV3* infection. Indeed, these 53R+ mononuclear phagocytes not only stained positive for HAM56 but also exhibited typical macrophage morphology (e.g., reniform nucleus, scattered granulation, ruffled membranes). Similar to epithelial cells infected by *FV3* [23], the cellular 53R-staining pattern of these macrophages was strictly cytosolic with punctate structures of different sizes (Fig. 6B–D). Whereas some macrophages exhibited faint positive 53R signal (Fig. 6B), others were strongly stained for 53R (Fig. 6C, D). In addition, there were no obvious signs of apoptosis (e.g., pyknotic nuclei) or marked cellular damage in the infected macrophage cells (Fig. 6 and data not shown). Intriguingly, no HAM negative cells were stained with the anti-53R Ab., indicating that *FV3* peritoneal reactivation was confined to HAM+ mononuclear phagocytes. Finally, no cells were stained by the anti-53R in PLs from uninfected, bacterially stimulated controls (Fig. 6E).

4. Inefficiency of peritoneal macrophages to produce infectious virus

Given our previous [14,15] and present (Fig. 6) observations indicating that *FV3* infection of macrophages is different from that of epithelial cells such as in the kidney, we investigated the ability of PLs to support *in vitro* viral replication and to produce infectious virus. For this purpose, we infected in parallel at an MOI of 1 equal numbers (1×10^6) of PLs obtained from uninfected bacterially elicited frogs and the *X. laevis* A6 kidney cell line (Fig. 7). To establish that the cells were infected, they were assayed for *FV3* vDNA Pol II gene expression as in Fig. 3. Whereas vDNA Pol II gene expression was detected in both cell types, indicating that both were infected, there were approximately 2 logs greater viral gene expression from the A6 cells at 24 h and 3 logs by 48 h as compared to PLs (Fig. 7A). Furthermore, plaque assay analysis revealed that *FV3* infection of PLs resulted in little to no virus production, whereas a significant increase in *FV3* production was seen in the A6 cells by 24 h (Fig. 7B). Notably, PL lysis and cell death remained negligible for 6–7 days (20–30%) after infection, whereas most A6 cells were lysed within this time frame (data not shown).

Owing to the apparent lack of *FV3* expansion in *X. laevis* PL cultures *in vitro* (Fig. 7), we next assessed whether virus was produced during HK *E. coli*-mediated *FV3* reactivation *in vivo*. PLs and kidneys from *FV3* infected and reactivated animals were harvested and assessed (Fig. 8). Consistently, a significant fraction of these animals exhibited *FV3* reactivation in PLs as determined by PCR (Fig. 8A). However, plaque assays revealed a complete absence of infectious viral particles within these cells. In contrast, kidney tissues from five randomly selected animals yielded notable infectious *FV3* particles (Fig. 8B). To confirm the inability of PLs to foster infectious *FV3 in vivo*, another pool of adult frogs was infected for 3, 6 and 30 days before PLs and kidneys were harvested for plaque assay (Fig. 8C). Notably, infectious virus was detectable in PLs harvested at 3 and 6 dpi but not at 35 dpi following inflammatory stimulation (Fig. 8C). In contrast, the

Table 2. Detection of viral DNA and viral transcription in *X. laevis* adult's PL cells lysates after *FV3* infection or *FV3* + Bacterial stimulation.

Treatment [a]	Experiments	Total Number of frogs	PCR [b]	RT-PCR [b]	Sign of infection	Death [c]
FV3 + *E. coli*	Exp. 1	10	7	7	2	3 (30%)
	Exp. 2	10	5	5	4	5 (50%)
	Exp. 3	15	11	11	5	7 (43%)
	Exp. 4	10	5	2	2	1 (10%)
	Total	**45**	**28**	**25**	**13**	**16 (36%)**
FV3 only	Exp. 1	10	3	3	ND	0 (0%)
	Exp. 2	10	1	0	ND	0 (0%)
	Exp. 3	20	2	3	3	4 (20%)
	Exp. 4	10	3	0	ND	0 (0%)
	Total	**50**	**9**	**6**	**3**	**4 (8%)**
E. Coli only	Exp. 1	10	ND	ND	1	1 (10%)
	Exp. 2	10	ND	ND	ND	1 (10%)
	Exp. 3	13	ND	ND	ND	0 (0%)
	Total	**33**	**ND**	**ND**	**1**	**2 (6%)**
APBS	Exp. 1	5	ND	ND	ND	0 (0%)
	Exp. 2	5	ND	ND	ND	0 (0%)
	Exp. 3	8	ND	ND	ND	0 (0%)
	Total	**18**	**ND**	**ND**	**ND**	**0 (0%)**

[a]Treatments: Adult frogs were treated by i.p. injection with: APBS only (30 days treatment); *E. coli* only (3 days treatment); *FV3* only (30 days treatment); or *FV3* + *E. coli* (30 days treatment with *FV3* preceding of 2 days of recovery and 3 days treatment with HK *E. coli*).
[b]*FV3* detection by the indicated method; ND: not detected.
[c]Death that resulted from the treatments. All frogs in each group were monitored and death was recorded daily for 60 days after each treatment.

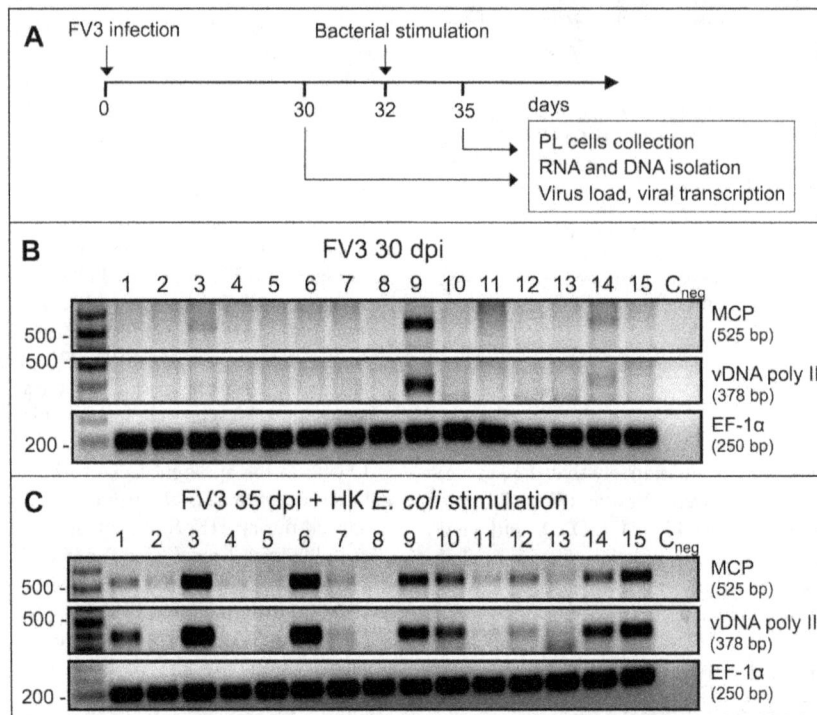

Figure 2. Bacterial stimulation-mediated reappearance of *FV3* DNA in PLs of adult frogs after viral clearance. (A) Experimental outline. (B) PCR assay on total DNA purified from PLs harvested from 15 different outbred frogs (Experiment 3 in Table 2) at 30 dpi, and (C) PCR assay on DNA purified from PLs collected from the same animals 3 days after bacterial stimulation (35 dpi). Presence of viral DNA was assed by PCR on 50 ng of total DNA using *FV3* specific primers for MCP and vDNA poly II as well as *X. laevis* Ef-1α as a loading control.

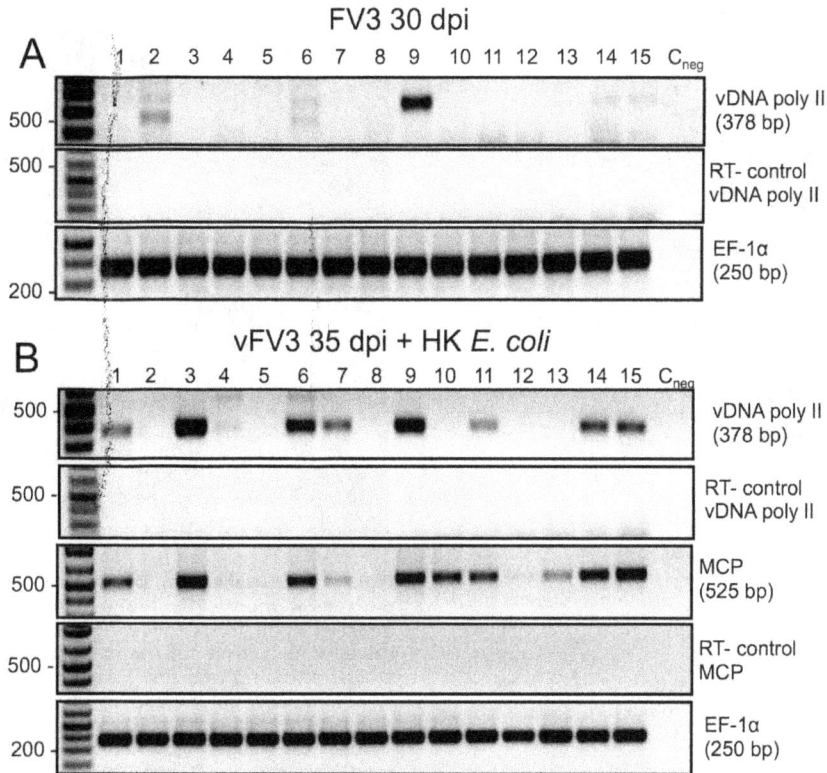

Figure 3. Detection of viral gene expression in PLs of frogs following bacterial stimulation. RT-PCR assay of DNase-treated RNA purified from PLs harvested from the same 15 different frogs used in Fig. 2 ((Experiment 3 in Table 2) at 30 dpi (A), and 3 days later after bacterial stimulation at 35 dpi (B) using *FV3* specific primers for vDNA pol and MCP as well as *X. laevis* Ef-1α as a loading control. RT minus controls were included to rule out contamination by genomic DNA.

kidney tissues contained significant PFU of *FV3* during the primary infection (3 & 6 dpi) and following reactivation with HK *E. coli*, 33 dpi (Fig. 8C).

These data further substantiates the poor ability of *FV3* harboring PLs to produce infectious virus progeny, suggesting that the kidney may also be the primary site of productive infection upon FV3 reactivation.

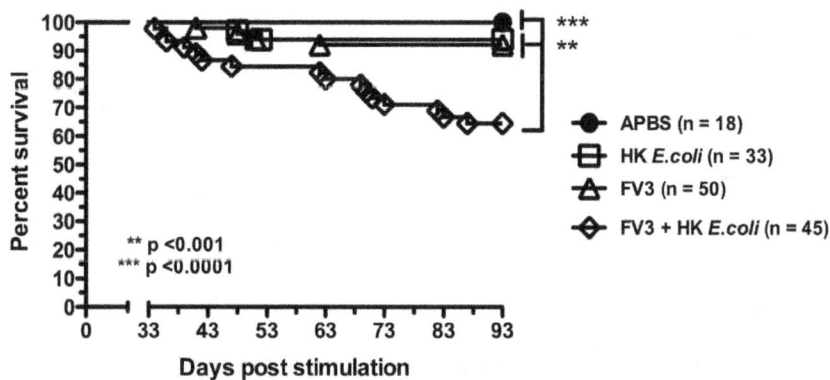

Figure 4. Survival of asymptomatic *FV3* infected adult frogs following bacterial stimulation. Kaplan-Meier curves represent outbred individual animals from three different experiments (35 total animals) that were infected with 1×10^6 PFU of *FV3*, subjected to a peritoneal lavage at 30 dpi, injected with heat-killed bacteria and subjected to another peritoneal lavage at 35 dpi, then monitored daily for signs of *FV3* infection and death for 60 days (*FV3*+HK *E. coli*). Control animals included a group of 18 uninfected animals injected with saline vehicle (APBS), a group of 33 animals shame-infected with APBS that underwent peritoneal lavages and bacterial stimulation (HK *E. coli*), and a group of 40 animals infected with 1×10^6 *FV3* (FV3). Statistical analysis was performed using the log-rank test (Mantel Cox) of a GraphPad Prism version 6.00 for Windows, La Jolla California USA, (URL: www.graphpad.com). The result are as follows: APBS vs HK *E. coli*, $P < 0.1$; APBS vs *FV3*, $P < 0.1$; APBS vs *FV3*+HK *E coli*, $P < 0.001$; HK *E. coli* P vs *FV3*+HK *E. coli*, $P < 0.001$.

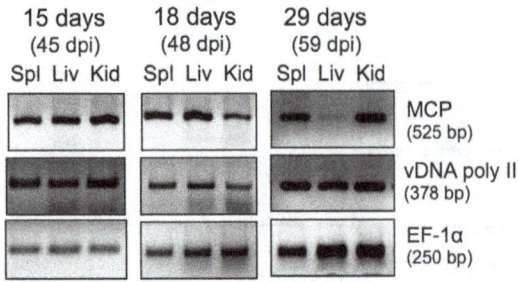

Figure 5. PCR diagnostic of asymptomatic *FV3* infected adult frogs that died following bacterial stimulation. PCR was performed on DNA extracted from spleen (Spl), liver (Liv) and kidneys (Kid) of a representative of frogs that died 15, 18 or 29 days after bacterial stimulation (45, 48 or 59 dpi, respectively) using primers specific for *FV3* MCP, vDNA poly II and EF-1α as control.

Discussion

This study represents the first report detailing concrete evidence of the roles of macrophage-lineage cells in the persistence of RV infections in otherwise resistant and asymptomatic hosts. Furthermore, our findings pertaining to the capacity of inflammatory stimuli such as bacterial challenge to reactivate and reestablish previously dormant ranavirus infections, often to the detriment of the amphibian hosts, reflect a previously unappreciated mechanism of RV dissemination.

Although macrophages have been found infected by RVs in amphibian [24,25] and reptile [26,27] species, little is known about the precise roles of these cells during RV infections. As in mammals, we have shown that *Xenopus* macrophages are actively involved in early host antiviral innate immune responses [14], and serve as antigen presenting cells able to activate T cells [28,29]. Interestingly, studies using *FV3* inoculations of rats as a hepatitis model have underlined the preferential tropism of *FV3* for liver macrophages (Kupffer cells, [30]). Notably, shortly after infection viral particles have been detected in phagocytic vacuoles and endocytic compartments of these macrophages [31]. Although mammalian cells grow at 37°C and are thus not permissive to ranaviral replication, these earlier studies suggest that mononuclear phagocytes represent cellular targets of RV infections, presumably due to their high phagocytic and endocytic activities. Our present work using the *Xenopus* animal model supports the notion that *FV3* infection of peritoneal macrophages is distinct from epithelial cell infiltration by this virus. In mammals, certain RNA viruses such as HIV or measles infect macrophage subsets to evade immunity and persist in a latent or quiescent state within their hosts [11,12]. However, this strategy is not typical of large DNA viruses such as *FV3*. Poxviruses such as vaccinia, which have similarities to RVs and are thought to be phylogenetically related [32], are not known to remain quiescent in host cells, but have evolved a number of genes targeting multiple host immune mechanisms including macrophage responses [33]. Herpesviruses like HSV-1 targets fibroblast for latency, whereas Epstein Barr virus uses B cells [34]. Our data showing the preponderant role of macrophages in long term quiescent infection of *Xenopus* by one of the RV main type *FV3* suggests that RVs have evolved new mechanisms to persist in their hosts.

We previously reported that *FV3* DNA was detected in a significant fraction of apparently healthy *X. laevis* adults obtained from various suppliers, suggesting that such asymptomatic carriers could serve as vectors of RV dissemination in the wild [15]. Presumably, physiological and/or immune perturbations may

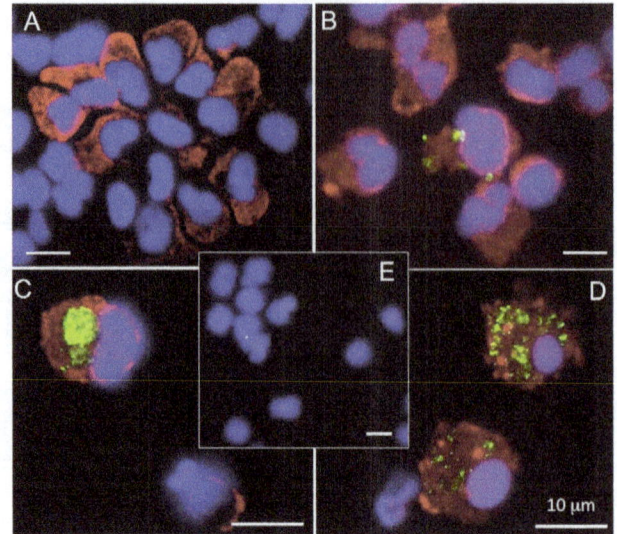

Figure 6. Visualization by immunofluorescence of infected peritoneal monocytic leukocytes from asymptomatic *FV3* infected adult frogs following bacterial stimulation. PLs were harvested from uninfected controls (A, E) or asymptomatic *FV3* infected outbred animals 3 days after bacterial stimulation (B, C D). Cells were cytocentrifuged on microscope slides, fixed with formaldehyde, permeabilized with ethanol, then stained with a rabbit anti-53R and Dylight 488-conjugated donkey anti-rabbit Abs (green) followed by anti-HAM56 mAb and Dylight 594-conjugated anti mouse Ab (red). Cells were then stained with the DNA dye Hoechst-33258 (Blue) mounted in anti-fade medium and visualized with a Leica DMIRB inverted fluorescence microscope. Bar represents 10 μm in each panel. (A) PLs from a bacterially stimulated, non-*FV3* infected frog stained with anti-HAM mAb; (B) PLs with low level of 53 specific signal from reactivated asymptomatic *FV3* infected animals; (C, D) PLs with high levels of 53 specific signal from reactivated asymptomatic *FV3* infected animals; (E) PLs from a bacterially stimulated, non-*FV3* infected frog stained with anti-53R Ab.

trigger productive reactivation of quiescent *FV3*, leading to high viral titer shedding. This is exemplified in the present study where an inflammatory stimulus in the form of HK *E. coli* resulted in prominent re-activation of *FV3* infection. Unlike LPS, which is not readily immuno-stimulatory to *Xenopus* [18,35], heat-killed bacterial stimulation within frog peritonea elicits robust accumulation of macrophages that display multiple features of activation including increased expression of inflammatory genes (Il-1β, TNFα), stress proteins (gp96) and scavenger receptors (CD91) [18,36]. Our gene expression data suggest that as in mammals, *X. laevis* coordinate the inflammatory recruitment of granulocytes, followed by macrophages, represented by marked PL expression increases of G-CSFR then the M-CSFR, respectively. The present study also suggests that heat-killed bacteria may serve not only as stimulus of *Xenopus* macrophage recruitment and activation, but may also facilitate *FV3* reactivation within a fraction of these cells. At present, the abundance and tissue distribution of *FV3* harboring macrophages following viral clearance is unclear, although our past work indicates that these cells may reside in the peritoneum and/or the kidney [14,23]. It is noteworthy that in our previous [14,15] and present studies we have failed to detect *FV3* in polymorphonuclear peritoneal leukocytes. This is intriguing considering the related myelopoietic origins of granulocytes and macrophages. However, granulocytes are typically short-lived and thus may represent poor viral reservoirs, whereas some

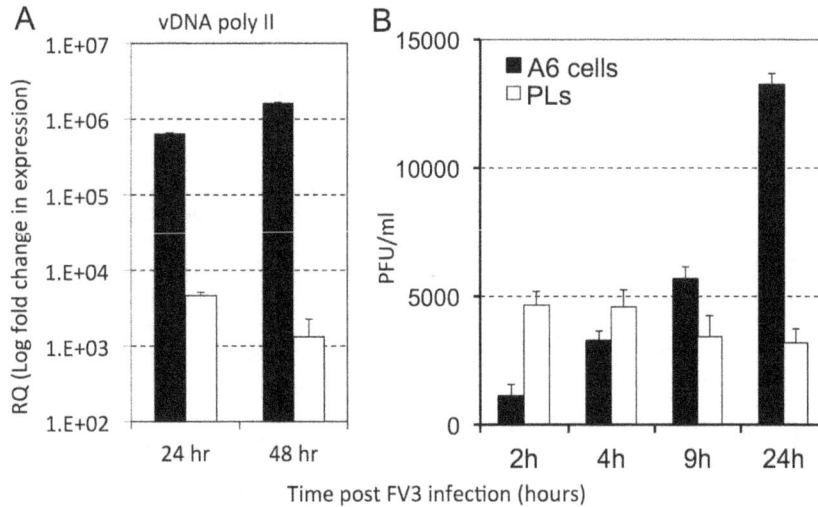

Figure 7. Comparison of viral gene expression and infectious virus produced by PLS and A6 kidney cell line infected in vitro with *FV3.* PLs from uninfected outbred animals and *Xenopus* A6 kidney cells were seeded at 1×10^6 cells/well and infected with a MOI of 1 for (A) 24 and 48 hrs or (B) 2, 4, 9, 24 hrs. (A) The PLs and A6 cultures infected for 24 and 48 hrs were assessed for *FV3* vDNA Pol II gene expression by the delta^deltaCT method qRT-PCR, using GAPDH as an endogenous control. (B) The *FV3* infectious burdens were enumerated by performing plaque assays on *FV3*-infected PLs and A6 culture lysates. Results are means ± SEM, N = 3.

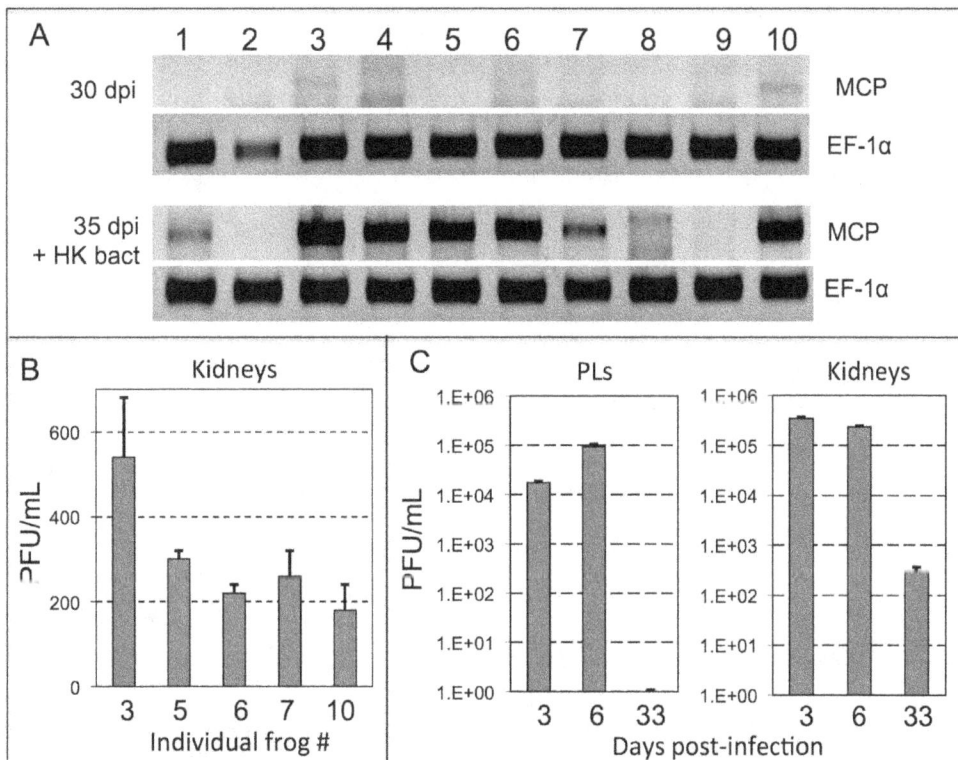

Figure 8. Detection of infectious virus in kidneys but not PLs of reactivated asymptomatic infection. (A) PCR assay on total DNA purified from PLs harvested from 10 different outbred frogs at 30 dpi and 35 dpi, (3 days after bacterial stimulation). Presence of viral DNA was assed by PCR on 50 ng of total DNA using *FV3* specific primers for MCP as well as *X. laevis* Ef-1α as a loading control. (B) Number of infectious *FV3* (PFU/ml/whole kidney) detected in kidney by plaque assay for frogs number (#) 3, 5, 6, 7, 10 from A sacrificed at 35 dpi. (C) Number of infectious *FV3* detected by plaque assay from PLs and kidneys of *FV3* infected frogs at 3, 6 and 33 dpi (3 individual for each time point).

macrophage subsets exhibiting uncanny longevity would be ideal for viral persistence.

Our present findings as well as a recent related work [37] converge to indicate that *X. laevis* macrophages effectively harbor *FV3*, but do not facilitate viral expansion or extensive progeny virus production. This may well be advantageous to the virus, where in absence of high intracellular titers, *FV3* may better evade host immune detection, avoid cell stress and activation, and otherwise disseminate and remain quiescent within its amphibian hosts. Presumably, under appropriate conditions, for example when a secondary infection would skew the immune response towards anti-bacterial rather than anti-viral immunity, *FV3* may leave its macrophage hiding place and re-infect its primary tropic cells, such as the kidney epithelia (as seen here).

Presumably, bacterial stimulation increases the proportion of macrophages harboring *FV3* through peritoneal recruitment/ accumulation, while concomitantly it elicits *FV3* reactivation. The precise mechanism involved in these processes remains to be elucidated. However, it is remarkable that the reactivation of these chronic quiescent RV infections appears to circumvent immune defenses, especially considering that *Xenopus* adults are inherently resistant to *FV3* and develop efficient immunological memory, resulting in faster and more potent viral clearance upon acute re-infection [8,9]. This implies that the route of *FV3* reactivation subverts the immunological barriers that established during the primary infection. Presumably, upon *FV3* re-challenge of previously infected animals with exogenous virus, the virus now encounters the established and expanded adaptive immune components, rapidly controlling and clearing the reinfection. Conversely, it is reasonable that RVs have evolved to bypass this established adaptive barrier from within the organism through the establishment of quiescence in subsets of immune (macrophage) cells and efficient reactivation following appropriate stimuli such as an immune response skewed away from viral clearance.

Our findings have relevance for RV infection of other amphibian species, considering the variable susceptibility observed across anurans, especially adult animals [7]. In the face of the amphibian declines, it is crucial to consider that resistant amphibian species with persistent asymptomatic RV infections may represent major, previously overlooked facets of RV dissemination. Indeed, in addition to co-infections of amphibians by RVs and other pathogens such as bacteria, fungi and parasites, chronic inflammation may also be induced by a variety of physiological stressors including habitat perturbation, resource competition and pollution. These various effects may well be compounding towards quiescent RV reactivation in wild amphibian populations. As such, the remarkable capacity of *FV3* and presumably other RVs to chronically persist in migrating reservoir hosts represent an additional avenue for infection dissemination; likely contributing to the rapid expansion of these pathogens and possibly the escalating amphibian decline.

Supporting Information

Figure S1 Detection of infectious virus in kidneys but not PLs of reactivated asymptomatic infection. PCR assay on total DNA purified from PBLs and erythrocytes from blood collected from 15 different frogs at 30 dpi, and from the same animals 3 days after bacterial stimulation (35 dpi). Presence of viral DNA was assed by PCR on 50 ng of total DNA using *FV3* specific primers for MCP and vDNA poly II as well as *X. laevis* Ef-1α as a loading control.

Acknowledgments

We thank Tina Martin for animal husbandry. We would like also to thank Qianlangyue Xu and Robert Bortz for their significant technical contribution to this work.

Author Contributions

Conceived and designed the experiments: JR LG ESE BW FA. Performed the experiments: JR LG ESE BW FA. Analyzed the data: JR LG ESE BW FA. Wrote the paper: JR LG ESE BW FA.

References

1. Robert J, Gregory Chinchar VG (2012) "Ranaviruses: an emerging threat to ectothermic vertebrates" report of the First International Symposium on Ranaviruses, Minneapolis MN July 8, 2011. Dev Comp Immunol 36: 259–261.
2. Gray MJ, Miller DL, Hoverman JT (2009) Ecology and pathology of amphibian ranaviruses. Dis Aquat Organ 87: 243–266.
3. Abrams AJ, Cannatella DC, Hillis DM, Sawyer SL (2013) Recent host-shifts in ranaviruses: signatures of positive selection in the viral genome. J Gen Virol 94: 2082–2093. doi: 2010.1099/vir.2080.052837-052830. Epub 052013 Jun 052819.
4. Jancovich JK, Bremont M, Touchman JW, Jacobs BL (2010) Evidence for multiple recent host species shifts among the Ranaviruses (family Iridoviridae). J Virol 84: 2636–2647.
5. Tan WG, Barkman TJ, Gregory Chinchar V, Essani K (2004) Comparative genomic analyses of frog virus 3, type species of the genus Ranavirus (family Iridoviridae). Virology 323: 70–84.
6. Lei XY, Ou T, Zhu RL, Zhang QY (2012) Sequencing and analysis of the complete genome of Rana grylio virus (RGV). Arch Virol 157: 1559–1564.
7. Grayfer L, Andino Fde J, Chen G, Chinchar GV, Robert J (2012) Immune evasion strategies of ranaviruses and innate immune responses to these emerging pathogens. Viruses 4: 1075–1092.
8. Gantress J, Maniero GD, Cohen N, Robert J (2003) Development and characterization of a model system to study amphibian immune responses to iridoviruses. Virology 311: 254–262.
9. Morales HD, Robert J (2007) Characterization of primary and memory CD8 T-cell responses against ranavirus (FV3) in Xenopus laevis. J Virol 81: 2240–2248.
10. Pluddemann A, Mukhopadhyay S, Gordon S (2011) Innate immunity to intracellular pathogens: macrophage receptors and responses to microbial entry. Immunol Rev 240: 11–24.
11. Duncan CJ, Sattentau QJ (2011) Viral determinants of HIV-1 macrophage tropism. Viruses 3: 2255–2279.
12. de Vries RD, Mesman AW, Geijtenbeek TB, Duprex WP, de Swart RL (2012) The pathogenesis of measles. Curr Opin Virol 2: 248–255.
13. Duncan CJ, Sattentau QJ (2011) Viral determinants of HIV-1 macrophage tropism. Viruses 3: 2255–2279.
14. Morales HD, Abramowitz L, Gertz J, Sowa J, Vogel A, et al. (2010) Innate immune responses and permissiveness to ranavirus infection of peritoneal leukocytes in the frog Xenopus laevis. J Virol 84: 4912–4922.
15. Robert J, Abramowitz L, Gantress J, Morales HD (2007) Xenopus laevis: a possible vector of Ranavirus infection? J Wildl Dis 43: 645–652.
16. Hadji-Azimi I, Coosemans V, Canicatti C (1987) Atlas of adult Xenopus laevis laevis hematology. Dev Comp Immunol 11: 807–874.
17. Robert J, Ohta Y (2009) Comparative and developmental study of the immune system in Xenopus. Dev Dyn 238: 1249–1270.
18. Marr S, Goyos A, Gantress J, Maniero GD, Robert J (2005) CD91 up-regulates upon immune stimulation in Xenopus adult but not larval peritoneal leukocytes. Immunogenetics 56: 735–742.
19. Marr S, Morales H, Bottaro A, Cooper M, Flajnik M, et al. (2007) Localization and differential expression of activation-induced cytidine deaminase in the amphibian Xenopus upon antigen stimulation and during early development. J Immunol 179: 6783–6789.
20. Whitley DS, Yu K, Sample RC, Sinning A, Henegar J, et al. (2010) Frog virus 3 ORF 53R, a putative myristoylated membrane protein, is essential for virus replication in vitro. Virology 405: 448–456.
21. Robert J, George E, De Jesus Andino F, Chen G (2011) Waterborne infectivity of the Ranavirus frog virus 3 in Xenopus laevis. Virology 417: 410–417.
22. Chen G, Ward BM, Yu KH, Chinchar VG, Robert J (2011) Improved knockout methodology reveals that frog virus 3 mutants lacking either the 18K immediate-early gene or the truncated vIF-2alpha gene are defective for replication and growth in vivo. J Virol 85: 11131–11138.
23. Robert J, Morales H, Buck W, Cohen N, Marr S, et al. (2005) Adaptive immunity and histopathology in frog virus 3-infected Xenopus. Virology 332: 667–675.
24. Cunningham AA, Tems CA, Russell PH (2008) Immunohistochemical demonstration of Ranavirus Antigen in the tissues of infected frogs (Rana

temporaria) with systemic haemorrhagic or cutaneous ulcerative disease. J Comp Pathol 138: 3–11. Epub 2007 Nov 2005.

25. Miller DL, Rajeev S, Gray MJ, Baldwin CA (2007) Frog virus 3 infection, cultured American bullfrogs. Emerg Infect Dis 13: 342–343.

26. Hyatt AD, Williamson M, Coupar BE, Middleton D, Hengstberger SG, et al. (2002) First identification of a ranavirus from green pythons (Chondropython viridis). J Wildl Dis 38: 239–252.

27. Allender MC, Fry MM, Irizarry AR, Craig L, Johnson AJ, et al. (2006) Intracytoplasmic inclusions in circulating leukocytes from an eastern box turtle (Terrapene carolina carolina) with iridoviral infection. J Wildl Dis 42: 677–684.

28. Morales H, Robert J (2008) In vivo and in vitro techniques for comparative study of antiviral T-cell responses in the amphibian Xenopus. Biol Proced Online 10: 1–8.

29. Robert J, Ramanayake T, Maniero GD, Morales H, Chida AS (2008) Phylogenetic conservation of glycoprotein 96 ability to interact with CD91 and facilitate antigen cross-presentation. J Immunol 180: 3176–3182.

30. Gut JP, Anton M, Bingen A, Vetter JM, Kirn A (1981) Frog virus 3 induces a fatal hepatitis in rats. Lab Invest 45: 218–228.

31. Gendrault JL, Steffan AM, Bingen A, Kirn A (1981) Penetration and uncoating of frog virus 3 (FV3) in cultured rat Kupffer cells. Virology 112: 375–384.

32. Iyer LM, Aravind L, Koonin EV (2001) Common origin of four diverse families of large eukaryotic DNA viruses. J Virol 75: 11720–11734.

33. Smith GL, Benfield CT, Maluquer de Motes C, Mazzon M, Ember SW, et al. (2013) Vaccinia virus immune evasion: mechanisms, virulence and immunogenicity. J Gen Virol 94: 2367–2392.

34. Weck KE, Barkon ML, Yoo LI, Speck SH, Virgin HI (1996) Mature B cells are required for acute splenic infection, but not for establishment of latency, by murine gammaherpesvirus 68. J Virol 70: 6775–6780.

35. Bleicher PA, Rollins-Smith LA, Jacobs DM, Cohen N (1983) Mitogenic responses of frog lymphocytes to crude and purified preparations of bacterial lipopolysaccharide (LPS). Dev Comp Immunol 7: 483–496.

36. De Jesus Andino F, Chen G, Li Z, Grayfer L, Robert J (2012) Susceptibility of Xenopus laevis tadpoles to infection by the ranavirus Frog-Virus 3 correlates with a reduced and delayed innate immune response in comparison with adult frogs. Virology 432: 435–443.

37. Grayfer L, Robert J (2014) Divergent Antiviral Roles of Amphibian (Xenopus laevis) M-CSF- and IL-34-Derived Macrophages. J Leuk Biol In press.

5

Increased Bone Marrow (BM) Plasma Level of Soluble CD30 and Correlations with BM Plasma Level of Interferon (IFN)-γ, CD4/CD8 T-Cell Ratio and Disease Severity in Aplastic Anemia

Qingqing Wu[◊][¶], Jizhou Zhang[◊][¶], Jun Shi, Meili Ge, Xingxin Li, Yingqi Shao, Jianfeng Yao, Yizhou Zheng*

Severe Aplastic Anemia Studying Program, State Key Laboratory of Experimental Hematology, Institute of Hematology & Blood Diseases Hospital, Chinese Academy of Medical Sciences & Peking Union Medical College, 288 Nanjing Road, Tianjin, 300020, P.R.CHINA

Abstract

Idiopathic aplastic anemia (AA) is an immune-mediated bone marrow failure syndrome. Immune abnormalities such as decreased lymphocyte counts, inverted CD4/CD8 T-cell ratio and increased IFN-γ-producing T cells have been found in AA. CD30, a surface protein belonging to the tumor necrosis factor receptor family and releasing from cell surface as a soluble form (sCD30) after activation, marks a subset of activated T cells secreting IFN-γ when exposed to allogeneic antigens. Our study found elevated BM plasma levels of sCD30 in patients with SAA, which were closely correlated with disease severity, including absolute lymphocyte count (ALC) and absolute netrophil count (ANC). We also noted that sCD30 levels were positively correlated with plasma IFN-γ levels and CD4/CD8 T-cell ratio in patients with SAA. In order to explain these phenomena, we stimulated T cells with alloantigen in vitro and found that CD30[+] T cells were the major source of IFN-γ, and induced CD30[+] T cells from patients with SAA produced significantly more IFN-γ than that from healthy individuals. In addition, increased proportion of CD8[+] T cells in AA showed enhanced allogeneic response by the fact that they expressed more CD30 during allogeneic stimulation. sCD30 levels decreased in patients responded to immunosuppressive therapy. In conclusion, elevated BM plasma levels of sCD30 reflected the enhanced CD30[+] T cell-mediated immune response in SAA. CD30 as a molecular marker that transiently expresses on IFN-γ-producing T cells, may participate in mediating bone marrow failure in AA, which also can facilitate our understanding of AA pathogenesis to identify new therapeutic targets.

Editor: Vassiliki A. Boussiotis, Beth Israel Deaconess Medical Center, Harvard Medical School, United States of America

Funding: This study was supported by the National Public Health Grant Research Foundation of China (no. 201202017) to Y.Z., http://www.nhfpc.gov.cn/zhuzhan/index.shtml; the Fundamental Research Funds for the Central Universities of China (no. 2012N05) to Y.Z., http://www.moe.gov.cn/; the National Basic Research Program (2010CB945204) to Y.Z., http://www.nsfc.gov.cn/; the National Natural Science Foundation of China (NNSFC, no. 81330015) to Z.H., http://www.nsfc.gov.cn/; and the NNSFC (no. 81300388) to M.G., http://www.nsfc.gov.cn/. The funders had no role in study design, data collection and analysis, decision to publish, or preparation of the manuscript.

Competing Interests: The authors have declared that no competing interests exist.

* Email: zheng_yizhou@hotmail.com

◊ These authors contributed equally to this work.

¶ QW and JZ are co-first authors on this work.

Introduction

Acquired aplastic anemia (AA) is an immune-mediated bone marrow (BM) failure syndrome characterized by persistent peripheral blood (PB) pancytopenia and BM hypoplasia [1]. Immune abnormalities such as decreased lymphocyte counts, inverted CD4/CD8 T-cell ratio and increased IFN-γ-producing T cells have been found in AA [2–4]. Autoreactive T cells activated by specific antigen(s) attacking CD34[+] multipotential hematopoietic cells directly [5], and producing type I cytokines such as IFN-γ [6], are thought to be the major villain responsible for destruction of BM hematopoiesis in AA. Effectiveness of immunosuppressive agents further supports the immune-mediated pathogenesis of AA.

Although accumulating laboratory and clinical data suggest that AA is an immune-mediated disorder, the T cell-mediated immunopathology in AA remains to be poorly understood. Recent evidence indicates that oligoclonal expanded cytoxic T cells which are suggestive of an antigen-driven clonal response exist in AA [5,7]. Furthermore, these oligoclones recognize and induce apoptosis of autologous myeloid cells [8]. However, the triggering autoantigens expressed by hematopoietic stem cells (HSC) in AA remain unknown. Only few reports identify autoantibodies in AA, and their pathological significance is unclear [9–12]. In a mouse model the single minor histocompatibility antigen H60 mismatch can trigger immune response and lead to massive BM destruction [13]. Other direct evidence to prove the existence of autoantigen in AA is still limited.

CD30, a cell-surface molecule belonging to the tumor necrosis factor receptor superfamily, is mainly expressed by activated T cells in the physiological condition [14]. CD30 is up-regulated on T cells exposed to allogeneic antigens, and these CD30[+] T cells are

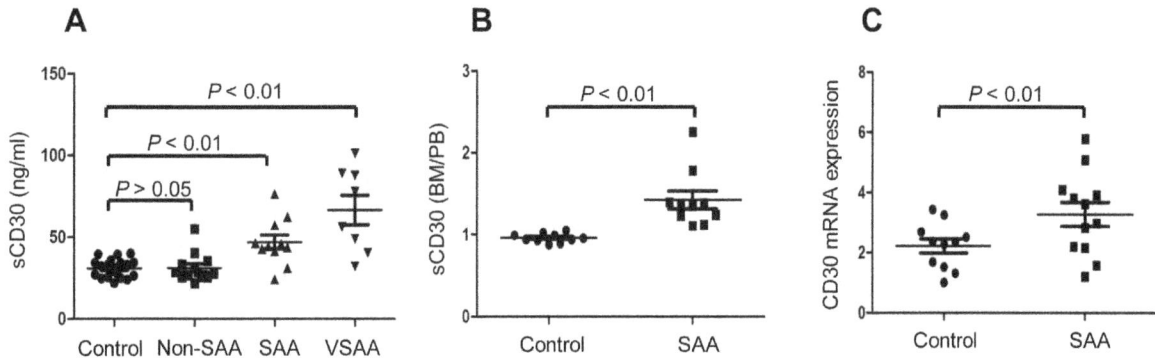

Figure 1. Plasma sCD30 levels and CD30 mRNA expressions in BMMCs from AA patients (n = 42) and healthy individuals (n = 20). (A) BM plasma sCD30 concentrations in healthy individuals (n = 20), Non-SAA patients (n = 13), SAA patients (n = 11) and VSAA patients (n = 8) were measured by ELSIA. (B) The ratios of BM plasma sCD30 level/PB plasma sCD30 level in SAA and VSAA patients (n = 11) and in healthy individuals (n = 11). (C) Relative expressions of CD30 in BMMNCs were measured by real-time PCR in *de novo* SAA patients (n = 12) and healthy individuals (n = 11).

a major source of IFN-γ [15–17]. Quickly after stimulation, surface CD30 is proteolytically cleaved by metalloproteinases and released into bloodstream as soluble CD30 (sCD30) [18]. Therefore, circulating sCD30 is thought to be reflective activation of the immune system.

Low serum levels of sCD30 are detected in healthy individuals [19]. In several classical autoimmune diseases, such as rheumatoid arthritis, atopic dermatitis and systemic lupus erythematosus, high levels of sCD30 have been found to represent the loss of tolerance to self-antigens [20–22]. More interestingly, sCD30 increases significantly in patients who developed acute graft versus host disease (GvHD) after allogeneic hematopoietic cell transplantation (HCT), which implies that elevated levels of sCD30 might be a potential biomarker of allograft rejection in HCT [23–24]. Brentuximab vedotin (SNG35), made by attaching the antitublin agent monomethyl auristatin E (MMAE) to the CD30-specific monoclonal antibody cAC10, has been proved to be efficient in inducing durable objective responses and resulting in tumor regression for CD30-positive lymphomas with only mild-to-moderate toxic effects [25–26]. The US Food and Drug Administration (FDA) has approved Brentuximab vedotin to be used in patients with relapsed/refractory Hodgkin lymphoma and anaplastic large cell lymphoma [27–28].

Thus, it's intriguing to probe whether CD30 is involved in over-production of IFN-γ by T cells given CD30+ T cells are the predominant proliferating and IFN-γ-producing cells in response to alloantigen. So, we carefully evaluated the role of CD30 in the pathogenesis of AA. Our findings suggested that CD30 as a cell surface marker that transiently expressed on activated T cells, might be associated with T cell-mediated bone marrow failure in AA, which could facilitate our understanding of AA pathogenesis to identify new therapeutic targets.

Materials and Methods

Patients and healthy individuals

We analysed samples of PB and BM from 56 patients with AA (median age 28 years, 29 male and 27 female), and 20 BM donors as healthy individuals (median age 27 years, 10 male and 10 female) after written informed consent in accordance with the Declaration of Helsinki, which was approved by the Ethics Committee of the Chinese Academy of Medical Sciences and Peking Union Medical College. The diagnosis and severity classifications of the cohort of patients with AA were established according to the international criteria [29–30], including 13 patients with non-severe AA (Non-SAA), 30 patients SAA and 13 patients very SAA (VSAA). Inherited bone marrow failures and clonal hematologic disorders were excluded from our study. Of 56 patients, 32 patients were analyzed at diagnosis, and 24 patients in complete response (CR) after immunosuppressive therapy (IST) of the combination of antithymocyte globulin (ATG) plus cyclosporine A (CSA). Serial samples pre- and post-ATG/CSA therapy were obtained from 6 patients with SAA. All patients were free from active infection at the time of sampling.

Cell culture

BM mononuclear cells (BMMCs) isolated by Ficoll-Hypaque (1.077 g/mL) density gradient centrifugation were used for the measurements of CD30 mRNA expression. In some experiments, CD3+ T cells were enriched from BMMCs using a commercial CD3+ human T cell isolation kit (Mitenyi Biotec) according to the manufacturer's instructions. CD3+ T cells were mixed at a ratio of 1:1 with autologous or allogenetic PB mononuclear cells pretreated with mitomycin C and seeded at 5×10^5 cells/mL. Cells were cultured for 7 days at 37°C with 5% CO_2 atmosphere, in an optimized serum-free cell culture medium (TexMACS Medium, Miltenyi Biotec) developed for the cultivation and expansion of human T cells, supplemented with 2 mmol/L penicillin/strepto-mycin. Every 24 h, cells and culture supernatants were collected and analysed by flow cytometry (FCM) and enzyme-linked immune sorbent assay (ELISA), respectively.

Quantitative real-time PCR

Total RNA was isolated from cells with Trizol reagent (Invitrogen) following the manufacturer's instructions. cDNA was synthesized from the purified RNA using a reverse transcription system (Promega) with random primers. Real-time PCR was performed using SYBR green PCR kit (Invitrogen). β-actin was used to normalize gene expression levels. PCR primer sequences were as follows: CD30 forward 5′-GACAAGGCTGTCAG-GAGGTG-3′, reverse 5′-ACTGGAGGTTGCTGGGGACA-3′; β-actin forward 5′- CTCTTCCAGCCTTCCTTCCT-3′, reverse 5′- AGCACTGTGTGTTGGCGTACAG-3′.

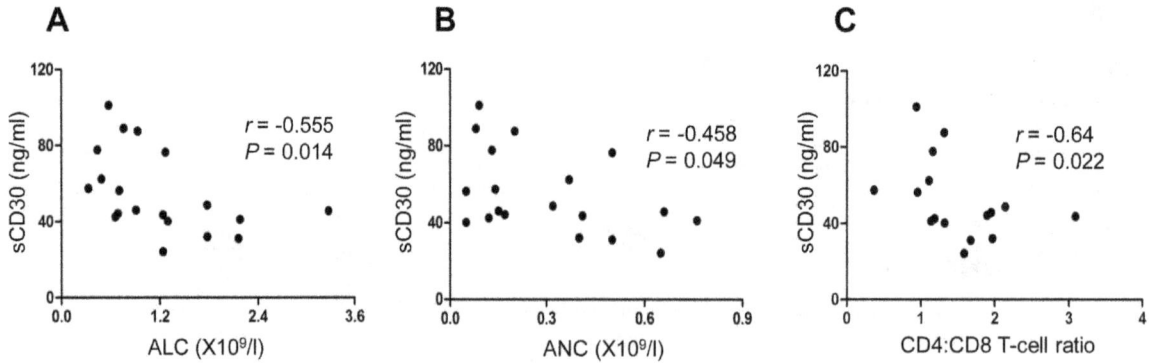

Figure 2. Correlations of BM plasma sCD30 levels with baseline ALC (A), ANC (B), or CD4/CD8 ratio (C) in AA patients (n = 19).

Flow cytometry and cell sorting

In the total 7 days mixed lymphocyte culture system, surface antigen of T cells were analysed by FCM every 24 h. Cultured cells were harvested and washed twice in PBS by centrifugation at 300 g for 5 min. Cells were then stained with the following antibodies: CD3-FITC (Biolegend), CD8-APC (Biolegend), CD30-PE (eBioscience), and the appropriate isotypic control according to the manufacturer's instructions. After incubation, cells were resuspended with 1% paraformaldehyde for FCM analysis. Cell sorting was performed by using BD FACS Canto II (BD Biosciences).

Cytokine ELISA

The plasma and culture supernatants were stored at $-80°C$ until ELISA was performed. The concentrations of sCD30 and IFN-γ were measured by Human sCD30 Instant ELISA kit (eBioscience) and Human IFN-γ ELISA kit (Boshide Biotech, China), respectively.

Statistics

Data were shown as mean ± SEM. The statistical differences were evaluated by the nonparametric Mann–Whitney U-test between unpaired data and by Wilcoxon matched pairs test for two paired variables. The Spearman's rank correlation test was used for correlation analysis. All analyses were performed using SPSS 16.0 software (SPSS Science). P values <0.05 were considered statistically significant.

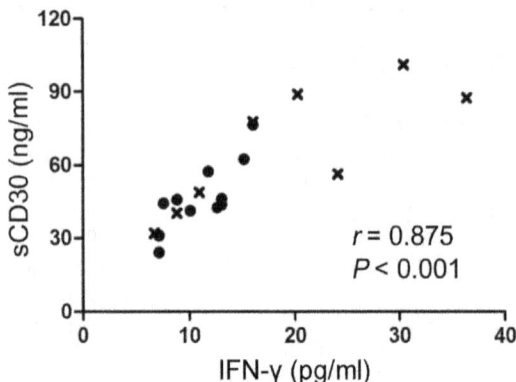

Figure 3. Correlation of BM IFN-γ levels with BM sCD30 levels in SAA patients (•, n = 11) and VSAA patients (×, n = 8).

Ethics Statement

We analysed samples of PB and BM from 56 patients with AA, and 20 BM donors as healthy individuals after written informed consent in accordance with the Declaration of Helsinki to the protocol obtained, which was approved by the Ethics Committee of the Chinese Academy of Medical Sciences and Peking Union Medical College.

Results

Quantitative measurement of sCD30 in AA patients

The comparisons of BM plasma sCD30 levels between *de novo* AA patients (including 13 Non-SAA, 15 SAA and 14 VSAA) and healthy individuals measured by ELISA were shown in Figure 1A. Plasma sCD30 levels were found to be positively correlated with the severity of AA, the median plasma sCD30 levels in healthy individuals, Non-SAA, SAA and VSAA patients were as of 30 ng/mL, 32 ng/mL, 46 ng/mL and 62 ng/mL, respectively.

Because CD30 was suggested to highly express in the target organs of certain autoimmune diseases, we compared sCD30 levels between PB and BM (the latter as the target organ in AA) from 12 SAA and VSAA patients and 11 healthy individuals. Data shown that sCD30 level in BM plasma was higher than its corresponding PB level in each patient with SAA, but healthy individuals had comparable levels of sCD30 between BM and PB, as shown by the significantly higher ratio of BM sCD30/PB sCD30 in patients with SAA in comparison with healthy individuals (Figure 1B). To further confirm CD30 expression in BM, we analysed the mRNA levels of CD30 in BMMCs by real-time PCR, which revealed significantly increased CD30 expression in patients with SAA (Figure 1C).

Correlations between BM plasma sCD30 levels and baseline PB counts

In consideration of alloactivated T cells are the major source of sCD30, we analysed the correlation between BM plasma sCD30 levels and baseline absolute lymphocyte count (ALC), absolute netrophil count (ANC) and absolute reticulocyte count (ARC) in patients with SAA (including VSAA). Our results showed specific inverse correlations between sCD30 levels and ALC (Figure 2A) or ANC (Figure 2B), although no correlation were found between sCD30 levels and ARC (Figure S4).

Interestingly, we also found an inverse correlation between sCD30 levels and CD4/CD8 T-cell ratio (Figure 2C), which suggested patient with a higher CD8$^+$ T cell proportion tended to have a higher plasma level of sCD30.

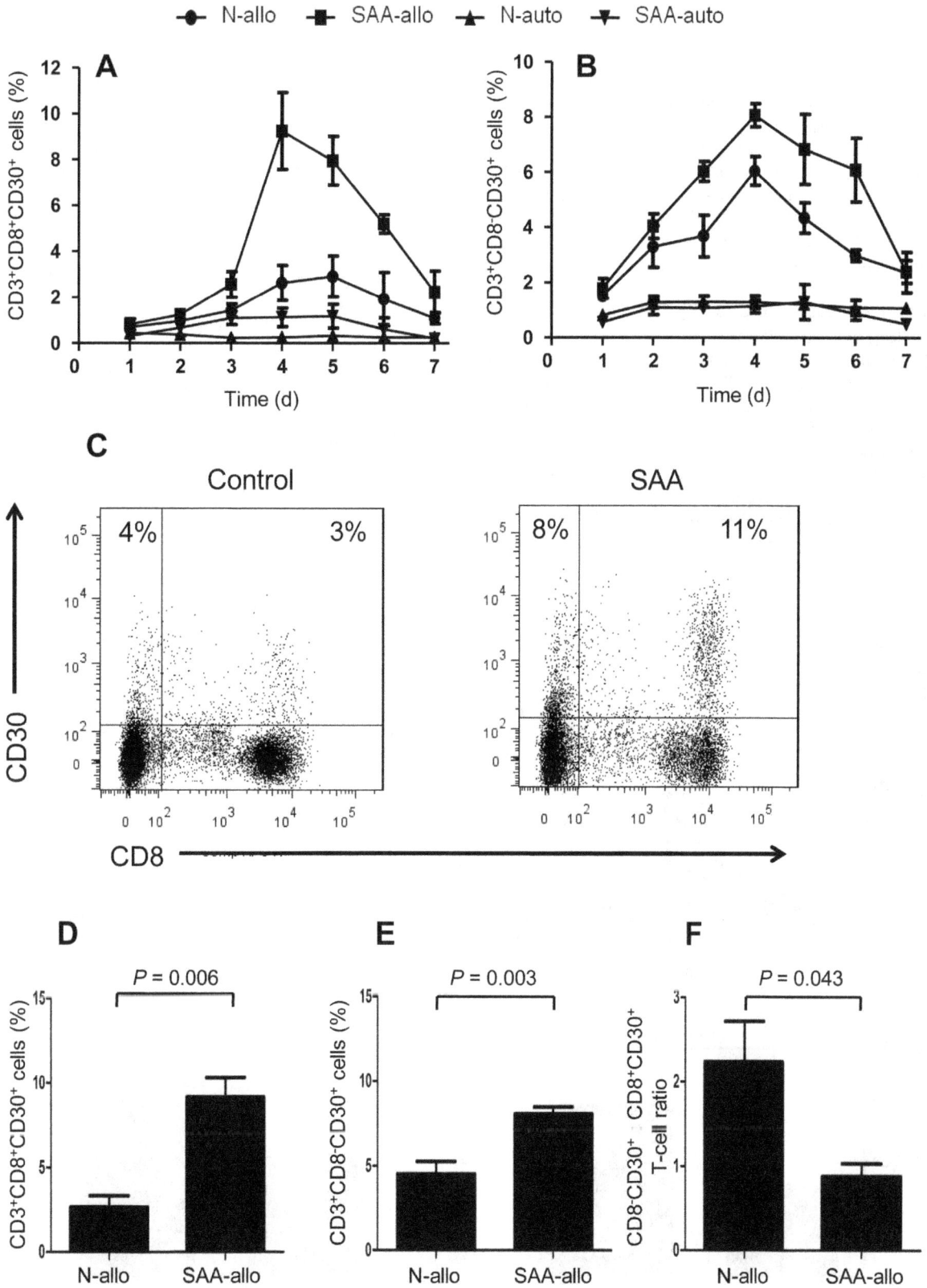

Figure 4. Allogeneic stimulation-induced surface expression of CD30 on T cells. BM CD3$^+$ T cells from healthy individuals and SAA patients were co-cultured with mitomycin C treated autologous or allogenetic mononuclear cells for a total of 7 days, kinetics of cell surface expression of CD30 by CD3$^+$CD8$^+$ T cells (A) and CD3$^+$CD8$^-$ T cells (B) were determined by FCM. Data represent mean ± SE of three independent experiments. (C) Representative FCM analyses of cell surface expression of CD30 by T cells from healthy individuals and SAA patients after allogeneic stimulation. Results at day 4 when the maximum CD30 expression reached were shown. (D) and (E) Cells surface expression of CD30 by allogeneic stimulated T-

cell subsets at day 4 were determined in 5 healthy individuals and 6 SAA patients. (F) CD3+CD8−CD30+: CD3+CD8+CD30+ T-cell ratios in healthy individuals and in SAA patients

Correlation between BM plasma sCD30 levels and BM plasma IFN-γ levels

CD30 was identified as a marker of IFN-γ-producing T cells, so we further determined BM plasma IFN-γ levels in patients with SAA (including VSAA), and found a positive correlation between sCD30 levels and IFN-γ levels (Figure 3), which indicated enhanced CD30 signaling might lead to increased production of IFN-γ in patients with SAA.

Cell surface expression of CD30 by SAA CD3+ T cells during allogeneic stimulation

We had found elevated BM sCD30 levels in SAA, so next we wanted to explore whether T cells from SAA patients expressed more CD30 when exposed to alloantigen compared to those from healthy individuals. To answer this issue, we determined the induction kinetics of CD30 expression on T-cell subsets from SAA patients and healthy individuals after autologous and allogeneic stimulations. The significantly increased percentages of CD30-expressing CD3+CD8+ (Figure 4A) and CD3+CD8− (Figure 4B) T cells in SAA patients as well as in healthy individuals after

allogeneic stimulation instead of autologous stimulation were observed. In both SAA patients and healthy individuals, cell surface expression of CD30 by T cells reached peak at day 4 or day 5 during allogeneic stimulation, then quickly decreased to a very low level. Importantly, the significantly higher percentages of CD30-expressing CD3+CD8+ and CD3+CD8− T cells in SAA patients than those in healthy individuals, especially at day 4 were also observed (Figures 4C-E). Furthermore, we found that CD3+CD8− T cells expressed more CD30 than CD3+CD8+ T cells in healthy individuals, whereas the expression levels of CD30 were comparable between CD3+CD8− T cells and CD3+CD8+ T cells in patients with SAA, as shown by the significantly higher CD3+CD8−CD30+: CD3+CD8+CD30+ T-cell ratios in healthy individuals in comparison with patients with SAA (Figure 4F).

Release of sCD30 and IFN-γ by SAA CD3+ T cells during allogeneic stimulation

Surface CD30 can be cleaved as soluble form, so we measured the kinetics of sCD30 and IFN-γ released into the culture supernatants by autologous and allogeneic stimulated CD3+ T cells. In line with CD30 expression on T cells, significantly

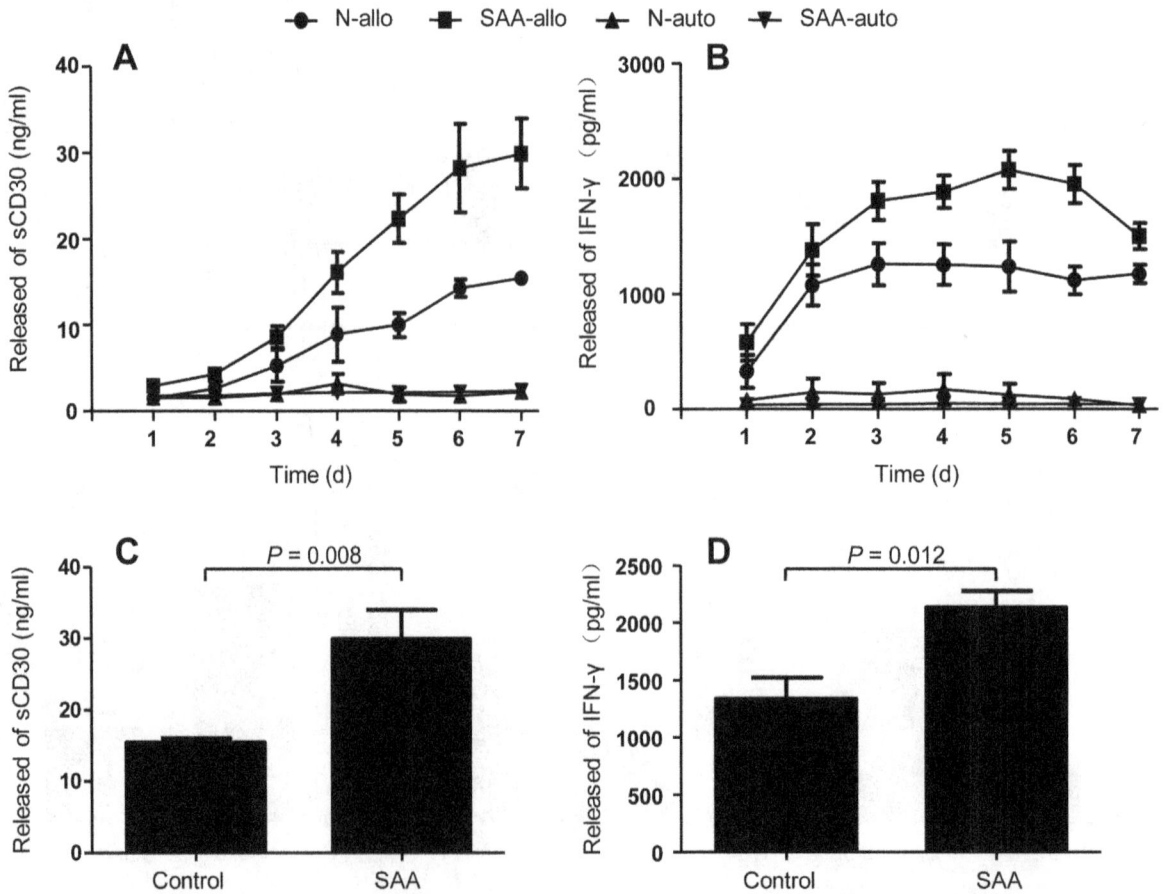

Figure 5. Allogeneic stimulation-induced release of sCD30 and IFN-γ by T cells. BM CD3+ T cells from healthy individuals and SAA patients were co-cultured with mitomycin C treated autologous or allogenetic mononuclear cells for a total of 7 days, kinetics of sCD30 (A) and IFN-γ (B) released into culture supernatants were analysed by ELISA. Data represent mean ± SE of three independent experiments. (C) and (D) Released sCD30 and IFN-γ by allogeneic stimulated T cells at day 4 were determined in 5 healthy individuals and 6 SAA patients.

Table 1. Maximum sCD30 level or IFN-γ level positively correlates with the percentage of CD30$^+$ T cells at day 4 but not day 7 after allogeneic stimulation.

| | CD30$^+$ T (%) | | | |
| | d4 | | d7 | |
	r	p	r	p
sCD30	0.886	0.019	0.23	0.661
IFN-γ 0.018	0.889	0.018	0.126	0.812

Spearman's rank correlation test.

increased levels of sCD30 were detected in culture supernatants from allogeneic stimulated T cells but not from autologous stimulated T cells (Figure 5A). After allogeneic stimulation, sCD30 levels were significant higher in patients with SAA than in healthy individuals (Figure 5C). Distinct correlation was observed between maximum sCD30 level (reached at day 7) and CD30 expression on T cells at day 4 instead of at day 7 (Table 1), when most CD30 had been cleaved from T cells surface.

Significantly elevated levels of IFN-γ were detected in allogeneic cultures but not in autologous cultures (Figure 5B). After allogeneic stimulation, IFN-γ levels were significantly higher in SAA patients than those in healthy individuals (Figure 5D). Once again, specific correlation between maximum IFN-γ levels (reached at day 4 or day 5) and CD30 expression on T cells was observed at day 4 instead of day 7 (Table 1).

Production of IFN-γ by allogeneic sitmulated CD30$^+$ T cells

To assess IFN-γ-producing capacity of induced CD30$^+$ T cells from SAA patients, allogeneic stimulated T cells were separated by FACS day 4 after culture. CD30$^+$ and CD30$^-$ T cells were separately cultured for additional 2 days, followed by determining the levels of IFN-γ in the culture supernatants by ELISA. CD30$^+$ T cells produced significant more IFN-γ than did CD30$^-$ cells in SAA patients as well as in healthy individuals (Figure 6). Importantly, induced CD30$^+$ T cells from SAA patients produced more IFN-γ than healthy individuals.

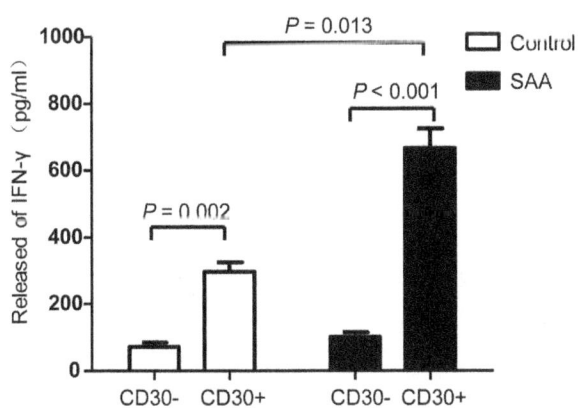

Figure 6. Relationship between CD30 and IFN-γ. After 4 days of culture, allogeneic stimulated T cells were sorted by FACS, CD30$^+$ and CD30$^-$ T cells were separately cultured for additional 2 days, then IFN-γ levels in the culture supernatants were determined by ELISA. Data represent mean ± SE of three independent experiments.

Association between IST and sCD30

In order to investigate the association between sCD30 and disease activity, we detected the sCD30 levels in patients with SAA (including VSAA) at diagnosis (n = 29) and in CR (n = 24). Patients in CR had significantly lower levels of sCD30 than patients at diagnosis (Figure 7A). BM samples pre- and post-IST were collected from 6 SAA patients who had responded to IST, all patients had significant decrease in sCD30 levels after successful IST (Figure 7B).

To test the direct effect of CsA on CD30 expression, we added CsA at 200 ng/mL to the allogeneic cultures. Surface CD30 expression on T cells, and levels of sCD30 and IFN-γ in culture supernatants were analysed at day 4. CsA significantly inhibited CD30 expression on CD3$^+$CD8$^-$ (Figure 7C) and CD3$^+$CD8$^+$ T cells (Figure 7D) of both SAA patients and healthy individuals. CsA also reduced sCD30 (Figure 7E) and IFN-γ (Figure 7F) in the culture supernatants from T cells of both SAA patients and healthy individuals.

Discussion

Elevated amounts of sCD30 in blood have been reported in many autoimmune diseases. This is the first study to investigate the role of CD30 in the pathogenesis of AA. We found increased BM plasma levels of sCD30 correlated well with disease severity, CD4/CD8 T-cell ratio and BM plasma levels of IFN-γ in SAA. More interestingly, higher plasma level of sCD30 in BM than in PB was observed in each SAA patient, but not in healthy individual. We also revealed an elevated CD30 expression at mRNA levels in BMMCs of patients with SAA compared with healthy individuals. These data suggested that CD30-associated T cell activation did exist, especially in BM as the target organ of immune attack in patients with SAA. In addition, T cells and in particular CD8$^+$ T cells from patients with SAA showed enhanced allogeneic response by the fact that immune cells from these patients could be induced by alloantigen to express more CD30 than that from healthy controls.

Though the physiological function of CD30 remains unclear, it is unambiguous that CD30 is not a general marker of activated T cells but plays a critical role in alloimmune response. CD30 was suggested to participate in eliminating autoreactive T cells in thymus and inducing T cell apoptosis in periphery in vivo [31–34]. Compared with anti-CD3 plus anti-CD28 antibodies and autologous antigen presenting cell (APC), allogeneic APC induced a greater proportion of CD30$^+$ cells which not only were the predominant proliferating T cells in response to alloantigen, but also represented a subset of T cells that were the primary source of IFN-γ in vitro [17]. These findings also agreed with the observation that BM plasma levels of sCD30 positively correlated with the levels of IFN-γ in patients with SAA.

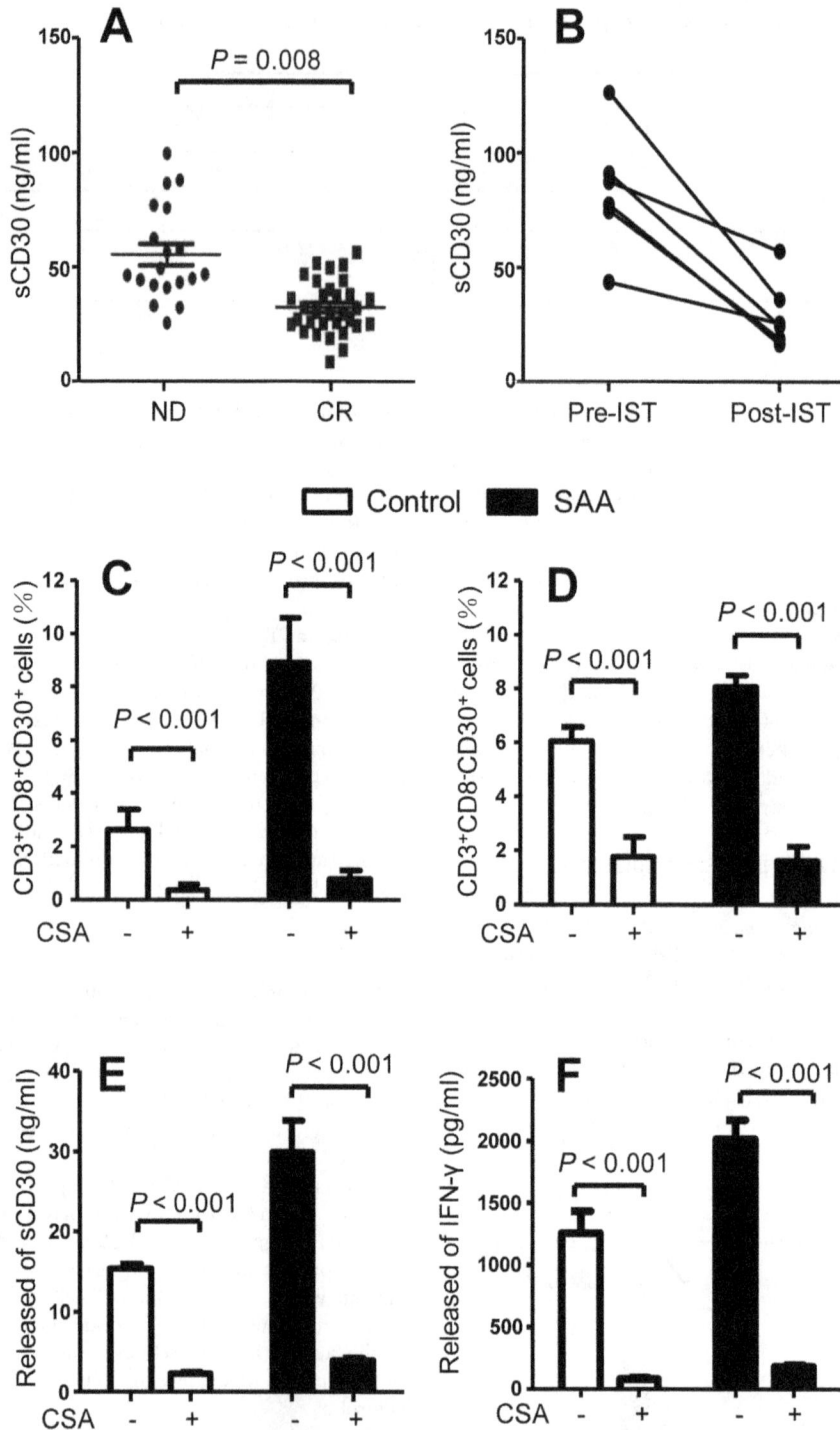

Figure 7. Relationship between BM plasma sCD30 levels and IST. (A) BM plasma sCD30 levels in SAA patients at diagnosis (n = 19) and in CR (n = 24). (B) BM samples pre- and post-IST were collected from 6 SAA patients, BM plasma sCD30 levels were determined by ELISA. CsA was added at 200 ng/mL to the allogeneic stimulated cultures, cells surface CD30 expressions (C and D) and released sCD30 (E) and IFN-γ (F) into culture supernatants were analysed at day 4 by FCM and ELISA, respectively. Data represent mean $\pm$ SE of three independent experiments.

Our *in vitro* stimulation experiments unveiled that the proportion of CD30+ cells increased and peaked at day 4, then decreased quickly, but the sCD30 levels increased in a time-dependent manner paralleled with high production of IFN-γ.

Significant correlation of maximum sCD30 level or maximum IFN-γ level with CD30 expression on T cells was observed at day 4, but no at day 7 when most surface CD30 had been cleaved and released as soluble CD30. This observation, consistent with previous studies [35], implied that surface CD30 was transiently expressed by activated T cells, but sCD30 could exist for a relatively longer period, and was easily quantified to reflect the maximum cell surface CD30 expression. It is intriguing to speculate that potent proliferating of CD30$^+$ T cells caused by autoantigens exist abundantly in the early phase of SAA, when the disease still hardly been aware because of lacking obvious clinical symptoms. These CD30$^+$ T cells may have a powerful ability to inhibit hematopoiesis because of enhanced production of IFN-γ. During the aggressive stage of SAA, drastic immune attack eliminates most hematopoietic cells baring autoantigens, leads to few new born CD30$^+$ T cells which only have a transient existence, but sCD30 cleaved from activated CD30$^+$ T cells can circulate in the bloodstream for a relative long time and reflect the degree of T cell activation. This may explain why we can't detect abundant expression of CD30 on T cell surface but elevated sCD30 levels in SAA.

Another interesting observation was the inverse correlation between plasma sCD30 levels and ALC. As we know most SAA patients show activated immune responses and decreased T cell counts. In addition, the baseline ALC is predictive of response at 6 months following IST [2]. The inverse correlation between sCD30 levels and ALC implied that CD30 participated in regulating apoptosis of T cells in SAA patients. However, the role of CD30 in human peripheral T cell apoptosis is still unclear. Only a few studies reported that CD30 regulated apoptosis in human blood eosinophils, anaplastic large cell lymphoma cells and murine CD8$^+$ T cells [34,36,37]. So If CD30 signaling affects the apoptosis of human T cells needs further study, especially in patients with SAA.

Disturbed T-cell subset balance with low CD4/CD8 T-cell ratio is present in many AA patients. We found the inverted CD4/CD8 T-cell ratio correlated with sCD30 levels in patients with SAA. This association was also reported in patients with common variable immunodeficiency [38]. We tried to explain this observation and found that while CD30 was predominantly expressed on CD3$^+$CD8$^-$ T cells in healthy individuals after allogeneic stimulation, the expression level of CD30 was comparable between CD3$^+$8$^-$ T cells and CD3$^+$CD8$^+$ T cells in AA. CD8$^+$ T cells from AA patients expressed more CD30 than that from healthy individuals. Although very preliminary, these findings suggested that activated CD8$^+$ T cells with increased proportion and enhanced allogeneic response might partly contribute to the elevated sCD30 in AA. In addition, we found that the release of IFN-γ reached plateau sooner than the release of sCD30 in allogeneic cultures. This could be explained by a very recent report that IFN-γ was able to trigger the release of sCD30 from allogeneic stimulated T lymphocytes [35]. So, while the CD30 pathway regulate the production of IFN-γ by T cells, IFN-γ may also function as a negative feedback modulator of T cell function by promoting CD30 release from T cells.

Correlations of sCD30 levels with disease activity/severity were reported in patients with systemic lupus erythematosus [22]. Increased levels of sCD30 in serum and synovial fluid were also observed in patients with rheumatoid arthritis [20]. So, sCD30 may be an indicator of immune activation in autoimmune diseases, including AA. Recently, CD30 has been investigated in acute GvHD after HCT [23–24]. The well-known pathophysiology of acute GvHD is clear that donor-derived T cells driven by antigen-present cell participated in the genesis of aGVHD, and minor histocomatibility antigens play a critical role [39]. As a marker of alloimmune responses, the elevated amounts of sCD30

in blood decreased after successful IST in SAA, which was similar with aGvHD. Brentuximab vedotin, an antibody-drug conjugates targeting CD30, has been approved by FDA for treatment of relapsed/refractory Hodgkin lymphoma and anaplastic large cell lymphoma [27–28]. Besides in hematopoietic cancers, Brentuximab vedotin is now being tested in prevention of GvHD after mismatched unrelated allogeneic HCT and treatment of refractory chronic GvHD. So, considering the increased expression of CD30 in many autoimmune diseases, and the treatment effect of CD30 antibody in type-I sensitized mice [40], this drug may have an application prospect in these diseases with elevated levels of sCD30.

Conclusion

In summary, we found that sCD30 plasma levels were increased in AA and correlated with disease severity, IFN-γ levels and CD4/CD8 T-cell ratio. T cells and in particular CD8$^+$ T cells which had increased proportion and enhanced allogeneic response partly contributed to the elevated levels of sCD30 and IFN-γ in AA. CD30 as a molecular marker that transiently express on IFN-γ-producing T cells, may participate in mediating bone marrow failure in AA. Our results shed more insight into the immune pathology involved in SAA. And in light of the importance of IFN-γ in the pathogenesis of SAA, CD30 may be a potent therapeutic target for SAA. CD30-directed drugs, for example, Brentuximab vedotin, should be tested *in vitro* and in AA mouse model for its ability to suppress activation of T cells by alloantigen.

Supporting Information

Figure S1   Expression of CD30 on T cells after allogeneic stimulation. Representative FCM analyses showed the kinetics of cell surface expression of CD30 by CD3$^+$CD8$^+$ T cells and CD3$^+$CD8$^-$ T cells after allogeneic stimulation. BM CD3$^+$ T cells from healthy individuals and SAA patients were co-cultured with mitomycin C treated allogenetic mononuclear cells for a total of 7 days.

Figure S2   CD30 positive T cells were mainly contained in the cell population with larger FSC and SSC. Representative FCM analyses showed the cell surface expression of CD30 on T cells at day 4 after allogeneic stimulation.

Figure S3   CsA inhibited the expression of CD30 on T cells after allogeneic stimulation. Representative FCM analyses showed the cell surface expression of CD30 on T cells at day 4 after allogeneic stimulation.

Author Contributions

Conceived and designed the experiments: JZ QW YZ. Performed the experiments: JZ QW JS MG XL. Analyzed the data: JZ QW JS MG XL. Contributed reagents/materials/analysis tools: MG XL YS JY. Wrote the paper: JZ QW YZ.

References

1. Brodsky RA, Jones RJ (2005) Aplastic anaemia. Lancet 365: 1647–1656.
2. Scheinberg P, Wu CO, Nunez O, Young NS (2009) Predicting response to immunosuppressive therapy and survival in severe aplastic anaemia. Br J Haematol 144: 206–216.
3. Zoumbos NC, Ferris WO, Hsu SM, Goodman S, Griffith P, et al. (1984) Analysis of lymphocyte subsets in patients with aplastic anaemia. Br J Haematol 58: 95–105.
4. Sloand E, Kim S, Maciejewski JP, Tisdale J, Follmann D, et al. (2002) Intracellular interferon-gamma in circulating and marrow T cells detected by flow cytometry and the response to immunosuppressive therapy in patients with aplastic anemia. Blood 100: 1185–1191
5. Risitano AM, Kook H, Zeng W, Chen G, Young NS, et al. (2002) Oligoclonal and polyclonal CD4 and CD8 lymphocytes in aplastic anemia and paroxysmal nocturnal hemoglobinuria measured by V beta CDR3 spectratyping and flow cytometry. Blood 100: 178–183.
6. Young NS, Scheinberg P, Calado RT (2008) Aplastic anemia. Curr Opin Hematol 15: 162–168.
7. Zeng W, Maciejewski JP, Chen G, Young NS (2001) Limited heterogeneity of T cell receptor BV usage in aplastic anemia. J Clin Invest 108: 765–773.
8. Risitano AM, Maciejewski JP, Green S, Plasilova M, Zeng W, et al. (2004) In-vivo dominant immune responses in aplastic anaemia: molecular tracking of putatively pathogenetic T-cell clones by TCR beta-CDR3 sequencing. Lancet 364: 355–364.
9. Hirano N, Butler MO, Von Bergwelt-Baildon MS, Maecker B, Schultze JL, et al. (2003) Autoantibodies frequently detected in patients with aplastic anemia. Blood 102: 4567–4575.
10. Hirano N, Butler MO, Guinan EC, Nadler LM, Kojima S (2005) Presence of anti-kinectin and anti-PMS1 antibodies in Japanese aplastic anaemia patients. Br J Haematol 128: 221–223.
11. Takamatsu H, Espinoza JL, Lu X, Qi Z, Okawa K, et al. (2009) Anti-moesin antibodies in the serum of patients with aplastic anemia stimulate peripheral blood mononuclear cells to secrete TNF-alpha and IFN-gamma. J Immunol 182: 703–710.
12. Goto M, Kuribayashi K, Takahashi Y, Kondoh T, Tanaka M, et al. (2013) Identification of autoantibodies expressed in acquired aplastic anaemia. Br J Haematol 160: 359–362.
13. Chen J, Ellison FM, Eckhaus MA, Smith AL, Keyvanfar K, et al. (2007) Minor antigen h60-mediated aplastic anemia is ameliorated by immunosuppression and the infusion of regulatory T cells. J Immunol 178: 4159–4168.
14. Ellis TM, Simms PE, Slivnick DJ, Jack HM, Fisher RI (1993) CD30 is a signal-transducing molecule that defines a subset of human activated CD45RO+ T cells. J Immunol 151: 2380–2389.
15. Alzona M, Jack HM, Fisher RI, Ellis TM (1994) CD30 defines a subset of activated human T cells that produce IFN-gamma and IL-5 and exhibit enhanced B cell helper activity. J Immunol 153: 2861–2867.
16. Martinez OM, Villanueva J, Abtahi S, Beatty PR, Esquivel CO, et al. (1998) CD30 expression identifies a functional alloreactive human T-lymphocyte subset. Transplantation 65: 1240–1247.
17. Chan KW, Hopke CD, Krams SM, Martinez OM (2002) CD30 expression identifies the predominant proliferating T lymphocyte population in human alloimmune responses. J Immunol 169: 1784–1791.
18. Hansen HP, Dietrich S, Kisseleva T, Mokros T, Mentlein R, et al. (2000) CD30 shedding from Karpas 299 lymphoma cells is mediated by TNF-alpha-converting enzyme. J Immunol 165: 6703–6709.
19. Schlaf G, Altermann WW, Rothhoff A, Seliger B (2007) Soluble CD30 serum level–an adequate marker for allograft rejection of solid organs? Histol Histopathol 22: 1269–1279.
20. Gerli R, Muscat C, Bistoni O, Falini B, Tomassini C, et al. (1995) High levels of the soluble form of CD30 molecule in rheumatoid arthritis (RA) are expression of CD30+ T cell involvement in the inflamed joints. Clin Exp Immunol 102: 547–550.
21. Dummer W, Brocker EB, Bastian BC (1997) Elevated serum levels of soluble CD30 are associated with atopic dermatitis, but not with respiratory atopic disorders and allergic contact dermatitis. Br J Dermatol 137: 185–187.
22. Caligaris-Cappio F, Bertero MT, Converso M, Stacchini A, Vinante F, et al. (1995) Circulating levels of soluble CD30, a marker of cells producing Th2-type cytokines, are increased in patients with systemic lupus erythematosus and correlate with disease activity. Clin Exp Rheumatol 13: 339–343.
23. Hubel K, Cremer B, Heuser E, von Strandmann EP, Hallek M, et al. (2010) A prospective study of serum soluble CD30 in allogeneic hematopoietic stem cell transplantation. Transpl Immunol 23: 215–219.
24. Chen YB, McDonough S, Hasserjian R, Chen H, Coughlin E, et al. (2012) Expression of CD30 in patients with acute graft-versus-host disease. Blood 120: 691–696.
25. Fanale MA, Forero-Torres A, Rosenblatt JD, Advani RH, Franklin AR, et al. (2012) A phase I weekly dosing study of brentuximab vedotin in patients with relapsed/refractory CD30-positive hematologic malignancies. Clin Cancer Res. 18: 248–255.
26. Younes A, Bartlett NL, Leonard JP, Kennedy DA, Lynch CM, et al. (2010) Brentuximab vedotin (SGN-35) for relapsed CD30-positive lymphomas. N Engl J Med 363: 1812–1821.
27. Sasse S, Rothe A, Goergen H, Eichenauer DA, Lohri A, et al. (2013) Brentuximab vedotin (SGN-35) in patients with transplant-naive relapsed/refractory Hodgkin lymphoma. Leuk Lymphoma 54: 2144–2148.
28. Pro B, Advani R, Brice P, Bartlett NL, Rosenblatt JD, et al. (2012) Brentuximab vedotin (SGN-35) in patients with relapsed or refractory systemic anaplastic large-cell lymphoma: results of a phase II study. J Clin Oncol 30: 2190–2196.
29. Camitta BM, Thomas ED, Nathan DG, Gale RP, Kopecky KJ, et al. (1979) A prospective study of androgens and bone marrow transplantation for treatment of severe aplastic anemia. Blood 53: 504–514.
30. Marsh JC, Ball SE, Cavenagh J, Darbyshire P, Dokal I, et al. (2009) Guidelines for the diagnosis and management of aplastic anaemia. Br J Haematol 147: 43–70.
31. Amakawa R, Hakem A, Kundig TM, Matsuyama T, Simard JJ, et al. (1996) Impaired negative selection of T cells in Hodgkin's disease antigen CD30-deficient mice. Cell 84: 551–562.
32. Chiarle R, Podda A, Prolla G, Podack ER, Thorbecke GJ, et al. (1999) CD30 overexpression enhances negative selection in the thymus and mediates programmed cell death via a Bcl-2-sensitive pathway. J Immunol 163: 194–205.
33. Zeiser R, Nguyen VH, Hou JZ, Beilhack A, Zambricki E, et al. (2007) Early CD30 signaling is critical for adoptively transferred CD4+CD25+ regulatory T cells in prevention of acute graft-versus-host disease. Blood 109: 2225–2233.
34. Telford WG, Nam SY, Podack ER, Miller RA (1997) CD30-regulated apoptosis in murine CD8+ T cells after cessation of TCR signals. Cell Immunol 182: 125–136.
35. Velasquez SY, Garcia LF, Opelz G, Alvarez CM, Susal C (2013) Release of soluble CD30 after allogeneic stimulation is mediated by memory T cells and regulated by IFN-gamma and IL-2. Transplantation 96: 154–161.
36. Berro AI, Perry GA, Agrawal DK (2004) Increased expression and activation of CD30 induce apoptosis in human blood eosinophils. J Immunol 173: 2174–2183.
37. Mir SS, Richter BW, Duckett CS (2000) Differential effects of CD30 activation in anaplastic large cell lymphoma and Hodgkin disease cells. Blood 96: 4307–4312.
38. Rezaei N, Haji-Molla-Hoseini M, Aghamohammadi A, Pourfathollah AA, Moghtadaie M, et al. (2008) Increased serum levels of soluble CD30 in patients with common variable immunodeficiency and its clinical implications. J Clin Immunol 28: 78–84.
39. Couriel D, Caldera H, Champlin R, Komanduri K (2004) Acute graft-versus-host disease: pathophysiology, clinical manifestations, and management. Cancer 101: 1936–1946.
40. Saraiva M, Smith P, Fallon PG, Alcami A (2002) Inhibition of type 1 cytokine-mediated inflammation by a soluble CD30 homologue encoded by ectromelia (mousepox) virus. J Exp Med 196: 829–839.

6

Cell Fate Decisions in Malignant Hematopoiesis: Leukemia Phenotype Is Determined by Distinct Functional Domains of the MN1 Oncogene

Courteney K. Lai[1,2], Yeonsook Moon[3], Florian Kuchenbauer[4,5], Daniel T. Starzcynowski[6], Bob Argiropoulos[7], Eric Yung[1], Philip Beer[1], Adrian Schwarzer[8], Amit Sharma[8], Gyeongsin Park[9], Malina Leung[1], Grace Lin[1], Sarah Vollett[1], Stephen Fung[1], Connie J. Eaves[1,2], Aly Karsan[10,11], Andrew P. Weng[1,11], R. Keith Humphries[1,2*¶], Michael Heuser[12¶]

1 Terry Fox Laboratory, BC Cancer Agency Research Centre, Vancouver, BC, Canada, 2 Department of Medicine, Faculty of Medicine, University of British Columbia, Vancouver, BC, Canada, 3 Department of Laboratory Medicine, Medical School of Inha University, Incheon, Korea, 4 Department of Internal Medicine III, University Hospital of Ulm, Ulm, Germany, 5 Institute of Experimental Cancer Research, Comprehensive Cancer Centre, University Hospital of Ulm, Ulm, Germany, 6 Department of Pediatrics, Cincinnati Children's Hospital Medical Center, Cincinnati, Ohio, United States of America, 7 Department of Medical Genetics, University of Calgary, Calgary, AB, Canada, 8 Institute of Experimental Hematology, Hannover Medical School, Hannover, Germany, 9 Department of Hospital Pathology, Catholic University of Korea, Seoul, Korea, 10 Genome Sciences Centre, BC Cancer Agency, Vancouver, BC, Canada, 11 Department of Pathology and Laboratory Medicine, University of British Columbia, Vancouver, BC, Canada, 12 Department of Hematology, Hemostasis, Oncology, and Stem Cell Transplantation, Hannover Medical School, Hannover, Germany

Abstract

Extensive molecular profiling of leukemias and preleukemic diseases has revealed that distinct clinical entities, like acute myeloid (AML) and T-lymphoblastic leukemia (T-ALL), share similar pathogenetic mutations. It is not well understood how the cell of origin, accompanying mutations, extracellular signals or structural differences in a mutated gene determine the phenotypic identity of leukemias. We dissected the functional aspects of different protein regions of the MN1 oncogene and their effect on the leukemic phenotype, building on the ability of MN1 to induce leukemia without accompanying mutations. We found that the most C-terminal region of MN1 was required to block myeloid differentiation at an early stage, and deletion of an extended C-terminal region resulted in loss of myeloid identity and cell differentiation along the T-cell lineage in vivo. Megakaryocytic/erythroid lineage differentiation was blocked by the N-terminal region. In addition, the N-terminus was required for proliferation and leukemogenesis in vitro and in vivo through upregulation of *HoxA9*, *HoxA10* and *Meis2*. Our results provide evidence that a single oncogene can modulate cellular identity of leukemic cells based on its active gene regions. It is therefore likely that different mutations in the same oncogene may impact cell fate decisions and phenotypic appearance of malignant diseases.

Editor: Ken Mills, Queen's University Belfast, United Kingdom

Funding: This study was supported by grants from the Terry Fox Foundation, Canada (http://www.terryfox.org/TerryFox/The_Terry_Fox_Foundation.html) (grant Nos. 18006 and 122869), the Cancer Research Society, Canada (http://www.crs-src.ca/), the Stem Cell Network of Canada (http://www.stemcellnetwork.ca/index.php?page=funding-opportunities), Deutsche Krebshilfe e.V (grant No. 109003, 110284, 110292, and 111267) (http://www.krebshilfe.de/metanavigation/english.html), grant No. DJCLS H09/1f, R 10/22, and R13/14 from the Deutsche-José-Carreras Leukämie-Stiftung e.V (http://www.carreras-stiftung.de/); grant No. M 47.1 from the H. W. & J. Hector Stiftung (http://www.hector-stiftung.de/), the German Federal Ministry of Education and Research grant 01EO0802 (IFB-Tx) (http://www.bmbf.de/en/14580.php), and DFG grants HE 5240/4-1, HE 5240/5-1 (http://www.dfg.de/en/research_funding/programmes/individual/research_grants/). CKL was supported by studentships from the Canadian Institute of Health Research (http://www.cihr-irsc.gc.ca/e/193.html#), the University of British Columbia (https://www.grad.ubc.ca/awards/four-year-doctoral-fellowship-4yf), and the BC Cancer Agency (http://www.bccancer.bc.ca/default.htm). FK was supported by grants from Deutsche Krebshilfe grant 109420 (Max-Eder program) (http://www.krebshilfe.de/metanavigation/english.html); fellowship 2010/04 by the European Hematology Association (http://www.ehaweb.org/career/career-development-grants/eha-research-fellowships-and-the-jose-carreras-foundation-eha-young-investigator-fellowship/); and by the Deutsche Forschungsgemeinschaft (grant D.3955 (SFB 1074)) (http://www.dfg.de/en/research_funding/programmes/individual/). PB was supported by an intermediate fellowship from the Kay Kendall Leukaemia Fund (http://www.kklf.org.uk/intermediate.html). GL was supported by a BC Cancer Studentship from the BC Cancer Agency (http://www.bccancer.bc.ca/default.htm). SV was supported by a studentship from the Stem Cell Network of Canada (http://www.stemcellnetwork.ca/index.php?page=co-op-award). The funders had no role in study design, data collection and analysis, decision to publish, or preparation of the manuscript.

* Email: khumphri@bccrc.ca

¶ RKH and MH are senior authors on this work.

Introduction

The postulated requirement for induction of leukemogenesis has long been the combination of class I and II mutations [1], although recent insights into the genetic composition of acute myeloid leukemia (AML) cells has revealed additional pathogenetic mechanisms including changes in epigenetic regulation. On average, 13 coding genes are mutated per AML genome [2], suggesting that several events are required for leukemogenesis. Despite the heterogeneity of cells that can give rise to AML, only a small proportion of AML cells show clonogenic activity in culture and only a small fraction of AML blast cells are able to confer disease to immune-deficient mice [3]. While such disease-propagating or leukemia-initiating cells (LICs) may be rare, they are not necessarily restricted to the most primitive cells within the hematopoietic hierarchy but rather, can include committed progenitor cells such as common myeloid progenitors (CMPs) or common lymphoid progenitors (CLPs) [4–7]. The high level of heterogeneity seen in AML and within an individual patient underscores the importance of understanding the molecular mechanisms underlying this disease and the functional consequences on leukemic cells.

While there is a high degree of cellular heterogeneity within the cells of an individual leukaemia [8], there is striking redundancy of mutated genes in distinct diseases like AML [9], T-lymphoblastic leukemia (T-ALL) [10], and primary myelofibrosis [11], including mutations in *DNMT3A* and several other genes. Explanations for how mutations in the same gene can cause different diseases may include: differing cells of origin [12] or cell-extrinsic signals [13], as illustrated by the ability of the MLL-AF9 fusion gene to cause myeloid and lymphoid leukemias; the influence of the microenvironment, such as the ability of abnormal stroma cells to induce myelodysplasia in hematopoietic stem cells (HSCs) [14]; and the ability of mutations to change the lineage potential of the oncogene and possibly the phenotype of the disease, as in EZH2 mutations in B-non-Hodgkin lymphoma and myeloid disorders [15,16]. The meningioma (disrupted in balanced translocation) 1 (*MN1*) model of leukemogenesis constitutes a simple and ideal model to test this latter hypothesis due to its ability to induce leukemia as a single hit through constitutive overexpression [17].

The ability of MN1 to induce rapid onset leukemia on its own highlights its central regulatory role in hematopoietic transformation. MN1 has been shown to be most highly expressed in murine CMPs, but is downregulated upon differentiation [17] and is capable of enhancing proliferation of human CD34+ cord blood cells [18]. High MN1 expression has been associated with both acute myeloid and lymphoid leukemias [19] as well as other AML characteristics such as inv(16) [20] or overexpression of EVI-1 [21]. Significantly, it also has been identified as an independent prognostic factor in patients with AML with normal cytogenetics, associated with shorter relapse-free survival, overall survival, and resistance to ATRA-induced differentiation [19,22–25]. As loss of MN1 expression has been shown to impair proliferation and significantly decrease clonogenic activity of human leukemic cells, it is a potential therapeutic target in AML patients [26].

MN1 has been shown to rapidly induce leukemia in mice [20,22]. We have recently shown that MN1 is capable of transforming single CMP cells as the cell of origin [17]. Significantly, GMPs required co-overexpression of *Meis1* for in vitro transformation, and the additional co-overexpression of HOXA9 or HOXA10 to induce leukemia in vivo [17]. Loss of MEIS1 expression abrogated leukemic activity in MN1 cells, suggesting that, combined with co-localization of MN1 and MEIS1 at a large proportion of MEIS1 target sites, MEIS1 and

its cofactor HOXA9 are essential to MN1 leukemogenesis [17]. In addition, MN1 cells are arrested at an immature stage of myelopoiesis and are highly resistant against all-trans retinoic acid (ATRA) [22], a potent inducer of myeloid differentiation, although ectopic CEBPα expression, which MN1 is thought to repress, can abrogate the leukemogenic activity of MN1 [18].

We hypothesize that multiple functions are encoded in this protein and can be localized to different regions. Thus, delineation and localisation of these functions at a structural level will provide insight into the key mechanisms required for leukemic transformation by a single central regulator such as MN1. Despite the established role of MN1 overexpression in leukemia, little is known about the protein itself. The MN1 protein is highly conserved between different species, but largely lacks recognised protein domains excepting two proline-glutamine stretches and a single 28 residue-long glutamine stretch. Here, we systematically localise known properties of MN1 leukemia using both *in vitro* and extensive *in vivo* studies to specific physical regions of wildtype MN1 through a detailed structure-function analysis of MN1. We demonstrate that the proliferative ability and self-renewal activity, and the inhibition of megakaryocyte/erythroid, myeloid, and lymphoid differentiation are localised to distinct regions within MN1 and provide evidence that different mutations of a single oncogene can induce distinct diseases such as myeloid and lymphoid leukemia and myeloproliferative disease.

Materials and Methods

Retroviral vectors and vector production

Retroviral vectors for expression of MN1 [22] and NU-P98HOXD13 (ND13) [27] have been previously described. Primers were designed for each MN1 mutant truncation construct to ensure the N- and C-termini of the final construct were flanked by *Not*I sites, then subcloned into the expression vector pSF91 [28] upstream of the internal ribosomal entry site (IRES) and the enhanced green fluorescent protein (GFP) gene. MN1 Strategy 1 constructs were generated by PCR amplification of the N- (proximal) and C-terminal (distal) regions of the construct with *Hind*III sites at the internal sites. The proximal and distal fragments were then subcloned into the pSF91-IRESeGFP vector. As a control, the pSF91 vector carrying only the IRES-enhanced GFP cassette was used. Constructs were validated by sequencing and correct expression and transmission were confirmed by qRT-PCR and PCR. Primer sequences can be found in Table S1. For HA-tagged constructs, full-length and MN1 mutant deletion constructs were cut to ensure the N- and C-termini of the final construct were flanked by *Bgl*II or *Bam*HI (for constructs lacking the N-terminal region) and *Not*I sites, respectively, then subcloned into the MSCV-IRES-GFP expression vector [29], and an HA-tag was cloned to the N-terminus of MN1 or the deletion constructs. Helper-free recombinant retrovirus was generated by using supernatants from the transfected ecotropic Phoenix packaging cell line to transduce the ecotropic GP + E86 packaging cell line [30].

Clonogenic progenitor assays

Colony-forming cells (CFCs) were assayed in methylcellulose (MethoCult M3434 or MegaCult-C, Catalog No. 04964; STEMCELL Technologies, Vancouver, BC, Canada). For each assay freshly isolated and transduced unsorted bone marrow cells were plated in duplicate in Methocult medium (1000 cells/well). Colonies were evaluated microscopically 10 days after plating using standard criteria. To assay megakaryocyte progenitor frequency, freshly isolated and transduced bone marrow cells were sorted for GFP expression, and 1×10^5 cells were suspended in MegaCult-C medium containing recombinant human thrombopoietin (50 ng/mL), recombinant human IL6 (20 ng/mL), recombinant human IL11 (50 ng/mL), and recombinant mouse IL3 (10 ng/mL), mixed with collagen and dispensed in chamber slides (all from STEMCELL Technologies, Vancouver, BC, Canada). Cultures were incubated at 37°C for 7 days. Slides were stained with acetylthiocholiniodide according to manufacturer's instructions, and colonies were counted manually under a microscope, as previously described [31].

Quantitative real-time RT-PCR

Total RNA from stored, frozen cell pellets was isolated using TRIZOL reagent (Life Technologies, Burlington, ON, Canada). Total RNA was converted into cDNA using the SuperScript VILO cDNA synthesis kit (Life Technologies, Burlington, ON, Canada) using 500 ng of total RNA. Quantitative real-time PCR was performed as previously described using the 7900 HT Fast Real-Time PCR system (Applied Biosystems, Foster City, CA, USA) [32] and Fast SYBR Green Master Mix (Life Technologies, Burlington, ON, Canada) [32]. Relative expression was determined with the $2^{-\Delta\Delta CT}$ method, and the housekeeping gene transcript $Abl1$ was used to normalize the results. Primers were manufactured by Life Technologies. Primer sequences can be found in Table S2.

Western blot analysis

For Western blot analysis, 1×10^6 cells were lysed with 150 μL lysis buffer (50 mM Tris-HCl [pH 8], 0,1% Tween-20, 0.1% SDS, 150 mM NaCl, 0.5 mM EDTA, 10 mM DTT, and 1 mM PMSF, plus protease inhibitor cocktail; Sigma, Oakville, ON, Canada) and incubated for 20 minutes on ice. NuPage LPS loading buffer (4x) and NuPage Sample Reducing Agent (10x) (Life Technologies, Burlington, ON, Canada) were added and samples were heated for 15 minutes at 95°C. Lysates were loaded onto 4%-12% NuPage Novex BIS-Tris SDS-polyacrylamide gels (Life Technologies, Burlington, ON, Canada) and electroblotted in MOPS transfer buffer to nitrocellulose membrane (Life Technologies, Burlington, ON, Canada). Rabbit polyclonal anti-HA (Abcam, Cambridge, England) or mouse monoclonal anti-beta-actin (abm, Richmond, BC, Canada) and Mouse TrueBlot ULTRA HRP-conjugated anti-mouse (Rockland Inc., Gilbertsville, PA, USA) or goat anti-rabbit IgG antibodies (Jackson ImmunoResearch Laboratories Inc., PA, USA) in 1:5000 dilutions of 0.1% Tween-20, 5% bovine serum albumin (BSA), Tris-buffered saline (TBS) were used for protein detection. Proteins were visualised using Clarity Western enhanced chemiluminescence (ECL) Substrate (Bio-Rad, Hercules, CA, USA).

ATRA cytotoxicity assay

To ensure that cells proliferated in vitro even if a MN1 mutation was non-functional, MN1 deletion constructs were transduced in bone marrow cells immortalized by retroviral expression of the fusion gene ND13. In vitro cytotoxicity assays were performed in Dulbecco's modified Eagle medium (DMEM) supplemented with 15% fetal bovine serum (FBS), 6 ng/mL murine interleukin 3 (mIL3), 10 ng/mL human interleukin 6 (hIL6), and 20 ng/mL murine stem-cell factor (mSCF; all from STEMCELL Technologies, Vancouver, BC, Canada). Cells were seeded at a cell density of 1×10^4/mL in a 96 well plate, and incubated under light-protective conditions. ATRA (Sigma, Oakville, ON, Canada) was dissolved in DMSO (Sigma) and added to the culture medium at the specified concentrations as 1/1000th of the final volume. After 64 hours, cells were stained with Alamar Blue (Sigma) for 8 hours

and fluorescence was measured with a Tecan Safire^2 microplate reader (Life Technologies, Burlington, ON, Canada). Viability was determined as percentage of DMSO-treated cells after background subtraction of fluorescence in wells with medium only. The 50% inhibitory concentration was determined as the concentration of ATRA that reduced cell viability to 50% of DMSO-treated cells.

Mice and retroviral infection of primary bone marrow cells and bone marrow transplantation

Primary mouse bone marrow cells from 5-fluorouracil treated C57BL/6J donor mice (Faulding, Underdaler, Australia) were prestimulated for 48 hours, transduced by co-cultivation with viral producers for 48 hours, then harvested and plated into CFC media or directly transplanted into lethally irradiated syngeneic recipient mice, as previously described [32]. Recipient mice were exposed to a single dose of 750 to 810 cGy total-body irradiation accompanied by a life-sparing dose of 1×10^5 freshly isolated bone marrow cells from syngeneic mice, and were monitored daily. Engraftment of transduced cells in peripheral blood was monitored every 4 weeks by fluorescence-activated cell-sorter (FACS) analysis and quantification of GFP-positive cells. Sick or moribund mice were sacrificed, spleens weighed, and red blood cells and white blood cells were counted using the scil Vet abc blood analyser (Vet Novations, Barrie, ON, Canada).

Ethics Statement

C57BL/6J mice were bred and maintained in the Animal Research Centre of the British Columbia Cancer Agency as approved by the University of British Columbia Animal Care Committee (the Institutional Animal Care and Use Committee, IACUC). Experimental studies were approved by the University of British Columbia Animal Care Committe under experimental protocol numbers A04-0380 and A09-0009, and all efforts were made to minimise suffering.

FACS analysis

Lineage distribution was determined by FACS analysis (FACSCalibur; Becton Dickinson, Mississauga, ON, Canada) as previously described [27]. Monoclonal antibodies used were phycoerythrin (PE)-labeled Gr1 (clone Ly6G-6C), B220 (CD45R), CD4, Ter119, and Sca-1 (Ly6A/E) and allophycocyanin (APC)-labeled CD11b, CD8, and c-kit (CD117) (BD Biosciences, Mississauga, ON, Canada).

Bone marrow morphology

Cytospin preparations were stained with Wright-Giemsa stain. Images were visualised using a Nikon Eclipse 80i microscope (Nikon, Mississauga, ON, Canada) and a 20x/0.40 numerical aperture objective, or a 100x/1.25 numerical aperture objective and Nikon Immersion Oil (Nikon). A Nikon Coolpix 995 camera (Nikon) was used to capture images.

Confocal microscopy

Twenty-four hours prior to fixation, micro growth glass cover slips (VWR International, Mississauga, ON, Canada) were coated in Cultrex Poly-L-Lysine (Trevigen, Gaithersburg, MD, USA). GP + E86 expressing cell lines expressing MN1, MN1Δ1, and MN1Δ5-7 were then plated. Cells were fixed in 4% paraformaldehyde in phosphate-buffered saline (PBS) for 10 minutes at room temperature, incubated with a 1:500 dilution of rabbit anti-HA primary antibody followed by a 1:300 dilution of anti-rabbit Alexa eFluor 594 secondary antibody (Life Technologies, Burlington, ON, Canada) and then stained with DAPI at 1 μg/mL (Sigma-

Aldrich, St Louis, MO, USA). Slides were then mounted with DABCO mounting medium (Sigma-Aldrich, St Louis, MO, USA) and Z-stack photographs were taken 0.13 μm apart using a Leica TCS SP5 Confocal microscope (100x objective). Images were captured using LAS AF software (Leica Microsystems, Inc., Exton, PA, USA) and deconvoluted using Real-time GPU-based 3D Deconvolution [33] and DeconvolutionLab [34] in ImageJ.

Gene expression profiling and gene set enrichment analysis

RNA was extracted using TRIZOL reagent (Life Technologies, Burlington, ON, Canada) from GFP+ cells that were sorted from mouse bone marrow cells four weeks after transplantation. Quality and integrity of the total RNA isolated was controlled by running all samples on an Agilent Technologies 2100 Bioanalyzer (Agilent Technologies, Mississauga, ON). Extracted RNA from MN1, MN1Δ1, and MN1Δ7 leukemia cells and Gr1+/CD11b+ bone marrow cells were hybridized to the Affymetrix GeneChip Mouse 430 2.0 (43.000 probes) microarray (n = 2) according to the manufacturer's instructions. Experiments were performed at the British Columbia Genome Sciences Centre, Vancouver, Canada. Gene expression can be found at the Gene Expression Omnibus database (GEO accession number GSE46990; http://www.ncbi.nlm.nih.gov/geo/query/acc.cgi?token=zhedbmoeuqcksli&acc=GSE46990). Data were analyzed using R and Bioconductor [35]. Quality was assessed with the ArrayQualityMetrics package [36]. Arrays were preprocessed using RMA [37]. Differentially expressed probesets were calculated with the LIMMA package [38] applying Benjamini-Hochberg multiple testing correction at an FDR of 0.05. For gene set enrichment the Broad Institute GSEA software package was used [39]. The datasets were collapsed into single genes and rank-ordered by signal to noise ratio. Gene set permutations were used to estimate statistical significance. Analyzed gene ontology sets were obtained from MSigDB v3.1 [39]. The gene set enrichment analysis software [39] (http://www.broad.mit.edu/gsea/index.jsp) was used to compare gene enrichment of Gene Ontology gene sets (dataset C5, available from the Molecular Signature database v3.1 [39]) between MN1Δ1 vs MN1 and MN1Δ7 vs. MN1.

Statistical analysis

Comparisons were performed by unpaired T-tests. The two-sided level of significance was set at P less than 0.05. Comparison of survival curves were performed using the Kaplan-Meier method and log-rank test. Statistical analyses were performed with Excel (Microsoft Canada, Mississauga, ON, Canada) and GraphPad Prism 6 (GraphPad Software, La Jolla, CA, USA).

Results

The N-terminal region of MN1 is required for immortalization of bone marrow cells in vitro

To elucidate the relationship between the structure of MN1 and the characteristics of MN1 leukemia, MN1 deletion mutants were generated in three strategies. Wildtype MN1 was divided into seven regions, each approximately 200 amino acids in length and numbered sequentially from the N-terminus. In an internal deletion series (strategy 1), distinct 200 amino acid regions were deleted (Figure 1A). Due to technical difficulties the construct lacking the third region from the N-terminus (MN1Δ3) did not express and was excluded from further analysis. Progressive N-terminal deletions (strategy 2) included six mutant constructs in which approximately 200 amino acid-regions were cumulatively deleted starting from the MN1 N-terminus. For progressive C-

terminal deletions (strategy 3), stretches of approximately 200 amino acids were cumulatively deleted starting from the MN1 C-terminus (Figure 1A). The size and expression of all mutant constructs was validated at the RNA and protein level. The expected protein was detected for all constructs lacking one or two regions and for the constructs MN1Δ1-4, MN1Δ3-7, and MN1Δ5-7 lacking three or more regions. The remaining constructs lacking three or more regions did not, however, yield detectable protein (Figure S1A–B).

Freshly isolated bone marrow cells were transduced with MN1 mutation constructs or control (CTL) vector and plated in CFC medium, and replating ability and proportion of transduced cells (GFP+) were measured. While GFP-positive cells were lost in CTL-transduced cells after the second replating, GFP-positive cells outgrew non-transduced cells for internal deletion constructs (strategy 1) and could be replated up to the fifth plating, with the exception of MN1Δ6, where no colonies grew after the fourth plating (Figure S2A–B). For progressive N-terminal deletions (strategy 2), only cells lacking the most N-terminal domain (MN1Δ1) immortalized bone marrow cells in vitro, and competitively outgrew non-transduced cells; deletion of larger MN1 N-terminal stretches resulted in loss of replating capacity (Figure S2C and D). Cumulative deletions from the C-terminus (strategy 3) could immortalize bone marrow cells up to MN1Δ3-7, in which only 317 N-terminal amino acids are retained (Figure S2E and F), including MN1Δ4-7 which showed colony replating ability despite protein being unable to be detected by Western blot (Figure S1). In summary, the N-terminus of MN1 is necessary and sufficient to immortalize bone marrow cells in vitro with select regions, such as amino acids 1008–1201 playing a significant role in in vitro immortalization.

The N-terminal domain of MN1 is required for its leukemogenic potential in vivo

MN1-transduced bone marrow cells were transplanted into lethally irradiated mice, and engraftment in peripheral blood was monitored monthly. Regardless of the mutation construct, mice showed at least minimal engraftment 4 weeks post-transplant (engraftment ≥1%). All internal deletion (strategy 1) constructs showed statistically significant higher engraftment than CTL mice with increasing engraftment over 16 weeks (Figure 1B). Progressive N-terminal deletion (strategy 2) constructs also showed engraftment at 4 weeks post-transplant, although engraftment levels did not significantly differ from control mice except for MN1Δ1, which showed higher early engraftment levels similar to full-length MN1. In addition, engraftment decreased over 16 weeks, suggesting that these constructs, including MN1Δ1, had defects in their proliferative and self-renewal capabilities and, thus, were unable to outcompete the co-transplanted normal bone marrow cells (Figure 1C and Table S3). Of the progressive C-terminal deletions (strategy 3), MN1Δ7 showed the highest engraftment levels, and MN1Δ6-7, MN1Δ5-7 and MN1Δ3-7 had significantly higher engraftment of transduced cells compared to CTL cells at 16 weeks (Figure 1D). The MN1 mutations that enhanced engraftment and proliferation in vivo also induced high WBC counts, anemia, and thrombocytopenia (Figures S3–S5, Tables S4–5).

All transplantation groups were fully characterized at time of sacrifice including bone marrow morphology with blast count, immunophenotype of GFP+ bone marrow cells, spleen weight and (for most constructs) secondary transplantations (Table S3). For mice succumbing to hematologic disease, the diagnosis is noted in Table S3 and supported by bone marrow morphology (Figure 1H). In summary, deletions including the first 221 N-terminal

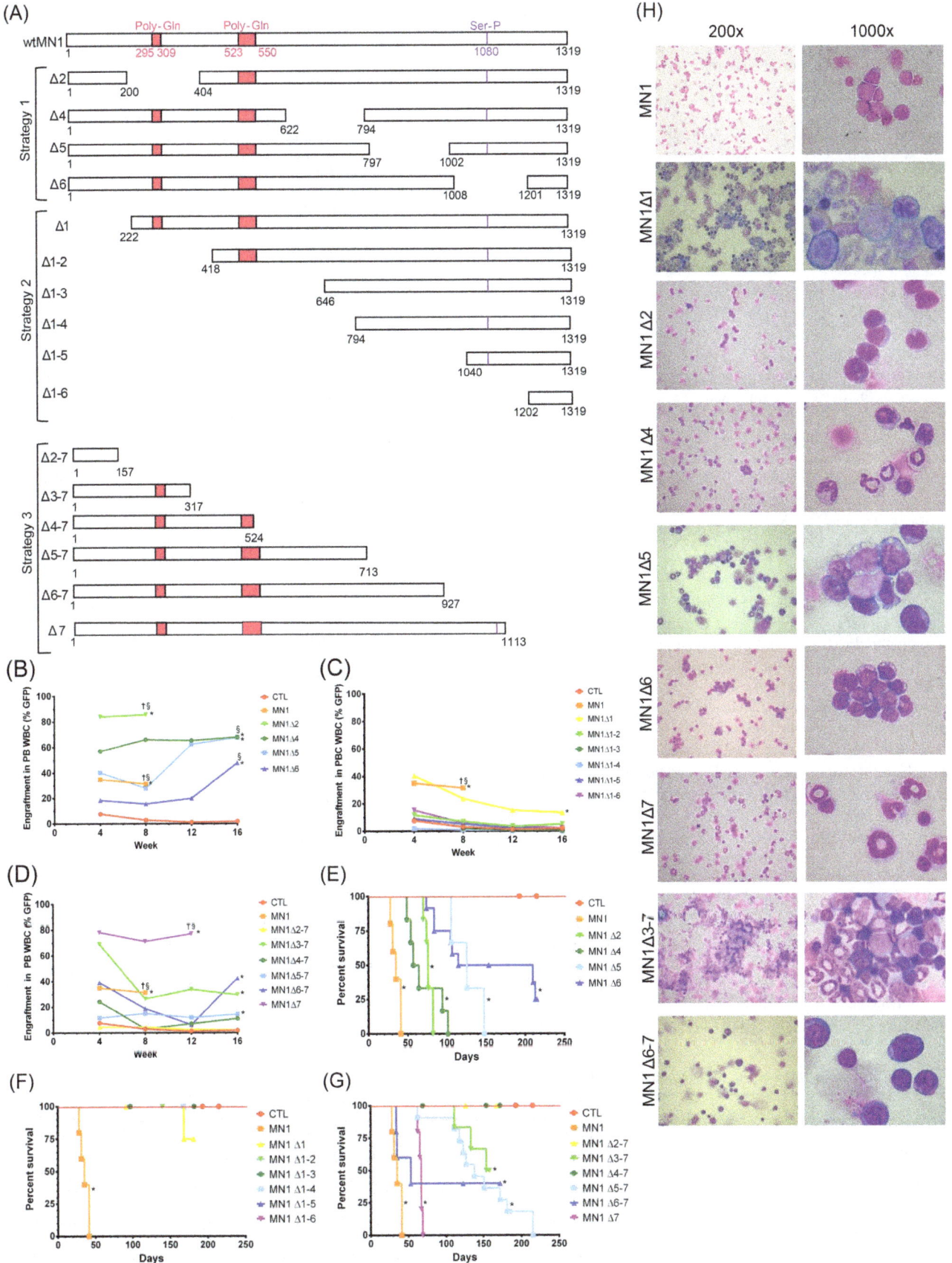

Figure 1. The N-terminal region of MN1 is required for its leukemogenic potential. (A) MN1 mutation constructs for structure-function analysis. In strategy 1 distinct stretches of approximately 200 amino acids were deleted throughout wildtype MN1. In strategy 2, stretches of approximately 200 amino acids were cumulatively deleted starting from the MN1 N-terminus. In strategy 3, stretches of approximately 200 amino acids were cumulatively deleted starting from the MN1 C-terminus. (B–D) Percentage of transgene-positive white blood cells engrafting in peripheral blood of transplanted mice at 4-week intervals. P values are given for the comparison of the indicated construct with CTL-transduced cells. The average engraftment is shown. Number of analysed mice and standard error can be found in Table S1. (E-G) Survival of mice receiving transplants of cells transduced with (E) strategy 1, (F) strategy 2, and (G) strategy 3 MN1 deletions. P values are given for the comparison of the indicated construct with CTL-transduced cells. The number of analysed mice is detailed in Table S1. (H) Morphology of bone marrow cells at death of diseased mice. The cells were Wright-Giemsa stained. Images were visualised using a Nikon Eclipse 80i microscope (Nikon, Mississauga, ON, Canada) and a 20x/0.40 numerical aperture objective, or a 100x/1.25 numerical aperture objective and Nikon Immersion Oil (Nikon). A Nikon Coolpix 995 camera (Nikon) was used to capture images. § engraftment in peripheral blood at the indicated time point or at death in cases where a mouse died before that time point. † all mice were dead at this time point due to disease. * indicates P<0.05, ** indicates P<0.001.

amino acids prevented MN1-induced AML, except one MN1Δ1 mouse that died with low engraftment, low WBC count, and a non-elevated blast count (Figure 1F). Confocal microscopy of cells expressing MN1Δ1 showed the protein present in both the cytoplasm and the nucleus to a similar extent as MN1, suggesting that loss of this region did not impact the ability of the mutant to localize to the nucleus. (Figure S6). Deletion of domains 2, 5, 6, or 7 did not affect the ability of MN1 to induce AML, although their loss significantly prolonged disease latency (Figure 1E). Deletion of domain 4 resulted in a rapid disease onset with low blast count, most likely a myelproliferative disease (Figure 1E and G). Combined deletion of domains 6 and 7 (MN1Δ6–7) at the C-terminus resulted in AML with 60% penetrance (Figure 1G). Interestingly, despite showing nuclear localization of the protein by confocal microscopy (Figure S6), deletion of domains 5–7 (MN1Δ5–7) at the C-terminus in two independent experiments resulted in T-lymphoblastic leukemia (see below). The minimal portion of MN1 with biologic function was MN1Δ3-7, corresponding to the 317 amino acids at the N-terminus, which induced a myeloproliferative disease with long latency and 50% penetrance (Figure 1G). In summary, these data suggest that the N-terminus of MN1 is required and sufficient for its proliferation-enhancing function in vivo (see also Table 1).

The N-terminal region of MN1 is required to block megakaryocyte/erythroid differentiation

Peripheral blood from mice transplanted with MN1-transduced bone marrow cells was also assayed at 4-week intervals to determine the engraftment of red blood cells. The majority of mutants showed decreasing red blood cell engraftment over the 16-week period or the lifetime of the mouse. MN1Δ2 and MN1Δ4 mice had high engraftment levels at 4 weeks corresponding to high WBC engraftment. Only two constructs, MN1Δ1 and MN1Δ5, showed an increase in red blood cell engraftment over time, although the absolute number of red blood cells and hemoglobin did not increase in these mice (Figure 2A–C). When comparing the ratio of transgene positive RBC to WBC, MN1Δ1 and to a

lesser extent MN1Δ5 were the only mutant constructs that showed a higher engraftment in red blood cells than white blood cells; a difference that increased over 16 weeks (Figure 2D–F). To assess the ability of MN1 deletion mutants to support megakaryocyte differentiation, we performed CFU-Mk assays of all internally-deleted (strategy 1) and select N- and C-terminally deleted (strategy 2 and 3) constructs. CTL cells, but not full-length MN1 cells, formed few, small CFU-Mk colonies. Similar to full-length MN1 cells, most MN1 deletion mutants were unable to form CFU-Mk colonies. However, N-terminally deleted (MN1Δ1) cells gave rise to 2 to 3-fold more colonies and larger colonies than control-transduced cells, sustained over two replatings (Figure 2G and H). A small number of colonies were also derived from MN1Δ6-transduced cells (Figure 2G). Together, these experiments suggest that the ability of MN1 to block erythroid-megakaryocyte differentiation can be localized to the N-terminus, with some contribution of domains 5 and 6 (see also Table 1).

The C-terminal region of MN1 is required to block myeloid differentiation

To assess the effect of MN1 deletions on resistance to ATRA, we transduced ND13 bone marrow cells, previously reported to immortalize cells in vitro [27], with all MN1 deletion mutants. ND13 control cells were sensitive to in vitro ATRA administration with an IC50 of 0.27 μM. ND13+MN1-transduced cells were highly resistant with an IC50 of 32.4 μM, while MN1-transduced cells were even more ATRA resistant with an IC50 beyond 100 μM. When distinct regions were internally deleted from MN1 (strategy1), loss of domains 2 or 4 had no effect on ATRA resistance (Figure 3A). However, loss of domain 5, 6, or 7 restored ATRA sensitivity of the cells (Figure 3B). Progressive N-terminal deletions (strategy 2) with 2 or more domains deleted from the N-terminus were sensitive to ATRA (Figure 3C and D). All constructs with cumulative deletions of the C-terminus (strategy 3) were sensitive to ATRA (Figure 3E and F), highlighting the importance of the most C-terminal 206 amino acids of MN1 for ATRA resistance. These data suggest that the MN1 C-terminus

Table 1. Role of MN1 regions in leukemia cell fate regulation.

Phenotype	Required Domain(s)	Dispensable Domain(s)	Deletions likely too large to have any effect
Proliferation/Self-Renewal	1	One of: 3, 4, 5, 6, 7	2–7, 1–2, 1–3,1–4, 1–5, 1–6
Myeloid Differentiation Block	2, 7	One of: 1, 4, 5, 6	
Megakaryocyte/Erythroid Differentiation Block	1	One of: 2, 4, 5, 6, 7, 3–7, 5–7	
ATRA resistance	5, 6, 7	One of: 1, 2, 4	
Lymphoid Differentiation Block	5–7	One of: 1, 2, 4	

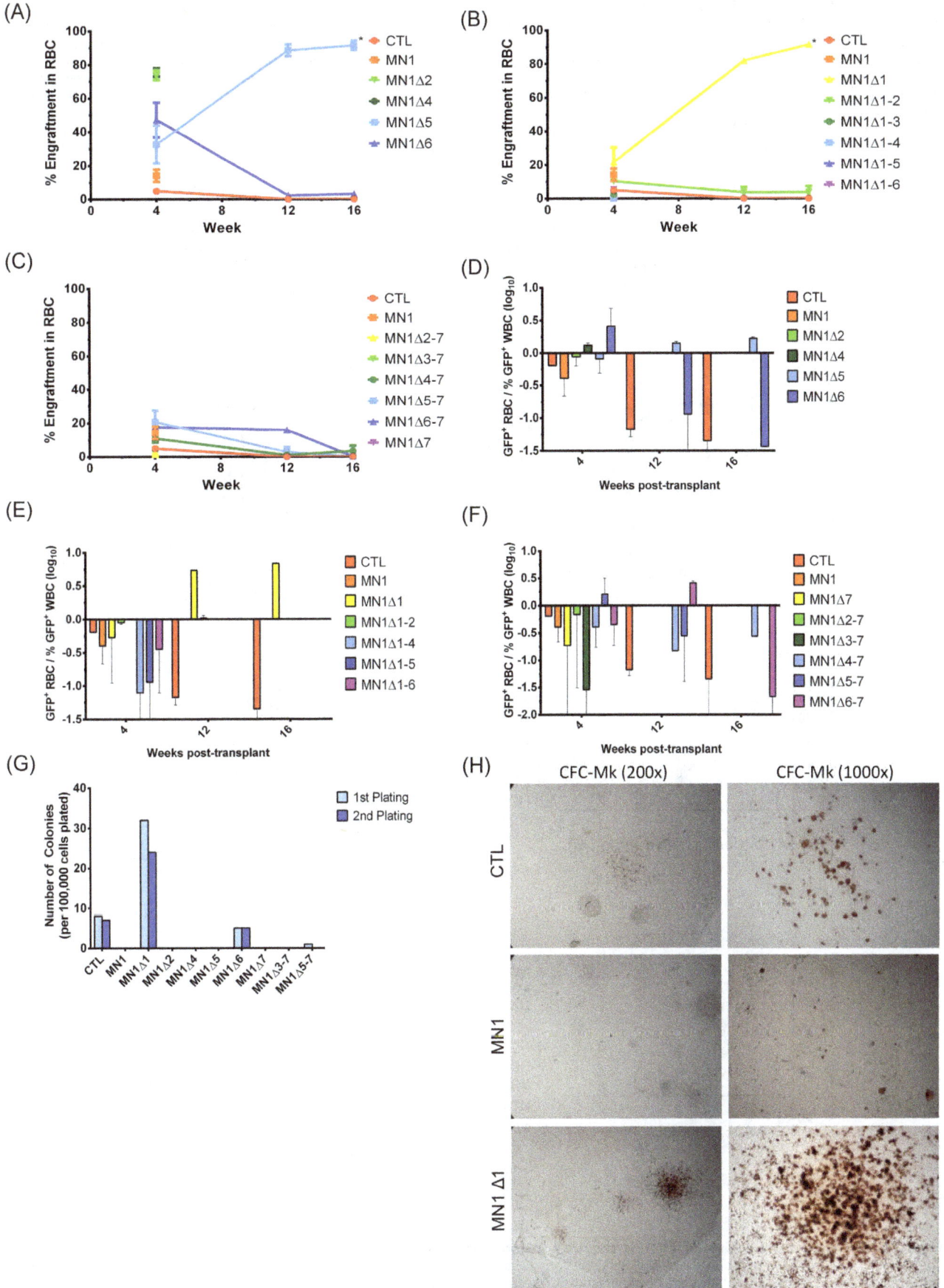

Figure 2. The N-terminal region of MN1 is required to block megakaryocyte/erythroid differentiation. (A–C) Percentage of transgene positive red blood cells engrafting in peripheral blood of transplanted mice at 4-week intervals. P values are calculated for the comparison of the indicated construct with CTL-transduced cells. The number of analysed mice and standard error is detailed in Table S3. (D–F) Proportion of red blood cells (RBC) compared to white blood cells (WBC) expressing (D) strategy 1, (E) strategy 2, or (F) strategy 3 MN1 deletion constructs after transplantation. P values are calculated for the comparison of the indicated construct with CTL-transduced cells. The number of analysed mice and standard error is detailed in Table S3. (G) Megakaryocyte colony-forming ability of mouse bone marrow cells transduced with MN1 deletion constructs (mean ± SD, n = 4). (H) Micrographs of representative CFC-Mk slides at the end of the first plating of bone marrow cells transduced with CTL vector, full-length MN1 or MN1Δ1. Images were visualised using a Nikon Eclipse 80i microscope (Nikon, Mississauga, ON, Canada) and a 20x/0.40 numerical aperture objective, or a 100x/1.25 numerical aperture objective and Nikon Immersion Oil (Nikon). A Nikon Coolpix 995 camera (Nikon) was used to capture images. * indicates P<0.05.

plays an important role in regulating resistance to ATRA in MN1 cells, with the MN1 N-terminus (amino acids 222–418) being important for maintaining functionality of the MN1 protein.

We performed gene expression profiling on GFP-positive bulk MN1-, MN1Δ1- and MN1Δ7-transduced bone marrow cells, and normal $Gr1^+CD11b^+$ differentiated myeloid cells sorted from bone marrow. Unsupervised hierarchical clustering showed that bulk C-terminally deleted MN1 cells (MN1Δ7, with an average 26.9% $GFP^+/Gr1^+/CD11b^+$ population) clustered with $Gr1^+CD11b^+$ normal myeloid cells, which have been previously shown to have

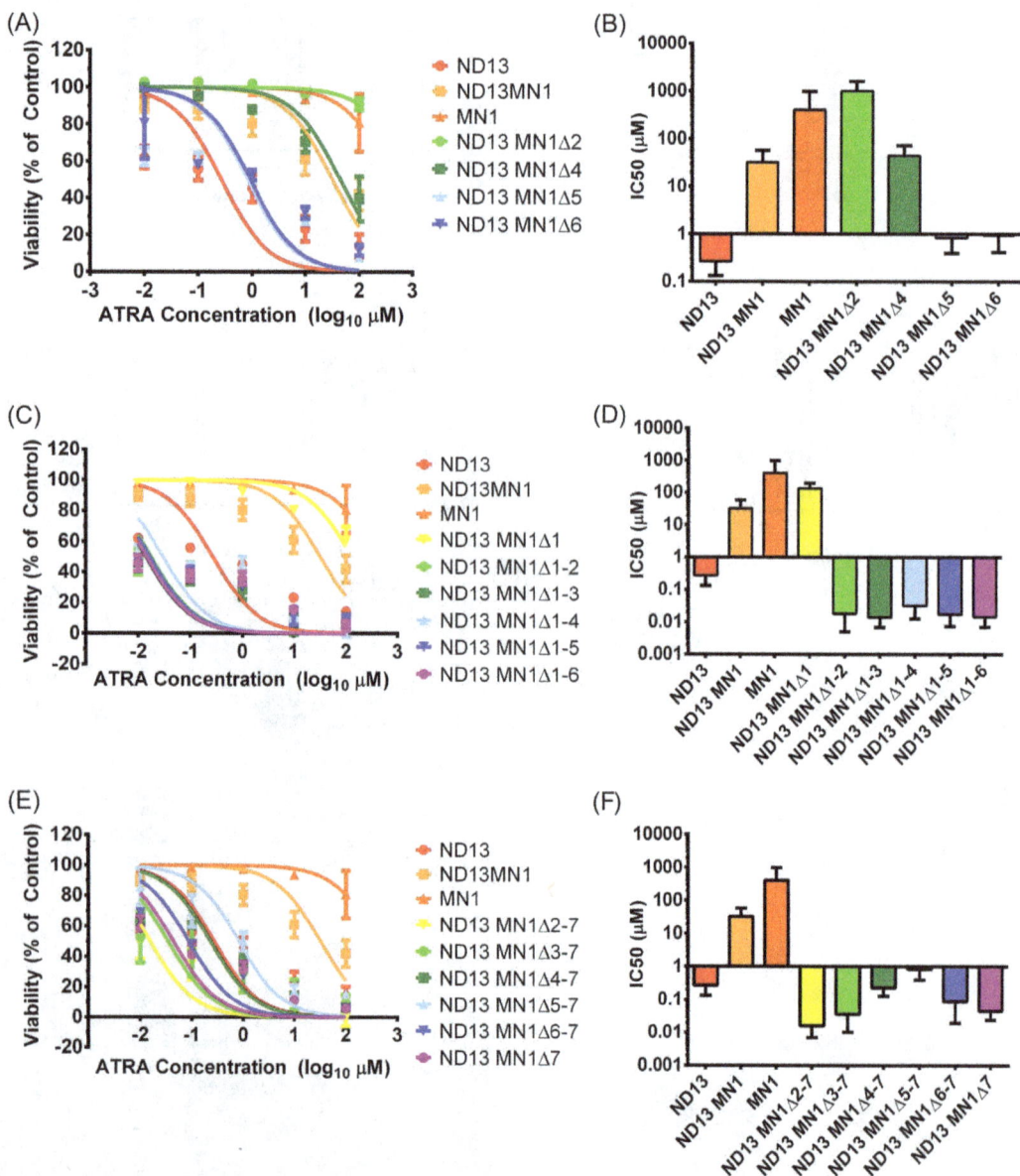

Figure 3. The C-terminal region of MN1 is required to block myeloid differentiation. (A–F) In vitro sensitivity to ATRA of ND13-immortalized cells that were transduced with MN1 deletion constructs. Dose-response curves are shown in the left panels (A, C, E) and IC50 values are shown in the right panels (B, D, F) for each deletion strategy (mean ± SD, n≥6).

low Mn1 expression [17]. Alternatively, N-terminally deleted MN1 cells (MN1Δ1, with an average 24.3% GFP$^+$/Gr1$^+$/CD11b$^+$ population) clustered with wildtype MN1 cells (Figure 4A). Comparison of the 60 most differentially expressed gene ontology gene sets between wildtype MN1 and MN1Δ1 or MN1Δ7 cells showed that those related to differentiation and metabolism were overrepresented in MN1Δ7 cells compared to MN1Δ1 cells (Figure 4B and Table S7). Conversely, gene sets related to signal transduction and cell structure were overrepresented in MN1Δ1 cells (Figure 4B and Table S8). The most differentially expressed genes in MN1Δ1 compared to MN1 cells were *HOXA9*, *HOXA10* and *MEIS2* (Table S9). These genes are among the most important genes driving self-renewal of HSCs, and their low expression in MN1Δ1 cells may explain their loss of leukemogenic potential. Several Krüppel-like factors were upregulated in MN1Δ1 cells, providing a link for their preferential erythroid differentiation. In MN1Δ7 cells 3 members of the eosinophil cationic protein (*Ecp* or *Ear1*, *2*, *3*) and eosinophil peroxidase were most differentially upregulated compared to MN1 cells (Table S10).

To compare the differentiation potential of cells transduced with different MN1 deletions, the immunophenotype of GFP positive cells in peripheral blood at week 4 post-transplant and in bone marrow at death was compared for all deletion constructs (Figures S7–S9). Expression of the progenitor cell marker cKit inversely correlated with those of the myeloid markers Gr1 and CD11b. Loss of the C-terminus and unexpectedly, also the loss of domain region 2, resulted in increased expression of myeloid markers Gr1 and CD11b, as well as mature neutrophils (MN1Δ7) and monocytic cells (MN1Δ2) besides blast cells in bone marrow smears of diseased mice (Figure 1H and Figures S7–S8). In summary, the C-terminal region is required to block myeloid differentiation and to induce resistance against ATRA, while domain 2 prevents myeloid differentiation but is dispensable for ATRA resistance (see also Table 1).

A 606 amino-acid C-terminal region of MN1 is required to prevent T-lymphoid differentiation

Combining deletion of the three most C-terminally located regions in MN1Δ5-7 resulted in delayed onset of leukemia with a median survival of 123 days (Figure 1G and Table S3). Interestingly, immunophenotypic analysis revealed CD4/CD8 double positive T cells within the GFP gate, and morphologic analysis showed blast cells in diseased mice in two independent experiments (Figure 5A–B), consistent with a diagnosis of T-lymphoblastic leukemia. Furthermore, these cells also induced T-ALL upon secondary transplantation (Figure 5C–D). Despite the differences in leukemic phenotype, MN1Δ5-7 was also shown to localise to the nucleus (Figure S6). In summary, these data suggest that the extended C-terminus of MN1 is required to block lymphoid differentiation and demonstrates the role of MN1 in regulating hematopoietic cell fate (see also Table 1 and Figure S9).

Discussion

In this study, we systematically determined the functional properties of MN1 deletion mutants to identify regions that encode the key leukemogenic functions of MN1. Our analyses demonstrate that a single gene can induce leukemia by a "double-hit", as the two functions promoting proliferation and inhibiting differentiation are encoded in structurally distinct regions. We also show that the myeloid or lymphoid lineage identity of leukemias can be determined by different mutations of the same oncogene, thus

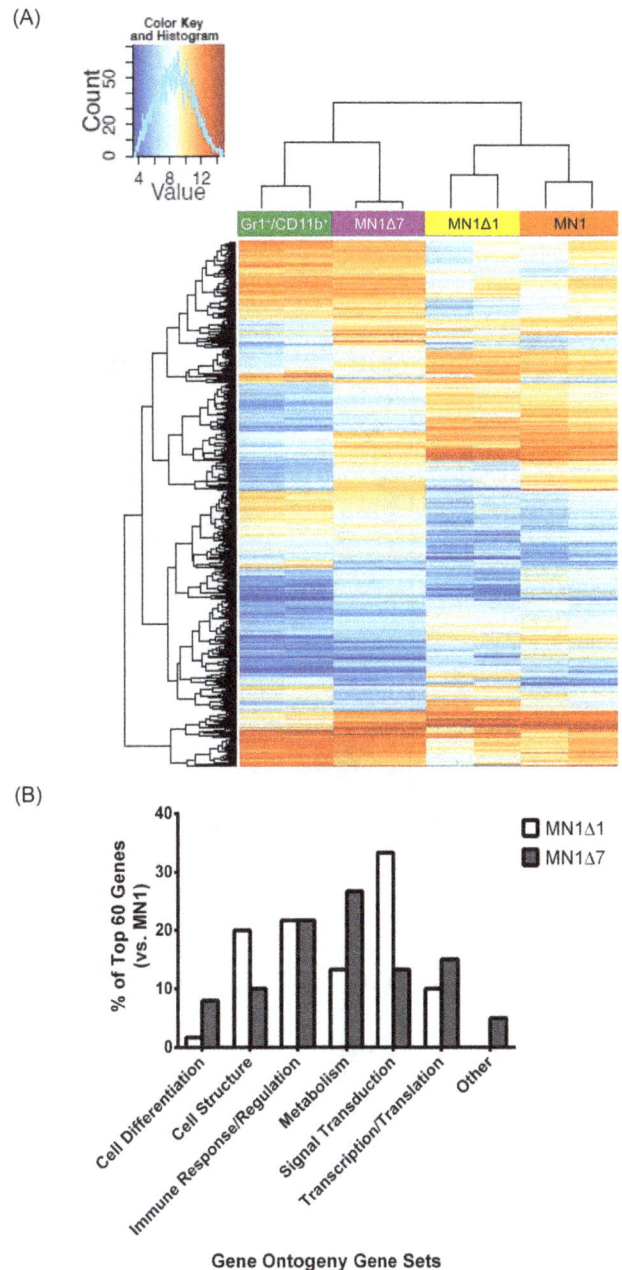

Figure 4. Hierarchical clustering of cells with N- and C-terminally deleted MN1. (A) Heat map of differentially regulated pathways for enhanced proliferation and blocked differentiation. (B) Comparison of top 60 enriched gene ontology gene sets for the comparison of MN1Δ1 and MN1Δ7 with wildtype MN1.

providing a potential explanation for the similar mutation spectrum in phenotypically distinct diseases like AML and T-ALL.

Deletion of the 221 most N-terminal amino acids (MN1Δ1) abolished the leukemogenicity of MN1 in vivo, as evidenced by decreased WBC engraftment in mice over time and failure to develop leukemia. However, the MN1Δ1 mutant provided both growth advantage and retention of ATRA resistance to bone marrow cells in vitro. We report the novel finding that MN1Δ1-transduced cells preferentially differentiated to the erythroid lineage in vivo and had an increased megakaryocyte differentiation

(A)

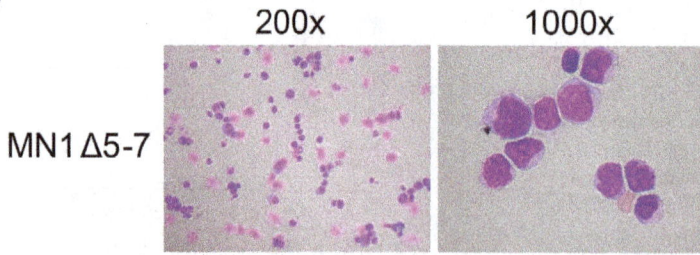

MN1Δ5-7

(B)

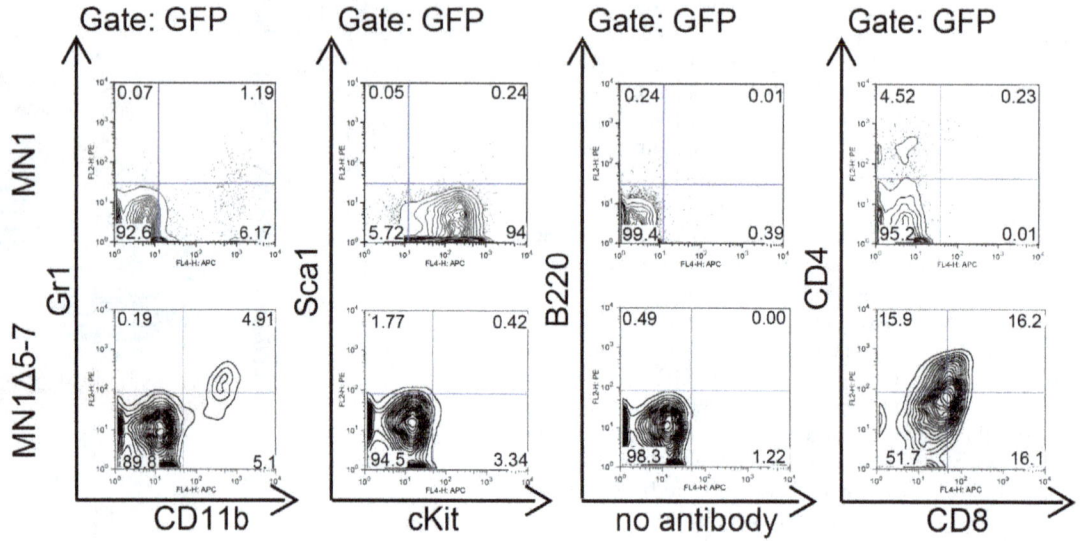

(C)

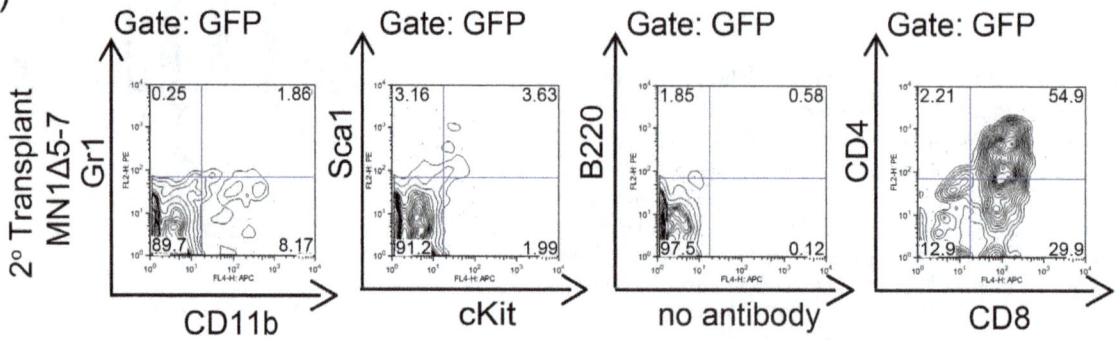

(D)

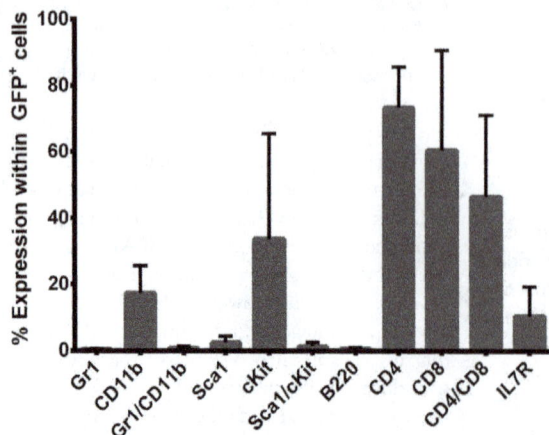

Figure 5. A 606 amino-acid C-terminal portion of MN1 prevents T-lymphoid differentiation. (A) Morphology of bone marrow cells from MN1Δ5-7 mice at death, showing a shift in leukemia from AML, as seen in MN1 leukemia, to an ALL leukemia upon loss of the C-terminal domains 5–7. (B) Representative immunophenotype of GFP+ MN1Δ5-7 bone marrow cells compared to wildtype MN1 bone marrow cells at death. (C) Representative immunophenotype of secondary transplants of GFP+ MN1Δ5-7 bone marrow cells at death. (D) Average cell surface marker expression for secondary transplants of GFP+ MN1Δ5-7 bone marrow cells at death (mean ± SEM, n = 3).

potential in vitro, suggesting that the most N-terminal sequence of MN1 is also critical in blocking megakaryocyte/erythroid differentiation (Figure 6). Consistent with the reduced proliferative ability of MN1Δ1 cells, expression levels of HOXA9, HOXA10, and MEIS2 were most differentially downregulated compared to full-length MN1. In addition, JUN and FOS, factors of the AP1 complex, were most upregulated together with Kruppel-like factors (KLF) 2, 3, 4 and 6, which play an important role in erythroid differentiation and bind DNA at CACCC motifs [40–43]. Interestingly, the CACCC motif has also been identified as a consensus motif for MN1 binding to DNA in an oligonucleotide selection assay [44,45].

Additional deletion of a region containing the first poly-Gln repeat (MN1Δ1-2) abolished any functional effect of MN1 in vitro and in vivo, despite the formation of protein. Conversely, the N-terminal sequence up to amino acid 317 (MN1Δ3-7) was sufficient to induce strong myeloproliferation with high WBC counts and large spleen with full myeloid differentiation potential, demonstrating that the MN1 N-terminus is driving proliferation in MN1 leukemia. We have previously shown that MN1 and MEIS1 share a high proportion of their regulatory chromatin sites and that MN1 leukemogenicity depends on MEIS1 [17]. Therefore, we speculate that the N-terminus is required for localization of MN1 to MEIS1 chromatin binding sites. In addition, van Wely *et al.* showed that MN1 interacts with P300 at amino acids 48 to 256, a region with considerable transcription activation function [44], the

majority of which overlaps with domain 1. Future studies will be required to demonstrate if interaction between the MN1 N-terminus and P300 is required for the N-terminal functions promoting proliferation and blocking megakaryocyte/erythroid differentiation.

Several levels of evidence suggested that the MN1 C-terminus is required to inhibit myeloid differentiation (Table 1). First, loss of individual domains 5, 6, or 7 restored sensitivity to ATRA in vitro. Second, myeloid surface markers Gr1 and CD11b were most highly expressed in cells transduced with MN1Δ7 in vivo. In addition, gene expression profiling showed a close relationship of MN1Δ7 cells to differentiated myeloid cells, and more differentiation-related gene sets were upregulated in MN1Δ7 than in MN1Δ1 cells. Third, cumulative loss of domains 5, 6 and 7 resulted in loss of myeloid identity (see below). Lastly, cumulative deletion of domains 3 to 7 (MN1Δ3-7) resulted in a myeloproliferative disease with full differentiation potential to mature neutrophils (Table 1). These data suggest that the C-terminal regions (MN1Δ5, 6, 7) are the critical regions mediating resistance to ATRA-cytotoxicity, with some contribution from amino acids 222–418 (Figure 6). Recent work by Sharma et al. which showed that *Ccl9* and *Irf8* were upregulated in both MN1Δ7 cells and the MN1 model fused to the transcriptional activation domain VP16 (MN1VP16), suggesting that phenotypic similarities between the two models may be rooted in underlying gene expression patterns [46]. Van Wely et al. showed that MN1 binds to retinoic-acid

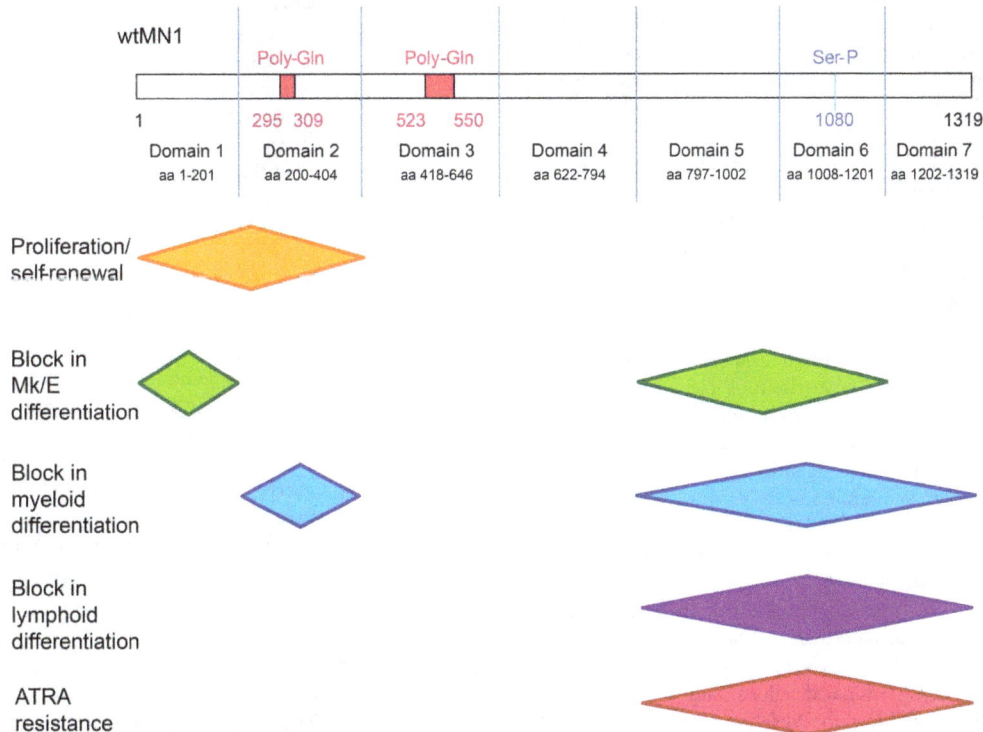

Figure 6. Functionally defined regions of MN1.

response elements by an oligonucleotide selection assay [44] and, combined with our data, we hypothesize that the MN1 C-terminus directs MN1 to retinoic acid response elements to regulate transcription. Although retroviral overexpression, as used in this study, is likely to lead to artificially high transcriptional expression of MN1 and the mutants, we found that AML patients with the highest MN1 expression had similar expression levels to our murine MN1-transduced cell lines with the lowest MN1 expression, suggesting that at least some of our cell lines are comparable to patient data (data not shown). In addition, previous studies have shown that MN1 induces resistance to ATRA-induced differentiation and cell death [22], and that high-level expression of MN1 predicts ATRA resistance in AML patients, suggesting its future use as a biomarker for ATRA treatment [22,47].

Deletion of a 606 amino acid fragment from the C-terminus reproducibly resulted in T-lymphoblastic leukemia with CD4- and CD8-double positive cells in mice. This suggests that the C-terminus of MN1 directs hematopoietic progenitor cells towards the myeloid lineage, but in its absence, allows differentiation towards the T cell lineage. Although this study cannot rule out that T-cell precursors may have been transduced by MN1Δ5-7, resulting in a bias or advantage towards lymphoid differentiation seen in the T-ALLs that developed, it is unlikely as findings were consistent in two independent experiments performed and supported by similar findings by an independent group [48]. Interestingly, mice lacking a portion of this 606 amino acid fragment, namely MN1Δ5 or MN1Δ7, developed AML. This suggests that amino acids 714–797 may be critical for myeloid differentiation, and it is only in their absence that lymphoid differentiation may occur. Kawagoe and Grosveld also described CD4/CD8 double positive T cell lymphomas in mice expressing the MN1/TEL fusion oncoprotein under the control of the AML1 promoter [49]. In this fusion protein, the 60 C-terminal amino acids of MN1 are lost due to the fusion to TEL [50]. As AML1 is also expressed in the T-lineage, these data suggest that overexpression of MN1 in T-progenitor cells can promote leukemogenesis, with Neumann and colleagues providing evidence of MN1 overexpression in T-lymphoblastic leukemias [51]. Taken together, we suggest that the C-terminus of MN1 encoded by amino acids 513–1319 (domains 5–7) instructs progenitor cells to the myeloid lineage and that in its absence progenitor cells can differentiate to the lymphoid lineage (Table 1).

During preparation of the present paper, one other group characterised functional MN1 regions, creating deletion constructs modelled off known MN1 protein domains in U937 cells [48]. Consistent with our data, Kandilci and colleagues reported decreased growth and colony-forming ability in vitro upon loss of the MN1 N-terminus. Kandilci et al. also showed that the loss of MN1 amino acids 570–1273 gave rise to T-cell lymphoma. This deleted region partially overlaps with our MN1Δ5-7 mutant, supporting the idea that the MN1 C-terminus promotes a myeloid-skew to MN1 leukemia. Finally, Kandilci et al. were also able to localise ATRA resistance to amino acids 18–458, but not 12–228, with their MN1-transduced U937 cells showing increased CD11b expression after 3 days of treatment. Interestingly, this region partially overlaps with domain 2 of our deletion mutants, providing support for our observation of increased CD11b expression in peripheral blood of animals transplanted with MN1Δ2. Kandilci et al. did not, however, report increased CD11b expression in C-terminal deletions, although this may be attributed to their most C-terminal deletion mutant retaining the 46 most C-terminal amino acids. It is possible that retention of these critical amino acids may have abrogated the differentiation effect seen in our complete deletions.

In summary, we characterized functional regions of the MN1 protein by a systematic mutation analysis and identified key regions that enhance proliferation and self-renewal, block myeloid, megakaryocytic/erythroid, and lymphoid differentiation, and induce resistance against ATRA. Our data support a critical function of MN1 as a key cell fate regulator in malignant hematopoiesis and provide a powerful new model for further dissection of the molecular events controlling transformation and the resulting leukemic phenotype.

Supporting Information

Figure S1   Expression levels of MN1 deletion constructs.
(A) Western blots illustrating the expression and size of protein products of the MN1 deletion constructs compared to full-length MN1. The figure is a composite of multiple gels with each lane representing a single construct stained with either anti-HA or anti-β-actin antibody. (B) Gel electrophoresis with PCR products illustrating the relative size of the MN1 deletion constructs compared to full-length MN1. (C–E) Expression levels of MN1 deletion constructs measured by qRT-PCR. MN1 deletion constructs were transduced in cells immortalized by NU-P98HOXD13 (ND13). Mean ± SD, n = 3.

Figure S2   Potential of MN1 variants to immortalize bone marrow cells in vitro. Left panels (A, C, E) show number of CFC colonies per plating in methylcellulose under myeloid cytokine conditions. 5-FU pretreated bone marrow cells were transduced with MN1 deletions and were plated after transduction without sorting of cells. Right panels (B, D, F) show percentage of GFP positive cells at the end of each round of plating.

Figure S3   White blood cell count in transplanted mice.
(A–C) White blood cell count (WBC) in peripheral blood of mice at 4-week intervals after transplantation. MN1 mutation constructs were used from (A) Strategy 1, (B) Strategy 2, and (C) Strategy 3. P values are given for the comparison of the indicated construct with CTL. The average WBC count is shown. Number of analyzed mice and standard error can be found in Table S5. § WBC count in peripheral blood at the indicated time point or at death in cases where a mouse died before that time point. † indicates that all mice were dead at this time point due to disease. * indicates P< 0.05.

Figure S4   Red blood cell count in transplanted mice. (A–C) Red blood cell count (RBC) in peripheral blood of mice at 4 week intervals after transplantation. MN1 mutation constructs were used from (A) Strategy 1, (B) Strategy 2, and (C) Strategy 3. P values are given for the comparison of the indicated construct with CTL. The average RBC count is shown. Number of analyzed mice and standard error can be found in Table S5. § RBC count in peripheral blood at the indicated time point or at death in cases where a mouse died before that time point. † indicates that all mice were dead at this time point due to disease. * indicates P< 0.05.

Figure S5   Platelet count in transplanted mice. (A–C) Platelet count in peripheral blood of mice at 4 week intervals after transplantation. MN1 mutation constructs were used from (A) Strategy 1, (B) Strategy 2, and (C) Strategy 3. P values are given for the comparison of the indicated construct with CTL. The average platelet count is shown. Number of analyzed mice and standard deviation can be found in Table S5. § Platelet count in peripheral blood at the indicated time point or at death in cases where a mouse died before that time point. † indicates that all mice were dead at this time point due to disease. * indicates P<0.05.

Figure S6 Confocal microscopy of MN1-transduced cells. Representative confocal microscopy images of GP + E86 cells transduced with (A) negative control, (B) MN1 tagged with an HA-tag, (C) MN1Δ1 with an HA-tag, and (D) MN1Δ5–7 with an HA-tag stained with (i) DAPI or (ii) anti-HA and (iii) DAPI and anti-HA merged.

Figure S7 Immunophenotype of MN1-transduced cells in transplanted mice – stem and progenitor markers. Percentage of GFP-expressing cells and expression of ckit and Sca1 in GFP+ cells in peripheral blood at 4 weeks and in bone marrow at death of mice receiving transplants of MN1-transduced cells. (A) Strategy 1, (B) Strategy 2, and (C) Strategy 3 MN1 constructs. Mean ± SEM. The number of analyzed mice is provided in Table S6.

Figure S8 Immunophenotype of MN1-transduced cells in transplanted mice – myeloid markers. Expression of myeloid markers in GFP+ cells in peripheral blood at 4 weeks and in bone marrow at death of mice receiving transplants of MN1-transduced cells. (A) Strategy 1, (B) Strategy 2, and (C) Strategy 3 MN1 constructs. Mean ± SEM. The number of analyzed mice is provided in Table S6.

Figure S9 Immunophenotype of MN1-transduced cells in transplanted mice – T-cell markers. Expression of T-cell markers in GFP+ cells in peripheral blood at 4 weeks and in bone marrow at death of mice receiving transplants of MN1-transduced cells. (A) Strategy 1, (B) Strategy 2, and (C) Strategy 3 MN1 constructs. Mean ± SEM. The number of analyzed mice is provided in Table S6.

Table S1 MN1 deletion mutant primer sequences.

Table S2 MN1 qPCR primer sequences.

Table S3 Characterisation of mouse phenotype after transplantation with MN1 deletion constructs.

Table S4 *In vivo* engraftment of cells transduced with MN1 deletion constructs.

Table S5 Peripheral blood counts in mice receiving transplants of cells transduced with MN1 deletion constructs.

Table S6 Immunophenotype of GFP-positive cells in peripheral blood of mice receiving transplants of cells transduced with MN1 deletion constructs.

Table S7 Gene ontology gene sets enriched in MN1Δ7 cells compared to MN1 cells.

Table S8 Gene ontology gene sets enriched in MN1Δ1 cells compared to MN1 cells.

Table S9 Differentially Expressed Genes in MN1Δ1 cells compared to MN1 cells.

Table S10 Differentially Expressed Genes in MN1Δ7 cells compared to MN1 cells.

Acknowledgments

We thank Patty Rosten, Christy Brookes, Justin Smrz, the staff of the Flow Cytometry Facility of the Terry Fox Laboratory, and the staff of the Animal Resource Centre of the BC Cancer Agency, and the staff of the Imaging Facility at the Child and Family Research Institute for their excellent technical assistance.

Author Contributions

Conceived and designed the experiments: CKL RKH MH. Performed the experiments: CKL YM FK DTS BA EY PB A. Schwarzer A. Sharma GP ML GL SV SF APW MH. Analyzed the data: CKL MY FK DTS BA EY PB A. Schwarzer A. Sharma GP ML GL SV SF CJE AK APW MH. Contributed reagents/materials/analysis tools: CKL YM FK DTS BA EY PB A. Schwarzer A. Sharma GP ML GL SV SF APW MH. Wrote the paper: CKL RKH MH.

References

1. Gilliland DG (2001) Hematologic malignancies. Curr Opin Hematol 8: 189–191.
2. Cancer Genome Atlas Research N (2013) Genomic and epigenomic landscapes of adult de novo acute myeloid leukemia. N Engl J Med 368: 2059–2074.
3. Dick JE (2000) Stem cell concepts renew cancer research. Blood 112: 4793–4807.
4. Kirstetter P, Schuster MB, Bereshchenko O, Moore S, Dvinge H, et al. (2008) Modeling of C/EBPalpha mutant acute myeloid leukemia reveals a common expression signature of committed myeloid leukemia-initiating cells. Cancer Cell 13: 299–310.
5. Deshpande AJ, Cusan M, Rawat VP, Reuter H, Krause A, et al. (2006) Acute myeloid leukemia is propagated by a leukemic stem cell with lymphoid characteristics in a mouse model of CALM/AF10-positive leukemia. Cancer Cell 10: 363–374.
6. Somervaille TC, Cleary ML (2006) Identification and characterization of leukemia stem cells in murine MLL-AF9 acute myeloid leukemia. Cancer Cell 10: 257–268.
7. Goardon N, Marchi E, Atzberger A, Quek L, Schuh A, et al. (2011) Coexistence of LMPP-like and GMP-like leukemia stem cells in acute myeloid leukemia. Cancer Cell 19: 138–152.
8. Heuser M, Sly LM, Argiropoulos B, Kuchenbauer F, Lai C, et al. (2009) Modeling the functional heterogeneity of leukemia stem cells: role of STAT5 in leukemia stem cell self-renewal. Blood 114: 3983–3993.
9. Thol F, Damm F, Ludeking A, Winschel C, Wagner K, et al. (2011) Incidence and prognostic influence of DNMT3A mutations in acute myeloid leukemia. J Clin Oncol 29: 2889–2896.
10. Neumann M, Heesch S, Schlee C, Schwartz S, Gokbuget N, et al. (2013) Whole-exome sequencing in adult ETP-ALL reveals a high rate of DNMT3A mutations. Blood 121: 4749–4752.
11. Vannucchi AM, Lasho TL, Guglielmelli P, Biamonte F, Pardanani A, et al. (2013) Mutations and prognosis in primary myelofibrosis. Leukemia 27: 1861–1869.
12. Horton SJ, Jaques J, Woolthuis C, van Dijk J, Mesuraca M, et al. (2013) MLL-AF9-mediated immortalization of human hematopoietic cells along different lineages changes during ontogeny. Leukemia 27: 1116–1126.
13. Wei J, Wunderlich M, Fox C, Alvarez S, Cigudosa JC, et al. (2008) Microenvironment determines lineage fate in a human model of MLL-AF9 leukemia. Cancer Cell 13: 483–495.
14. Raaijmakers MH, Mukherjee S, Guo S, Zhang S, Kobayashi T, et al. (2010) Bone progenitor dysfunction induces myelodysplasia and secondary leukaemia. Nature 464: 852–857.

15. Morin RD, Johnson NA, Severson TM, Mungall AJ, An J, et al. (2010) Somatic mutations altering EZH2 (Tyr641) in follicular and diffuse large B-cell lymphomas of germinal-center origin. Nat Genet 42: 181–185.

16. Ernst T, Chase AJ, Score J, Hidalgo-Curtis CE, Bryant C, et al. (2010) Inactivating mutations of the histone methyltransferase gene EZH2 in myeloid disorders. Nat Genet 42: 722–726.

17. Heuser M, Yun H, Berg T, Yung E, Argiropoulos B, et al. (2011) Cell of origin in AML: susceptibility to MN1-induced transformation is regulated by the MEIS1/AbdB-like HOX protein complex. Cancer Cell 20: 39–52.

18. Kandilci A, Grosveld GC (2009) Reintroduction of CEBPA in MN1-overexpressing hematopoietic cells prevents their hyperproliferation and restores myeloid differentiation. Blood 114: 1596–1606.

19. Heuser M, Beutel G, Krauter J, Dohner K, von Neuhoff N, et al. (2006) High meningioma 1 (MN1) expression as a predictor for poor outcome in acute myeloid leukemia with normal cytogenetics. Blood 108: 3898–3905.

20. Carella C, Bonten J, Sirma S, Kranenburg TA, Terranova S, et al. (2007) MN1 overexpression is an important step in the development of inv(16) AML. Leukemia 21: 1679–1690.

21. Valk PJ, Verhaak RG, Beijen MA, Erpelinck CA, Barjesteh van Waalwijk van Doorn-Khosrovani S, et al. (2004) Prognostically useful gene-expression profiles in acute myeloid leukemia. N Engl J Med 350: 1617–1628.

22. Heuser M, Argiropoulos B, Kuchenbauer F, Yung E, Piper J, et al. (2007) MN1 overexpression induces acute myeloid leukemia in mice and predicts ATRA resistance in patients with AML. Blood 110: 1639–1647.

23. Langer C, Marcucci G, Holland KB, Radmacher MD, Maharry K, et al. (2009) Prognostic importance of MN1 transcript levels, and biologic insights from MN1-associated gene and microRNA expression signatures in cytogenetically normal acute myeloid leukemia: a cancer and leukemia group B study. J Clin Oncol 27: 3198–3204.

24. Schwind S, Marcucci G, Kohlschmidt J, Radmacher MD, Mrozek K, et al. (2011) Low expression of MN1 associates with better treatment response in older patients with de novo cytogenetically normal acute myeloid leukemia. Blood 118: 4188–4198.

25. Haferlach C, Kern W, Schindela S, Kohlmann A, Alpermann T, et al. (2011) Gene expression of BAALC, CDKN1B, ERG, and MN1 adds independent prognostic information to cytogenetics and molecular mutations in adult acute myeloid leukemia. Genes Chromosomes Cancer 51: 257–265.

26. Liu T, Jankovic D, Brault L, Ehret S, Baty F, et al. (2010) Functional characterization of high levels of meningioma 1 as collaborating oncogene in acute leukemia. Leukemia 24: 601–612.

27. Pineault N, Buske C, Feuring-Buske M, Abramovich C, Rosten P, et al. (2003) Induction of acute myeloid leukemia in mice by the human leukemia-specific fusion gene NUP98-HOXD13 in concert with Meis1. Blood 101: 4529–4538.

28. Schambach A, Wodrich H, Hildinger M, Bohne J, Krausslich HG, et al. (2000) Context dependence of different modules for posttranscriptional enhancement of gene expression from retroviral vectors. Mol Ther 2: 435–445.

29. Antonchuk J, Sauvageau G, Humphries RK (2002) HOXB4-induced expansion of adult hematopoietic stem cells ex vivo. Cell 109: 39–45.

30. Gurevich RM, Aplan PD, Humphries RK (2004) NUP98-topoisomerase I acute myeloid leukemia-associated fusion gene has potent leukemogenic activities independent of an engineered catalytic site mutation. Blood 104: 1127–1136.

31. Starczynowski DT, Kuchenbauer F, Argiropoulos B, Sung S, Morin R, et al. (2010) Identification of miR-145 and miR-146a as mediators of the 5q-syndrome phenotype. Nat Med 16: 49–58.

32. Heuser M, Yap DB, Leung M, de Algara TR, Tafech A, et al. (2009) Loss of MLL5 results in pleiotropic hematopoietic defects, reduced neutrophil immune function, and extreme sensitivity to DNA demethylation. Blood 113: 1432–1443.

33. Bruce MA, Butte MJ (2013) Real-time GPU-based 3D Deconvolution. Opt Express 21: 4766–4773.

34. Vonesch C, Unser M (2008) A fast thresholded landweber algorithm for wavelet-regularized multidimensional deconvolution. IEEE Trans Image Process 17: 539–549.

35. Gentleman RC, Carey VJ, Bates DM, Bolstad B, Dettling M, et al. (2004) Bioconductor: open software development for computational biology and bioinformatics. Genome Biol 5: R80.

36. Kauffmann A, Gentleman R, Huber W (2009) arrayQualityMetrics–a bioconductor package for quality assessment of microarray data. Bioinformatics 25: 415–416.

37. Gautier L, Cope L, Bolstad BM, Irizarry RA (2004) affy–analysis of Affymetrix GeneChip data at the probe level. Bioinformatics 20: 307–315.

38. Smyth G (2005) Limma: linear models for microarray data.; Gentleman R, Carey V, Dudoit S, Irizarry R, and Huber W., editor. New York: Springer.

39. Subramanian A, Tamayo P, Mootha VK, Mukherjee S, Ebert BL, et al. (2005) Gene set enrichment analysis: a knowledge-based approach for interpreting genome-wide expression profiles. Proc Natl Acad Sci U S A 102: 15545–15550.

40. Jacobs-Helber SM, Sawyer ST (2004) Jun N-terminal kinase promotes proliferation of immature erythroid cells and erythropoietin-dependent cell lines. Blood 104: 696–703.

41. Funnell AP, Norton LJ, Mak KS, Burdach J, Artuz CM, et al. (2012) The CACCC-binding protein KLF3/BKLF represses a subset of KLF1/EKLF target genes and is required for proper erythroid maturation in vivo. Mol Cell Biol 32: 3281–3292.

42. Kalra IS, Alam MM, Choudhary PK, Pace BS (2011) Kruppel-like Factor 4 activates HBG gene expression in primary erythroid cells. Br J Haematol 154: 248–259.

43. Marini MG, Porcu L, Asunis I, Loi MG, Ristaldi MS, et al. (2010) Regulation of the human HBA genes by KLF4 in erythroid cell lines. Br J Haematol 149: 748–758.

44. van Wely KH, Molijn AC, Buijs A, Meester-Smoor MA, Aarnoudse AJ, et al. (2003) The MN1 oncoprotein synergizes with coactivators RAC3 and p300 in RAR-RXR-mediated transcription. Oncogene 22: 699–709.

45. Meester-Smoor MA, Molijn AC, Zhao Y, Groen NA, Groffen CA, et al. (2007) The MN1 oncoprotein activates transcription of the IGFBP5 promoter through a CACCC-rich consensus sequence. J Mol Endocrinol 38: 113–125.

46. Sharma A YH, Jyotsana N, Chaturvedi A, Schwarzer A, Yung E, et al. (2014) Constitutive Irf8 expression inhibits AML by activation of repressed immune response signaling. Leukemia.

47. Burnett AK, Hills RK, Green C, Jenkinson S, Koo K, et al. (2010) The impact on outcome of the addition of all-trans retinoic acid to intensive chemotherapy in younger patients with nonacute promyelocytic acute myeloid leukemia: overall results and results in genotypic subgroups defined by mutations in NPM1, FLT3, and CEBPA. Blood 115: 948–956.

48. Kandilci A, Surtel J, Janke L, Neale G, Terranova S, et al. (2013) Mapping of MN1 sequences necessary for myeloid transformation. PLoS One 8: e61706.

49. Kawagoe H, Grosveld GC (2005) MN1-TEL myeloid oncoprotein expressed in multipotent progenitors perturbs both myeloid and lymphoid growth and causes T-lymphoid tumors in mice. Blood 106: 4278–4286.

50. Buijs A, Sherr S, van Baal S, van Bezouw S, van der Plas D, et al. (1995) Translocation (12;22) (p13;q11) in myeloproliferative disorders results in fusion of the ETS-like TEL gene on 12p13 to the MN1 gene on 22q11. Oncogene 10: 1511–1519.

51. Neumann M, Heesch S, Gokbuget N, Schwartz S, Schlee C, et al. (2012) Clinical and molecular characterization of early T-cell precursor leukemia: a high-risk subgroup in adult T-ALL with a high frequency of FLT3 mutations. Blood Cancer J 2: e55.

7

IL-17A and Serum Amyloid A Are Elevated in a Cigarette Smoke Cessation Model Associated with the Persistence of Pigmented Macrophages, Neutrophils and Activated NK Cells

Michelle J. Hansen*, **Sheau Pyng J. Chan**, **Shenna Y. Langenbach**, **Lovisa F. Dousha**, **Jessica E. Jones**, **Selcuk Yatmaz**, **Huei Jiunn Seow**, **Ross Vlahos**, **Gary P. Anderson**, **Steven Bozinovski**

Lung Health Research Centre, Department of Pharmacology and Therapeutics, The University of Melbourne, Victoria, Australia

Abstract

While global success in cessation advocacy has seen smoking rates fall in many developed countries, persistent lung inflammation in ex-smokers is an increasingly important clinical problem whose mechanistic basis remains poorly understood. In this study, candidate effector mechanisms were assessed in mice exposed to cigarette smoke (CS) for 4 months following cessation from long term CS exposure. BALF neutrophils, $CD4^+$ and $CD8^+$ T cells and lung innate NK cells remained significantly elevated following smoking cessation. Analysis of neutrophil mobilization markers showed a transition from acute mediators (MIP-2α, KC and G-CSF) to sustained drivers of neutrophil and macrophage recruitment and activation (IL-17A and Serum Amyoid A (SAA)). Follicle-like lymphoid aggregates formed with CS exposure and persisted with cessation, where they were in close anatomical proximity to pigmented macrophages, whose number actually increased 3-fold following CS cessation. This was associated with the elastolytic protease, MMP-12 (macrophage metallo-elastase) which remained significantly elevated post-cessation. Both GM-CSF and CSF-1 were significantly increased in the CS cessation group relative to the control group. In conclusion, we show that smoking cessation mediates a transition to accumulation of pigmented macrophages, which may contribute to the expanded macrophage population observed in COPD. These macrophages together with IL-17A, SAA and innate NK cells are identified here as candidate persistence determinants and, we suggest, may represent specific targets for therapies directed towards the amelioration of chronic airway inflammation.

Editor: Thomas H. Thatcher, University of Rochester Medical Center, United States of America

Funding: This work was supported by NHMRC (National Health and Medical Research Council) Australia (www.NHMRC.gov.au), project grant number 628492. The funders had no role in study design, data collection and analysis, decision to publish, or preparation of the manuscript.

Competing Interests: The authors have declared that no competing interests exist.

* Email: mjhansen@unimelb.edu.au

Introduction

Chronic Obstructive Pulmonary Disease (COPD) is a debilitating lung condition that is characterized by chronic airway inflammation. COPD is now the third cause of death worldwide and kills more than 3.5 million people per year. About 85% of all COPD is caused by inhalation of irritants mostly cigarette smoke (active and passive), ambient air pollutants and poor indoor air quality caused by biomass cooking and heating fumes. Inflammation induced by these irritants contributes to key pathological processes in COPD including small airway narrowing, destruction of alveolar walls (emphysema) and mucous hypersecretion (reviewed in [1]). Innate immune cells including macrophages and neutrophils accumulate and are considered essential for disease progression [2], as are immune cells of the adaptive response including $CD8^+$ T cells [3]. $CD4^+$ T cells and B cells also aggregate and can organize into lymphoid follicles, the percentage of which increases with progression of COPD [2]. The close association of de novo lymphoid follicles with persistence and severity of COPD strongly suggests their contribution to deleterious autoimmunity in the airways although beneficial effects in terms of mounting a rapid immune response to respiratory pathogens have not been formally excluded. The combined activity of the these inflammatory cells is thought to drive the accelerated decline in lung function that is a hallmark of the disease.

Cigarette smoke (CS) cessation currently remains the single most effective strategy to reduce the accelerated decline in lung function attributable to COPD. At least in developed countries there is clear evidence that smoking rates have fallen, in part due to effective cessation strategies. However, cross-sectional and longitudinal studies have shown that in individuals with established disease, airway inflammation does not fully resolve with CS cessation [4,5] and post cessation persistent lung disease is an increasingly important clinical problem. In particular, airway and sputum neutrophils persist and in some cases, increase with cessation [4–6]. Neutrophilic inflammation is particularly damaging in COPD due to a deficiency in efferocytosis (clearance of moribund cells) mediated by excessive oxidative stress [7,8], which can lead to excessive degranulation of necrotic neutrophils. Activated neutrophils release neutrophil elastase and other serine proteases, which increases with the severity of COPD and these processes are intrinsically insensitive to inhaled glucocorticosteroids [9]. Neutrophil elastase degrades extracellular matrix components including elastin, collagens I–IV and fibrinogen and the degree of elastase localized to lung elastic fibers correlates with the degree of emphysema [10]. Neutrophil elastase can also promote mucin production [11] and activate TLR4-dependent production of IL-8 via epidermal growth factor receptor (EGFR) transactivation mechanisms [12].

Macrophages also accumulate in COPD airways and are positively associated with disease severity [2]. Importantly, depletion of macrophages protected against the development of emphysema in a chronic smoke exposure model; demonstrating a pathogenic role for this immune cell [13]. Furthermore, it is now recognized that macrophages acquire a distinct phenotype associated with the progressive induction of M2-related programs as a consequence of smoke exposure and COPD [14]. Macrophages can initiate neutrophilic inflammation as they are a major source of neutrophil chemokines. Several neutrophil chemokines such as IL-8 (CXCL8), KC (CXCL1) and MIP-2α (CXCL2) are implicated in COPD as they are elevated in CS exposure models [15] and during exacerbations [16]. In addition, Interleukin-17A (IL-17A) can promote neutrophil mobilization through its regulation of leukocyte growth factors and cytokines. Immunoreactive IL-17A+ cells increase in frequency in the submucosa of COPD patients [17] and IL-17A expression is elevated in CS exposure models, where mice lacking IL-17RA were protected from developing emphysema [18]. Serum Amyloid A (SAA) can also mobilize neutrophils into the airways, and SAA is elevated in COPD lung tissue [19] and is related to neutrophilic lung infiltration [20]. In this study, a CS cessation model was used to identify which molecular markers most closely relate to the persistence of innate immune responses. We identify IL-17A and SAA inflammatory cytokine networks in the persistence of inflammation following CS cessation and suggest that targeting these networks may be of therapeutic benefit in augmenting the benefit of smoking cessation in this disease group.

Materials and Methods

Animals

Specific pathogen-free male BALB/c mice obtained from the Animal Resource Centre (Perth, Australia) arrived at 6 weeks of age were housed at in sterile micro-isolator cages, and maintained on a 12:12 h light/dark cycle. This study was carried out in strict accordance with the National Health and Medical Research Council (NHMRC) of Australia. All procedures were approved by the Animal Experimentation Ethics Committee of the University of Melbourne.

Treatment

After a one week acclimatization period, mice were randomly divided into 4 groups (n = 14–18 per group) that were matched for body weight. Two groups of animals were exposed to cigarette smoke (CS) and two groups were sham exposed according to our published protocol [21,22]. Briefly, animals underwent whole body exposure to the smoke of 1 filtered cigarette inside an 18 liter plastic chamber (Winfield Red, 16 mg or less of tar, 1.2 mg or less

of nicotine and 15 mg or less of CO, Philip Morris) over 15 min with a 5 minute recovery interval and this was then repeated such that mice received 2 cigarettes over a 30 min period. Smoke was generated in 50-ml tidal volumes over 10 seconds by use of timed draw-back. The mean total suspended particulate (TSP) mass concentration in the chamber containing cigarette smoke generated from one cigarette, measured from 3 min 13 s to 15 min, was 419 mg/m^3 as previously published [22]. This exposure protocol was repeated three times a day (8 am, 12 pm and 4 pm exposures) for 6 days a week and generates carboxyhemoglobin levels within the range observed in human smokers [22]. Sham animals were handled identically without cigarette smoke exposure. After 16 weeks of CS one group of mice was sacrificed, as described below. The remaining groups were then sacrificed after a period without CS of 4 and 12 weeks. Body weight was measured twice per week.

Tissue Collection

The study protocol included 4 groups (n = 11–14 per group). Mice were weighed and given an anesthetic overdose (ketamine and xylazine, 180 and 32 mg/kg i.p., respectively) and allocated to the following experimental protocols. Cohort 1 (n = 8) were subjected to bronchoalveolar lavage (BAL). Briefly, lungs from each mouse were lavaged in situ with 0.4 ml PBS, followed by three 0.3 mL of PBS, with 1 ml of BAL fluid (BALF) recovered from each animal. Smoke exposure had no effect on the recovered volume as previously shown [22]. Whole lungs were perfused free of blood via right ventricular perfusion with 10 ml of saline, rapidly excised en bloc, blotted. The large left lobe was snap frozen in liquid nitrogen and stored at −80°C for QPCR analysis. The remaining lung tissue was retained and subjected to flow cytometry analysis as detailed in the flow cytometry methods section. Cohort 2 (n = 5–6) were subjected to histology as detailed in the histology methods section.

Cellular Inflammatory Response

Bronchoalveolar lavage fluid (BALF) was collected as previously described [22]. Cytospins were prepared at 400 rpm for 10 min on a Cytospin 3 (Shandon, UK). Cytospin slides were stained with DiffQuik (Dade Baxter, Australia) and 500 cells per slide were by standard morphological criteria.

Flow Cytometry

BALF cells were resuspended in FACS buffer (PBS 1% FCS). Lungs were perfused with ice-cold PBS to remove excess blood before single cell suspensions were obtained using collagenase. Briefly, whole lungs were digested with RPMI containing collagenase D (1 mg/mL) and DNase I (Roche, Mannheim, Germany) and cells were washed and recovered by centrifugation. Erythrocytes were lysed by incubation with RBC lysis buffer. To avoid non-specific binding of Abs to FcRγ, FACS Buffer containing anti-mouse CD16/32 mAb (Mouse BD Fc Block) (2.4G2, BD) was added to all primary stains. Cells were labeled with fluorophore-conjugated antibodies at pre-optimized dilutions to CD3-FITC, CD4-PE, CD8-PE, CD49b-PE (NK/NK T marker) and CD69-FITC (all from Becton Dickinson) for 1 h at 4°C and then washed twice in FACS buffer and resuspended in a final volume of 0.5 ml of FACS buffer. Data was acquired on a BD FACSCalibur flow cytometer (Becton Dickinson) and typically up to 10^5 viable cell events were collected for analysis. A strict gating strategy was used to determine different immune cell populations as follows: single cell gate (FSC-H vs FSC-A), live cells (propidium iodide exclusion), granularity/size cell gate (FSC-A vs SSC-A) and specific surface marker gates. Flowjo software (version 7.2.4, Tree Star, OR) was used to generate plots for data analysis.

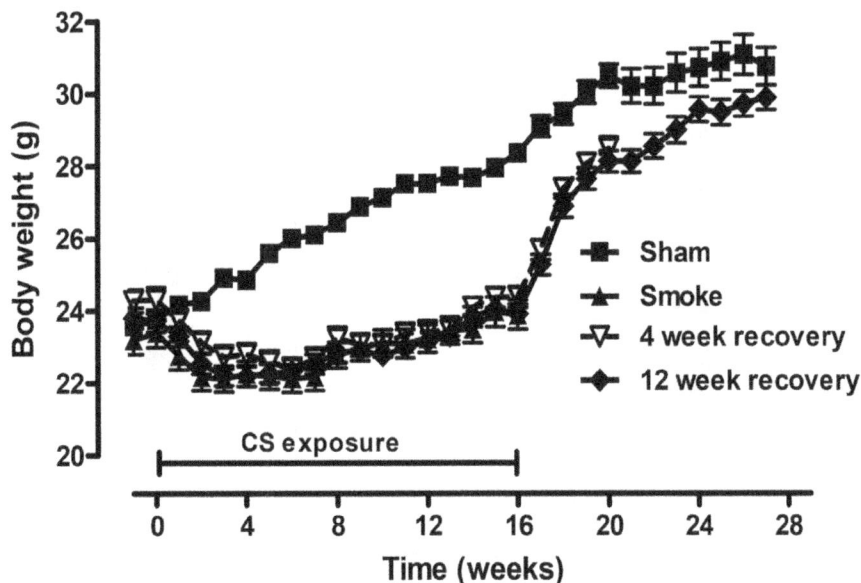

Figure 1. Smoke-induced weight loss was reversed 12 weeks after CS cessation. Male BALB/c mice were either exposed to 6 cigarettes/day, 6 days/week (■) or sham handled (▲) for 16 weeks. After smoke exposure, groups of mice were then exposed to room air without cigarette smoke for either 4 weeks (▽) or 12 weeks (◆). For all groups body weight was determined weekly. Data are shown as mean ± SE for n = 14–18 per treatment group.

Histology

Mouse lungs (n = 5–6 per group) were perfusion fixed *in situ* via a tracheal cannula with 10% neutral buffered formalin (NBF) at 25 cm H_2O pressure. After 10 min, the trachea was ligated and the lungs were left *in situ* for 1 hr, then removed and immersed in 10% NBF for at least 24 hr and then embedded in paraffin. After paraffin embedding, 4 µm sections were prepared and stained with hematoxylin and eosin. The number of pigmented macrophages was counted by a treatment-blind observer at x200 magnification, with at least 8 fields captured per sample for analysis using ImageJ software. Assessment of the number of lymphoid follicles per mm^2 of lung tissue was determined as previously published [23].

Quantitative RT-PCR

Total RNA was isolated from lung tissue using an RNeasy kit (Qiagen, MD, USA) and was used as a template to generate first-strand cDNA synthesis using SuperScript III (Invitrogen, CA, USA). TaqMan low density arrays (Applied Biosystem, CA, USA) were used for determining gene expression of individual samples using an ABI 7900 HT Sequence Detection System (Applied Biosystems). Gene expression was quantified using 18S rRNA as an internal control as previously described [22].

Statistical Analyses

Results are expressed as mean ± SE. All data were analyzed using two-way ANOVA and when statistical significance was achieved a *post hoc* Bonferroni test for multiple comparisons was used to compare between treatment groups. All statistical analyses were performed with GraphPad Prism for Windows (version 6.02). In all cases, probability values less than 0.05 (P<0.05) were considered statistically significant.

Results

Cessation of CS exposure restored body weight

As previously reported [24,25] mice exposed to CS failed to gain as much body weight as the Sham handled mice and were 15% lighter at the conclusion of the 16 week exposure period (P< 0.05; Figure 1). After smoking cessation mice rapidly gained weight but remained significantly lighter by 6% after 4 weeks of recovery (P<0.05). By 12 weeks of recovery the body weight of mice previously exposed to CS was no different to the sham handled mice. Since the systemic effects of cigarette smoke resolve by 12 weeks, the cellular and molecular markers were characterized at this time point. In addition, following 16 weeks of smoke exposure, no significant increase in airspace enlargement was observed in BALB/c mice, which is consistent with previous studies that show an increase in mean linear intercept and destructive index in longer term chronic exposure models (i.e. 6 months) [26].

Neutrophil and lymphocyte cell number remained elevated after 12 weeks of CS cessation

Mice exposed to CS for 16 weeks (6 cigarettes/day, 6 days/week) had a significant increase in total, macrophage and neutrophil number in BALF compared to sham mice (P<0.05, Figure 2A–C). Following 12 weeks of CS cessation BALF macrophage and total cell number decreased to sham levels. Peak neutrophil numbers in CS exposed mice declined by approximately 10-fold in the 12 weeks CS cessation group, however remained significantly elevated by 5-fold compared to Sham mice (P<0.05, Figure 2C). FACS analysis was used to determine the number of Ly6G+ neutrophils in the lung tissue, which showed that tissue neutrophils accumulated with CS exposure, resulting in a 1.6-fold increase above sham exposed mice (Figure 2D). Unlike neutrophil numbers in the BALF, tissue associated neutrophil numbers in the CS cessation group normalized to sham levels (Figure 2D).

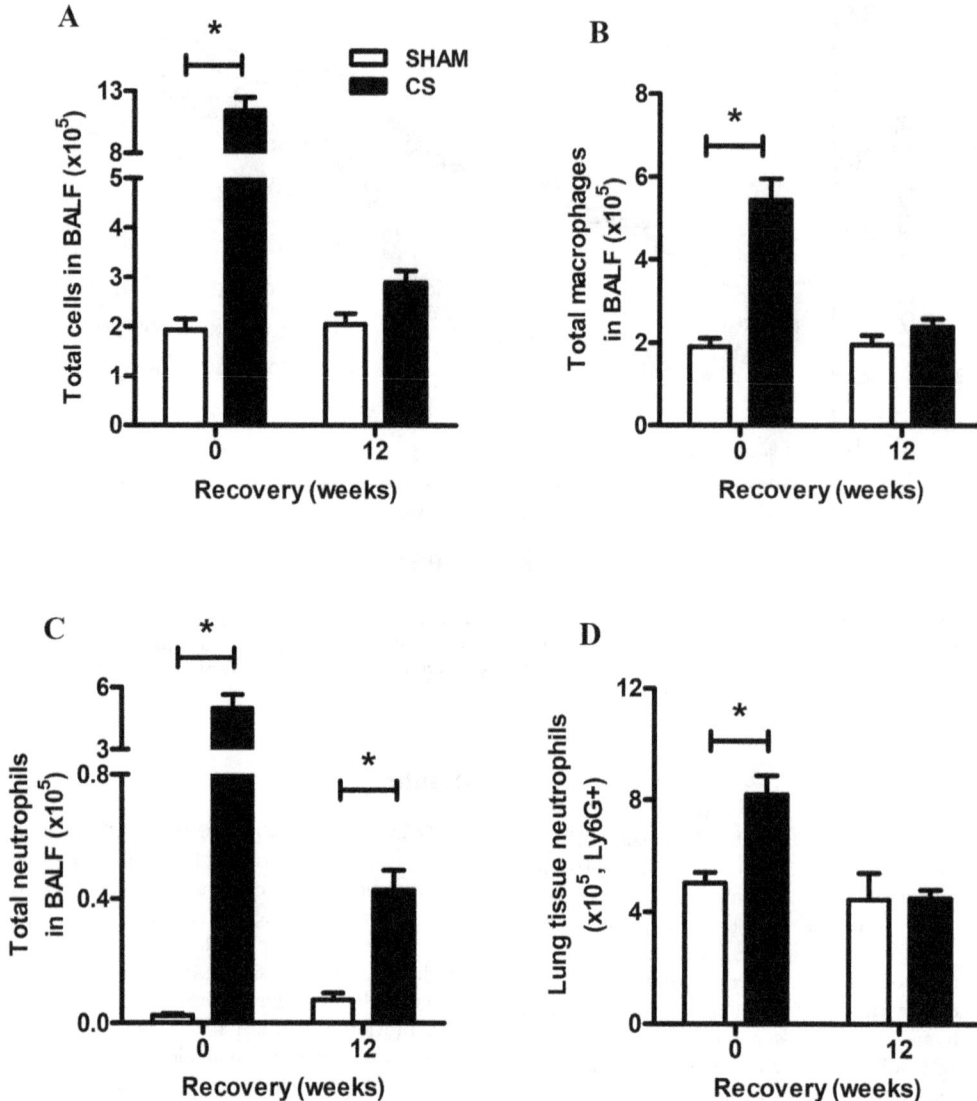

Figure 2. Effect of sub-chronic smoke exposure and 12 weeks of CS cessation on BALF cellularity and lung neutrophilia. Male BALB/c mice were either exposed to 6 cigarettes/day, 6 days/week (■) or sham handled (□) for 16 weeks. After smoke exposure a group of mice was then exposed to room air without cigarette smoke for 12 weeks. Total cells (A), macrophages (B) and neutrophils (C) were determined in BALF. Data are shown as mean ± SE for n = 8–11 per treatment group. (D) Single cell suspension of the lungs was used to determine neutrophil numbers in the lung tissue by flow cytometry. Data were analysed by two-way ANOVA and when significance was achieved a *post hoc* Bonferroni test was performed. #P<0.05 significant *post hoc* effect of CS compared to sham animals at the same recovery time-point.

FACS analysis was used to determine CD3+ CD4+ and activated CD69+CD8+ T cell number in BALF and lung tissue (Figure 3A–F). In lung tissue, CS had no effect on CD4+ T cell numbers and no change in frequency was observed in the cessation groups (Figure 3A). CD4+ T cells were also analyzed in the BALF compartment following 12 weeks CS recovery, demonstrating a 1.6-fold increase above Sham exposed mice (Figure 3B). Activated CD8+ T cells were also quantified by flow cytometry in the lung tissue, demonstrating a significant 2.3-fold increase in CS-exposed mice above Sham controls (Figure 3C). There was also a trend towards increased CD8+ T cell numbers in the CS cessation group (1.5-fold); however this failed to reach statistical significance. Analysis of BALF CD8+ T cells numbers demonstrated a 2.4-fold increase in the recovery group compared to the Sham controls (Figure 3D). In addition, activated NK cells were quantified in the lung and BAL compartment demonstrating

a 2-fold increase in the lung tissue that was maintained in the CS cessation group (Figure 3E). In contrast there was no increase in activated NK cells in the BAL compartment (Figure 3F).

Cigarette smoke exposure induced lymphoid aggregates and the prolonged elevation in pigmented macrophages

Hematoxylin and eosin staining of lung sections revealed the presence of structures consistent with the formation of lymphoid aggregates, a hallmark of chronic inflammation in CS exposed mice, which persisted following 12 weeks of cessation (Figure 4A). Quantification of the number of tertiary lymphoid aggregates demonstrated that these structures appeared with 16 weeks of CS exposure and consistent with a recent study [23], persisted in the cessation group where numbers appeared to slightly increase over time (Figure 4B). The lymphoid aggregates were anatomically located in close proximity to pigmented macrophages. The

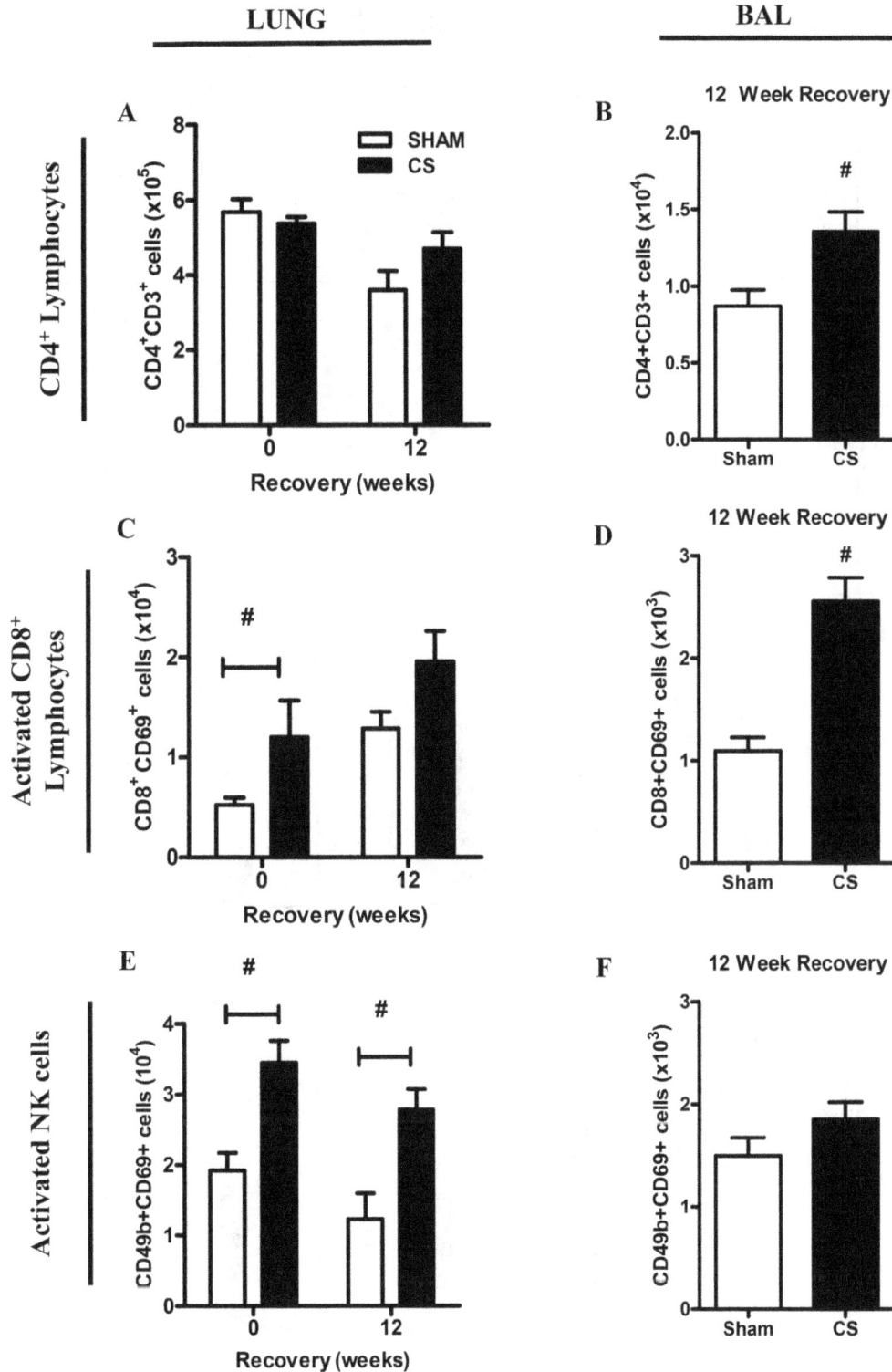

Figure 3. Effect of sub-chronic smoke exposure and 12 weeks of CS cessation on BALF and lung CD4[+] and activated CD8[+] lymphocytes. Male BALB/c mice were either exposed to 6 cigarettes/day, 6 days/week (■) or sham handled (□) for 16 weeks. After smoke exposure a group of mice was then exposed to room air without cigarette smoke for 12 weeks. CD4[+]CD3[+] lymphocyte number was determined in individual lung single cell suspensions (A) and BALF cells (B) using FACS analysis. Activated CD8[+]CD69[+] lymphocyte number was determined in individual lung single cell suspensions (C) and BALF cells (D) using FACS analysis. In addition, activated NK cell numbers were quantified in individual lung single cell suspensions (E) and BALF cells (F). Data are shown as mean ± SE for n = 7–8 per treatment group. Data were analysed by two-way ANOVA and when significance was achieved a *post hoc* Bonferroni test was performed. #P<0.05 significant *post hoc* effect of CS compared to sham animals at the same recovery time-point.

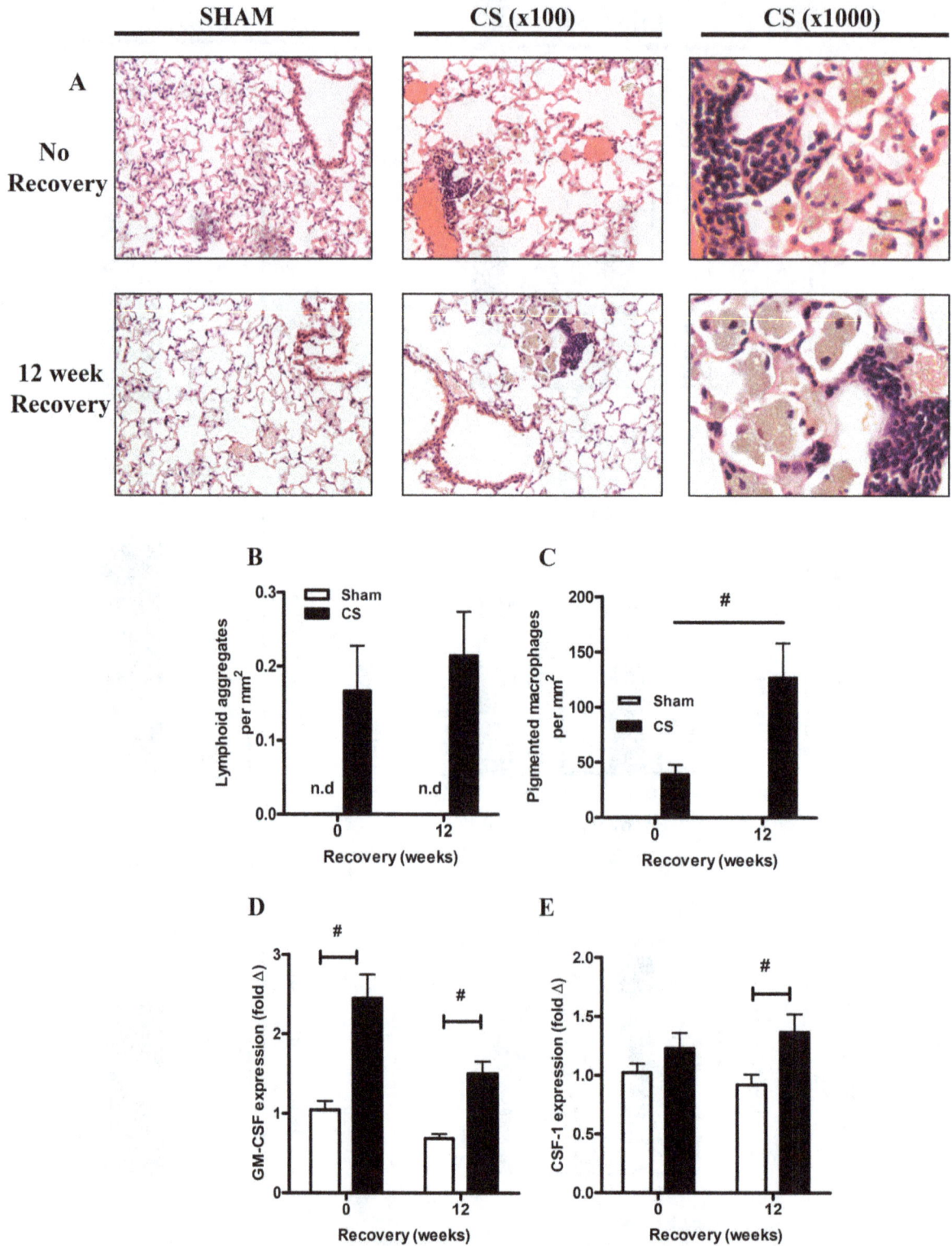

Figure 4. Sub-chronic smoke exposure resulted in the prolonged presence of pigmented macrophages. Representative histological staining of hematoxylin and eosin sections from sham and CS exposed mice and after 12 weeks of recovery (A). Magnification, x100 and x1000. The histological sections were scored for the number of lymphoid aggregates (B). The histological sections were scored for the presence of pigmented macrophages (C). Gene expression of the macrophage survival cytokines GM-CSF (D) and CSF-1 (E) was determined by Q-PCR, normalized to 18S rRNA and expressed as a fold change relative to the Sham no recovery group. Data are shown as mean $\pm$ SE for n = 7–8 per treatment group for QPCR and n = 4–6 for immunhistochemistry. Data were analysed by two-way ANOVA and when significance was achieved a *post hoc* Bonferroni test was performed. #P<0.05 significant *post hoc* effect.

A

B

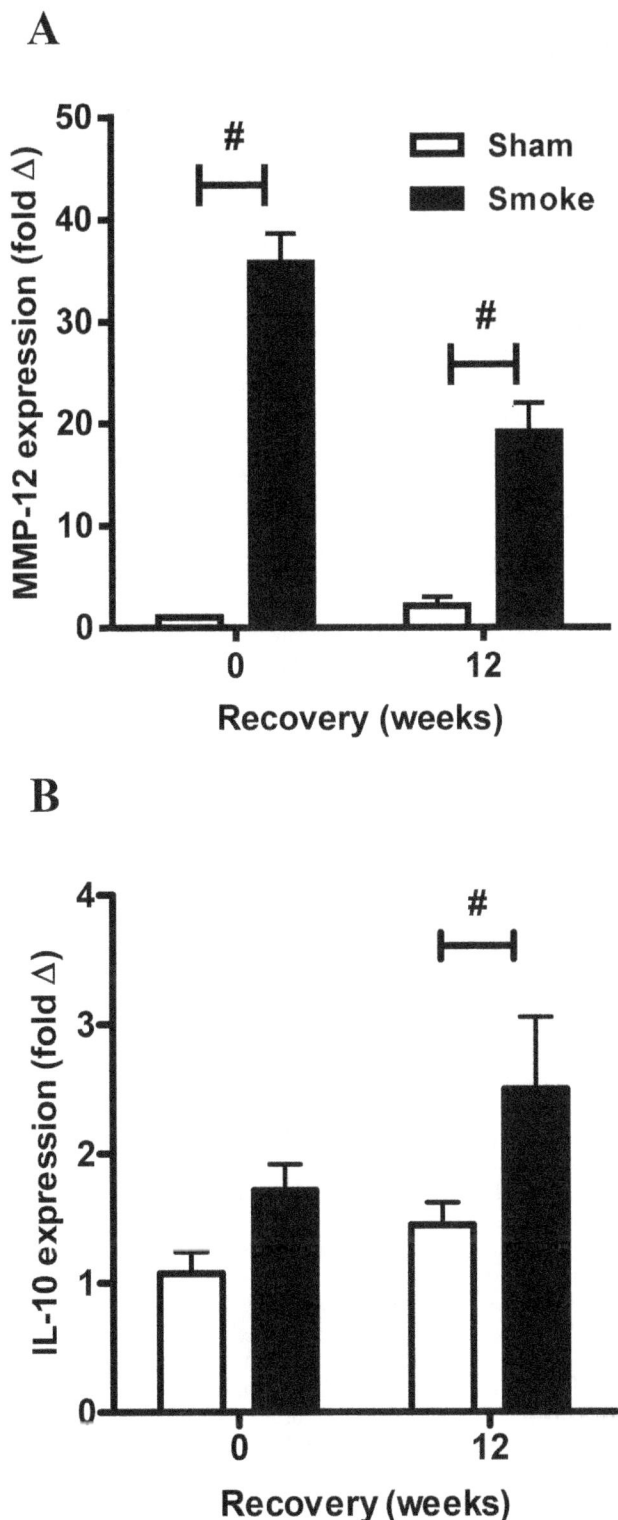

Figure 5. Effect of sub-chronic smoke exposure and 12 weeks of CS cessation on alternative macrophage marker mRNA expression in lung tissue. Male BALB/c mice were either exposed to 6 cigarettes/day, 6 days/week (■) or sham handled (□) for 16 weeks. After smoke exposure a group of mice was then exposed to room air without cigarette smoke for 12 weeks. Gene expression of the alternative macrophage markers, MMP-12 (A) and IL-10 (B) was determined by Q-PCR, normalized to 18S rRNA and expressed as a fold change relative to the Sham 0 weeks recovery group. Data are shown as mean $\pm$ SE for n = 7-8 per treatment group. Data were analysed by two-way ANOVA and when significance was achieved a *post hoc* Bonferroni test was performed. #P<0.05 significant *post hoc* effect.

accumulation of brown pigmented macrophages in the CS mice was quantified by a blind observer. CS exposure induced a significant increase in pigmented macrophages compared to sham mice (P<0.05, Figure 4C). Cessation resulted in a further 3-fold increase in the numbers of pigmented macrophages when compared to mice analyzed immediately after the 16 weeks of CS exposure (P<0.05, Figure 4C). Gene expression analysis of macrophage colony stimulating factors known to promote the survival and proliferation of leukocytes demonstrated that CS exposure caused a significant induction of GM-CSF mRNA compared to sham animals and this increase persisted following 12 weeks of cessation (P<0.05, Figure 4D). The mRNA expression of CSF-1 was also significantly induced after 12 weeks of CS cessation (P<0.05, Figure 4E).

Differential effects of CS cessation on markers of alternative macrophage activation and neutrophil mobilization

Expression of markers of alternative macrophage activation, MMP-12 and IL-10, was examined by QPCR of the lung tissue. CS caused a marked induction of MMP-12 gene expression (36-fold) and this remained significantly elevated by 19-fold after 12 weeks of cessation compared to sham animals (P<0.05, Figure 5A). IL-10 mRNA expression was also significantly elevated in the CS group after 12 weeks of smoking cessation compared to sham mice (P<0.05, Figure 5B).

The mRNA expression of neutrophil mobilization mediators was also examined. CS exposure significantly increased the mRNA expression of MIP-2α, KC and G-CSF compared to sham mice (P<0.05, Figure 6). 12 weeks of CS cessation resulted in a significant reduction in the mRNA expression of MIP-2α (2.3-fold), KC (2.3-fold) and G-CSF (2.1-fold) when compared to mice that were analyzed immediately following CS (P<0.05). Expression of the alternative neutrophil mobilizing mediators, IL17A and SAA, significantly increased by 9-fold and 33-fold above sham exposed mice respectively (P<0.05, Figure 7). IL-17A transcript levels did not decrease with CS cessation, where there was a 13-fold increase in the CS cessation group (Figure 7A). Although there was a trend towards reduced expression of SAA transcript in the CS cessation group (17-fold above sham), this was not significantly different to levels in CS exposed mice (Figure 7B). In addition, the well characterized T_H17 polarising cytokines IL-6 (Figure 7C) and IL23 (Figure 7D) were measured by QPCR in the lung tissue. IL-6 levels were increased by 16 weeks of CS exposure; however there was no difference in IL-6 expression in the CS cessation arm. IL23 levels did not significantly increase with 16 weeks CS exposure.

Discussion

COPD is a disease that displays a complex immunological profile associated with the engagement of innate and adaptive cellular processes in response to chronic CS exposure. Immune cells of both the innate and adaptive response persisted in our CS cessation model and this was previously associated with a modest reduction of alveolar enlargement and increased pulmonary compliance [27]. The innate response is particularly active in COPD, where macrophages and neutrophils accumulate in COPD airways [28], and neutrophilic inflammation fails to fully

A

B

C

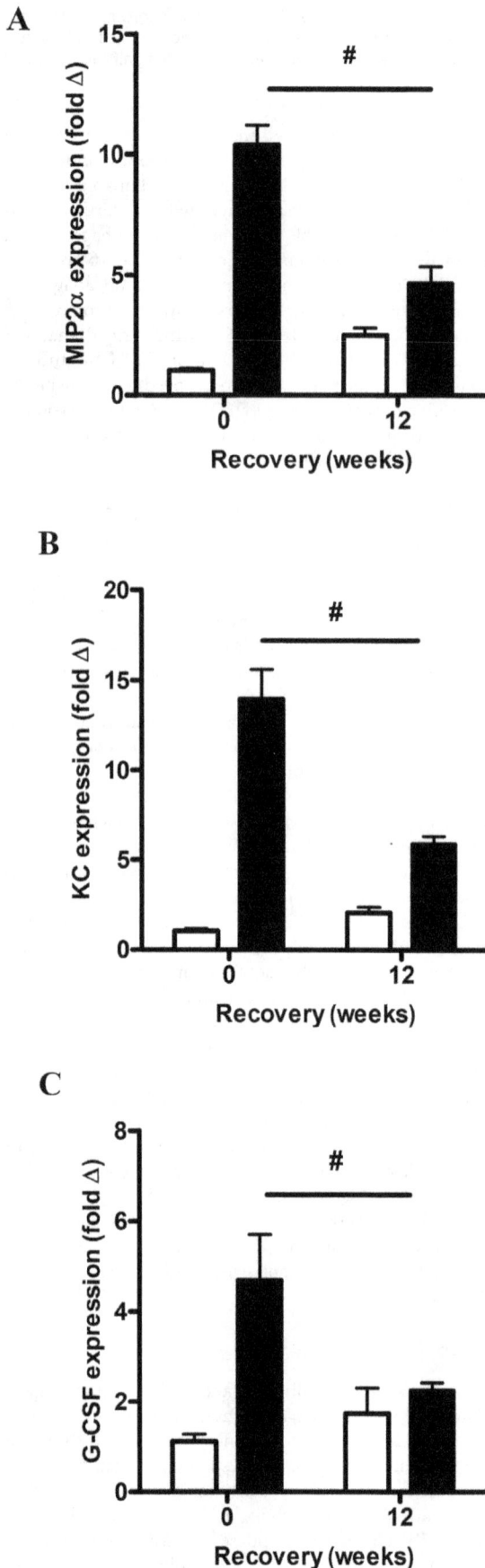

Figure 6. Effect of sub-chronic smoke exposure and 12 weeks of CS cessation on classic neutrophil mobilization mediators. Male BALB/c mice were either exposed to 6 cigarettes/day, 6 days/week (■) or sham handled (□) for 16 weeks. After smoke exposure a group of mice was then exposed to room air without cigarette smoke for 12 weeks. Gene expression of MIP-2α (A), KC (B) and G-CSF (C) was determined by Q-PCR, normalized to 18S rRNA and expressed as a fold change relative to the Sham group. Data are shown as mean ± SE for n = 7–8 per treatment group. Data were analysed by two-way ANOVA and when significance was achieved a *post hoc* Bonferroni test was performed. #P<0.05 significant *post hoc* effect.

resolve in response to CS cessation [4,5]. Our experimental model displayed a similar response to CS cessation where neutrophilic inflammation in the BAL compartment reduced with cessation but failed to fully resolve to control levels. In contrast, tissue neutrophils declined to control levels with CS cessation, which was consistent with the decline in G-CSF, a major hematopoietic growth factor required for mobilization and maturation of granulocyte precursors. Given the short-lived nature of blood derived neutrophils, the low level persistence of neutrophils in the BAL compartment is characteristic of an inflammatory response that has failed to fully resolve.

In addition, the adaptive response was also engaged, where increased CD4+ and CD8+ lymphocyte numbers in the BALF compartment remained elevated following CS cessation. Although total lymphocyte numbers in lung tissue were not significantly increased in the CS cessation group, there was an accumulation of lymphoid follicle-like structures in response to CS exposure that persisted in the cessation group. This is consistent with a recent report, where the persistence of lymphoid aggregates was associated with increased anti-nuclear autoantibody (ANA) production [23]. The role of these organized structures remain to be fully resolved, however therapeutic targeting of lymphoid follicle formation in mice chronically exposed to CS failed to suppress airway remodeling and alveolar enlargement [29]. There was also an increase in innate lymphoid NK cells in CS exposed mice, which persisted in the cessation group. This is consistent with the observed increase in NK cells in the induced sputum of COPD patients [30]. In a chronic CS challenge model, NK cells were shown to be more primed to release inflammatory mediators including IL-12 and IL-18 [31]. It has also been shown that the NK cell group 2D (NKG2D) ligand is increased in response to CS-exposure [32], which can sustain activation of cytotoxic T cells including NK cells.

CS models consistently show increased macrophage numbers in the BALF compartment (reviewed in [33]) and elevated macrophage numbers have been observed in other CS cessation models [27]. Here, we observed the persistence of pigmented macrophage populations that typically clustered together in regions adjacent to lymphoid aggregates. The presence of pigmented macrophages is thought to be related to the accumulation of CS products ingested by resident lung macrophages. To the best of our knowledge, this is the first study to quantify pigmented macrophages and demonstrate an increase with CS cessation. In conjunction with increased pigmented macrophage numbers, leukocyte colony stimulating factors, GM-CSF and CSF-1 transcript were significantly increased in the CS cessation group. Both CSFs are known to promote survival, proliferation and differentiation of myeloid lineages, and the findings presented here suggest that pigmented macrophages may proliferate in response to increased CSF expression. Whether these pigmented macrophages represent a distinct phenotype in COPD that contribute to disease pathobiology remains to be determined. There is however, growing evidence that macrophages do not conform to the classic M1/M2

A

B

C

D

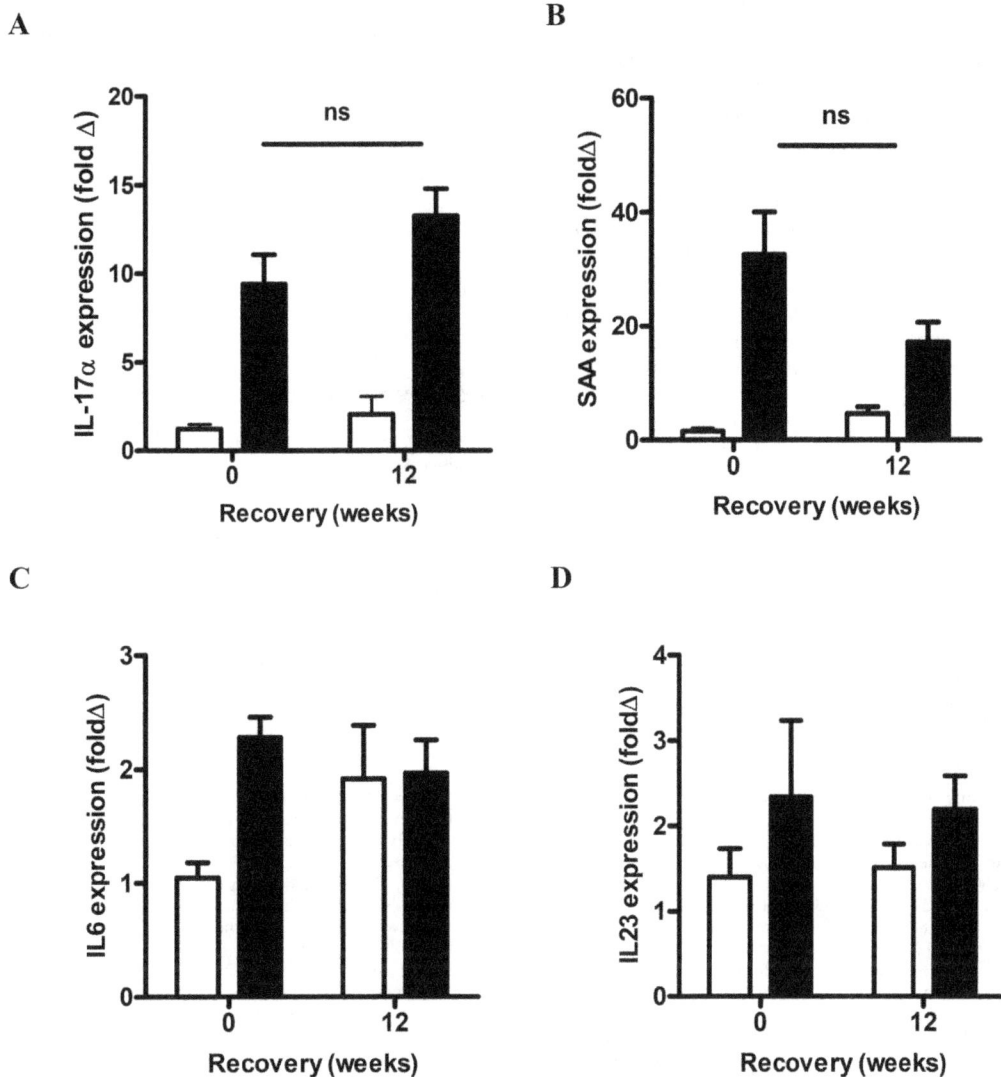

Figure 7. Effect of sub-chronic smoke exposure and 12 weeks of CS cessation on IL-17A and SAA expression. Male BALB/c mice were either exposed to 6 cigarettes/day, 6 days/week (■) or sham handled (□) for 16 weeks. After smoke exposure a group of mice was then exposed to room air without cigarette smoke for 12 weeks. Gene expression of IL-17A (A), SAA (B), IL-6 (C) and IL23 (D) was determined by Q-PCR, normalized to 18S rRNA and expressed as a fold change relative to the Sham group. Data are shown as mean ± SE for n = 6–8 per treatment group. Data were analyzed by two-way ANOVA and when significance was achieved a *post hoc* Bonferroni test was performed.

dichotomy in COPD [14,34]. In this study, IL-10 and MMP-12 expression were used as markers for differential macrophage polarization as previously reported [34], and increased expression suggest that alternative macrophage populations persist and contribute to chronic inflammation.

Previous global expression studies have shown that the majority of CS-inducible genes decline with cessation [35]. In our study, there was a focus on genes involved in neutrophil mobilization that are known to be upregulated in COPD. We have shown that IL-17A and SAA were not significantly reduced in the CS cessation group, in contrast to MIP-2α, KC and G-CSF that significantly declined with recovery. Our previous studies have demonstrated intense SAA immunoreactivity [19] and a positive correlation with neutrophilic airway inflammation [20] in the lungs of COPD patients. SAA is also a ligand for the GPCR termed ALX/FPR2, where SAA is a potent chemotactic factor that mediates phagocyte migration via this receptor [36]. SAA also promotes airway

neutrophilic inflammation in a manner that is opposed by the eicosanoid, LipoxinA4 [19]. Lipoxins and resolvins are alternative lipid-based ALX/FPR2 ligands that can oppose the actions of SAA and actively promote the resolution of inflammation (reviewed in [37,38]). Hence, the relative abundance of alternative ALX/FPR2 ligands may contribute to the impairment of resolution, where increased SAA may skew the balance towards a pro-inflammatory state.

SAA has also been shown to promote airway neutrophil recruitment via IL-17A dependent mechanisms [20]. There is also emerging evidence for an important role for IL-17A in COPD. IL-17A+ cells have been shown to be increased in the bronchial submucosa of chronic smokers and stable COPD subjects [17,39]. Furthermore, genetic ablation of the IL-17R in experimental CS models protected the mice against the development of emphysema [18], hence identifying IL-17A as a major inflammatory cytokine that can drive pathological inflammation. Recent studies also demonstrate that neutrophilic inflammation induced by CS exposure is potently suppressed in mice deficient in IL-17A [40] and in response to neutralisation with a blocking antibody [41]. Furthermore, inhibition of IL-17A signaling in an experimental COPD model also suppressed accumulation of macrophages in response to CS exposure [18]. Our finding of persistent IL-17A expression in the CS cessation group is consistent with a recent study that identified an increase in the frequency of IL-17A expressing CD4$^+$ (T$_H$17) and CD8$^+$ (T$_C$17) T cells in CS exposed mice [42]. In our study, known T$_H$17 cytokines were also quantified by QPCR and showed that IL-6, but not IL23 was significantly increased in response to CS exposure. This finding is consistent with our previous study that investigated T$_H$17 cytokine expression in response to SAA stimulation, where IL-6 was predominately induced [20]. Although SAA levels were not significantly reduced with CS cessation, there was a trend towards reduced expression relative to the non-cessation group and IL-6 levels were not increased in the CS cessation group. This data suggests that SAA and IL-6 can be sufficient to initiate polarization and maturation of IL-17A expressing cellular populations in CS exposed lungs, however once established, IL-17A$^+$ cells may be maintained in the mucosa independently of T$_H$17 cytokines.

In addition to classic T$_H$17 pathways, there is also emerging evidence for alternative innate cellular sources of IL-17A in inflammatory lung models. This may be particularly relevant to COPD as NOD. SCID mice deficient in B and T cells still develop airspace enlargement in response to chronic CS exposure, to suggest a more prominent role for innate immune responses [43]. Indeed, innate sources of IL-17A have been identified in inflammatory lung models including macrophages, neutrophils, NK cells and γδ T cells [20,44] and the predominant source of IL-17A in COPD is yet to be defined. In conclusion, this study has investigated innate and adaptive responses following CS cessation and has identified the IL-17A and SAA innate cytokine networks as markers of persistent inflammatory responses. The targeting of the IL-17A axis may represent a novel therapeutic strategy to promote the resolution of inflammation following CS cessation.

Acknowledgments

The authors would like to thank Debbie Allen, Oliver Ferdinando and Lindsay Kosack for their technical assistance.

Author Contributions

Conceived and designed the experiments: MH SB GA RV. Performed the experiments: SC SL LD JJ HS SY. Analyzed the data: MH SB GA RV SC SL JJ HS. Contributed to the writing of the manuscript: MH SB GA RV.

References

1. Barnes PJ (2008) Immunology of asthma and chronic obstructive pulmonary disease. Nat Rev Immunol 8: 183–192.
2. Hogg JC, Chu F, Utokaparch S, Woods R, Elliott WM, et al. (2004) The nature of small-airway obstruction in chronic obstructive pulmonary disease. N Engl J Med 350: 2645–2653.
3. Saetta M, Di Stefano A, Turato G, Facchini FM, Corbino L, et al. (1998) CD8$^+$ T-lymphocytes in peripheral airways of smokers with chronic obstructive pulmonary disease. Am J Respir Crit Care Med 157: 822–826.
4. Rutgers SR, Postma DS, ten Hacken NH, Kauffman HF, van Der Mark TW, et al. (2000) Ongoing airway inflammation in patients with COPD who Do not currently smoke. Chest 117: 262S.
5. Willemse BW, ten Hacken NH, Rutgers B, Lesman-Leegte IG, Postma DS, et al. (2005) Effect of 1-year smoking cessation on airway inflammation in COPD and asymptomatic smokers. Eur Respir J 26: 835–845.
6. Stanescu D, Sanna A, Veriter C, Kostianev S, Calcagni PG, et al. (1996) Airways obstruction, chronic expectoration, and rapid decline of FEV1 in smokers are associated with increased levels of sputum neutrophils. Thorax 51: 267–271.
7. Bozinovski S, Vlahos R, Zhang Y, Lah LC, Seow HJ, et al. (2011) Carbonylation caused by cigarette smoke extract is associated with defective macrophage immunity. Am J Respir Cell Mol Biol 45: 229–236.
8. Hodge S, Hodge G, Ahern J, Jersmann H, Holmes M, et al. (2007) Smoking alters alveolar macrophage recognition and phagocytic ability: implications in chronic obstructive pulmonary disease. Am J Respir Cell Mol Biol 37: 748–755.
9. Vlahos R, Wark PA, Anderson GP, Bozinovski S (2012) Glucocorticosteroids differentially regulate MMP-9 and neutrophil elastase in COPD. PLoS One 7: e33277.
10. Damiano VV, Tsang A, Kucich U, Abrams WR, Rosenbloom J, et al. (1986) Immunolocalization of elastase in human emphysematous lungs. J Clin Invest 78: 482–493.
11. Shao MX, Nadel JA (2005) Neutrophil elastase induces MUC5AC mucin production in human airway epithelial cells via a cascade involving protein kinase C, reactive oxygen species, and TNF-alpha-converting enzyme. J Immunol 175: 4009–4016.
12. Walsh DE, Greene CM, Carroll TP, Taggart CC, Gallagher PM, et al. (2001) Interleukin-8 up-regulation by neutrophil elastase is mediated by MyD88/ IRAK/TRAF-6 in human bronchial epithelium. J Biol Chem 276: 35494–35499.
13. Beckett EL, Stevens RL, Jarnicki AG, Kim RY, Hanish I, et al. (2013) A new short-term mouse model of chronic obstructive pulmonary disease identifies a role for mast cell tryptase in pathogenesis. J Allergy Clin Immunol 131: 752–762.
14. Shaykhiev R, Krause A, Salit J, Strulovici-Barel Y, Harvey BG, et al. (2009) Smoking-dependent reprogramming of alveolar macrophage polarization: implication for pathogenesis of chronic obstructive pulmonary disease. J Immunol 183: 2867–2883.
15. Stevenson CS, Coote K, Webster R, Johnston H, Atherton HC, et al. (2005) Characterization of cigarette smoke-induced inflammatory and mucus hyper-secretory changes in rat lung and the role of CXCR2 ligands in mediating this effect. Am J Physiol Lung Cell Mol Physiol 288: L514–522.
16. Qiu Y, Zhu J, Bandi V, Atmar RL, Hattotuwa K, et al. (2003) Biopsy neutrophilia, neutrophil chemokine and receptor gene expression in severe exacerbations of chronic obstructive pulmonary disease. Am J Respir Crit Care Med 168: 968–975.
17. Di Stefano A, Caramori G, Gnemmi I, Contoli M, Vicari C, et al. (2009) T helper type 17-related cytokine expression is increased in the bronchial mucosa of stable chronic obstructive pulmonary disease patients. Clin Exp Immunol 157: 316–324.
18. Chen K, Pociask DA, McAleer JP, Chan YR, Alcorn JF, et al. (2011) IL-17RA is required for CCL2 expression, macrophage recruitment, and emphysema in response to cigarette smoke. PLoS One 6: e20333.
19. Bozinovski S, Uddin M, Vlahos R, Thompson M, McQualter JL, et al. (2012) Serum amyloid A opposes lipoxin A(4) to mediate glucocorticoid refractory lung inflammation in chronic obstructive pulmonary disease. Proc Natl Acad Sci U S A 109: 935–940.
20. Anthony D, Seow HJ, Uddin M, Thompson M, Dousha L, et al. (2013) Serum amyloid A promotes lung neutrophilia by increasing IL-17A levels in the mucosa and gammadelta T cells. Am J Respir Crit Care Med 188: 179–186.
21. Hansen MJ, Chen H, Jones JE, Langenbach SY, Vlahos R, et al. (2013) The lung inflammation and skeletal muscle wasting induced by subchronic cigarette smoke exposure are not altered by a high-fat diet in mice. PLoS One 8: e80471.
22. Vlahos R, Bozinovski S, Jones JE, Powell J, Gras J, et al. (2006) Differential protease, innate immunity, and NF-kappaB induction profiles during lung inflammation induced by subchronic cigarette smoke exposure in mice. Am J Physiol Lung Cell Mol Physiol 290: L931–945.
23. Morissette MC, Jobse BN, Thayaparan D, Nikota JK, Shen P, et al. (2014) Persistence of pulmonary tertiary lymphoid tissues and anti-nuclear antibodies following cessation of cigarette smoke exposure. Respir Res 15: 49.
24. Chen H, Hansen MJ, Jones JE, Vlahos R, Bozinovski S, et al. (2007) Regulation of hypothalamic NPY by diet and smoking. Peptides 28: 384–389.
25. Chen H, Vlahos R, Bozinovski S, Jones J, Anderson GP, et al. (2005) Effect of short-term cigarette smoke exposure on body weight, appetite and brain neuropeptide Y in mice. Neuropsychopharmacology 30: 713–719.
26. Motz GT, Eppert BL, Sun G, Wesselkamper SC, Linke MJ, et al. (2008) Persistence of lung CD8 T cell oligoclonal expansions upon smoking cessation in a mouse model of cigarette smoke-induced emphysema. J Immunol 181: 8036–8043.
27. Braber S, Henricks PA, Nijkamp FP, Kraneveld AD, Folkerts G (2010) Inflammatory changes in the airways of mice caused by cigarette smoke exposure are only partially reversed after smoking cessation. Respir Res 11: 99.
28. Hogg JC (2004) Pathophysiology of airflow limitation in chronic obstructive pulmonary disease. Lancet 364: 709–721.

29. Bracke KR, Verhamme FM, Seys LJ, Bantsimba-Malanda C, Cunoosamy DM, et al. (2013) Role of CXCL13 in cigarette smoke-induced lymphoid follicle formation and chronic obstructive pulmonary disease. Am J Respir Crit Care Med 188: 343–355.

30. Urbanowicz RA, Lamb JR, Todd I, Corne JM, Fairclough LC (2010) Enhanced effector function of cytotoxic cells in the induced sputum of COPD patients. Respir Res 11: 76.

31. Motz GT, Eppert BL, Wortham BW, Amos-Kroohs RM, Flury JL, et al. (2010) Chronic cigarette smoke exposure primes NK cell activation in a mouse model of chronic obstructive pulmonary disease. J Immunol 184: 4460–4469.

32. Borchers MT, Wesselkamper SC, Curull V, Ramirez-Sarmiento A, Sanchez-Font A, et al. (2009) Sustained CTL activation by murine pulmonary epithelial cells promotes the development of COPD-like disease. J Clin Invest 119: 636–649.

33. Vlahos R, Bozinovski S (2014) Recent advances in pre-clinical mouse models of COPD. Clin Sci (Lond) 126: 253–265.

34. Woodruff PG, Koth LL, Yang YH, Rodriguez MW, Favoreto S, et al. (2005) A distinctive alveolar macrophage activation state induced by cigarette smoking. Am J Respir Crit Care Med 172: 1383–1392.

35. Halappanavar S, Russell M, Stampfli MR, Williams A, Yauk CL (2009) Induction of the interleukin 6/signal transducer and activator of transcription pathway in the lungs of mice sub-chronically exposed to mainstream tobacco smoke. BMC Med Genomics 2: 56.

36. Su SB, Gong W, Gao JL, Shen W, Murphy PM, et al. (1999) A seven-transmembrane, G protein-coupled receptor, FPRL1, mediates the chemotactic activity of serum amyloid A for human phagocytic cells. J Exp Med 189: 395–402.

37. Levy BD, Vachier I, Serhan CN (2012) Resolution of inflammation in asthma. Clin Chest Med 33: 559–570.

38. Serhan CN, Chiang N, Van Dyke TE (2008) Resolving inflammation: dual anti-inflammatory and pro-resolution lipid mediators. Nat Rev Immunol 8: 349–361.

39. Doe C, Bafadhel M, Siddiqui S, Desai D, Mistry V, et al. (2010) Expression of the T helper 17-associated cytokines IL-17A and IL-17F in asthma and COPD. Chest 138: 1140–1147.

40. Chang Y, Al-Alwan L, Audusseau S, Chouiali F, Carlevaro-Fita J, et al. (2014) Genetic deletion of IL-17A reduces cigarette smoke-induced inflammation and alveolar type II cell apoptosis. Am J Physiol Lung Cell Mol Physiol 306: L132–143.

41. Shen N, Wang J, Zhao M, Pei F, He B (2011) Anti-interleukin-17 antibodies attenuate airway inflammation in tobacco-smoke-exposed mice. Inhal Toxicol 23: 212–218.

42. Duan M-C, Tang H-J, Zhong X-N, Huang Y (2013) Persistence of Th17/Tc17 Cell Expression upon Smoking Cessation in Mice with Cigarette Smoke-Induced Emphysema. Clinical and Developmental Immunology 2013: 11.

43. D'Hulst A I, Maes T, Bracke KR, Demedts IK, Tournoy KG, et al. (2005) Cigarette smoke-induced pulmonary emphysema in scid-mice. Is the acquired immune system required? Respir Res 6: 147.

44. Essilfie AT, Simpson JL, Horvat JC, Preston JA, Dunkley ML, et al. (2011) Haemophilus influenzae infection drives IL-17-mediated neutrophilic allergic airways disease. PLoS Pathog 7: e1002244.

8

Global Characterization of Differential Gene Expression Profiles in Mouse Vγ1⁺ and Vγ4⁺ γδ T Cells

Peng Dong¹, Siya Zhang¹, Menghua Cai¹, Ning Kang¹, Yu Hu¹, Lianxian Cui¹, Jianmin Zhang¹,²*, Wei He¹*

1 Department of Immunology, Institute of Basic Medical Sciences, Chinese Academy of Medical Sciences and School of Basic Medicine, Peking Union Medical College, State Key Laboratory of Medical Molecular Biology, Beijing, China, 2 Neuroregeneration and Stem Cell Programs, Institute for Cell Engineering, Department of Neurology, Johns Hopkins University School of Medicine, Baltimore, MD, United States of America

Abstract

Peripheral γδ T cells in mice are classified into two major subpopulations, Vγ1⁺ and Vγ4⁺, based on the composition of T cell receptors. However, their intrinsic differences remain unclear. In this study, we analyzed gene expression profiles of the two subsets using Illumina HiSeq 2000 Sequencer. We identified 1995 transcripts related to the activation of Vγ1⁺ γδ T cells, and 2158 transcripts related to the activation of Vγ4⁺ γδ T cells. We identified 24 transcripts differentially expressed between the two subsets in resting condition, and 20 after PMA/Ionomycin treatment. We found that both cell types maintained phenotypes producing IFN-γ, TNF-α, TGF-β and IL-10. However, Vγ1⁺ γδ T cells produced more Th2 type cytokines, such as IL-4 and IL-5, while Vγ4⁺ γδ T cells preferentially produced IL-17. Our study provides a comprehensive gene expression profile of mouse peripheral Vγ1⁺ and Vγ4⁺ γδ T cells that describes the inherent differences between them.

Editor: Domingos Henrique, Instituto de Medicina Molecular, Portugal

Funding: This study was supported by the Health Research Special Program, Ministry of Science and Technology of the People's Republic of China (Grant No. 20130217). The funder had no role in study design, data collection and analysis, decision to publish, or preparation of the manuscript.

Competing Interests: The authors have declared that no competing interests exist.

* Email: heweiimu@public.bta.net.cn (WH); jzhang42@gmail.com (JZ)

Introduction

γδ T cells were discovered more than 30 years ago. Although considerable progress has been made in characterizing their biological significance, much remains unknown. γδ T cells arise earlier than αβ T cells during thymic ontogeny, predominately at the early stage of fetal development [1]. After birth, however, γδ T cells make up a minor fraction of circulating T lymphocytes in rodents and humans. Similar to αβ T cells, γδ T cells also have a diverse repertoire of T cell receptors (TCR) derived through somatic rearrangement of V, D and J gene segments. Although few V, D and J gene elements are responsible for genetic rearrangement, additional diversity is added to the γ and δ chains via junctional diversification processes [2].

γδ T cells exert diverse functions, however, individual subsets within the population appear to be biased toward specialized functions [1]. Mouse peripheral lymphoid γδ T cells are classified into two major subsets, Vγ1⁺ and Vγ4⁺ γδ T cells, depending on their TCR expression [1,3,4]. Vγ1⁺ and Vγ4⁺ γδ T cells perform distinct functions in many disease models. For example, Vγ1⁺ γδ T cells produce IL-4 and IFN-γ in the liver [5], and Vγ4⁺ γδ T cells produce IFN-γ or IL-17 depending on the studied models [6]. Vγ1⁺ and Vγ4⁺ γδ T cells function as oppositional pairs in diseases including coxsackievirus B3 infection [7], West Nile virus infection [4], airway hyperresponsiveness [8,9], macrophage homeostasis [10] and ovalbumin induced IgE production [11]. However, the functional relatedness of Vγ1⁺ and Vγ4⁺ γδ T cells remains unresolved, partly due to a lack of comprehensive analysis and comparison of gene expression. Although, gene-expression profiles of emergent γδTCR⁺ thymocytes have been reported [12], a comprehensive analysis of peripheral Vγ1⁺ and Vγ4⁺ γδ T cells functional differences has not been reported. This is likely due to the limited number of cells that can be obtained from healthy mice.

In this study, we expanded Vγ1⁺ and Vγ4⁺ γδ T cells simultaneously from the same pool of mouse splenocytes. We comprehensively analyzed gene expression profiles using Illumina's sequencing technology. We identified 1995 transcripts related to the activation of Vγ1⁺ γδ T cells, and 2158 transcripts were related to the activation of Vγ4⁺ γδ T cells. Interestingly, only 24 transcripts were differentially expressed between two subsets in resting condition, and 20 transcripts after PMA/Ionomycin-induced activation. Both cells produced high levels of IFN-γ, TNF-α, TGF-β and IL-10. However, Vγ1⁺ γδ T cells produced more Th2 type cytokines, while Vγ4⁺ γδ T cells tended to produce more IL-17. These findings describe the inherent differences between Vγ1⁺ and Vγ4⁺ γδ T cells.

Materials and Methods

Mice

Male C57BL/6J mice aged 6–8 weeks were purchased from the National Institute for Food and Drug Control. All mice were maintained under specific pathogen-free conditions in the Experimental Animal Center, Institute of Basic Medical Sciences, Chinese Academy of Medical Sciences. All animal experiments were approved by and performed in accordance with the guidelines of the international Agency for Research on Cancer's Animal Care and Use Committee and IBMS/PUMC's Animal Care and Use Committee.

Expansion of Vγ1$^+$ and Vγ4$^+$ γδ T cells

Vγ1$^+$ and Vγ4$^+$ γδ T cells were expanded from splenocytes as described previously [13]. Briefly, flat-bottom 24 well plates were coated with 500μl purified anti-mouse TCRγ/δ antibody (UC7–13D5, 1μg/ml; Biolegend) at 37°C for 2 hours. Splenocytes were collected from six male C57BL/6J mice to decrease individual variation. Erythrocytes were lysed in Tris-NH4Cl buffer. Cells were then loaded onto a sterile nylon wool column, sealed and incubated at 37°C with 5% CO2 for 45 minutes. 5×10^7 cells were eluted and added to the Ab-coated wells (4×10^6 cells/well) and cultured in RPMI 1640 medium (Gibco BRL) supplemented with 10% fetal calf serum and IL-2 (200 IU/ml). After 8 days of expansion, the proportion of γδ T cells reached approximately 80% as determined by Flow Cytometry.

Cell sorting and stimulation

1.0×10^7 Vγ1$^+$ and 1.2×10^7 Vγ4$^+$ γδ T cells were sorted by Flow Cytometric Cell Sorting (FACS) with PE conjugated anti-mouse TCR Vγ1.1/Cr4 antibody (2.11, Biolegend) and APC conjugated anti-mouse TCR Vγ2 antibody (UC3–10A6, Biolegend). The purity of sorted cells was more than 99%. 5×10^6 cells per well were seeded into 6-well culture plates at a concentration of 1×10^6/ml and rested overnight at 37°C in 5% CO2 in RPMI with 10% FCS. Cells were stimulated for 4 h with PBS or 20 ng/ml of PMA (Sigma) and 0.5μg/ml of Ionomycin (Sigma). Cells were washed with PBS and pelleted by centrifugation. Total RNA from each sample was extracted by Trizol reagent (Invitrogen) according to the manufacturer's instructions. The quality of total RNA from each sample was confirmed and comparable, based on results of Agilent Technologies 2100 Bioanalyzer.

Processing samples for Illumina sequencing

We prepared the Illumina libraries according to the manufacturer's instructions. Briefly, mRNAs were extracted from total RNA by mRNA enrichment kit (Life technologies, USA) followed by fragmentation of mRNA into 250–350 bp sizes. The first strand cDNAs were synthesized using reverse transcriptase and random primers. Second strand cDNAs were synthesized using DNA

Polymerase I followed by the addition of a single A base at the ends for the ligation to the adapters. After purification, the final cDNA library was created by PCR. Finally, 400–500 bp products were used for cluster generation, 36 bp single-end sequencing was performed using Illumina HiSeq 2000 Sequencer according to the manufacturer's instructions (Beijing Berry Genomics Co. Ltd. China). The RNA-Seq raw data files have been deposited in NCBI's Sequence Read Archive (SRA) and are accessible through SRA Series accession number SRP042029.

Analysis of RNA-seq data

We performed base calling using CASAVA 1.7 software (Illumina). Low quality and polluted adapter reads were filtered; clean reads were stored on fastq files. The sequence reads were aligned to the mouse genome (mm9), and gene expression was calculated by RPKM value. Differentially expressed transcripts were identified using General Chi-square test analysis. Q values were obtained by the "BH" method [14]. NIH DAVID web server was used for the functional annotation clustering analysis of differentially expressed transcripts.

Quantitative RT-PCR

Several genes from Vγ1$^+$ and Vγ4$^+$ γδ T cells were selected for verification from biological replicates with real-time quantitative PCR. RNA was extracted as described above. 500 ng of total RNA was reverse transcribed using PrimeScript RT reagent Kit with gDNA Eraser (Takara Bio). Gene-specific primers are listed in (Table 1). The real-time quantitative PCR was performed on the StepOnePlus Real-Time PCR System (Life Technologies) using SYBR green labeling (SYBR Premix Ex Taq II; Takara Bio). A cycle threshold (Ct) was assigned at the beginning of the logarithmic phase of PCR amplification and relative quantitation was done using the $2^{-\Delta\Delta Ct}$ method. β-actin was used for normalization control.

Cytokines

Cells were stimulated 4 h with PBS or PMA and Ionomycin then pelleted by centrifugation. Determined cytokine concentration in cell-free supernatants by enzyme linked immunosorbent assay (ELISA; R&D Systems) as described previously [15] and MILLIPLEX MAP Mouse Cytokine Kit (MT17MAG47

Table 1. Gene-specific primers for real-time quantitative PCR.

Specificity	Primer orientation	Sequence (5′ → 3′)
IL-4	Forward	ACGGAGATGGATGTGCCAAAC
	Reverse	AGCACCTTGGAAGCCCTACAGA
IL-5	Forward	TGAGGCTTCCTGTCCCTACTCATAA
	Reverse	TTGGAATAGCATTTCCACAGTACCC
IL-17A	Forward	CTGATCAGGACGCGCAAAC
	Reverse	TCGCTGCTGCCTTCACTGTA
IL-17F	Forward	ATGAAGTGCACCCGTGAAACAG
	Reverse	CTCAGAATGGCAAGTCCCAACA
SCART 2	Forward	GGATCAGGGCCTTTGTGGA
	Reverse	TGCCATTGACCAGTCGGAAC
beta-actin	Forward	CATCCGTAAAGACCTCTATGCCAAC
	Reverse	ATGGAGCCACCGATCCACA

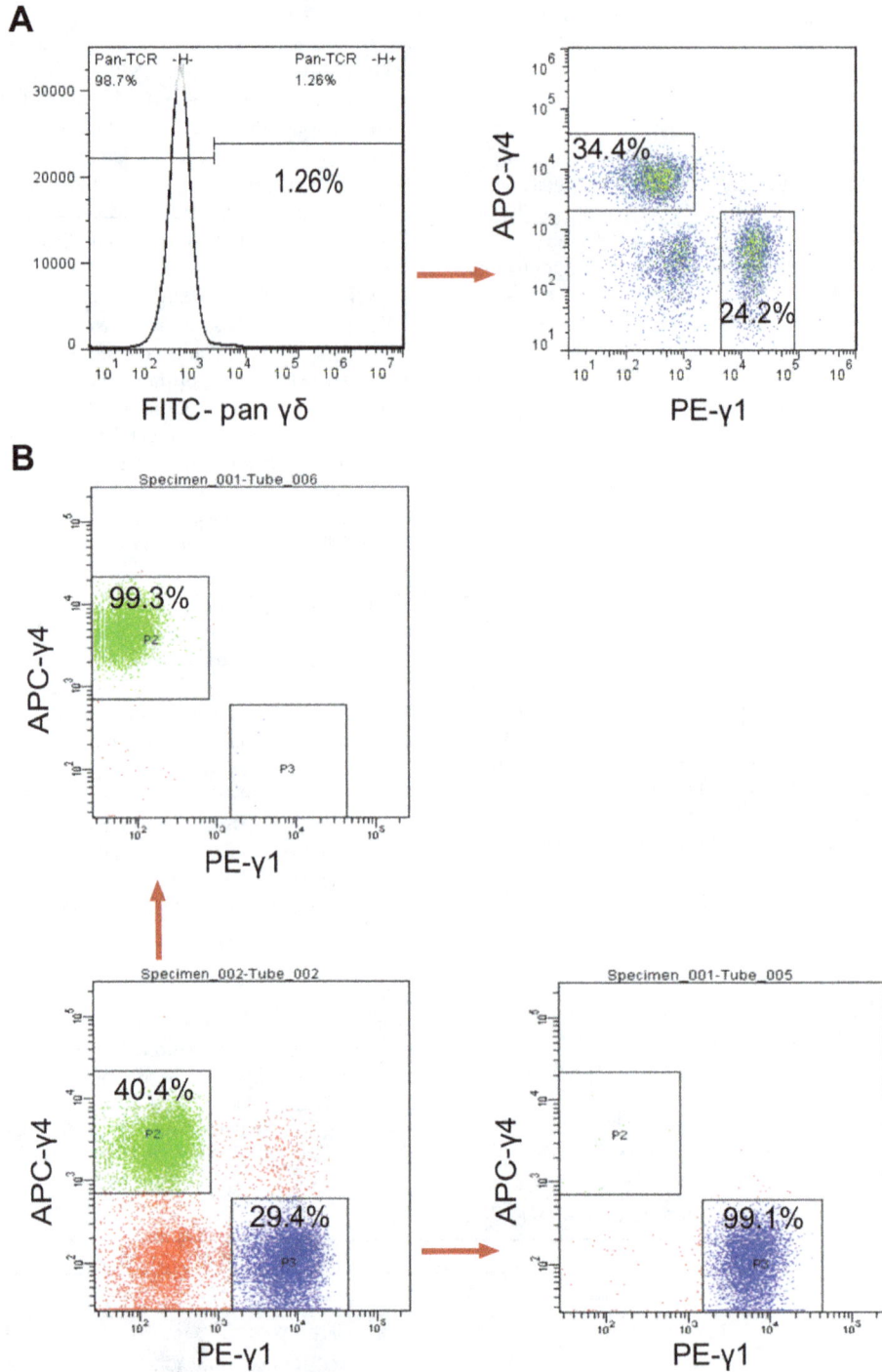

Figure 1. Vγ1+ and Vγ4+ γδ T cells are the major subpopulations in the spleen. (A) γδ T cells account for approximately 1.5% of total splenocytes. Isolated fresh Vγ1⁺ and Vγ4⁺ γδ T cells comprised approximately 35% and 25% of γδ T cells respectively. (B) 1.5×10⁸ cells were expanded simultaneously from a single pool of mouse splenocytes with purified pan anti-mouse TCR γδ antibody (UC7–13D5). After 8 days, Vγ1⁺ and Vγ4⁺ γδ T cells comprised approximately 40% and 30% of the expanded cells, respectively. 1.0×10⁷ Vγ1⁺ γδ T cells were sorted by FACS with PE conjugated anti-mouse TCR Vγ1.1/Cr4 antibody and 1.2×10⁷ Vγ4⁺ γδ T cells were sorted by FACS with APC conjugated anti-mouse TCR Vγ2 antibody. Purity of sorted cells was >99%. Data are representative of four independent experiments.

Table 2. Sequencing reads and mapping rates of each sample.

Sample Info	Total Reads	Mapped Reads	Ratio
γ1-PBS	22,672,055	20,190,322	89.05%
γ1-PMA/Ion	28,235,208	24,381,541	86.35%
γ4-PBS	33,529,245	29,854,538	89.04%
γ4-PMA/Ion	34,338,657	30,274,218	88.16%

γ1-PBS, Vγ1⁺ γδ T cells treated with PBS; γ1-PMA/Ion, Vγ1⁺ γδ T cells treated with PMA and Ionomycin; γ4-PBS, Vγ4⁺ γδ T cells treated with PBS; γ4-PMA/Ion, Vγ4⁺ γδ T cells treated with PMA and Ionomycin.

K–PX25; Merck Millipore) according to the manufacturer's instructions.

Results

Expansion and isolation of Vγ1⁺ and Vγ4⁺ γδ T cells from mouse splenocytes

γδ T cells account for approximately 1~2% of total splenocytes in healthy mice and Vγ1⁺ and Vγ4⁺ γδ T cells comprised approximately 35% and 25% respectively (Figure 1A). Therefore, we expanded the cells from mouse spleens in vitro for RNA-seq analysis. Although Vγ1⁺ and Vγ4⁺ γδ T cells can be expanded separately with sorted splenic γδ T cells using anti-Vγ1 and anti-Vγ4 Abs [16,17], potentially important biological interactions between the subsets during culture would be neglected. We therefore established a primary culture method to expand the cells simultaneously from the same pool of mouse splenocytes with pan anti-mouse TCR γδ antibodies (UC7–13D5) and IL-2. After 8 days of expansion, the proportion of γδ T cells reached approximately 80%, Vγ1⁺ and Vγ4⁺ γδ T cells comprised approximately 40% and 30% of the expanded cells, respectively (Figure 1B). No significant change was observed in the ratio of γ1 cells to γ4 cells in the in vitro expanded γδ T cells when compared with that of freshly isolated γδ T cells (in vivo subsets). γδ T cells were not screwed to one preferential subset after in vitro expansion, suggesting that in vitro expanded γδ T cells with anti-mouse TCRγδ antibodies plus IL-2 were still representative of in vivo subsets of γδ T cells. Expanded Vγ1⁺ and Vγ4⁺ γδ T cells were then sorted by FACS with PE-conjugated anti-mouse TCR Vγ1.1/Cr4 antibody and APC conjugated anti-mouse TCR Vγ2

antibody. We found the purities of sorted Vγ1⁺ and Vγ4⁺ γδ T cells were more than 99% (Figure 1B).

cDNA library preparation for RNA sequencing from resting and activated Vγ1⁺ and Vγ4⁺ γδ T cells

In order to compare gene expression profiles between subsets in both the resting and activated state, sorted cells were rested overnight at 37°C then stimulated 4 h with either PBS (control) or 20 ng/ml of PMA+0.5 μg/ml of Ionomycin (activated) before mRNA extraction and fragmentation. After cDNA synthesis, adapter ligation and PCR amplification, four cDNA libraries were constructed for the resting and activated γδ T cell subsets. 400–500 bp-sized products were used for cluster generation and 36 bp single-end sequencing was performed by using Illumina HiSeq 2000 Sequencer. Approximately 28 million clean reads were obtained from each sample. More than 88% of reads were mapped to the mouse genome using the default setting in TopHat, suggesting high quality of RNA-seq (Table 2). Cufflinks with default settings were used to assemble the mapped reads against the ENSEMBL gene structure annotation, and estimated expression levels for each transcript. More than 18,286 genes were detected. 25.4–26.1% of genes showed expression levels changed by at least four fold while the majority of genes changed less than four fold (Figure 2, Dataset S1).

Differential gene expression between Vγ1⁺ and Vγ4⁺ γδ T cells

RNA-seq results show Vγ1⁺ and Vγ4⁺ γδ T cells share similar transcript profiles in both the resting and activated subsets. We identified 24 transcripts with differential expression between the

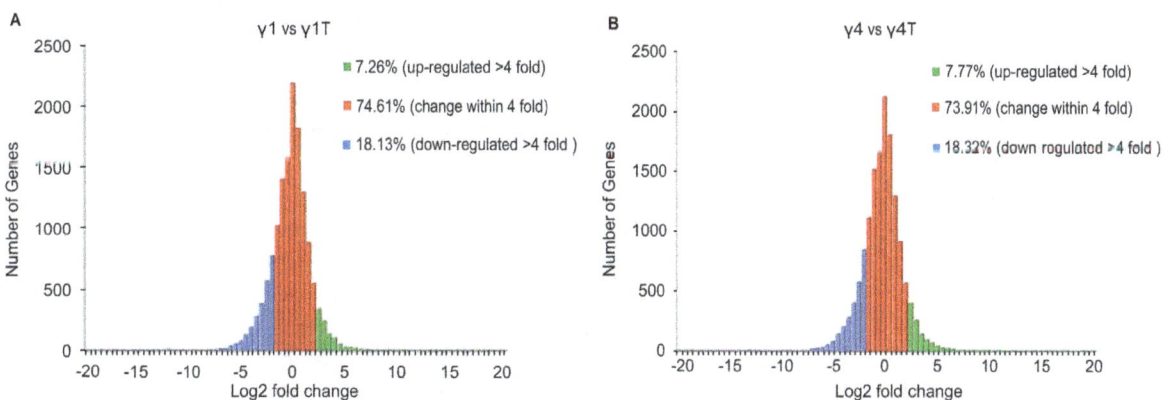

Figure 2. The distribution of gene expression. The 'x' axis represents Log fold-change of differentially expressed genes. The 'y' axis represents number of genes. Red region represents genes with expression within 4-fold change; green and blue regions represent genes with more than 4-fold change either up or down regulated, respectively. Library pairs: A, resting Vγ1⁺ vs activated Vγ1⁺ γδ T cells; B, resting Vγ4⁺ vs activated Vγ4⁺ γδ T cells.

resting Vγ1$^+$ and Vγ4$^+$ γδ T cells (Table 3). We used the Database for Annotation, Visualization and Integrated Discovery (DAVID), an on-line functional annotation tool for gene enrichment analysis, to gain further insight into biological pathways associated with the differentially expressed gene transcripts. We found most of the differentially expressed genes in the resting subsets related to chemokines, transcription and the plasma membrane (Table 3). Resting Vγ1$^+$ γδ T cells expressed higher levels of XCL1 and CCL1 compared with Vγ4$^+$ γδ T cells, suggesting Vγ1$^+$ γδ T cells possess higher chemotactic activity for lymphocytes and monocytes. Vγ4$^+$ γδ T cells displayed higher levels of *Rorc*, *Sox13* and *Scart2* expression. In addition, high levels of *Bclaf1* and *Atf2* were expressed in Vγ4$^+$ γδ T cells while *Arnt2*, *Hmga1* and *Zfp386* were preferentially expressed in Vγ1$^+$ γδ T cells.

In the PMA/Ionomycin-activated Vγ1$^+$ and Vγ4$^+$ γδ T cells, we found 20 differentially expressed genes, most of which are related to cytokines, cell differentiation, transcription and translation (Table 4). Activated Vγ1$^+$ γδ T cells expressed higher levels of IL-4 and IL-5. Vγ4$^+$ γδ T cells secreted more IL-17A and IL-17F. Alternatively spliced transcript variants *Smurf1*, *Pphln1*, *Ilf3* and *Sema6d* were preferentially expressed in Vγ4$^+$ γδ T cells. Vγ1$^+$ γδ T cells preferentially expressed *Bcl11b*, *Hmga1* and a

second spliced transcript variant of *Sema6d*. These results taken together indicate that a very small number of genes are sufficient to define the characteristics of these two subsets of γδ T cells.

Validation of differentially expressed genes in Vγ1$^+$ and Vγ4$^+$ γδ T cells

We measured expression levels in both subsets by PCR to verify whether the genes identified via RNA-sequencing were differentially expressed in Vγ1$^+$ and Vγ4$^+$ γδ T cells. Several genes from both subsets were randomly selected for verification (Figure 3). Consistent with the RNA-seq results, *Scart2* mRNA was only detectable in Vγ4$^+$ γδ T cells (Figure 3E). Real-time quantitative PCR confirmed that expression levels of IL-4 and IL-5 mRNA were significantly higher in PMA/Ionomycin-activated Vγ1$^+$ γδ T cells compared with activated Vγ4$^+$ γδ T cells (Figure 3A and 3B), whereas the expression levels of IL-17A and IL-17F mRNA were significantly higher in activated Vγ4$^+$ γδ T cells (Figure 3C and 3D). ELISA results confirmed that IL-4 was mainly expressed in activated Vγ1$^+$ γδ T cells whereas IL-17 was predominately expressed in activated Vγ4$^+$ γδ T cells (Figure 4A and 4B). Together, all of the genes randomly selected for expression

Table 3. 24 transcripts expressed differently between resting Vγ1$^+$ and Vγ4$^+$ γδ T cells.

Category	GN	AN	γ1 RPKM	γ4 RPKM	Gene function
Chemokine					
	XCL1	NM_008510	340.582	59.158	Chemotactic activity
	CCL1	NM_011329	84.8039	11.7718	Chemotactic activity
Transcription					
	*BCLAF1	NM_001025392	0.10265	8.85303	Transcriptional repressor
	RORC	NM_011281	0.0844492	0.761408	Orphan nuclear receptor
	SOX13	NM_011439	0.909818	4.99875	Ttranscription factor
	*ATF2	NM_009715	0.702722	4.69872	Transcriptional activator
	*ARNT2	NM_007488	0.799234	0.135113	Recognizes xenobiotic response element (XRE)
	*HMGA1	NM_001039356	5.3784	0.84425	Regulation of inducible gene transcription
	*ZFP386	NM_019565	20.4163	0.927052	Transcriptional regulation
Plasma membrane					
	*CD74	NM_001042605	3.99813	0.540024	Antigen processing
	*CTC1	NM_001013256	0.062176	6.89298	Uncharacterized
	*ABI1	NM_145994	0.0359843	6.83637	Cytoskeletal reorganization and EGFR signaling
	*CACNB3	NM_001044741	0.410331	4.17596	The beta subunit of calcium channels
	*SYT13	NM_183369	1.88579	0.141228	Vesicle trafficking
	*SLC17A6	NM_080853	0.80135	0.0264333	Mediates the uptake of glutamate
	*TMEM219	NM_028389	0.071877	43.5973	Unknown
Miscellaneous					
	SCART2	NM_175533	0.22478	3.02098	Scavenger receptor
	*SENP7	NM_001003972	0.178749	7.79658	Protease
	*ENTPD5	NM_007647	8.35339	0.00516434	Promote reglycosylation
	*FAR1	NM_026143	0.900286	6.64512	Fatty Acyl CoA Reductase 1
	*GOLGA2	NM_133852	0.942965	7.61176	Maintaining cis-Golgi structure
	*ITIH5	NM_172471	2.98889	0.530132	Tumor suppressor
	*PPHLN1	NM_001083114	4.76635	0.114948	Epidermal integrity and barrier formation
	*BC003331	NM_001077237	5.03977	0.527241	LAG1-Interacting Protein

GN, Gene name; AN, Accession Number; γ1 RPKM, the RPKM value of gene in resting Vγ1$^+$ γδ T cells; γ4 RPKM, the RPKM value of gene in resting Vγ4$^+$ γδ T cells; "*", Gene's alternatively spliced transcript variants.

Table 4. 20 transcripts expressed differently between activated Vγ1$^+$ and Vγ4$^+$ γδ T cells.

Category	GN	AN	γ1 RPKM	γ4 RPKM	Gene function
Cytokine					
	IL-17A	NM_010552	0.360943	5.13468	Inflammation
	IL-17F	NM_145856	0.0597255	2.86449	Inflammation
	IL −4	NM_021283	3.25878	0.126145	B-cell activation
	IL- 5	NM_010558	3.89427	0.355691	Differentiation of late-developing B-cells
Cell differentiation					
	*BCL11B	NM_021399	0.980076	0.0949643	Regulator of thymocyte development
	SCART2	NM_175533	0.064865	0.562434	Scavenger receptor
	*SMURF1	NM_029438	0.00711406	6.66404	E3 ubiquitin-protein ligase
	*PPHLN1	NM_175363	0.0117361	8.20294	Epidermal integrity and barrier formation
	*SEMA6D	NM_199238	0.18461	6.73579	Neuronal connections
	*SEMA6D	NM_199240	3.96619	0.503894	Neuronal connections
Transcription/Translation					
	*HMGA1	NM_001039356	5.04288	0.0149135	Regulation of inducible gene transcription
	*ILF3	NM_001042707	0.0338755	6.4809	Regulate gene expression
	*ZFP692	NM_001040686	0.0424843	5.96934	Transcriptional regulation
	*GM5633	XM_001480560	27.59	0.0958007	mRNA turnover and ribosome assembly
	*TXNL4A	NM_001042408	0.577893	19.5602	Pre-mRNA splicing
Miscellaneous					
	*DCUN1D2	NM_001042651	0.459734	3.03555	DCN1-Like Protein 2
	*GNAS	NR_003258	23.7675	2.81557	G protein α subunit
	*CEACAM1	NM_001039186	0.870669	0.0859013	Immunoglobulin per family
	*NOLC1	NM_001039353	2.11695	18.0875	Lipid transporter activity
	*PLEC	NM_201392	0.00166738	1.77384	Intermediate Filament Binding Protein
	*SYTL3	NM_183369	0.146591	4.75764	Vesicle trafficking

GN, Gene name; AN, Accession Number; γ1 RPKM, the RPKM value of gene in activated Vγ1$^+$ γδ T cells; γ4 RPKM, the RPKM value of gene in activated Vγ4$^+$ γδ T cells; "*", Gene's alternatively spliced transcript variants.

analysis were consistent with RNA-seq results, confirming differential expression in Vγ1$^+$ and Vγ4$^+$ γδ T cells.

Gene expression in the resting compared with PMA/Ionomycin-activated state

PMA/Ionomycin treatment induces a robust non-TCR mediated response in γδ T cells [18]. As expected, we found both Vγ1$^+$ and Vγ4$^+$ γδ T cells responded robustly to PMA/Ionomycin treatment, as reflected in the total number of genes that significantly changed in each subset. 1,995 transcripts were differentially expressed between the resting and activated Vγ1$^+$ γδ T cells, with 560 up-regulated and 1435 down-regulated genes (q<0.05) (Figure 5A, Dataset S2). 2,158 transcripts were differentially expressed between resting and activated Vγ4$^+$ γδ T cells, with 622 up-regulated and 1536 down-regulated genes (q<0.05) (Figure 5A,Dataset S3). For a global perspective on gene dynamics, two heat maps of the 1,995 and 2,158 differentially expressed gene transcripts were generated using hierarchical clustering analysis (Figure 5B).

DAVID functional annotation clustering analysis showed the 1,995 transcripts identified via activation of Vγ1$^+$ γδ T cells were enriched for 32 KEGG pathways (p<0.05) (Table 5). 2,158 transcripts identified via activation of Vγ4$^+$ γδ T cells were enriched for 29 KEGG pathways (p<0.05) (Table 6). Our comparison of the KEGG pathways between the two subsets showed they share most of the same signal pathways including cytokine-cytokine receptor interaction, Jak-STAT signaling pathway, hematopoietic cell lineage, apoptosis, and pathways in cancer. Interestingly, both Vγ1$^+$ and Vγ4$^+$ γδ T cells showed connections to the intestinal immune network for IgA production, biosynthesis of unsaturated fatty acids, glycosphingolipid biosynthesis, glutathione metabolism, and purine and pyrimidine metabolism.

We analyzed the expression levels of some common representative markers in resting Vγ1$^+$ and Vγ4$^+$ γδ T cells (Table 7). Both subsets expressed high levels of the β and γ chains in the cytokine receptor genes IL-2R, IL-7R and interferon gamma receptor 1. We measured medium expression levels of interferon (alpha and beta) receptor 1 and 2, α and β chains of IL-10R, IL-18 receptor 1,

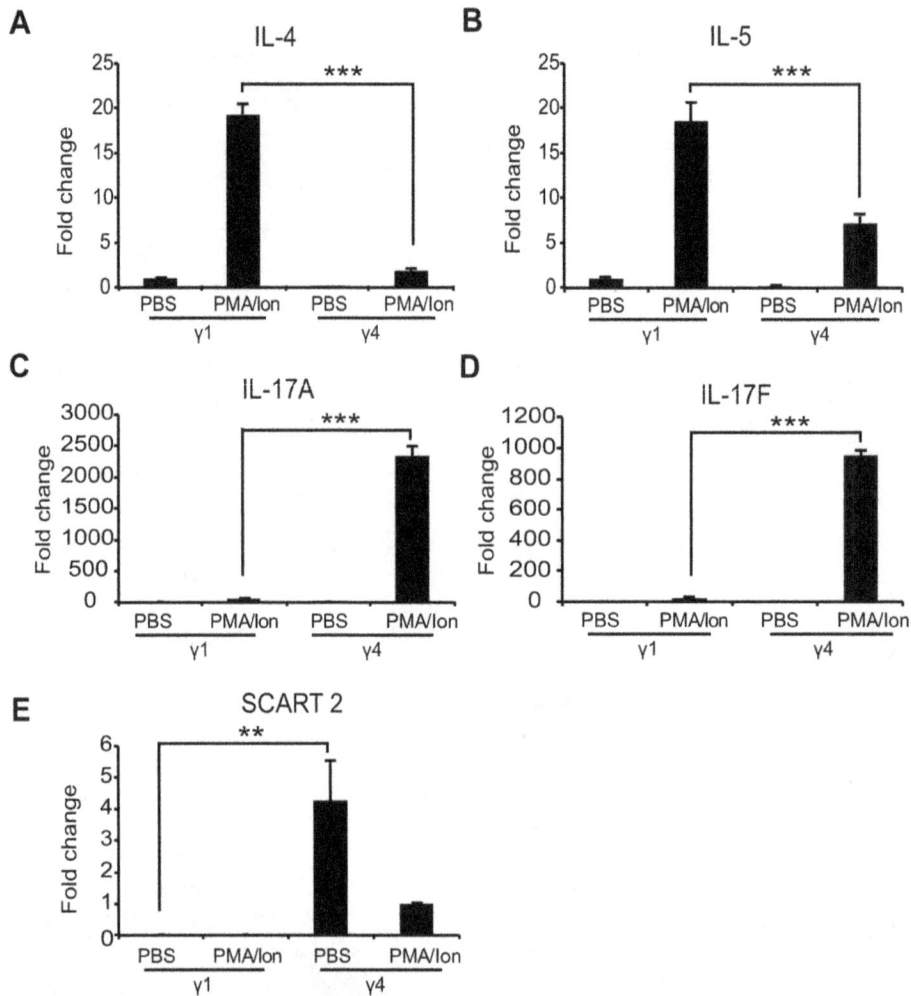

Figure 3. Gene verification with real-time quantitative PCR. Several genes from Vγ1⁺ and Vγ4⁺ γδ T cells were selected for verification against biological replicates using real-time quantitative PCR (A-E). Expression data for each gene were normalized against β-actin. Data shown are the means ± SD (error bars). (* p≤0.05, ** p≤0.01, *** p≤0.001, unpaired two-tailed Student's t-test). Data are representative of three independent experiments.

IL-18 receptor beta, IL-21R, α chain of IL-27R, beta receptor II of transforming growth factor and IL-4R. Both Vγ1⁺ and Vγ4⁺ γδ T cells expressed high levels of TGF-β, known to down-regulate immune response and a key regulator of T cell and Th17 differentiation [19–21]. Additionally, both Vγ1⁺ and Vγ4⁺ γδ T cells expressed IL-16. In contrast, IFN-γ, TNFα and LTA were expressed at relatively low levels during the resting condition. Several conventional T cell surface antigens were highly expressed in Vγ1⁺ and Vγ4⁺ γδ T cells, including CD2, CD3, CD7, CD27, CD37, CD47, CD48, CD52, CD53, CD82 and CD97. However, some surface markers, including CD25, CD44, and CD69 were expressed at low levels.

Resting Vγ1⁺ and Vγ4⁺ γδ T cells expressed high levels of Fas ligand and the granzymes *Gzma* and *Gzmb*. NK cells associated receptors including NKG2A, CD94 and NKG2D were also highly expressed by both resting subsets (Table 7). Interestingly, several integrins were highly expressed including *Itgb7* (Ly69), *Itgb2* (Cd18), *Itgal* (Cd11a), *Itgae* (Cd103) and *Itgb1* (Cd29) (Table 7). However, none of the TLRs showed high expression levels in either subset. In fact, TLR1, TLR6 and TLR12 were the only three detected, and with very low expression levels.

PMA/Ionomycin treatment activates Vγ1⁺ and Vγ4⁺ γδ T cells, upregulating T cell activation markers CD25, CD69 and CD44 along with several cytokines. Therefore, we analyzed the expression of these representative markers in activated Vγ1⁺ and Vγ4⁺ γδ T cells. As expected, PMA/Ionomycin treatment induced expression of XCL1, CCL3, CCL4, CCL1, IFN-γ, Lta, Csf2, TNF-α, IL-2, *Gzmb* and *Gzmc* (Table 8). MILLIPLEX results further confirmed that both Vγ1⁺ and Vγ4⁺ γδ T cells produced high levels of TNF-α, IL-2 and IFN-γ after PMA/Ionomycin treatment (Figure 4C, 4D and 4E). This is consistent with the hypothesis that γδ T cells acquire a pre-activated status poised to actively transcribe genes related to effector functions. Interestingly, IL-10, a Th1 cytokine down-regulator, was also highly expressed by both Vγ1⁺ and Vγ4⁺ γδ T cells (Table 8).

We analyzed the expression levels of transcription factors related to Th cell differentiation and cytokine secretion (Dataset S4). Both Vγ1⁺ and Vγ4⁺ γδ T cells expressed high levels of *Gata3, T-bet, Eomes, Foxp1, Stat1, Stat3, Stat4, Stat5a, Stat5b, Stat6, Runx3, Irf1, Ikzf1, Ikzf3, Ets1, Junb* and *Batf* at resting condition. After PMA/Ionomycin treatment, the expression levels of *Stat5a* and *Irf4* were upregulated significantly. The expression levels of *T-bet, Eomes, Foxp1, Stat5b, Gfi1* and *Junb* were

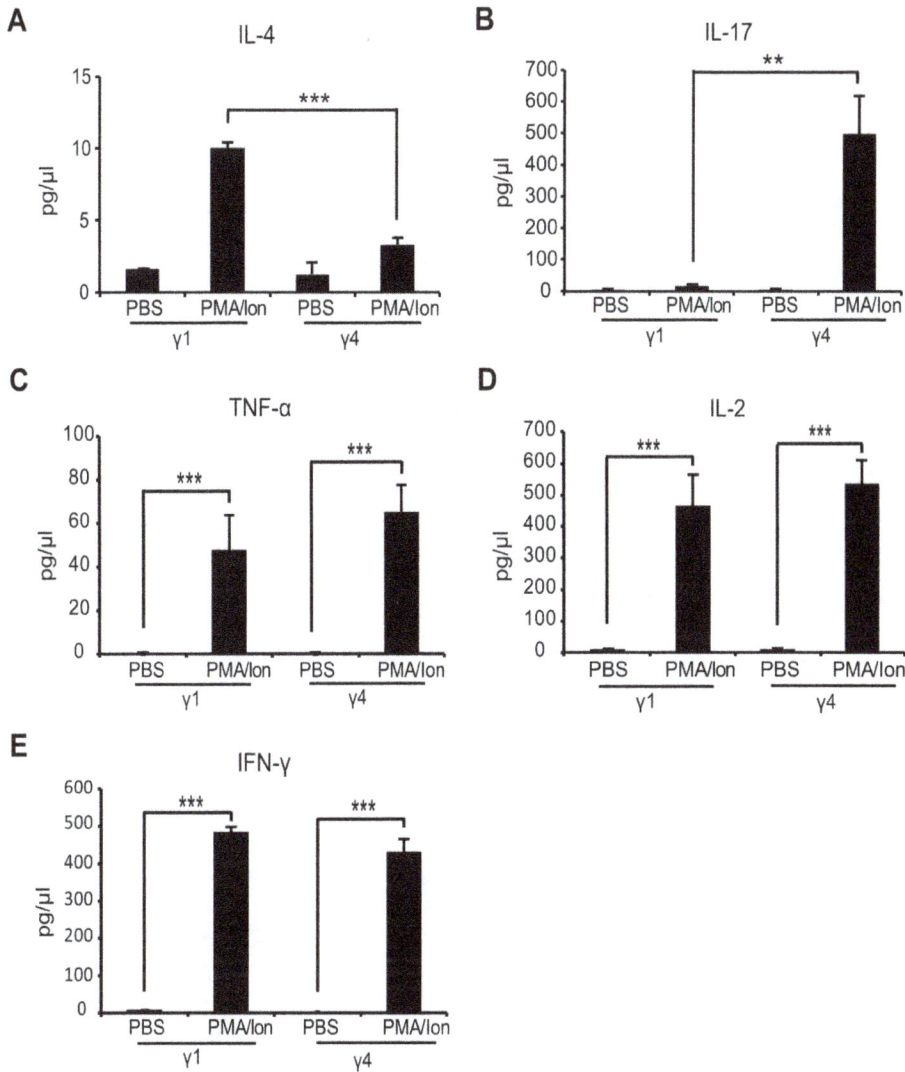

Figure 4. Cytokine expression. ELISA results of (A) IL-4 and (B) IL-17 after PBS or PMA and Ionomycin treatment. MILLIPLEX results of (C) TNF-α, (D) IL-2 and (E) IFN-γ after PBS or PMA and Ionomycin treatment. Data shown are mean ± SD (error bars). (* p≤0.05, ** p≤0.01, *** p≤0.001, unpaired two-tailed Student's t-test). Data are representative of three independent experiments.

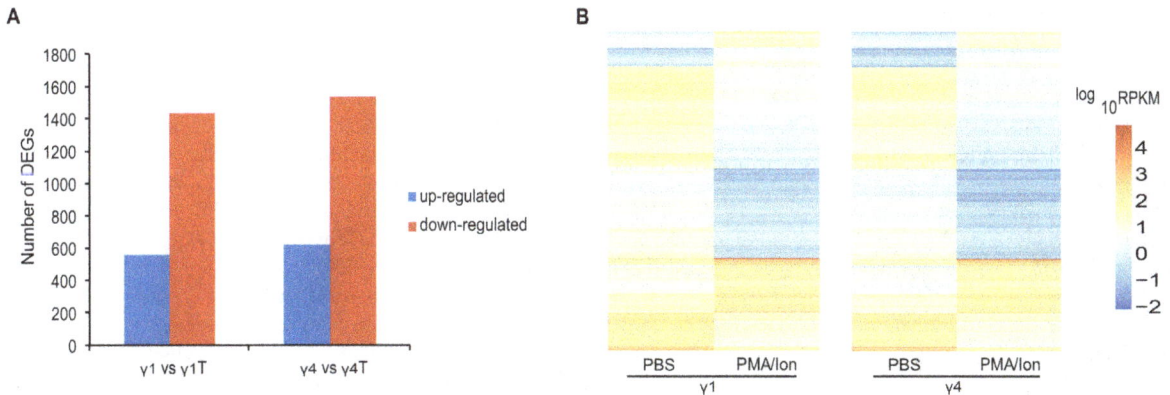

Figure 5. Changes in gene expression profile among Vγ1⁺ and Vγ4⁺ γδ T cells. (A) The number of up and down regulated genes between resting and activated Vγ1⁺ and Vγ4⁺ γδ T cells. (B) Heat maps of 1,995 (Vγ1⁺) and 2,158 (Vγ4⁺) differentially expressed transcripts associated with activated cells using hierarchical clustering analysis. γ1 vs γ1 T, resting Vγ1⁺ vs activated Vγ1⁺ γδ T cells; γ4 vs γ4T, resting Vγ4⁺ vs activated Vγ4⁺ γδ T cells; RPKM, Reads Per Kilo bases per Million reads.

Table 5. Significantly changed genes between resting and activated Vγ1$^+$ γδ T cells enriched for KEGG pathways.

Term	Count	P-Value
Cytokine-cytokine receptor interaction	45	1.50E-05
Jak-STAT signaling pathway	29	3.80E-04
Hematopoietic cell lineage	19	6.80E-04
Glutathione metabolism	14	8.20E-04
Apoptosis	19	1.10E-03
Intestinal immune network for IgA production	14	1.20E-03
Prostate cancer	19	1.60E-03
Small cell lung cancer	18	2.10E-03
Pathways in cancer	46	4.40E-03
p53 signaling pathway	15	4.40E-03
Bladder cancer	11	4.70E-03
Glycosphingolipid biosynthesis	8	5.40E-03
Pyrimidine metabolism	18	7.80E-03
Endometrial cancer	12	8.10E-03
Arrhythmogenic right ventricular cardiomyopathy	15	9.50E-03
Natural killer cell mediated cytotoxicity	21	9.80E-03
One carbon pool by folate	6	1.30E-02
Type I diabetes mellitus	13	1.30E-02
Colorectal cancer	16	1.40E-02
Melanoma	14	1.40E-02
Glioma	13	1.50E-02
Allograft rejection	12	1.80E-02
Chemokine signaling pathway	27	2.00E-02
Phosphatidylinositol signaling system	14	2.20E-02
ABC transporters	10	2.30E-02
Non-small cell lung cancer	11	2.80E-02
Asthma	8	3.10E-02
Insulin signaling pathway	21	3.40E-02
Biosynthesis of unsaturated fatty acids	7	3.70E-02
Fc gamma R-mediated phagocytosis	16	4.10E-02
Graft-versus-host disease	11	4.30E-02
ECM-receptor interaction	14	4.60E-02

Database for Annotation, Visualization and Integrated Discovery (DAVID), was used to analyze biological pathways associated with the differentially expressed gene transcripts. 1,995 transcripts that were identified to be related to the activation of Vγ1$^+$ γδ T cells were enriched for 32 KEGG pathways (p<0.05). KEGG, Kyoto Encyclopedia of Genes and Genomes.

upregulated slightly. Interestingly, the expression levels of *Gata3*, *Irf4* and *Gfi1* were slightly higher in Vγ1$^+$ γδ T cells than Vγ4$^+$ γδ T cells after PMA/Ionomycin treatment.

Taken together, these findings indicate that both Vγ1$^+$ and Vγ4$^+$ γδ T cells maintain phenotypes producing IFN-γ, TNFα, TGF-β and IL-10. However, Vγ1$^+$ γδ T cells tend to produce Th2 type cytokine while Vγ4$^+$ γδ T cells preferentially produce IL-17 (Figure 6).

Discussion

Phylogenetic analysis suggests γδ T cells are precursors to modern B and αβ T cells [22]. γδ T cells are divided into subsets based on composition of T cell receptors. Interestingly, γδ T cell subsets demonstrate bias in carrying out particular functions [1]. Previously, Jutila et al. analyzed gene expression profiles of bovine

CD8$^+$ and CD8$^-$ γδ T cells using microarray and serial analysis of gene expression (SAGE) technology. They concluded inherent gene expression differences in subsets defined their distinct functional responses [23,24]. In addition, Kress et al. found considerable inherent differences in gene expression among subsets of post PMA/Ionomycin or LPS treatment of circulating Vδ1 and Vδ2 subsets in humans [18].

Vγ1$^+$ and Vγ4$^+$ γδ T cells are major subpopulations of peripheral γδ T cells in mice. Although global gene expression profiles of all emergent γδ thymocyte subsets have been reported by the Immunological Genome (ImmGen) Project and much knowledge has been obtained about the early divergence of gene expression programs between different γδ thymocyte subsets [12], a comprehensive gene expression profiles analysis of peripheral Vγ1$^+$ and Vγ4$^+$ γδ T cells isn't available. A major hurdle has been

Table 6. Significantly changed genes between resting and activated Vγ4$^+$ γδ T cells enriched for KEGG pathways.

Term	Count	P-Value
Cytokine-cytokine receptor interaction	50	1.00E-06
Biosynthesis of unsaturated fatty acids	10	8.50E-04
Hematopoietic cell lineage	19	1.30E-03
Intestinal immune network for IgA production	14	2.00E-03
Jak-STAT signaling pathway	28	2.00E-03
Pathways in cancer	49	2.90E-03
Prostate cancer	19	3.00E-03
Small cell lung cancer	18	3.90E-03
Colorectal cancer	18	4.40E-03
Arrhythmogenic right ventricular cardiomyopathy	16	6.50E-03
Glycosphingolipid biosynthesis	8	7.30E-03
p53 signaling pathway	15	7.40E-03
Dilated cardiomyopathy	18	8.80E-03
Apoptosis	17	1.10E-02
Endometrial cancer	12	1.20E-02
Chemokine signaling pathway	29	1.30E-02
Non-small cell lung cancer	12	1.60E-02
One carbon pool by folate	6	1.70E-02
Melanoma	14	2.20E-02
Glioma	13	2.30E-02
Amyotrophic lateral sclerosis (ALS)	12	2.40E-02
Pyrimidine metabolism	17	2.80E-02
Glutathione metabolism	11	3.10E-02
Toll-like receptor signaling pathway	17	3.60E-02
Chronic myeloid leukemia	14	3.70E-02
Purine metabolism	24	3.90E-02
Regulation of actin cytoskeleton	31	4.10E-02
Endocytosis	29	4.50E-02
Type I diabetes mellitus	12	4.60E-02

Database for Annotation, Visualization and Integrated Discovery (DAVID), was used to analyze biological pathways associated with the differentially expressed gene transcripts. 2,158 transcripts that were identified to be related to the activation of Vγ4$^+$ γδ T cells were enriched for 29 KEGG pathways (p<0.05). KEGG, Kyoto Encyclopedia of Genes and Genomes.

the limited number of cells that can be obtained from healthy mice.

In this study, we resolved the limited cell count issue by establishing a primary culture method expanding Vγ1$^+$ and Vγ4$^+$ γδ T cells simultaneously from a single pool of mouse splenocytes. Our results proved that *in vitro* TCR-induced expansion for a week did not significantly change the proportion of Vγ1$^+$ and Vγ4$^+$ γδ T cells. We provide a comprehensive gene expression profile of mouse peripheral Vγ1$^+$ and Vγ4$^+$ γδ T cells in the resting and activated state. Although Vγ1$^+$ and Vγ4$^+$ γδ T cells share similar transcript profiles, we identified subset specific genes defining characteristics of each subset.

We identified 24 transcripts differentially expressed in resting Vγ1$^+$ and Vγ4$^+$ γδ T cells, and 20 transcripts differentially expressed after PMA/Ionomycin treatment. Consistent with γδ thymocytes, expression levels of *Rorc*, *Sox13* and *Scart2* were higher in Vγ4$^+$ γδ T cells compared with Vγ1$^+$ γδ T cells [12]. *Rorc* expression is reported in γδ T cells, Th22 cells, NKT cells, CD4$^+$ CD8$^+$ thymocytes, and others that do not belong to the T or B cell lineage [25–28]. *Rorc* is recognized as a lineage-specific

transcription factor of Th17 and is also required for IL-17 production [29]. Transcription factor *Sox13* serves a general role in the differentiation of γδ T cells [30]. Moreover, Gray et al. reported that *Sox13* was indispensable for the maturation of Vγ4$^+$ Th17 cells [31,32]. Scavenger receptor *Scart2* is a marker of γδ T cells prepared to secrete IL-17A [12,31,33,34]. Our data showing Vγ1$^+$ γδ T cells compared with Vγ1$^+$ γδ T cells produce significantly more IL-17A and IL-17F after PMA/Ionomycin treatment are also consistent with findings in γδ thymocytes [12]. Our findings show Vγ1$^+$ γδ T cells produce significantly more IL-4 and IL-5 after PMA/Ionomycin treatment compared with Vγ4$^+$ γδ T cells. This finding is consistent with earlier reports showing Vγ1$^+$ γδ T cells preferentially produce IL-4, and the depletion of Vγ1$^+$ subset cells increases host resistance against *Listeria monocytogenes* infection [35]. It is important to note that Vγ1$^+$ γδ T cells suppress Vγ4$^+$ γδ T cell mediated antitumor function through IL-4 [36].

Alternative splicing plays an important role in increasing functional diversity of eukaryotes. Compared with the ImmGen Project, one of the advantages of RNA-seq is able to quantify

Table 7. Expression levels for specific genes identified by RNA-seq in both resting Vγ1⁺ and Vγ4⁺ γδ T cells.

Category	Expression levels			
	++++	+++	++	+
Cytokine/chemokine/similar				
	CCL4	XCL1	CCL1	CCR1
	CCL5	Il16	CCL3	CCR10
	CCR2	Ifnar1	CCR7	CCR4
	CCR5	Ifnar2	CXCR4	CCR8
	CXCR3	Il10ra	Csf1	CCRk
	CXCR6	Il10rb	Ifng	CCRl2
	Il2rb	Il18RAP	Tnf	Il18
	Il7R	Il21r	Lta	Tgfb
	Ifngr1	Il27ra	Il12rb1	Il11ra1
	Il2rg	Il4ra	Il15ra	Il15ra
	Tgfb1	TnfrSF1B	Il3ra	Il17rd
		Tgfbr2	Ifnar1	Il1rap
		Il18r1		Il20rb
				Il4i1
Surface antigens				
	Cd2	Cd164	Cd1d1	Cd1d2
	Cd27	Cd247	Cd226	Cd200
	Cd37	Cd96	Cd244	Cd320
	Cd3d	CTLA4	Cd274	Cd38
	Cd3e		Cd28	Cd3eap
	Cd3g		Cd5	Cd55
	Cd47		Cd6	Cd63
	Cd48		Cd68	Cd69
	Cd52		Cd72	Cd74
	Cd53		Cd79b	Cd79a
	Cd7		Cd80	Cd81
	Cd82		Cd84	Cd93
	Cd97		Cd8a	
			Cd8b1	
			Cd9	
			Cd25	
			Cd44	
			Cd62L	
NK cell related				
	Klrc1; NKG2A	KLRK1; NKG2D	Klrb1c; NKRP1A	
	KLRD1; CD94		Klrc2; NKG2C	
	Cd160; BY55		Klrc3; NKG2E	
Integrin				
	ITGB7; Ly69	ITGA4; Cd49D	ITGAX; Cd11c	ITGAD; Cd11d
	ITGB2; Cd18	ITGB3; Cd61	ITGAM; Cd11b	ITGA6; Cd49f
	ITGAL; Cd11a		ITGAV; Cd51	ITGA3; Cd49C
	ITGAE; Cd103			ITGA2; Cd49b
	ITGB1; Cd29			ITGB5
Miscellaneous				
	Gzma	Gzmc	Fasl	Tlr1

Table 7. Cont.

	Expression levels			
Category	++++	+++	++	+
	Gzmb	Gzmk		Tlr12
				Tlr6

According to the expression abundance, transcripts with RPKM value over 1 were divided into 4 categories: "+" (1–10 RPKM), "++"(10–50 RPKM), "+++" (50–100 RPKM), and "++++"(>100 RPKM). RPKM, Reads Per Kilo bases per Million reads.

individual transcript isoforms and identify differentially expressed transcripts between Vγ1$^+$ and Vγ4$^+$ γδ T cells. We found *Bclaf1* and *Atf2* were preferentially expressed in Vγ4$^+$ γδ T cells while *Hmga1* and *Bcl11b* were preferentially expressed in Vγ1$^+$ γδ T cells. As a transcriptional repressor, *Bclaf1* interacts with several members of the *Bcl2* protein family and plays a role in the regulation of apoptosis and DNA repair [37,38]. *Bclaf1* also plays an important role in lymphocyte homeostasis and activation [39]. *Atf2* transcription factor is a member of the leucine zipper family of DNA binding proteins and forms a homodimer or a

Table 8. Expression levels of significantly changed genes identified by RNA-seq in both Vγ1$^+$ and Vγ4$^+$ γδ T cells after PMA/Inomycin treatment.

	Expression levels				
Category	++++	+++	++	+	−
Cytokine/chemokine/similar					
	XCL1	CCL9	CXCR3	CXCL14	CXCR4
	CCL3	Tnfsf11	CCR2	CCR7	CCR8
	CCL4	Il2	Il13	Ifngr1	CCR10
	CCL1	Tnfrsf8	Tnfrsf12a	Tnfaip8l2	CX3CR1
	Ifng	Tnfsf9	Ifnar1	Il10rb	Tnfrsf11b
	Tnfrsf9		Vegfa	Il1rl1	Tnfrsf23
	Lta			Il1r2	Tnfrsf26
	Csf2			Ifnar2	Tgfb1i1
	Tnfa			Il16	Il11ra1
	Tnfsf14			Il10ra	Tnfrsf13c
	Tnfrsf4			Il1rap	Tnfsf12
	Il10			Il7r	Il17rd
				Il1rl1	il-18
				Il33	
				Tnfaip8l1	
Surface antigens					
	Cd44	Cd274	Cd63	Cd83	Cd1d1
	Cd25	Cd7	Cd96	Cd24a	Cd200r1
		Cd69	Cd320	Cd79b	Cd79a
			Cd70	Cd93	Cd1d2
					Cd200r4
					Cd55
NK cell related					
			KLRD1	Klrb1c	Klrb1d
Miscellaneous					
	Gzmb		Gzme	Gzmk	Tlr1
	Gzmc		Gzmf		Tlr6
					Tlr12

According to the expression abundance, transcripts were divided into 5 categories: "−" (<1 RPKM), "+" (1–10 RPKM), "++"(10–50 RPKM), "+++" (50–100 RPKM), and "++++"(>100 RPKM). RPKM, Reads Per Kilo bases per Million reads.

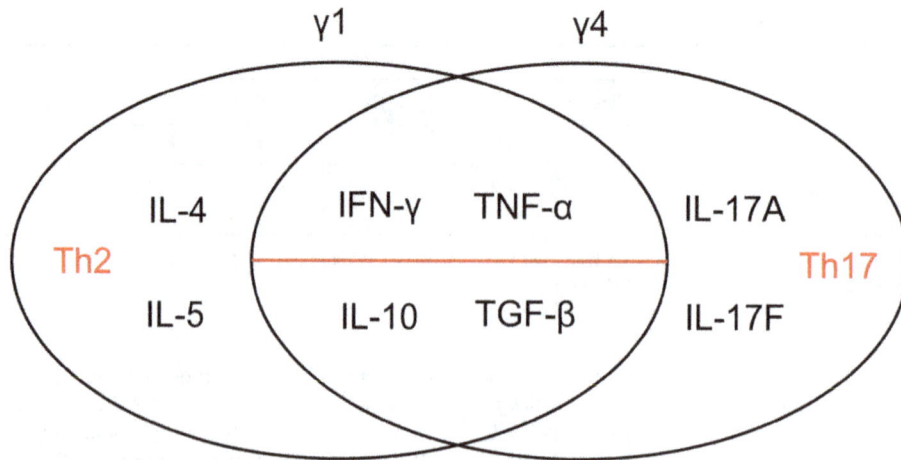

Figure 6. Cytokines secreted by Vγ1⁺ and Vγ4⁺ γδ T cells. Both subsets of γδ T cells produce IFN-γ, TNFα, TGF-β and IL-10. Vγ1+ γδ T cells tend to produce Th2 type cytokines IL-4 and IL-5 while Vγ4⁺ γδ T cells tend to produce IL-17.

heterodimer with *c-Jun*, stimulating cAMP responsive element (CRE) dependent transcription. *Atf2* expression is lower in CD8⁺ T cells compared with CD4⁺ T cells, a functional explanation to the differential response to glucocorticoids between CD8⁺ and CD4⁺ T cells [40]. As an architectural chromatin factor, *Hmga1* binds preferentially to the minor groove of AT rich regions in double stranded DNA. It is involved in many cellular processes including regulation of inducible gene transcription, insulin resistance, diabetes and malignant transformation [41,42]. Nakao et al. revealed a new role for *Hmga1* in transcriptional silencing in T cell lineages and leukemic cells [43]. However, the roles of *Bclaf1*, *Atf2* and *Hmga1* in γδ T cells have not been reported. *Bcl11b* is a T-cell specific gene and required for T-lineage commitment. Aberrant expression of *Bcl11b* contributes to human T-ALL [44]. In contrast with ImmGen Project results showing *Bcl11b* was preferentially expressed in Vγ4⁺ γδ thymocytes [12], we identified one transcript isoform of *Bcl11b* preferentially expressed in activated Vγ1⁺ γδ T cells. The role of the transcript isoform of *Bcl11b* in Vγ1⁺ γδ T cells needs further study.

Many of the differentially expressed gene transcripts identified in activated Vγ1⁺ and Vγ4⁺ γδ T cells shared similar signaling pathways. We found higher expression of IL-4 and IL-5 in activated Vγ1⁺ γδ T cells. This suggests a role in asthma given that Vγ4⁺ γδ T cells suppress airway hyperresponsiveness, compared with Vγ1⁺ γδ T cells that enhance airway hyperresponsiveness and raise levels of Th2 cytokines and eosinophils infiltration in the airways [8,9,45].

Both resting Vγ1⁺ and Vγ4⁺ γδ T cells exhibited high levels of transcripts for several chemokines and chemokine receptors, including CCL4, CCL5, CCR2, CCR5 and CXCR3. These data highlight the role of Vγ1⁺ and Vγ4⁺ γδ T cells in immunoregulatory and inflammatory processes. For example, CCL4 (MIP-1beta) and CCL5 (RANTES) are both Th1-associated chemokines that bind to CCR5. Up-regulation of CCR5 ligands may play a role in the recruitment process of blood monocytes, memory T helper cells and eosinophils. CCR2 is expressed on both Vγ1⁺ and Vγ4⁺ γδ T cells, and is necessary for the accumulation of γδ TILs to the tumor bed [46]. It is interesting to note that CXCR6 was previously thought to be expressed in human Vδ2 cells, but not Vδ1 cells [18]. However, we found high CXCR6 levels in both Vγ1⁺ and Vγ4⁺ γδ T cells. CXCR6 plays a critical role in NK cell memory of haptens and viruses [47]. Whether CXCR6 plays a

role in Vγ1⁺ and Vγ4⁺ γδ T memory cells needs further examination.

Integrins play key roles in immune responses, leukocyte trafficking and many human diseases. Most integrin related research has been focused on αβ T cells, with little published on γδ T cells. Our results show several integrins were highly expressed in Vγ1⁺ and Vγ4⁺ γδ T cells. For example, *Itgae* (Cd103), implicated in epithelial T cell retention, is highly expressed on Vγ1⁺ and Vγ4⁺ γδ T cells [48]. *Itgae* contributes to clustering and activation of Vγ 5 TCRs expressed by epidermal T cells [49]. Signals mediated by integrins play important roles in the activation of T cells [50]. Therefore, we suggest stimulating integrin expression provides a costimulation signal, increasing the sensitivity of γδ T cell activation.

PMA/Ionomycin induces a robust non-TCR mediated response in Vγ1⁺ and Vγ4⁺ γδ T cells. We show after PMA/Ionomycin treatment several activation markers of T cells were upregulated including CD25, CD69 and CD44, along with most cytokine genes in both subsets. In addition, activated Vγ1⁺ and Vγ4⁺ γδ T cells produced high levels of XCL1, CCL3, CCL4, CCL1, IFN-γ, TNFα, Lta, Csf2 and IL-10. IFN-γ and TNFα are Th1 type cytokines. Previous reports show Vγ4⁺ γδ T cells are the major γδ T subset producing IFN-γ, and they steer CD4⁺ T cells toward a dominant Th1 cell response [7,51,52]. Moreover, He et al. reported that CD44 rich Vγ4⁺ γδ T cells produced significantly more IFN-γ compared with Vγ1⁺ γδ T cells, partly due to the high expression level of eomesodermin [16]. In contrast, Matsuzaki et al. reported that Vγ1⁺ γδ T cells were the major γδ T subset producing IFN-γ in response to *L. monocytogenes* infection [53]. The opposing results are likely due to different disease models and treatment methods. A separate study reported higher levels of IL-10 in human Vδ1 cells compared with Vδ2 cells [18]. However, our results show both Vγ1⁺ and Vγ4⁺ γδ T cells produce high levels of IL-10.

Narayan et al. reported that Vγ4⁺ γδ thymocytes expressed high levels of *Stat4*, *Maf*, *Gata3* and *Eomes* compared with Vγ1⁺ γδ thymocytes [12]. However, our results show both Vγ1⁺ and Vγ4⁺ γδ T cells expressed high levels of these transcription factors and the levels of *Gata3* were slightly higher in Vγ1⁺ γδ T cells compared with Vγ4⁺ γδ T cells after PMA/Ionomycin treatment. *Gata3* is critical for Th2 cell differentiation and required for IL-4 production. The higher level of *Gata3* expression in Vγ1⁺ γδ T cells is consistent with the phenotype of Vγ1$^+$ γδ T cells producing more IL-4 than Vγ4$^+$ γδ T cells. T-bet is a major factor for Th1 cell differentiation and IFN-γ production [54]. *Eomes* is also involved in Th1 differentiation and IFN-γ production [55]. The upregulation of *T-bet* and *Eomes* is consistent with the phenotype of both Vγ1$^+$ and Vγ4$^+$ γδ T cells that produce high levels of IFN-γ. The difference between our results with the ImmGen Project may be due to the source of γδ T cells. The cells used in the ImmGen Project are γδ thymocytes, however the cells in our study were peripheral γδ T cells derived from the spleen.

Taken together, this study shows both Vγ1$^+$ and Vγ4$^+$ γδ T cells maintain inflammatory and regulatory phenotypes. Both demonstrate an inflammatory cell phenotype via IFN-γ and TNFα expression. And, both display a regulatory cell phenotype via TGF-β and IL-10 production. Vγ1$^+$ γδ T cells produced more Th2 type cytokines, while Vγ4$^+$ γδ T cells tended to produce more IL-17. Thus, Th2 type cytokines may explain how Vγ1$^+$ γδ T cells affect anti-inflammatory functions in different infection models, and describe the enhancing effect on airway hyperresponsiveness (AHR) [56]. IL-17 cytokines support the pro-inflammatory function of Vγ4$^+$ γδ T cells in the infection models and the inhibitory effect on airway hyperresponsiveness (AHR). Although this study was performed in Vγ1$^+$ and Vγ4$^+$ γδ T cells expanded *in vitro*, which may not fully represent the true status of Vγ1$^+$ and Vγ4$^+$ γδ T cells *in vivo*, our results support the hypothesis that distinct γδ TCR types direct cells to acquire a certain type of functional programming during thymic development [57].

Complementary to the ImmGen Project, this report provides a comprehensive gene expression profile of mouse peripheral Vγ1$^+$ and Vγ4$^+$ γδ T cells following PMA/Ionomycin treatment. Although both γδ T cell populations have similar transcript profiles, subset-specific transcripts define distinct characteristics and describe the inherent differences between Vγ1$^+$ and Vγ4$^+$ γδ T cells.

Acknowledgments

We thank Fang Hua, Yuli Zhu and Dan Wu for technical assistance and helpful discussion. We thank the flow cytometry facility at the Peking University Health Science Center for cell sorting and data analysis support.

Author Contributions

Conceived and designed the experiments: WH SZ JZ PD. Performed the experiments: PD SZ MC. Analyzed the data: WH PD LC. Contributed reagents/materials/analysis tools: PD SZ NK YH. Contributed to the writing of the manuscript: WH JZ PD.

References

1. Bonneville M, O'Brien RL, Born WK (2010) γδ T cell effector functions: a blend of innate programming and acquired plasticity. Nature Reviews Immunology 10: 467–478.
2. Kaufmann S (1996) gamma/delta and other unconventional T lymphocytes: what do they see and what do they do? Proceedings of the National Academy of Sciences 93: 2272–2279.
3. Carding SR, Egan PJ (2002) γδ T cells: functional plasticity and heterogeneity. Nature reviews immunology 2: 336–345.
4. Welte T, Lamb J, Anderson JF, Born WK, O'Brien RL, et al. (2008) Role of two distinct γδ T cell subsets during West Nile virus infection. FEMS Immunology & Medical Microbiology 53: 275–283.
5. Gerber DJ, Azuara V, Levraud J-P, Huang SY, Lembezat M-P, et al. (1999) IL-4-producing γδ T cells that express a very restricted TCR repertoire are preferentially localized in liver and spleen. The Journal of Immunology 163: 3076–3082.
6. Huber S, Shi C, Budd RC (2002) γδ T cells promote a Th1 response during coxsackievirus B3 infection in vivo: role of Fas and Fas ligand. Journal of virology 76: 6487–6494.
7. Huber S, Sartini D, Exley M (2002) Vγ4+ T cells promote autoimmune CD8+ cytolytic T-lymphocyte activation in coxsackievirus B3-induced myocarditis in mice: role for CD4+ Th1 cells. Journal of virology 76: 10785–10790.
8. Hahn Y-S, Taube C, Jin N, Sharp L, Wands J, et al. (2004) Different potentials of γδ T cell subsets in regulating airway responsiveness: Vγ1 cells, but not Vγ4+ cells, promote airway hyperreactivity, Th2 cytokines, and airway inflammation. The Journal of Immunology 172: 2894–2902.
9. Hahn Y-S, Taube C, Jin N, Takeda K, Park J-W, et al. (2003) Vγ4+ γδ T cells regulate airway hyperreactivity to methacholine in ovalbumin-sensitized and challenged mice. The Journal of Immunology 171: 3170–3178.
10. Tramonti D, Andrew EM, Rhodes K, Newton DJ, Carding SR (2006) Evidence for the opposing roles of different γδ T cell subsets in macrophage homeostasis. European journal of immunology 36: 1729–1738.
11. Huang Y, Jin N, Roark CL, Aydintug MK, Wands J, et al. (2009) The influence of IgE-enhancing and IgE-suppressive γδ T cells changes with exposure to inhaled ovalbumin. The Journal of Immunology 183: 849–855.
12. Narayan K, Sylvia KE, Malhotra N, Yin CC, Martens G, et al. (2012) Intrathymic programming of effector fates in three molecularly distinct [gamma][delta] T cell subtypes. Nature immunology 13: 511–518.
13. Kang N, Tang L, Li X, Wu D, Li W, et al. (2009) Identification and characterization of Foxp3< sup>+</ sup> γδ T cells in mouse and human. Immunology letters 125: 105–113.
14. Benjamini Y, Hochberg Y (1995) Controlling the false discovery rate: a practical and powerful approach to multiple testing. Journal of the Royal Statistical Society Series B (Methodological): 289–300.
15. Kong Y, Cao W, Xi X, Ma C, Cui L, et al. (2009) The NKG2D ligand ULBP4 binds to TCRγ9/δ2 and induces cytotoxicity to tumor cells through both TCRγδ and NKG2D. Blood 114: 310–317.
16. He W, Hao J, Dong S, Gao Y, Tao J, et al. (2010) Naturally activated Vγ4 γδ T cells play a protective role in tumor immunity through expression of eomesodermin. The Journal of Immunology 185: 126–133.
17. Zhao N, Hao J, Ni Y, Luo W, Liang R, et al. (2011) Vγ4 γδ T cell-derived IL-17A negatively regulates NKT cell function in Con A-induced fulminant hepatitis. The Journal of Immunology 187: 5007–5014.
18. Kress E, Hedges JF, Jutila MA (2006) Distinct gene expression in human Vδ1 and Vδ2 γδ T cells following non-TCR agonist stimulation. Molecular Immunology 43: 2002–2011.
19. Chen W, Jin W, Hardegen N, Lei K-j, Li L, et al. (2003) Conversion of peripheral CD4+ CD25− naive T cells to CD4+ CD25+ regulatory T cells by TGF-β induction of transcription factor Foxp3. The Journal of experimental medicine 198: 1875–1886.
20. Mangan PR, Harrington LE, O'Quinn DB, Helms WS, Bullard DC, et al. (2006) Transforming growth factor-β induces development of the TH17 lineage. Nature 441: 231–234.
21. Veldhoen M, Hocking RJ, Atkins CJ, Locksley RM, Stockinger B (2006) TGFβ in the context of an inflammatory cytokine milieu supports de novo differentiation of IL-17-producing T cells. Immunity 24: 179–189.
22. Richards M, Nelson J (2000) The evolution of vertebrate antigen receptors: a phylogenetic approach. Molecular biology and evolution 17: 146–155.
23. Hedges JF, Cockrell D, Jackiw L, Meissner N, Jutila MA (2003) Differential mRNA expression in circulating γδ T lymphocyte subsets defines unique tissue-specific functions. Journal of leukocyte biology 73: 306–314.
24. Meissner N, Radke J, Hedges JF, White M, Behnke M, et al. (2003) Serial analysis of gene expression in circulating γδ T cell subsets defines distinct immunoregulatory phenotypes and unexpected gene expression profiles. The Journal of Immunology 170: 356–364.
25. Duhen T, Geiger R, Jarrossay D, Lanzavecchia A, Sallusto F (2009) Production of interleukin 22 but not interleukin 17 by a subset of human skin-homing memory T cells. Nature immunology 10: 857–863.
26. Eberl G, Marmon S, Sunshine M-J, Rennert PD, Choi Y, et al. (2004) An essential function for the nuclear receptor RORγt in the generation of fetal lymphoid tissue inducer cells. Nature immunology 5: 64–73.

27. Jetten AM (2009) Retinoid-related orphan receptors (RORs): critical roles in development, immunity, circadian rhythm, and cellular metabolism. Nucl Recept Signal 7.

28. Trifari S, Kaplan CD, Tran EH, Crellin NK, Spits H (2009) Identification of a human helper T cell population that has abundant production of interleukin 22 and is distinct from TH-17, TH1 and TH2 cells. Nature immunology 10: 864–871.

29. Ivanov II, McKenzie BS, Zhou L, Tadokoro CE, Lepelley A, et al. (2006) The Orphan Nuclear Receptor RORγt Directs the Differentiation Program of Proinflammatory IL-17< sup>+</sup> T Helper Cells. Cell 126: 1121–1133.

30. Melichar HJ, Narayan K, Der SD, Hiraoka Y, Gardiol N, et al. (2007) Regulation of γδ Versus αß T Lymphocyte Differentiation by the Transcription Factor SOX13. Science 315: 230–233.

31. Gray EE, Ramírez-Valle F, Xu Y, Wu S, Wu Z, et al. (2013) Deficiency in IL-17-committed V [gamma] 4+[gamma][delta] T cells in a spontaneous Sox13-mutant CD45. 1+ congenic mouse substrain provides protection from dermatitis. Nature immunology 14: 584–592.

32. Malhotra N, Narayan K, Cho OH, Sylvia KE, Yin C, et al. (2013) A network of high-mobility group box transcription factors programs innate interleukin-17 production. Immunity 38: 681–693.

33. Kisielow J, Kopf M, Karjalainen K (2008) SCART scavenger receptors identify a novel subset of adult γδ T cells. The Journal of Immunology 181: 1710–1716.

34. Ribot JC, Pang DJ, Neves JF, Peperzak V, Roberts SJ, et al. (2009) CD27 is a thymic determinant of the balance between interferon-γ-and interleukin 17–producing γδ T cell subsets. Nature immunology 10: 427–436.

35. O'Brien RL, Yin X, Huber SA, Ikuta K, Born WK (2000) Depletion of a γδ T cell subset can increase host resistance to a bacterial infection. The Journal of Immunology 165: 6472–6479.

36. Hao J, Dong S, Xia S, He W, Jia H, et al. (2011) Regulatory role of Vγ1 γδ T cells in tumor immunity through IL-4 production. The Journal of Immunology 187: 4979–4986.

37. Liu H, Lu Z-G, Miki Y, Yoshida K (2007) Protein kinase C δ induces transcription of the TP53 tumor suppressor gene by controlling death-promoting factor Btf in the apoptotic response to DNA damage. Molecular and cellular biology 27: 8480–8491.

38. Lee Y, Yu Y, Gunawardena H, Xie L, Chen X (2012) BCLAF1 is a radiation-induced H2AX-interacting partner involved in γH2AX-mediated regulation of apoptosis and DNA repair. Cell death & disease 3: e359.

39. McPherson JP, Sarras H, Lemmers B, Tamblyn L, Migon E, et al. (2009) Essential role for Bclaf1 in lung development and immune system function. Cell Death & Differentiation 16: 331–339.

40. Li L-b, Leung DY, Strand MJ, Goleva E (2007) ATF2 impairs glucocorticoid receptor–mediated transactivation in human CD8+ T cells. Blood 110: 1570–1577.

41. Fedele M, Fidanza V, Battista S, Pentimalli F, Klein-Szanto AJ, et al. (2006) Haploinsufficiency of the Hmga1 gene causes cardiac hypertrophy and myelo-lymphoproliferative disorders in mice. Cancer research 66: 2536–2543.

42. Resar LM (2010) The high mobility group A1 gene: transforming inflammatory signals into cancer? Cancer research 70: 436–439.

43. Xi Y, Watanabe S, Hino Y, Sakamoto C, Nakatsu Y, et al. (2012) Hmga1 is differentially expressed and mediates silencing of the CD4/CD8 loci in T cell lineages and leukemic cells. Cancer science 103: 439–447.

44. Li L, Zhang JA, Dose M, Kueh HY, Mosadeghi R, et al. (2013) A far downstream enhancer for murine Bcl11b controls its T-cell specific expression. Blood 122: 902–911.

45. Lahn M, Kanehiro A, Takeda K, Terry J, Hahn Y-S, et al. (2002) MHC class I-dependent Vγ4+ pulmonary T cells regulate αβ T cell-independent airway responsiveness. Proceedings of the National Academy of Sciences 99: 8850–8855.

46. Lança T, Costa MF, Gonçalves-Sousa N, Rei M, Grosso AR, et al. (2013) Protective Role of the Inflammatory CCR2/CCL2 Chemokine Pathway through Recruitment of Type 1 Cytotoxic γδ T Lymphocytes to Tumor Beds. The Journal of Immunology 190: 6673–6680.

47. Paust S, Gill HS, Wang B-Z, Flynn MP, Moseman EA, et al. (2010) Critical role for the chemokine receptor CXCR6 in NK cell-mediated antigen-specific memory of haptens and viruses. Nature immunology 11: 1127–1135.

48. Cepek KL, Shaw SK, Parker CM, Russell GJ, Morrow JS, et al. (1994) Adhesion between epithelial cells and T lymphocytes mediated by E-cadherin and the αEβ7 integrin.

49. Timerbaev A, Sturup S (2012) Analytical approaches for assaying metallodrugs in biological samples: Recent methodological developments and future trends. Current drug metabolism 13: 272–283.

50. Brownlie RJ, Zamoyska R (2013) T cell receptor signalling networks: branched, diversified and bounded. Nature Reviews Immunology 13: 257–269.

51. Huber SA, Graveline D, Born WK, O'Brien RL (2001) Cytokine production by Vγ+-T-cell subsets is an important factor determining CD4+-Th-cell phenotype and susceptibility of BALB/c mice to coxsackievirus B3-induced myocarditis. Journal of virology 75: 5860–5869.

52. Huber SA, Graveline D, Newell MK, Born WK, O'Brien RL (2000) Vγ1+ T cells suppress and Vγ4+ T cells promote susceptibility to coxsackievirus B3-induced myocarditis in mice. The Journal of Immunology 165: 4174–4181.

53. Matsuzaki G, Yamada H, Kishihara K, Yoshikai Y, Nomoto K (2002) Mechanism of murine Vγ1+ γ δ T cell-mediated innate immune response against Listeria monocytogenes infection. European journal of immunology 32: 928–935.

54. Szabo SJ, Kim ST, Costa GL, Zhang X, Fathman CG, et al. (2000) A novel transcription factor, T-bet, directs Th1 lineage commitment. Cell 100: 655–669.

55. Suto A, Wurster AL, Reiner SL, Grusby MJ (2006) IL-21 inhibits IFN-γ production in developing Th1 cells through the repression of Eomesodermin expression. The Journal of Immunology 177: 3721–3727.

56. Jin N, Roark CL, Miyahara N, Taube C, Aydintug MK, et al. (2009) Allergic airway hyperresponsiveness-enhancing γδ T cells develop in normal untreated mice and fail to produce IL-4/13, unlike Th2 and NKT cells. The Journal of Immunology 182: 2002–2010.

57. O'Brien RL, Born WK (2010) γδ T cell subsets: A link between TCR and function? Elsevier. pp. 193–198.

9

Regulator of G-Protein Signaling 18 Controls Both Platelet Generation and Function

Nathalie Delesque-Touchard[1]*, Caroline Pendaries[1], Cécile Volle-Challier[1], Laurence Millet[1], Véronique Salel[1], Caroline Hervé[1], Anne-Marie Pflieger[1], Laurence Berthou-Soulie[2], Catherine Prades[2], Tania Sorg[3], Jean-Marc Herbert[1], Pierre Savi[1], Françoise Bono[1]

1 Early to Candidate (E2C), Sanofi, Toulouse, France, 2 SCP Biologics, Sanofi, Vitry-Sur-Seine, France, 3 Department of Scientific Operations PhenoPro, Mouse Clinical Institute (MCI), Strasbourg, France

Abstract

RGS18 is a myeloerythroid lineage-specific regulator of G-protein signaling, highly expressed in megakaryocytes (MKs) and platelets. In the present study, we describe the first generation of a RGS18 knockout mouse model (RGS18-/-). Interesting phenotypic differences between RGS18-/- and wild-type (WT) mice were identified, and show that RGS18 plays a significant role in both platelet generation and function. RGS18 deficiency produced a gain of function phenotype in platelets. In resting platelets, the level of CD62P expression was increased in RGS18-/- mice. This increase correlated with a higher level of plasmatic serotonin concentration. RGS18-/- platelets displayed a higher sensitivity to activation *in vitro*. RGS18 deficiency markedly increased thrombus formation *in vivo*. In addition, RGS18-/- mice presented a mild thrombocytopenia, accompanied with a marked deficit in MK number in the bone marrow. Analysis of MK maturation *in vitro* and *in vivo* revealed a defective megakaryopoiesis in RGS18-/- mice, with a lower bone marrow content of only the most committed MK precursors. Finally, RGS18 deficiency was correlated to a defect of platelet recovery *in vivo* under acute conditions of thrombocytopenia. Thus, we highlight a role for RGS18 in platelet generation and function, and provide additional insights into the physiology of RGS18.

Editor: Dermot Cox, Royal College of Surgeons, Ireland

Funding: In addition, the authors received no specific funding for this work. Sanofi provided support in the form of salaries for authors ND-T, C. Pendaries, CV-C, LM, VS, CH, A-MP, LB-S, C. Prades, J-MH, PS and FB. Sanofi had a role in study design, data collection and analysis, decision to publish, or preparation of the manuscript.

Competing Interests: ND-T, C. Pendaries, CV-C, LM, VS, CH, A-MP, LB-S, C. Prades, J-MH, PS and FB are employed by Sanofi. There are no patents, products in development or marketed products to declare.

* Email: nathalie.delesque-touchard@sanofi.com

Introduction

From the bone-marrow, where megakaryopoiesis and thrombopoiesis occur (i.e. proliferation, differentiation, migration, maturation of megakaryocytes and proplatelets into platelets) to injured tissue, where platelets get activated, there are many signaling pathways largely dependent on G protein-coupled receptors (GPCRs) involved. GPCRs are by far the most extensively validated class of therapeutic targets. Over half of the existing drugs currently on the market are GPCR ligands. However, only a small fraction of these receptors are targeted by drugs [1,2]. Drug discovery efforts for GPCR ligands have traditionally focused on targeting the orthosteric binding site of the receptors. One of the key issues in this regard is that the orthosteric binding sites across members of a single GPCR subfamily are often highly conserved, making it difficult to achieve high selectivity for specific GPCR subtypes. During the last decade, the idea of targeting allosteric sites – so called allo-targeting - as a novel approach to GPCR drug discovery has become a predominant approach [3]. Rather than targeting receptors directly, one could modulate signaling cascades downstream of receptor activation.

It is now well recognized that the regulators of G protein signaling (RGS) play essential roles in GPCR signaling [4]. RGS proteins are a family of cellular proteins with a conserved RGS domain (also called RGS-box) of about 120 amino-acid residues. RGS proteins specifically interact with the α subunits of G proteins, greatly enhance the intrinsic GTPase activities of Gα, and accelerate the hydrolysis of GTP to GDP by Gα, thus converting G proteins from a GTP-bound active state to a GDP-bound inactive state and terminating G protein-mediated signaling [5]. There are over 20 members in the mammalian RGS family. Based on sequence similarities and features of structural domains, they have been classified into 9 subfamilies [6]. *In vitro* and *in vivo* studies have provided strong evidence supporting that RGS proteins display remarkable specificity and selectivity in their regulation of GPCR-mediated physiological events [7]. The spatiotemporal-specific expression of RGS proteins and their target components, as well as the specific protein-protein recognition and interaction through their characteristic structural domains and functional motifs, are continually emerging as determinants for RGS selectivity and specificity. Recent research data are converging to highlight RGS proteins as attractive targets for the development of potential future therapeutics [8,9]. An RGS inhibitor would be expected to enhance GPCR signaling, and should do so in a tissue- or pathway-specific manner. Modulating RGS activity would then be a useful therapeutic strategy to control GPCR signaling in a unique way.

In 2001, several groups independently identified RGS18, and all agreed that RGS18 expression appears to be relatively restricted to bone marrow-derived cells [10–12]. RGS18 was found abundantly and predominantly expressed in platelets and, to a less extent in megakaryocytes (MKs) and leukocytes, but not in erythrocytes. In addition to RGS18, human MKs also highly express RGS16 [12,13]. RGS16 and RGS18 have their respective transcripts upregulated during MK differentiation and RGS16 was shown to act as a negative regulator of CXCR4 signaling in MKs [13]. However, in contrast to the restricted expression profile of RGS18, RGS16 is widely expressed. The expression patterns of RGS transcripts have been evaluated in platelets, and RGS18 was found to have the highest expression level, followed by RGS6, RGS10, and RGS16 [14–16]. The functional significance of RGS proteins in platelets has recently been validated in a mouse model expressing a serine to glycine substitution at position 184 in the α subunit of Gi2, the G protein that couples to platelet P2Y12 receptors for ADP [17]. The mutant Gαi2 was shown to be unable to interact with RGS, and loss of Gαi2: RGS interactions produced a gain of function in platelet activation. Most platelet agonists (thrombin, ADP, TXA2 …) activate members of the GPCR family, making G proteins and RGS proteins logical targets for regulation. On the basis of the abundant and specific expression pattern of RGS18 in platelets and MKs, we hypothesized that it might be a key regulator of GPCR signaling in these cells and to address this question, we have generated and phenotyped mice lacking a functional RGS18 gene.

Here we report that RGS18 deficiency produces a prothrombotic phenotype in mice, shifting the dose-response curve for platelet aggregation induced by thrombin to the left *in vitro* and increasing thrombus formation at sites of arteriovenous shunt *in vivo*. Moreover, we also show that RGS18 deficiency is sufficient to prime platelet activation even before an agonist is added. In addition, RGS18-/- mice present a mild thrombocytopenia, accompanied by a reduced number of megakaryocytes (MK) in their bone marrow. Analysis of MK maturation *in vitro* and *in vivo* reveals that RGS18-/- mice display a defective megakaryopoiesis. Finally, RGS18 was shown to display a thrombocytopoietic activity, as revealed by deficient platelet recovery in RGS18-/- mice under acute thrombocytopenia conditions.

Methods

Generation of RGS18 mutant mice

RGS18 knockout mice were generated at the MCI (Mouse Clinical Institute/Institut Clinique de la Souris, Strasbourg, France). The targeting vector was constructed as described follows: a 1kb PCR fragment encompassing exon 4 was cloned (PCR done on embryonic stem (ES) cell genomic DNA 129S2/SvPas genetic background) into an MCI proprietary vector, resulting in step 1 plasmid. This MCI vector has a floxed neomycin resistance cassette. Two PCR fragments of 4.2 kb corresponding to the 5′ homologous arm and 3 kb corresponding to the 3′ homologous arm were amplified and cloned successively into the step 1 plasmid to generate the final targeting construct. The linearized construct was electroporated into 129S2/SvPas mouse ES cells. After selection, targeted clones were identified by PCR using external primers and further confirmed by Southern

blot with 5′ and 3′ external probes. The positive ES clones were injected into C57BL/6J blastocysts, and male derived chimeras gave germline transmission. First L3 mice were successively bred with Flp and Cre transgenic mice (on C57BL/6 genetic background) to generate heterozygous mice with a deleted neomycin cassette and an inactivated RGS18 locus. Mice were then backcrossed for 4 consecutive generations to C57BL/6J genetic background. Deletion of exon 4 was confirmed at the DNA and transcript level.

Animals

C57BL/6J mice (Charles River Laboratories, Wilmington, MA, USA) weighing between 27 to 34 g were used throughout the study. The animals were kept on standard diet *ad libitum* and had free access to tap water. For the length of the experiment, the animals were maintained at an external temperature of 21°C +/−10%. The housing air was changed 15 to 20 times per hour. The animals were used after one week of quarantine. This protocol was approved by the "Comité d'Ethique Pour les Animaux de Laboratoire" (Animal Care and Use Committee) of Sanofi R&D.

In silico analysis of RGS18 promoter

The RGS18 promoter sequence (from −1000 bps to +100 bps) of human, mouse, rat, cow and dog were taken from Ensembl. Sequences were aligned and analyzed for phylogenetic conserved transcription factor binding sites (TFBS) using MatInspector and frameWorker programs from Genomatix software suite.

Peripheral blood cell counting

Mice were anesthetized by using isoflurane gas (Aerrane; Baxter, Lessines, Belgium). Peripheral blood samples were obtained from the retro-orbital plexus with 75 mm EDTA capillary tubes (Sarstedt, Montreal, Canada). Complete blood cell counts were performed with the VetABC animal cell counter (Horiba ABX SAS, Montpellier, France).

von Willebrand factor (vWF) staining on bone marrow sections

Femora were fixed in formalin, decalcified in Dc3 (Labonord, Temple-mars, France) and embedded in paraffin. Sections (5 μm) were deparaffined, rehydrated through serially diluted ethanol solutions to distilled water. After trypsin (Invitrogen, Carlsbad, CA, USA) treatment (10 minutes at 37°C), immunohistochemistry was performed using the Autostainer (Dako, Carpinteria, CA, USA). Endogenous peroxidase activity was quenched with 3% (wt/vol) hydrogen peroxide, and the sections were blocked with 10% (vol/vol) normal goat serum. The von Willebrand factor (Dako) staining (12.4 μg/ml) was carried out with a standard 3-stage immunoperoxidase method using the Vectastain Elite ABC peroxidase kit (Vector Laboratories, Peterborough, UK). Diaminobenzidine was used as chromogen. Counterstaining was performed with hematoxylin. For each section, the surface of the bone marrow was measured with the 4x objective (Nikon Eclipse E800) and the number of positive vWF MKs was counted using the 20x objective. Morpho Expert software (Explora Nova, La Rochelle, France) was used for the quantification.

Flow cytometric analysis

Blood samples were collected by retro-orbital puncture on hirudin at the final concentration of 20 μg/ml. Cells were incubated with FITC rat anti-mouse CD41 (BD Biosciences, San Jose, CA, USA; 100 ng/μl) or with FITC rat anti-mouse CD42b (Emfret Analytics, Eibelstadt, Germany; diluted to 1:5) for

10 minutes at room temperature. To measure basal platelet activation, cells were stained with rat anti-mouse P-Selectin (Emfret; diluted to 1:5) for 10 minutes at 37°C. After staining, cells were fixed with Cellfix (BD Biosciences) according to the manufacturer's instructions, and analyzed with CyanADP cytometer (Dako). MKs and platelets were discriminated according to their forward and side scatter parameters. To quantify splenic MKs and platelets, cells were isolated by homogenization of mice spleen in IMDM medium containing 2% heat-inactivated FBS using the Ribolyzer instrument (Hybaid, Teddington, UK). 100μl of the homogenate were stained and red blood cells were lysed with EasyLyse reagent (Dako) before cytometer analysis.

In vitro colony assays

Mice were lethally injected intraperitoneally with sodium pentobarbital (150 mg/kg). Bone marrow cells were flushed from femora and tibias with IMDM medium containing 2% heat-inactivated FBS. Single-cell suspensions were prepared under sterile conditions and enriched for Lineage-depleted (Lin⁻) cells using a Spin Sep mouse hematopoietic progenitor negative selection kit (StemCell Technologies, Vancouver, Canada). Lin⁻ marrow cells (5.10^4) were then cultured in double chamber slides with Mega-Cult-C media (StemCell Technologies) in presence of rmIl-3 (Peprotech, Rocky Hill, NJ, USA; 10 ng/ml), rmIl-6 (Peprotech; 3 ng/ml) and rhTPO (Peprotech; 50 ng/ml). After 11 days of culture, the slides were dehydrated and colonies were stained with FITC rat anti-mouse CD41 (BD Biosciences). Slides were scored microscopically, and MK colonies (CFU-MKs) were defined as colonies with at least 3-4MKs.

Ploidy analysis of CD41⁺ bone marrow megakaryocytes

Bone marrow suspensions were prepared in a phosphate-buffered saline (PBS)-bovine serum albumin (BSA) buffer (PBS containing 0.5% BSA). Cells (5.10^6) were labeled for 30 min at 4°C with 1.25 μg of a fluorescein isothiocyanate (FITC)-conjugated monoclonal antibody against CD41 (rat anti-mouse glycoprotein IIb; Pharmingen) and gently washed twice in PBS-BSA. The pellet was resuspended in 200 μl of PBS and 4 ml of a cold solution of 70% ethanol in PBS was added. After incubation for 1 h at 4°C, the suspension was centrifuged, the cells were resuspended in 100 μl of PBS and propidium iodide (Sigma-Aldrich, Gillingham, UK; 2 mL [50 μg/mL]) and RNAase (Sigma; 100 μg/ml) in PBS were added for 30 min at 37°C. The ploidy distribution in the CD41+ population was determined by two-color flow cytometry (BD FACSCanto; BD Biosciences).

Platelet depletion

Mice were given a sterile intraperitoneal injection of anti-mouse Gp1bα (Emfret; 2μg/g). 4 hours later, mice were tailed bled to determine baseline blood cell count. Then, platelet count was measured at 48, 72, 96, and 168 hours post injection by retro-orbital sampling.

Thrombocytopenia was also produced by the intraperitoneal injection of busulfan (Myleran; Burroughs-Wellcome, Research Triangle, NC, USA). Busulfan was injected to mice intraperitoneally at 30 mg/kg (in a 25% polyethylene glycol-400 solution) at day 0. Platelet counts were performed following the same procedure as described earlier at days 7, 11, 15, and 24.

Platelet Clearance

Mice platelets were biotinylated *in vivo* by infusion with NHS-biotin (Calbiochem, La Jolla, CA, USA). 10 mg NHS-biotin/kg body weight were dissolved in DMSO, then diluted into sterile saline solution at 1 mg/ml. The solution was slowly injected via the lateral tail vein of mice with a 26G1/2 needle. Blood collection was realized by retro-orbital sampling at days 1, 2, 3, 4 and 7 after biotin injection. Samples were stained with FITC rat anti-mouse CD41 (BD Biosciences; 100 ng/μl) and then incubated with PE-Streptavidin (Calbiochem; diluted to 1:3). The platelet biotinylation rate was analyzed by flow cytometry (CyanADP, FITC staining).

Platelet-rich Plasma (PRP) Preparation

Venous blood was collected into tubes containing a 3.8% trisodium citrate solution (9:1 vol/vol). Platelet-rich plasma (PRP) was obtained by centrifuging blood samples at 200×g for 10 min and left for 30 min at 37°C prior to stimulation.

Serotonin release assay

An aliquot of PRP was centrifuged at 2000×g for 10 min to obtain platelet-free plasma (PFP). 100 μl of PFP were used in the serotonin ELISA kit (Labor Diagnostika Nord Gmbh, Nordhorn, Germany) for the measurement of free (not bound to platelets) serotonin according to the manufacturer's instructions.

αIIbβ3 Activation

Platelet activation was determined according to the method of Bergmeier [18]. Platelets in PRP were stimulated at 37°C for 3 minutes using ADP (2.5 μM), collagen (10 μg/ml), or increasing doses of TRAP (125 μM-500 μM). Platelets were then stained with JON/A-PE32 (Emfret Analytics, Wuerzburg, Germany) for 10 minutes at room temperature and analyzed by flow cytometry.

Aggregometry

Platelet aggregation was determined according to the Born method [19] on a dual-channel Chrono-Log aggregometer (Chrono-log, Havertown, PA, USA). The experiment was performed at 37°C under constant stirring conditions (1200 rpm). Increasing concentrations of thrombin (0.01–1 UI/ml) were added to PRP and light transmission was recorded over 6 minutes.

Silk thread arterio-venous shunt model

Two 6 cm-long polyethylene tubing (0.28 and 0.61 mm inner and outer diameter, respectively) linked to a central part (3 cm-long; 0.58 and 0.96 mm inner and out diameter, respectively) containing a 3 cm-long silk thread and filled with saline solution were placed between the right carotid artery and the left jugular vein in anaesthetized animals (xylazine 20 mg/kg + ketamine 100 mg/kg ip). The central part of the shunt was removed after 10 minutes of blood circulation and the silk thread carrying the thrombus was pulled out. The wet weight of the thrombus was determined.

Experimental tail transection bleeding model

Mice were anesthetized by intraperitoneal injection of xylazine (20 mg/kg) with ketamine (100 mg/kg). The bleeding time was determined according to Dejana et al. [20] adapted for mice, by transection of the tail 2 mm from the tip. Blood was carefully blotted on a filter paper every 15 sec during the two first minutes and every 30 sec thereafter. The observation period was limited to 45 minutes. Hemostasis was considered to be achieved when no more bloodstaining was observed over 1 min. Raw data correspond to the bleeding time in minutes.

Table 1. Peripheral blood cell counts in WT and RGS18-/- mice.

	WT	RGS18-/-	P values
Platelets	1291.3	1119.1	<0.0001 (***)
MPV	4.94	5.05	0.0031 (**)
Red Blood cells	9.53	9.71	NS
White Blood cells	8.65	9.07	NS
Lymphocytes	6.054	6.496	NS
Monocytes	0.35	0.37	NS
Granulocytes	2.24	2.2	NS

Blood collected by retro-orbital venous puncture was analyzed in a VetABC animal cell counter. All counts are thousands per microliter, except for red blood cells which are millions per microliter. *P<.05; **P<.01; ***P<.001.

Statistical analysis

Results are presented as means ± SD. The data were analyzed by using a 1-way analysis of variance (ANOVA) with Student t test or Dunnett test. P values less than .05 were considered to be statistically significant.

Results

Generation of RGS18 mutant mice

To determine the role of RGS18 *in vivo*, RGS18 mutant mice were generated. In order to disrupt the RGS18 gene by homologous recombination in ES cells, a targeting vector was designed, with a selectable neomycin resistance cassette (Figure S1). After electroporation of the targeting vector into 129S2/SvPas ES cells, several independent clones exhibiting the expected homologous disruption of *RGS18* were used to generate chimeric mice by blastocyst injection (see Materials and Methods). Chimeric males were used for germline transmission of the targeted RGS18 allele. Adult mice carrying disrupted alleles of the RGS18 gene were viable, healthy, and displayed no visible physical abnormalities. The production colony provided normal ratios of WT and knockout males and females. The MCI performed the phenotype analysis of RGS18-/- mice; the metabolic or functional assessments performed are described in the "Information S1" document: metabolic exploration (Table S1), cardiovascular investigations (Table S2), necropsy and histological analysis (Table S3), and behavioral characterization (Table S4). No significant difference was observed between WT and RGS18-KO mice (data not shown), except during behavioral phenotyping where mutant mice displayed behavior that could be interpreted as an increase in reactivity/anxiety and increased pain sensibility (see Table S5, Figure S2 and Figure S3).

In silico analysis of RGS18 promoter

To further characterize RGS18 function, an *in silico* prediction of regulatory elements in the proximal promoter region was performed. 18 transcription factor binding sites conserved in at least 4 species were identified, and 11 of them are described as regulators of hematopoietic gene expression. More specifically, within the 200 bps from the transcriptional start site, 5 cis-regulatory elements corresponding to transcription factors, known to play a role in the development of hematopoietic cell lineages, were found (Figure S4). These binding sites correspond to the transcription factor GATA1, described as essential for erythroid and megakaryocyte development; RUNX1, (located close to GATA1) whose collaboration with GATA1 is required for megakaryocyte differentiation [21]; EVI1, frequently found in myeloid leukemias and whose expression is also associated with progression of megakaryocyte differentiation [22]; STAT3, which among its numerous diverse gene functions has been described to play a role in early stage of megakaryopoiesis too [23]; and MEIS1, known to play an important role in megakaryocytic-specific genes [24]. The identification of these predicted regulatory elements, associated with their co-localisation in the proximal promoter of RGS18 suggests a possible regulation of its gene expression during megakaryopoiesis.

Mice lacking RGS18 present a mild thrombocytopenia

Analysis of peripheral blood samples of RGS18-/- mice and normal littermates for their hematologic profile showed that RGS18-/- mice were moderately thrombocytopenic: a mean of ~15% reduction in platelet counts was observed in RGS18-/- mice with respect to WT mice (Table 1). All other blood parameters analyzed, including red blood cells and total white blood cells, were normal in RGS18-/- mice. Interestingly, the mean platelet volume was significantly increased from an average of 4.94 μm^3 in WT mice to 5.05 μm^3 in RGS18-/- mice. These data suggested that RGS18 might be implicated in megakaryopoiesis/thrombopoiesis.

One of the direct causes of thrombocytopenia is a reduction in the number of megakaryocytes (MK) in the bone marrow. We therefore examined MK counts in femora after staining of bone marrow sections for Von Willebrand Factor, a sensitive marker for identification of marrow MKs [25]. As shown in Figure 1, the number of MKs per μm^2 was markedly decreased in RGS18-/- mice.

In mice, in addition to bone marrow, the spleen is an important alternative hematopoietic organ. Indeed, MKs rarely appear in the spleen of normal adult mice, but are often found in the spleen when megakaryopoiesis in bone marrow is disrupted [26,27]. Therefore, we also examined the number of splenic MKs in RGS18-/- mice. Although MK counts were slightly increased in the spleens of RGS18-/- mice (0.87±0.07, n=6, in RGS18-/- mice versus 0.72±0.08, n=6, in WT mice), the difference was not found to be statistically significant (Figure S5).

A

WT   RGS18 -/-

B

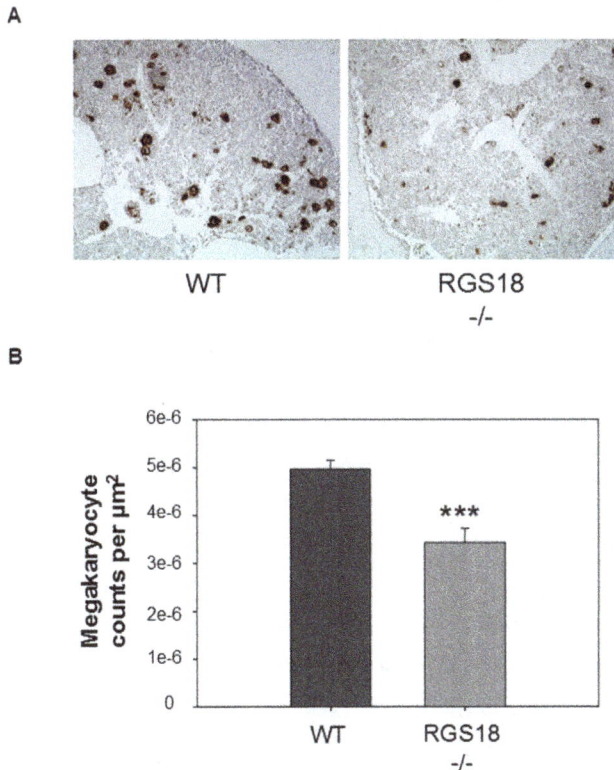

Figure 1. Bone marrow MKs in RGS18-/- mice. (A) Representative vWF immunostaining images of frozen femur sections from 9-week-old WT and RGS18-/- mice. Positively stained MKs from 6 bone marrow sections per mice (n=3 per group) were scored under a microscope. Images were obtained using ECLIPSE E800 microscope (Nikon, Tokyo, Japan) equipped with a 4x objective (Nikon Eclipse E800). The number of positive vWF MKs was counted by using the 20x objective. Morpho Expert software (Explora Nova, La Rochelle, France) was used to acquire and process images. (B) Cumulative analysis of the numbers of MKs per square millimeter is shown. ***$P<.001$.

Defective megakaryopoiesis in RGS18-/- mice

To further characterize megakaryopoiesis in the absence of RGS18, MK progenitor cells from bone marrow of RGS18-/- and WT mice were first assayed in clonogenic culture. *In vitro* colony assays in presence of a cocktail of cytokines regulating mega-karyopoiesis showed that the number of MK progenitors (CFU-Meg) was clearly higher in WT mice than in RGS18-/- mice (Figure 2A), indicating that RGS18 deficiency in MK progenitors affects their *in vitro* maturation potential.

To confirm these results, we next examined the *in vivo* maturation potential of bone marrow MKs. Bone marrow cells were stained for CD42b and MKs were identified by flow cytometry. We observed that the level of MKs from bone marrow of WT mice was in accordance with litterature data (<1%). However, the percentage of MKs was significantly decreased in RGS18-/- mice (Figure 2B), as previously observed in the histologic analysis of bone marrow sections.

Finally, we analyzed the ploidy distribution of bone marrow MKs. Ploidy, a distinctive characteristic of differentiated MKs, was measured by flow cytometry using propidium iodide fluorescence. Interestingly, we found that the frequency of early MK progenitors with 2N DNA content in RGS18-/- mice was similar to that of WT mice, while the proportion of more committed MK

precursors with >2N DNA content was markedly decreased in RGS18-/- mice (Figure 2C), indicating a direct correlation between RGS18 and MK maturation.

RGS18 deficiency induces a defect in platelet generation after acute thrombocytopenia

To evaluate the involvement of RGS18 in thrombocytopoietic activity *in vivo*, experiments of acute thrombocytopenia were conducted in RGS18-/- mice and their normal littermates. In the first model, a complement-mediated immune thrombocytopenia was induced by an intraperitoneal injection of an anti-mouse GpIb antibody, based on the method of Nieswandt et al. [28]. As shown in Figure 3A, GpIb antibody injection led to a dramatic decrease (>95%) in platelet counts within 4 hours in RGS18-/- and WT mice. Platelet recovery was measured at 48 h, 72 h, 96 h, and 168 h post-injection. As previously observed, recovery of platelet counts was achieved between 96 h and 168 h, and a defective platelet recovery was clearly observed in RGS18-/- mice (Figure 3A).

In the second model of thrombocytopenia, mice were myelosuppressed by intraperitoneal injection of busulfan, a cancer chemotherapy agent. The busulfan-treated mice showed platelet nadir around day 11, and then the platelet number gradually recovered to approximately 100% by day 24 in WT mice (Figure 3B). RGS18-/- mice showed a lower platelet number at the nadir and a significantly reduced platelet recovery over the experimental period compared to WT mice (Figure 3B).

RGS18-/- mice display a platelet destructive disorder

In addition to a defective platelet production by the bone marrow, thrombocytopenia could also reflect an increased rate of platelet removal from the blood. Abnormalities in different processes can lead to this, i.e. increased trapping of platelets by the spleen, diminished platelet survival, or platelet consumption. Thus, we first examined if the observed thrombocytopenia in RGS18-/- mice could be caused by a splenic sequestration of the platelets. As shown in Figure 4A, the spleens of the RGS18-/- mice did not contain an increased number of platelets. Platelet counts were significantly decreased compared with those of the WT mice (p = 0.031), in a parallel with the respective number of circulating platelets in WT and RGS18-/- mice. We consistently did not observe any splenomegaly in the RGS18-/- mice (data not shown).

To determine whether alterations in platelet half-life could contribute to thrombocytopenia in mice lacking RGS18, *in vivo* labeling studies of blood cells were performed by biotinylation. Flow cytometry analysis revealed no difference in the rate of platelet clearance from the circulation in RGS18-/- mice compared to WT controls (Figure 4B), indicating that the lower level of circulating RGS18-/- platelets is not the result of diminished platelet survival.

Finally, we investigated whether platelets from RGS18-/- mice could be consumed by spontaneous aggregation. Spontaneous platelet aggregation (SPA) was evaluated by flow cytometry on whole blood with no platelet agonists added. Analysis of circulating platelet aggregates showed that the RGS18-/- mice presented more spontaneous platelet aggregates than WT mice (Figure 4C), suggesting that the observed thrombocytopenia in RGS18-/- mice could be the reflect of both a defective megakaryopoiesis and a spontaneously enhanced platelet aggreg-ability.

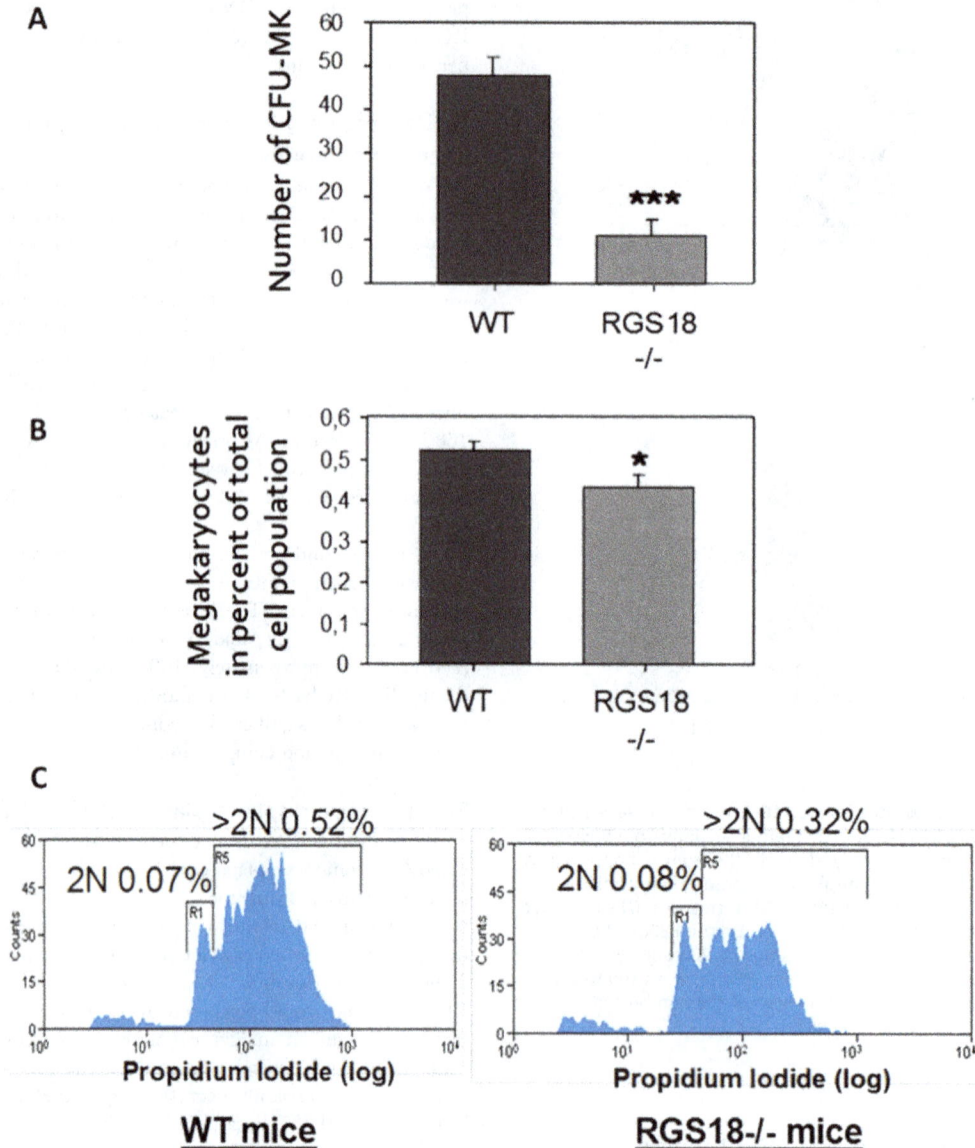

Figure 2. RGS18-/- mice present a defective megakaryopoiesis. (A) *In vitro* MK maturation. Lin⁻ bone marrow cells (5×10^4 cells/chamber) from 9/10-week-old WT and RGS18-/- mice (n = 5 per group) were cultured in Mega-Cult-C media containing 50 ng/mL rhTPO, 10 ng/ml rmIL3, and 3 ng/ml rmIL6 in double-chamber slides at 37°C for 11 days. Slides were then dehydrated and stained with CD41. Slides were scored microscopically, and MK colonies (CFU-MKs) were defined as colonies containing at least 3-4MKs. (B) *In vivo* MK maturation. Bone marrow cells from 9-week-old WT and RGS18-/- mice (n = 6 per group) were stained for CD42b, and MKs were identified by flow cytometry on the basis of size and CD42b positivity. Percentages of total bone marrow cell population are shown. (C) MK ploidy analysis. Bone marrow cells from 9-week-old WT and RGS18-/- mice (n = 6 per group) were stained for CD41 in presence of propidium iodide (PI). MKs were identified by flow cytometry on the basis of size and CD41 positivity. DNA cell content was evaluated on the basis of PI fluorescence intensity. Percentages of total bone marrow cell population with DNA content >2N are shown. *P<.05; **P<.01; ***P<.001.

RGS18 deficiency induces a prothrombotic phenotype in mice

To further investigate whether RGS18-/- mice could present thrombogenic disorders, we first analyzed the basal platelet activation state by measuring platelet activation markers. Serotonin has been shown to play a central role in the haemostatic process, and its release is considered to be the most reliable biological assay for platelet activation [29]. The quantitative determination of serotonin in plasma by enzyme immunoassay measurement showed increased levels in RGS18-/- mice, with concentrations being approximately 53% higher than those

measured from plasma samples of the WT mice (Figure 5A). CD62P (P-selectin) is a constituent of alpha granules and is released to the platelet surface upon activation, a process parallel to secretion of serotonin [30]. Basal platelet activation was thus assessed by flow cytometry on whole blood measuring surface CD62P expression with no platelet agonists added. Figure 5B shows a mean of ~54% increase in basal CD62P expression on RGS18-/- platelets with respect to WT platelets, indicating that RGS18 deficiency primes platelet activation even in the absence of an added platelet agonist.

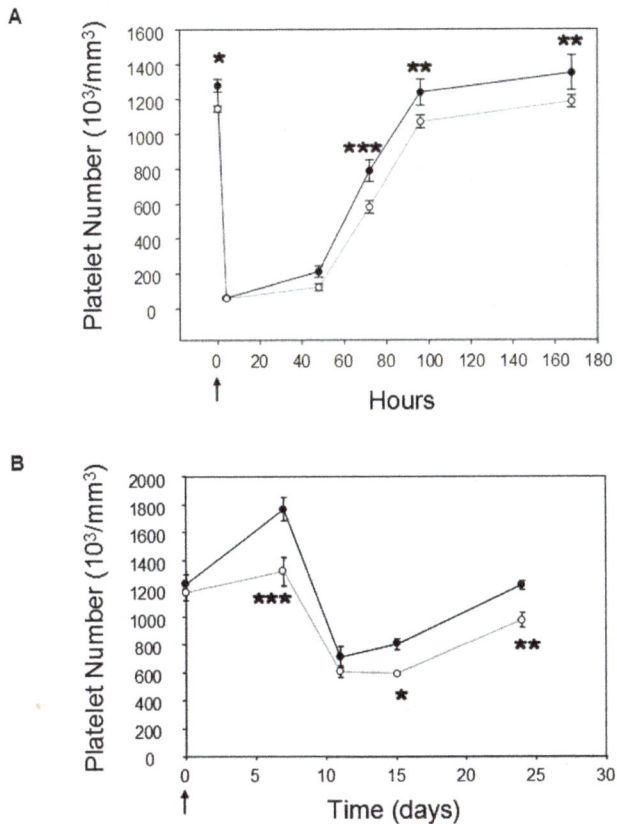

Figure 3. RGS18-/- mice present a defective thrombopoiesis after acute thrombocytopenia. (A) Complement-mediated immune thrombocytopenia. 10-week-old WT (n = 8; black circle) and RGS18-/- mice (n = 8; open circle) were given a sterile intraperitoneal injection of anti-mouse αGpIb antibody (2 μg/g of mouse) at T0 (Arrow). Platelet counts were measured at 4, 48, 72, 96, and 168 hours after injection. (B) Busulfan-induced thrombocytopenia. Busulfan was injected to 9/13-week-old WT (n = 15; black circle) and RGS18-/- mice (n = 14; open circle) intraperitoneally at 30 mg/kg (day 0; arrow). Platelet counts were measured at 7, 11, 15, and 24 days after injection. *P<.05; **P<.01; ***P<.001.

By analyzing basal and TRAP-activated platelets using 2-DE gel electrophoresis, RGS18 has recently been found to be phosphorylated on Ser49 in response to TRAP activation [31]. To determine whether RGS18 could also regulate PAR signaling in platelets, we next examined the platelet activation responses to TRAP and thrombin in WT and RGS18-/- mice. Platelet activation was assessed by flow cytometry measuring surface expression of activated integrin αIIbβ3. As shown in Figure 5C, murine TRAP (PAR-4 peptide activator) dose-dependently induced an activation-dependent conformational change in integrin αIIbβ3 on platelets from WT littermates, and an enhanced response was observed in RGS18-/- mice as early as the concentration of 0.25 mM of mTRAP. Similarly, the response to thrombin was found to be increased in RGS18-/- mice, as assessed using *in vitro* platelet aggregation assays (data not shown).

RGS18-/- mice show enhanced platelet function *in vivo*

Platelets are known to play a central role in both arterial and venous thrombosis. To determine whether RGS18 deficiency affects platelet function *in vivo*, we used the silk thread arteriovenous shunt thrombosis model, which has been characterized as a

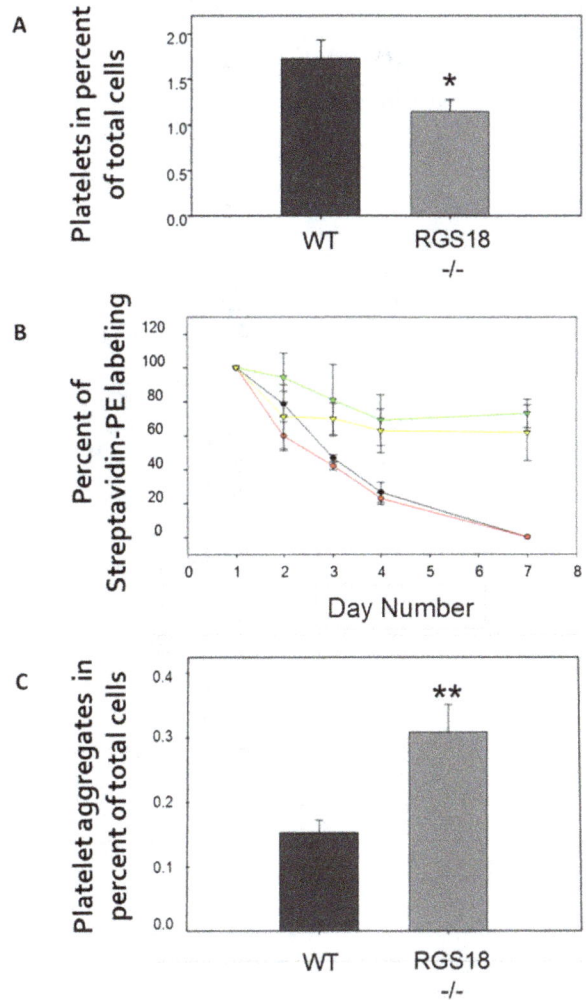

Figure 4. Rate analysis of platelet removal from blood. (A) Splenic sequestration of platelets. Crushed spleens from 9/13-week-old WT and RGS18-/- mice (n = 6 per group) were stained for CD42b, and platelets were identified by flow cytometry on the basis of size and CD42b positivity. Percentages of total splenic cell population are shown. (B) Clearance of platelets. Blood cells from 7-week-old mice were biotinylated *in vivo* by infusion of NHS-biotin, and then blood samples were collected at the time indicated. Biotinylated platelets from WT (black line) and RGS18-/- (red line) mice (n = 9 per group) were identified by flow cytometry on whole blood using PE-Streptavidin and CD41 staining. The stability of the biotinylation was assessed by examining the *in vivo* biotinylated CD41⁻ blood cells in WT (green line) and RGS18-/- (yellow line) mice (n = 9 per group). (C) Spontaneous platelet aggregation. Whole blood cells from 9/11-week-old WT and RGS18-/- mice (n = 12 per group) were stained for CD42b, and platelets were identified by flow cytometry on the basis of size and CD42b positivity. Platelet aggregates were monitored by extending the platelet gate so as to include the platelet "smearings" having elevated FSC and FITC fluorescence. Percentages of total cell population are shown. *P<.05; **P<.01.

"mixed" thrombosis model in rats [32]. In this model, both the activation of platelets (often linked to arterial thrombosis) and the coagulation cascade (commonly associated with venous thrombosis) are known to contribute to the thrombus formation. Since RGS18-/- platelets displayed an enhanced basal aggregability, thrombus formation was measured after a very short time of blood circulation. Analysis of thrombus weight after a 5 min-blood flow

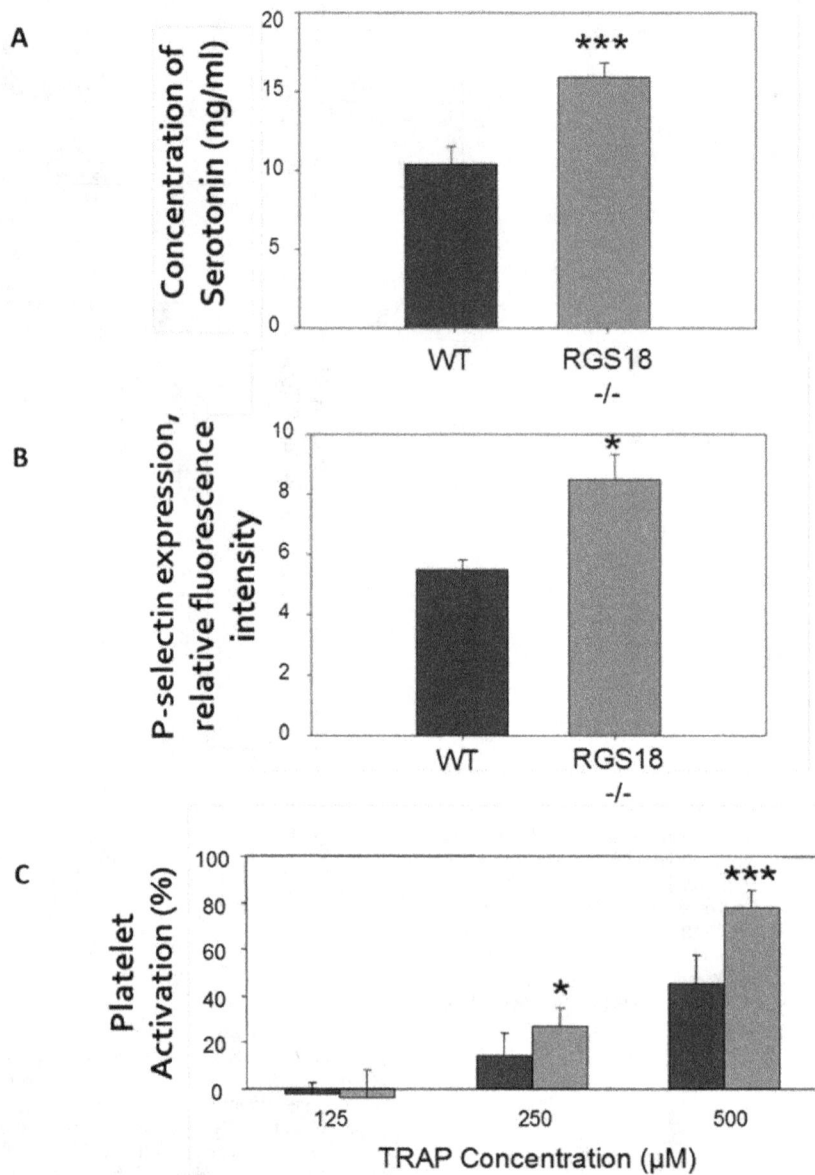

Figure 5. RGS18 deficiency induces a prothrombotic phenotype in mice. (A) Serum levels of serotonin. Blood from 10-week-old WT and RGS18-/- mice (n = 9 per group) was collected, and the quantitative determination of serotonin in serum was performed by enzyme immunoassay (ELISA). Concentrations of serotonin (ng/ml) are shown. (B) P-selectin (CD62P) expression on platelets. Whole blood cells from 12-week-old WT and RGS18-/- mice (n = 6 per group) were stained for CD62P, and platelets were identified by flow cytometry on the basis of size and CD42b positivity. Fluorescence intensities of platelet CD62P are shown. (C) Platelet activation in response to TRAP. Platelet-rich plasma (PRP) from 9/11-week-old WT and RGS18-/- mice (n = 6 per group) was prepared, and incubated at 37°C during 3 minutes with different concentrations of TRAP (μM). Platelet activation was measured by flow cytometry detection of activated integrin αIIbβ3. Percentages of platelet activation are shown. *P<.05; ***P<.001.

showed that RGS18 deficiency markedly increased platelet accumulation, with thrombi being more than 2 times larger in RGS18-/- mice than those of WT mice (Figure 6).

In agreement with the prothrombotic phenotype of the RGS18-/- mice, there was no evidence of spontaneous bleeding in these mice (data not shown).

Discussion

RGS18 has been described in 2001 as a myeloerythroid lineage-specific regulator of G-protein signaling, highly expressed in MKs and platelets. Several studies report that the RGS18 transcript is specifically detected in haematopoietic progenitor and myeloerythroid lineage cells, and that they are most highly abundant in MKs and platelets [10–12]. In accordance with this expression pattern, our results show that RGS18 is important for MK biology and that RGS18 deficiency produces a defective megakaryopoiesis, affecting the maturation potential of MK progenitors *in vitro* as well as *in vivo*. Moreover, RGS18 deficiency induces a chronic thrombocytopenia in mice and a defect in platelet recovery and formation after acute thrombocytopenia. Together, these results

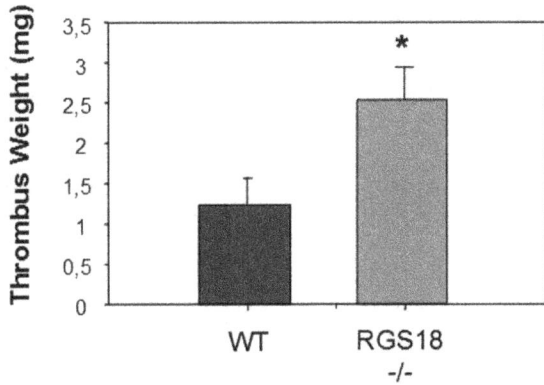

Figure 6. RGS18 deficiency increases thrombus formation at sites of arterio-venous shunt *in vivo*. An arterio-venous shunt was achieved as described on 11/13-week-old WT and RGS18-/- mice (n = 14 per group) and thrombus weight was determined after 10 minutes of blood circulation. *P<.05.

suggest that RGS18 plays a physiological role in hematopoiesis, in particular taking an active part in megakaryopoiesis and platelet generation. It is interesting to note that Louwette and colleagues recently reported that lentiviral RGS18 overexpression during *in vitro* differentiation of mouse Sca1$^+$ hematopoietic stem cells induced an increase in MK proliferation and that RGS18 depletion in zebrafish resulted in thrombocytopenia [33].

In 2005, Berthebaud and colleagues proposed that RGS16 might be a negative regulator of SDF-1/CXCR4 signaling in MKs [13]. They observed that overexpression of RGS16, but not of RGS18, in MO7e cells inhibited SDF1-induced migration, and down-regulation of RGS16 by RNA interference in MO7e cells and in primary MKs promoted SDF1-induced chemotaxis. In contrast with their results obtained with RGS18, we did indeed observe a functional role of RGS18 in MK migration (Figure S6). Actually, RGS18 downregulation by RNA interference in Dami cells comes with an increase of SDF1-induced Dami cell migration. The apparent discrepancy between these two sets of results could arise not only from the use of different megakaryoblastic cell lines, but also from the different technical strategies used to evaluate the role of RGS18 in MK cell migration – namely RGS18 overexpression versus silencing. To date, RGS18 expression levels in MK cells have been always reported to be strong and much higher than RGS16 expression levels [12,13,15]. Therefore, overexpressing RGS18 in cells where its expression level is already very strong might not be the most appropriate approach for observing subsequent effects. Furthermore, our results are well supported by a study from Nagata and colleagues who found that SDF-1 binding to its receptor CXCR4 affected the binding capacity of RGS18 to Gαi, but not Gαq, in MKs [10]. Based on these different observations, RGS18 might control MK migration to regulate megakaryopoiesis by attenuating CXCR4 signaling, suggesting that a functional redundancy among RGS16 and RGS18 might exist in MKs.

RGS1, 2, 3, 6, 9, 10, 16, 18, and 19 transcripts are shown to be detected in human platelets [14] and RGS2, 3, 5, 6, 10, 14, 16, and 18 transcripts are present in rat platelets [15]. At the protein level, only RGS10 and RGS18 have been detected in human platelets [31,34]. Functionally, these two RGS proteins have been found: (a) to be differentially phosphorylated after TRAP stimulation of platelets [31], (b) to be associated with spinophilin (SPL) in resting platelets [34], and (c) to be released from SPL after

platelet activation by thrombin [34]. Therefore, a functional redundancy among RGS family members might exist in platelets. At the bone marrow level, mRNA transcripts of RGS1, 2, 8, 10, 12, 14, 16, 18, and 19 are detected in mice, and no difference in their expression level is observed in extracts from either RGS18-deficient mice and WT mice (Figure S7). Because RGS18-deficient mice are viable, elucidating whether RGS10 partly compensates for RGS18 function in our RGS18 knockout model is a question that will need to be addressed.

In addition to the regulatory role of RGS18 in MK biology, our results show that RGS18 deficiency produces a gain of function phenotype in platelets, shifting the dose-response curve for platelet aggregation induced by thrombin to the left *in vitro* and increasing thrombus formation at sites of arteriovenous shunt *in vivo*. Moreover, we also show that RGS18 deficiency is sufficient to prime platelet activation even before an agonist is added. Collectively, these observations show for the first time the functional significance of RGS18 in platelets and suggest that its physiological role is to limit platelet activation and accumulation during thrombus formation.

In accordance with our results, Signarvic and colleagues recently demonstrated the active role of RGS proteins in regulating platelet responsiveness [17]. Platelets from mice with a G184S substitution in Giα2 that blocks RGS/Gi2 interactions, showed increased responsiveness to agonists *in vitro* and increased accumulation after vascular injury *in vivo*. This increased responsiveness was not limited to Gi2-coupled receptor agonists such as ADP. Giα2 (G184S) substitution also produced increased responses to PAR4 and TxA2 receptor agonists, although signaling downstream of these receptors in platelets is usually attributed to Gq and (to a lesser extent) G12 family members rather than to direct activation of Gi family members. In contrast to these results, we observe that RGS18 deficiency produces a pathway-selective gain of function in platelets. RGS18-deficient platelets respond significantly better than controls at low concentrations of either thrombin (PAR-1 receptor agonist) or TRAP (PAR-4 receptor agonist), whose receptors are both Gq-coupled receptors. On the other hand, RGS18 deficiency does not produce a shift in the dose-response curve for platelet aggregation induced by ADP (Figure S8). The Gi-coupled P2Y12 receptor is the major ADP receptor in platelets, and an increased response of RGS18-deficient platelets at suboptimal ADP concentration is what would be expected if RGS18 protein restrains this Gi-dependent signaling pathway. In investigating possible changes induced by RGS18 deficiency in platelet responsiveness not related to agonists coupled to G-protein pathways, we also found no difference in platelet aggregation induced by collagen between RGS18-deficient and WT platelets (Figure S8). Thus, we can assume that RGS18 retains specificity for pathways known to be mediated by Gq and does not spill over to predominantly Gi-driven events in platelets. To further establish that RGS18 regulation of platelet function is strictly confined to Gq-mediated events, it will be important to evaluate its role in RGS18-deficient platelet responsiveness to TxA2.

Nevertheless, our assumption is strongly supported by latest results of Ma and colleagues who described an association of spinophilin (SPL) with RGS18 in resting platelets and more especially an agonist-selective dissociation of this complex during platelet activation [34]. In their study, dissociation of the SPL/RGS18 complex occurred when human platelets were incubated with the two potent activators of Gq-mediated events, thrombin and TxA2, but not in presence of ADP or collagen. Similarly, we observed an increase of platelet responsiveness when RGS18-deficient platelets are incubated with thrombin or TRAP, but not in presence of ADP or collagen. Both studies converge on the idea that RGS18 might at least control PARs signaling. In 2004, Garcia and colleagues had already observed that PAR receptor signaling induced the phosphorylation of Serine 49 of RGS18 in platelets [31]. More recently, Gegenbauer and colleagues also showed that RGS18 is phosphorylated on S49 and S218 in platelets, and that phosphorylation of S49 increased with platelet activation by thrombin [35,36]. Furthermore, they also showed that RGS18 inhibited Gq-mediated Ca^{2+} release from intracellular stores. In agreement with this, we observe, in the megakaryocytic Dami cells, that downregulation of RGS18 by RNA interference strongly increases intracellular Ca^{2+} release as early as the concentration of 0.1 UI/ml of thrombin (Figure S9). Altogether these data suggest that RGS18 might control calcium signaling to limit platelet activation by attenuating Gq signaling pathways in platelets, in particular that of PAR receptors.

In conclusion, by generating RGS18 knockout mice for the first time and describing their phenotype, we have helped to advance in the understanding of the role of RGS proteins on MK differentiation and platelet generation *in vivo*. RGS proteins play essential regulatory roles in the signaling of G protein-coupled receptors and display remarkable specificity and selectivity in their regulation of GPCR-mediated physiological events. GPCRs constitute the largest family of receptors in the genome and are the targets for at least 50% of current medicines. For many G protein-coupled receptors, intense efforts to develop orthosteric drugs have failed to yield highly selective ligands. In recent years, major advances have been made and established allosteric GPCR modulators as a novel approach to regulate this important class of drug targets. In particular, these allosteric modulators have provided novel tools and drug leads for multiple receptors for which efforts aimed at discovery of orthosteric ligands had been unsuccessful. In parallel, research data have highlighted RGS proteins as attractive targets for the development of potential future therapeutics that would control GPCR signaling in a tissue- or pathway-specific manner. Here we have demonstrated the functional importance of endogenous RGS18 *in vivo*, showing that RGS18 is a key regulator of GPCR signaling in MKs and platelets, controlling both platelet generation and platelet function. Numerous RGS knockout mice have been generated [37]. These models have provided essential information for our understanding of the physiological role of RGS proteins but in many cases, reported effects are modest [38,39]. In the present study, we describe readily detectable effects in RGS18-deficient mice but nevertheless with only a mild phenotype. The most likely explication is a functional redundancy with other RGS proteins. It is evident that at least RGS10 and RGS16 present some degree of functional redundancy with RGS18 *in vitro* in platelets and megakaryocytes, respectively [31,34,13]; which might partially compensate for RGS18 deficiency in the different cellular contexts and thus explaining the minimal phenotype observed in mutant mice. From a clinical perspective, it is not clear whether increasing RGS18 function could protect from cardiovascular or hematological diseases. Yet what can be said at this point with some degree of assurance is that enhancers rather than inhibitors may be more useful in RGS18 drug development; emerging data show reductions in RGS protein expression or function in several pathophysiological states, and strategies to increase RGS function are now emerging [40].

Supporting Information

Figure S1 Targeting vector with a selectable neomycin resistance cassette (F_NEO) designed to disrupt the RGS18 gene.

Figure S2 Acoustic startle reactivity (A) and pre-pulse inhibition (B) in WT and RGS18-/- mice.

Figure S3 Anxiety assessment of RGS18-/- mice using the open field test.

Figure S4 In silico analysis of RGS18 Promoter.

Figure S5 Splenic MKs in RGS18 -/- mice.

Figure S6 RGS18 silencing increases MK cell migration.

Figure S7 RGS gene expression in bone marrow extracts.

Figure S8 Platelet activation in response to ADP and collagen.

Figure S9 Effect of RGS18 silencing on intracellular calcium release in MK cells.

Table S1 List of tests performed for metabolic exploration.

Table S2 List of tests performed for cardiovascular investigation.

Table S3 Necropsy and histological analysis.

Table S4 List of tests performed for behavioral characterization.

Table S5 Evaluation of pain sensitivity in WT and RGS18-/- mice.

Acknowledgments

We are grateful to the MCI for generation of Sanofi RGS18 knockout mice.

Author Contributions

Conceived and designed the experiments: ND-T PS. Performed the experiments: CH LM VS C. Pendaries A-MP LB-S. Analyzed the data: ND-T LM C. Prades CV-C TS PS. Wrote the paper: CV-C FB J-MH ND-T.

References

1. Esbenshade T (2005) G protein-coupled receptors as targets for drug discovery. G proein-coupled receptors in drug discovery. Taylor and Francis: 15–36.

2. Roth BL, Kroeze WK (2006) Screening the receptorome yields validated molecular targets for drug discovery. Curr Pharm Des 12: 1785–1795.

3. Conn PJ, Christopoulos A, Lindsley CW (2009) Allosteric modulators of GPCRs: a novel approach for the treatment of CNS disorders. Nat Rev 8: 41–54.

4. Bansal G, Druey KM, Xie Z (2007) R4 RGS proteins: regulation of G-protein signaling and beyond. Pharmacol Ther 116: 473–495.

5. Ross EM, Wilkie TM (2000) GTPase-activating proteins for heterotrimeric G proteins: regulators of G protein signaling (RGS) and RGS-like proteins. Annu Rev Biochem 69: 795–827.

6. Siderovski DP, Willard FS (2005) The GAPs, GEFs, and GDIs of heterotrimeric G-protein alpha subunits. Int J Biol Sci 1: 51–66.

7. Xie GX, Palmer PP (2007) How regulators of G protein signaling achieve selective regulation. J Mol Biol 366: 349–365.

8. Sjögren B (2011) Regulator of G protein signaling proteins as drug targets: current state and future possibilities. Adv Pharmacol 62: 315–347.

9. Kimple AJ, Bosch DE, Giguère PM, Siderovski DP (2011) Regulators of G-protein signaling and their Gα substrates: promises and challenges in their use as drug discovery targets. Pharmacol Rev 63: 728–749.

10. Nagata Y, Oda M, Nakata H, Shozaki Y, Kozasa T, et al. (2001) A novel regulator of G-protein signaling bearing GAP activity for Gαi and Gαq in megakaryocytes. Blood 97: 3051–3060.

11. Park IK, Klug CA, Li K, Jerabek L, Li L, et al. (2001) Molecular cloning and characterization of a novel regulator of G-protein signaling from mouse hematopoietic stem cells. J Biol Chem 276: 915–923.

12. Yowe D, Weich N, Prabhudas M, Poisson L, Errada P, et al. (2001) RGS18 is a myeloerythroid lineage-specific regulator of G-protein-signalling molecule highly expressed in megakaryocytes. Biochem J 359: 109–118.

13. Berthebaud M, Rivière C, Jarrier P, Foudi A, Zhang Y, et al. (2005) RGS16 is a negative regulator of SDF.1-CXCR4 signaling in megakaryocytes. Blood 106: 2962–2968.

14. Gagnon AW, Murray DL, Leadley RJ (2002) Cloning and characterization of a novel regulator of G protein signalling in human platelets. Cell Signal 14: 595–606.

15. Kim SD, Sung HJ, Park SK, Kim TW, Park SC, et al. (2006) The expression patterns of RGS transcripts in platelets. Platelets 17: 493–497.

16. Rowley JW, Oler A, Tolley ND, Hunter BN, Low EN, et al. (2011) Genome wide RNA-seq analysis of human and mouse platelet transcriptomes. Blood 118: e101–e111.

17. Signarvic RS, Cierniewska A, Stalker TJ, Fong KP, Chatterjee MS, et al. (2010) RGS/Gi2alpha interactions modulate platelet accumulation and thrombus formation at sites of vascular injury. Blood 116: 6092–6100.

18. Bergmeier W, Schulte V, Brockhoff G, Bier U, Zirngibl H, et al. (2002) Flow cytometric detection of activated mouse integrin alphaIIbbeta3 with a novel monoclonal antibody. Cytometry 48: 80–86.

19. Born GV (1962) Aggregation of blood platelets by adenosine diphosphate and its reversal. Nature 194: 927.

20. Dejana E, Callioni A, Quintana A, de Gaetano G (1979) Bleeding time in laboratory animals. II. A comparison of different assay conditions in rats. Thromb Res 15: 191–197.

21. Elagib KE, Racke FK, Mogass M, Khetawat R, Delehanty LL, et al. (2003) RUNX1 and GATA-1 coexpression and cooperation in megakaryocytic differentiation. Blood 101: 4333–4341.

22. Shimizu S, Nagasawa T, Katoh O, Komatsu N, Yokota J, et al. (2002) EVI1 is expressed in megakaryocyte cell lineage and enforced expression of EVI1 in UT-7/GM cells induces megakaryocyte differentiation. Biochem Biophys Res Commun 292: 609–616.

23. Kirito K, Osawa M, Morita H, Shimizu R, Yamamoto M, et al. (2002) A functional role of STAT3 in in vivo megakaryopoiesis. Blood 99: 3220–3227.

24. Okada Y, Nagai R, Sato T, Matsuura E, Minami T, et al. (2003) Homeodomain proteins MEIS1 and PBXs regulate the lineage-specific transcription of the platelet factor 4 gene. Blood 101: 4748–4756.

25. Tomer A (2004) Human marrow megakaryocyte differentiation: multiparameter correlative analysis identifies von Willebrand factor as a sensitive and distinctive marker for early (2N and 4N) megakaryocytes. Blood 104: 2722–2727.

26. Davis RE, Stenberg PE, Levin J, Beckstead JH (1997) Localization of megakaryocytes in normal mice and following administration of platelet antiserum, 5-fluorouracil, or radiostrontium: evidence for the site of platelet production. Exp Hematol 25: 638–648.

27. Slayton WB, Georgelas A, Pierce LJ, Elenitoba-Johnson KS, Perry SS, et al. (2002) The spleen is a major site of megakaryopoiesis following transplantation of murine hematopoietic stem cells. Blood 100: 3975–3982.

28. Nieswandt B, Bergmeier W, Rackebrandt K, Gessner JE, Zirngibl H (2000) Identification of critical antigen-specific mechanisms in the development of immune thrombocytopenic purpura in mice. Blood 96: 2520–2527.

29. Gobbi G, Mirandola P, Tazzari P, Ricci F, Caimi L, et al. (2003) Flow cytometry detection of serotonin content and release in resting and activated platelets. Br J Haematol 121: 892–896.

30. Larsen E, Celi A, Gilbert GE, Furie BC, Erban JK, et al. (1989) PADGEM protein: a receptor that mediates the interaction of activated platelets with neutrophils and monocytes. Cell 59: 305–312.

31. Garcia A, Prabhakar S, Hughan S, Anderson TW, Brock CJ, et al. (2004) Differential proteome analysis of TRAP-activated platelets: involvement of DOK-2 and phosphorylation of RGS proteins. Blood 103: 2088–2095.

32. Peters RF, Lees CM, Mitchell KA, Tweed MF, Talbot MD, et al. (1991) The characterisation of thrombus development in an improved model of arterio-venous shunt thrombosis in the rat and the effects of recombinant desulphato-hirudin (CGP 39393), heparin and iloprost. Thromb Haemost 65: 268–274.

33. Louwette S, Labarque V, Wittevrongel C, Thys C, Metz J, et al. (2012) Regulator of G-protein signaling 18 controls megakaryopoiesis and the cilia-mediated vertebrate mechanosensory system. FASEB J 26: 2125–2136.

34. Ma P, Cierniewska A, Signarvic R, Cieslak M, Kong H, et al. (2012) A newly identified complex of spinophilin and the tyrosine phosphatase, SHP-1, modulates platelet activation by regulating G protein-dependent signaling. Blood 119: 1935–1945.

35. Gegenbauer K, Elia G, Blanco-Fernandez A, Smolenski A (2012) Regulator of G-protein signaling 18 integrates activating and inhibitory signaling in platelets. Blood 119: 3799–3807.

36. Gegenbauer K, Nagy Z, Smolenski A (1013) Cyclic nucleotide dependent dephosphorylation of regulator of G-protein signaling in human platelets. PlosOne 8: e80251.

37. Kaur K, Kehrl JM, Charbeneau RA, Neubig RR (2011) RGS-insensitive Gα subunits: probes of Gα subtype-selective signaling and physiological functions of RGS proteins. Methods Mol Biol 756: 75–98.

38. Grillet N, Pattyn A, Contet C, Kieffer BL, Goridis C, et al. (2005) Generation and characterization of Rgs4 mutant mice. Mol Cell Biol 25: 4221–4228.

39. Serafimidis I, Heximer S, Beis D, Gavalas A (2011) G protein-coupled receptor signaling and sphingosine-1-phosphate play a phylogenetically conserved role in endocrine pancreas morphogenesis. Mol Cell Biol 31: 4442–4453.

40. Sjögen B, Neubig RR (2010) Thinking outside of the 'RGS box': a new approaches to therapeutic targeting of regulators of G protein signaling. Mol Pharmacol 78: 550–557.

10

A Non-Invasive Laboratory Panel as a Diagnostic and Prognostic Biomarker for Thrombotic Microangiopathy: Development and Application in a Chinese Cohort Study

Tao Zhang[1], Huimei Chen[1,2]*, Shaoshan Liang[1], Dacheng Chen[1], Chunxia Zheng[1], Caihong Zeng[1], Haitao Zhang[1], Zhihong Liu[1]*

1 National Clinical Research Center of Kidney Diseases, Jinling Hospital, Nanjing University School of Medicine, Nanjing 210002, P. R. China, 2 Jiangsu Key Laboratory of Molecular Medicine, Nanjing University School of Medicine, Nanjing, 210093, P. R. China

Abstract

Background: Thrombotic microangiopathy (TMA) in the kidney is a histopathologic lesion that occurs in a number of clinical settings and is often associated with poor renal prognosis. The standard test for the diagnosis of TMA is the renal biopsy; noninvasive parameters such as potential biomarkers have not been developed.

Methods: We analyzed routine parameters in a cohort of 220 patients with suspected TMA and developed a diagnostic laboratory panel by logistic regression. The levels of candidate markers were validated using an independent cohort (n = 46), a cohort of systemic lupus erythematosus (SLE) (n = 157) and an expanded cohort (n = 113), as well as 9 patients with repeat biopsies.

Results: Of the 220 patients in the derivation cohort, 51 patients with biopsy-proven TMA presented with a worse renal prognosis than those with no TMA (P = 0.002). Platelet and L-lactate dehydrogenase (LDH) levels showed an acceptable diagnostic value of TMA (AUC = 0.739 and 0.756, respectively). A panel of 4 variables - creatinine, platelets, ADAMTS13 (a disintegrin and metalloprotease with thrombospondin type 1 repeats 13) activity and LDH - can effectively discriminate patients with TMA (AUC = 0.800). In the validation cohort, the platelet and LDH levels and the 4-variable panel signature robustly distinguished patients with TMA. The discrimination effects of these three markers were confirmed in patients with SLE. Moreover, LDH levels and the 4-variable panel signature also showed discrimination values in an expanded set. Among patients undergoing repeat biopsy, increased LDH levels and panel signatures were associated with TMA status when paired evaluations were performed. Importantly, only the 4-variable panel was an independent prognostic marker for renal outcome (hazard ratio = 3.549; P<0.001).

Conclusions: The noninvasive laboratory diagnostic panel is better for the early detection and prognosis of TMA compared with a single parameter, and may provide a promising biomarker for clinical application.

Editor: Nancy Lan Guo, West Virginia University, United States of America

Funding: This work was supported in part by National Basic Research Program of China 973 Program No.2012CB517600 (No.2012CB517606) (to Z.L.)(http://www.973.gov.cn/AreaMana.aspx), National Natural Science Foundation (NSF) Grant 81370788 (to H.C.) (http://www.nsfc.gov.cn/), The National Key Technology R&D Program (2011BAI10B04) (to Z.L.) (http://kjzc.jhgl.org/) and Six Talent Peaks Project of Jiangsu Province (2012-WSN-071) (to H.C.) (http://archives.nuist.edu.cn/rcgf/). The funders had no role in study design, data collection and analysis, decision to publish, or preparation of the manuscript.

Competing Interests: The authors have declared that no competing interests exist.

* Email: chenhuimei@nju.edu.cn (HC); liuzhihong@nju.edu.cn (ZL)

Introduction

Thrombotic microangiopathy (TMA) is a pathological lesion that results in thrombosis in capillaries and arterioles, due to an endothelial injury [1–3]. TMA lesions in the kidney usually present in two different forms with considerable overlap: (1) glomerular involvement with capillary thrombi, capillary loops with double contours and mesangiolysis with microhemorrhage, that is most frequently seen in patients with hemolytic uremic syndrome; or (2) predominant arteriolar involvement with thrombi and fibrinoid necrosis, particularly in thrombotic thrombocytopenic purpura and malignant hypertension [4,5].

TMA lesions occur in a number of other kidney diseases as well, including IgA nephropathy, systemic lupus erythematosus (SLE), antiphospholipid antibody syndrome, systemic sclerosis, preeclampsia, infections, medications and post transplantation [2,6,7]. The presence of TMA in the kidney has been proven to be associated with poor renal prognosis [8,9]. Nephrologists often face a typical situation in which patients are suspected of having TMA lesions on the basis of renal disorders. In such cases, it is difficult to decide on an early therapy before the results of a renal biopsy are obtained [10]. While the interpretation of the renal biopsy has become more standardized and the invasive procedure safer over time, bleeding and subsequent functional impairment nevertheless still occur, especially in the patients with coagulopathy [11].

Heterogeneous disorders with TMA are usually characterized by microangiopathic hemolytic anemia (MAHA) [12], thrombocytopenia and/or ischemic organ failure. It is questionable as to whether these abnormalities can predict TMA, since they are also observed in patients without TMA, and studies have been inconsistent [13,14]. Hence, we enrolled cohorts of patients with renal damage and MAHA and/or thrombocytopenia to determine whether a single parameter or a diagnostic panel could predict the histological TMA. In addition, the association between the noninvasive prediction and a poor renal outcome was further investigated.

Methods

Ethics statement

The study was approved by the Ethics Committee of Jinling Hospital. Because this study was retrospective, the Ethics Committee agreed to waive the requirement for the informed consent, and the data were analyzed anonymously.

Patient selection and study design

We enrolled a cohort of suspected patients from the Research Institute of Nephrology, Jinling Hospital, Nanjing University School of Medicine, PR China during July 2011 to July 2012 (n = 266). The enrollment criteria were: renal damage (proteinuria, hematuria or renal dysfunction) and microangiopathic hemolytic anemia (hemoglobin level below 120 g/L for males, 110 g/L for females, at least 5 schistocytes per high power field in a peripheral blood smear, elevated LDH above 240 u/L [normal 60–240 u/L]) or thrombocytopenia (platelet counts below 100×10^9/L of blood at any time in the course of the disease) [15]. Patients were randomly divided into two cohorts: (1) derivation cohort (n = 220) and (2) validation cohort (n = 46).

In addition, 157 patients diagnosed with SLE were selected from the suspected patients, and 113 patients were enrolled in an expanded group for external validation. SLE was defined according to the 1997 American College of Rheumatology revised criteria for SLE [16]. The independent patients were enrolled in the expanded group according to the criteria: (1) renal damage (proteinuria, hematuria or renal dysfunction) and (2) fever (temperature of >38°C, no infection), elevated LDH (more than 240 u/L) or non-renal anemia. The information and profiles of patients during the follow-up sessions were also reviewed through October 2013.

Definitions

TMA in the kidney was defined by the histologic feature of occlusive fibrin-platelet thrombi in at least one glomerulus or one arteriole, with one or more of the following: (1) glomerular endothelial swelling and detachment, capillary wall thickening and double contour formation, mesangial lysis with microhemorrhage, and erythrocytolysis, and/or (2) obliterative arteriolopathy defined as luminal occlusion with mural myxoid or fibrinoid change, thickening of the vessel wall, with or without erythrocytolysis, luminal thrombosis and concentric spindle cell proliferation or hypercellularity [2,5].

All patients accepted adjunctive treatments, including protecting the organ function, symptomatic and immunosuppressive treatment. Glomerularfiltration rate was estimated (eGFR) using the simplified MDRD (Modification of Diet in Renal Disease) formula. End stage renal disease (ESRD) was defined as eGFR< 15 mL/min/1.73 m^2 or a need for permanent dialysis therapy.

During follow-up, the combined event defined as ESRD or a doubling of the serum creatinine level and death. The renal survival rate was defined as the percentage of patients who had preservation of renal function independent of ESRD and death, while the survival rate was defined as the percentage of live patients.

Laboratory features

Physical exams and routine laboratory tests were performed on the suspected patients. Serum ADAMTS13 activity was measured by the Fluorescence Resonance Energy Transfer (FRET) assay (United States Patent No.7270976) [17]. Serum anti-ADAMTS13 IgG antibodies (Sekisui Diagnostics, USA), vWF (von Willebrand factor) (Sunbiote, Shanghai, China), thrombomodulin (Diaclone Research, Besancon, France), E-selectin (R&D Systems, Minneapolis, Minnesota, USA) and soluble vascular cellular adhesion molecule-1 (sVCAM-1, VCAM) (R&D Systems, Minneapolis, Minnesota, USA) were measured using enzyme linked immunosorbent assays. The concentrations of endothelial cells in the circulation were sorted using a magnetic microbead sorting system (MACS, Miltenyi Biotec, Germany), according to the manufacturer's instructions [18].

Statistical analysis

All data were given a numerical code and statistical analysis was performed using SPSS software, version 19.0 or RMS software, version 2.12.2. Comparisons of proportions or mean values between patients with or without TMA in the kidney were calculated by the Mann-Whitney test or chi-square (χ2) test.

Logistic regression was used to identify 6 parameters - hemoglobin, platelets, serum creatinine, LDH, ADAMTS13 activity and THBD - that discriminated between patients with and without TMA in the kidney. Regression estimated from this panel defined a diagnostic signature or individual predictors, and the greatest area under the receiver-operating-characteristic (ROC) curve as the best-fitting model was used. The area under the curve (AUC) was calculated, and sensitivity and specificity were used to evaluate the ability of these to discriminate TMA in the kidney. The best sub-set panel was then fit to 1000 additional bootstrap samples. Cross-validated measures of discrimination (i.e., the AUC), model fit (i.e., calibration-curve intercept and slope) and a locally estimated scatterplot-smoothed (loess) calibration plot were obtained [19].

Cumulative incidence of poor renal outcome was calculated using Kaplan-Meier survival probabilities (1- survival probabilities) and comparisons were made using the log-rank test. Cox regression was performed to test the association of the pathologic findings and the 4-variable panel signature with the renal outcome. A two-tailed P value less than 0.05 is considered to be statistically significant.

Results

In the derivation cohort of 220 patients, 51 (23.2%) patients were histologically proven to have TMA by renal biopsy. Compared with patients without TMA, the patients with TMA presented a worse renal outcome (P = 0.002, log-rank test; Figure 1) at the 12-month follow-up, with a renal survival rate of 54.9% (P = 0.015; Table 1).

Correlation between laboratory parameters and TMA lesions

The levels of serum creatinine, LDH and thrombomodulin (THBD) were significantly higher in patients with TMA than those

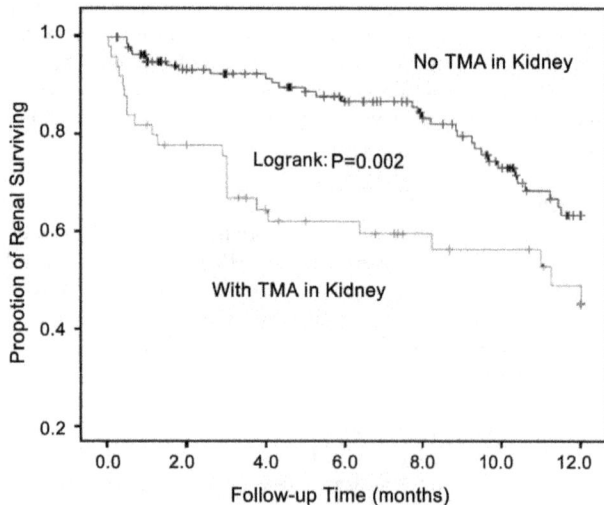

Figure 1. Comparison of renal outcome in suspected patients.
After 12 months of follow-up, the patients with TMA had a worse
outcome of renal survival than those without TMA (Log rank: P = 0.002).

without TMA, while levels of hemoglobin, platelets and
ADAMTS13 activity were remarkably lower (all P<0.05;
Table 1). With a cutoff of 0.05 (P value, in Table 1), 6 laboratory
parameters were included in the next binary logistic regression
analysis. The ROC curve showed that these 6 parameters
individually can distinguish patients with TMA in the derivation
set (all P<0.05; Figure 2A). Only the platelet and LDH levels
showed acceptable discrimination values (0.7≤AUC<0.8), while
levels of hemoglobin, serum creatinine, ADAMTS13 activity and
THBD had low discrimination accuracy (0.5≤AUC<0.7). With
the use of the cutoff point of 97.5×10^9/L, platelets had 82.4%
sensitivity and 60.9% specificity, and with the cutoff point of
289 u/L, LDH had 67.3% sensitivity and 74.1% specificity (Table
S1 in File S1).

In an independent validation cohort, platelet and LDH levels
also could discriminate patients with TMA from those without
TMA (Figure 2B; Table S2 in File S1). Thus, the levels of platelets
and LDH showed acceptable predictive probabilities of patients
with TMA in the kidney.

Correlation between the 4-variable panel and TMA lesions

Furthermore, multiple logistic regression analysis in the
derivation set indicated that levels of serum creatinine (SCr),
platelets (PLT), LDH and ADAMTS13 activity were valid
predictors of renal TMA lesions (all P<0.05; Table 2), with the
final panel signature:

$$-0.371 - 0.002 \times ADAMTS13 activity$$
$$+ 0.140 \times SCr + 0.004 \times LDH - 0.010 \times PLT$$

The units of measurement are as listed in Table 1. In the
equation, −0.371 was the intercept, and −0.002, 0.140, 0.004 and
−0.010 were the slopes (coefficients), respectively, for the
ADAMTS13 activity, SCr (mg/dL), LDH and PLT values in
the best-fitting logistic-regression model. The intercept and slopes
have no intrinsic units of measurement.

The ROC curve showed that this 4-variable model yielded an
AUC of 0.800 (95% confidence interval [CI], 0.723 to 0.877; P<
0.001), suggesting a good discrimination between patients with
TMA in the kidney and those without TMA (Figure 3A). With the
use of the cutoff point of 0.248, this diagnostic panel has 81.6%
sensitivity and 66.9% specificity. The diagnostic panel for the
prediction of TMA was validated in the independent cohort, with
an AUC of 0.815 (P<0.001; Figure 3B). The use of the cut-off of
0.248 predicted the presence of TMA with 80.0% sensitivity and
61.5% specificity.

Bootstrap validation of this 4-variable panel yielded a cross-
validated estimate of the AUC of 0.777, which is an estimate of the
expected value of the AUC in the combined derivation and
validation cohorts. The calibration-curve intercept and slope were
0.07 and 0.64, respectively. It was revealed that the predicted
probabilities of a biopsy showing TMA in the kidney tended to be
relatively higher than the actual probabilities (Figure 3C). The
loess-smoothed estimates of the unadjusted and cross-validated
calibration curves were overlaid on a diagonal reference line
representing good model calibration (P = 0.489). The close
correspondence of the two curves to the reference line shows
good fit and reflects the above interpretation of the intercept and
slope estimates of the calibration curve (Figure 3C).

Evaluation of LDH, platelet and the 4- variable panel in extra cohorts

Since renal TMA lesions occur in a number of kidney diseases,
we focused on a specific condition and 157 renal patients
diagnosed with SLE were selected in extra validation (Table S3
in File S1). All levels of platelets, LDH and the 4-variable panel
could discriminate patients with TMA in SLE. The ability of
discrimination in the 4-variable panel was higher than the levels of
platelets and LDH, with an AUC of 0.872 (Figure 4A). With the
use of the cutoff point of 0.248, the diagnostic panel has 74.1%
sensitivity and 83.6% specificity.

To further enhance the application of these markers, we
enrolled another independent group of 113 patients and determined the association between the levels of LDH, platelets and the
4-variable panel and TMA lesions (Table S4 in File S1). ROC
curve analysis showed that the levels of LDH and the 4-variable
panel yielded an AUC of 0.843 and 0.825, showing a good
discrimination of TMA (both P<0.001; Figure 4B). However,
platelet levels could not predict patients with TMA lesions in this
cohort (P = 0.068).

Evaluation of LDH and the 4-variable panel in patients with repeat biopsy

We then analyzed, in a subset of 9 patients who underwent
repeat renal biopsy, levels of LDH and the 4-variable panel in
paired blood samples taken at the time of the first and second
biopsy (Table S5 in File S1). It is interesting to note that the 4-
variable panel signature plummeted from 0.248 or higher in the
same subset of patients when they presented with TMA at the first
biopsy, but with no TMA at second biopsy (Figure 5A). On the
contrary, for the only patient who had no TMA at first biopsy but
exhibited TMA at the second biopsy, the 4-variable panel
dramatically increased to greater than 0.248. For the other 5
patients, the 4-variable signature was significantly decreased after
treatment (P = 0.030), although they each presented without TMA
at the two biopsies and the signature was 0.248 or less.

A similar pattern of LDH changes were observed in the patients
with repeat biopsy, and increased LDH levels were associated with
TMA status (Figure 5B). However, an LDH value of 289 u/L was

Table 1. Clinical laboratory data for suspected patients in derivation cohort (n = 220).

	TMA	No TMA	P Value
Number of patients	**51**	**169**	
Age (year)	26 (963)	28 (1370)	0.450
Male (n, %)	10 (19.6)	45 (26.6)	0.310
Clinical diagnosis			
HUS/TTP (n, %)	15 (29.4)	0 (0)	<0.001
Primary glomerulonephritis & acute interstitial nephritis (n, %)	0 (0)	22 (13.0)	0.003
Autoimmune diseases (n, %)	29 (56.9)	144 (85.2)	<0.001
SLE (n, %)	27/29 (93.1)	130/144 (90.3)	1.000
Pregnancy/postpartum (n, %)	5 (9.8)	1 (0.6)	0.003
Malignant hypertension (n, %)	1 (2.0)	0 (0)	0.232
Post-transplantation (n, %)	1 (2.0)	2 (1.2)	0.549
Laboratory profiles			
Urine protein (g/24 h)	1.5 (0.310.6)	2.5 (0.29.8)	0.073
Erythrocyturia (×10^4/mL)	18 (110000)	24 (19000)	0.364
Hemoglobin (g/L)	74.2±16.1	87.1±21.6	<0.001
Platelets (×10^9/L)	73 (10275)	108 (34441)	<0.001
Serum creatinine (umol/L)	347.2 (52.21697.5)	162.7 (33.61556.0)	<0.001
Globulin (g/L)	22.0±5.7	23.3±6.6	0.289
C3 (g/L)	0.62±0.29	0.57±0.30	0.219
C4 (g/L)	0.16±0.10	0.14±0.10	0.098
L-lactate dehydrogenase (u/L)	418 (1292920)	267 (64878)	<0.001
ADAMTS13 antibody (Au/mL)	16.6 (2.184.9)	16.6 (1.681.3)	0.862
ADAMTS13 activity (ng/mL)	616±331	772±255	0.001
NEC (/ml)	19.7±6.8	20.7±8.9	0.654
E-selectin (ng/mL)	65.2±37.3	73.1±72.8	0.636
VCAM (ng/mL)	2011±1070	2460±1340	0.073
Thrombomodulin (ng/mL)	6.3±4.3	4.4±2.8	<0.001
vWF (%)	184±127	215±120	0.080
After 12-months of follow up			
Renal survival rate (%)	54.9 (28/51)	74.6 (126/169)	0.015
Survival rate (%)	94.1 (48/51)	98.2 (166/169)	0.138

Values are expressed as medians (range), means ± standard deviation or percentages. P values were calculated by Mann-Whitney U test, Fisher's exact test or chi-square test as appropriate. HUS: hemolytic uremic syndrome; TTP: thrombotic thrombocytopenic purpura; SLE: systemic lupus erythematosus; C3: Complement component 3; C4: Complement component 4; ADAMTS13: A Disintegrin and Metalloprotease with ThromboSpondin type 1 repeats 13; NEC: normal endothelial cells; VCAM: vascular cell adhesion molecule; vWF: von Willebrand factor.

not a good cut-off level to discriminate TMA status in this group of patients.

Association of LDH levels and the 4-variable panel with renal survival

To further evaluate whether LDH levels and the 4-variable panel can serve as a predictor of renal survival in patients with suspected TMA, we performed a Kaplan-Meier survival analysis. As suspected, patients with a higher 4-variable panel signature had a statistically significant worse renal outcome (P<0.001, log-rank test; Figure 6A). However, the pattern of increased LDH concentrations was not associated with a poorer renal outcome (P = 0.183, log-rank test; Figure 6B).

Furthermore, the renal survival was only 53.9% in patients with a panel signature of more than 0.248, but was 79.5% in patients with a panel signature of less than 0.248. The Cox proportional

hazard survival regression model revealed that TMA lesions increased the risk for a poor renal outcome, with a hazard ratio of 2.235 (95% CI 1.306 to 3.826, P = 0.003), while a panel signature 0.248 or greater had a hazard ratio of 3.549 (95% CI 2.034 to 3.549, P<0.001). These two diagnostic factors showed a similar predictive effect on renal outcome (P = 0.964).

Discussion

Histological TMA in the kidney has been frequently described in association with a large number of underlying diseases [20–22]. Although the causes of TMA in the kidney are unclear, it has been reported that there is a significantly worse renal outcome among patients with TMA [16,22]. Kaplan et al. [23] reported that death rates were as high as 25% and progression to ESRD occurred in half of the patients with TMA within 10 years after diagnosis. In agreement with published studies [24], we confirmed that patients

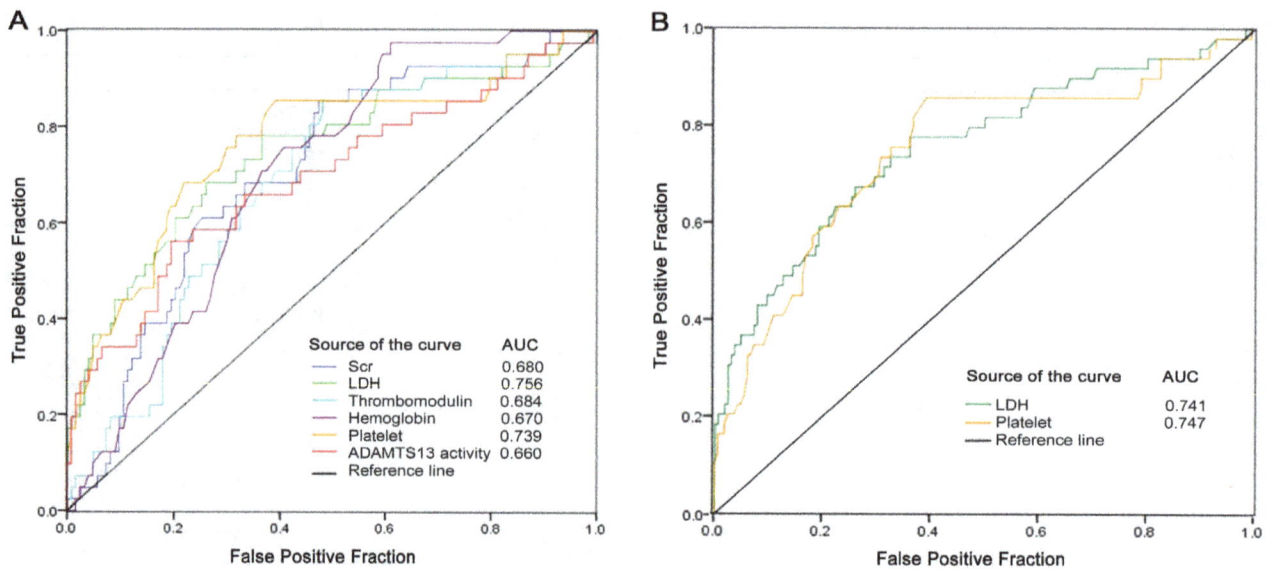

Figure 2. Receiver operating characteristic curves of laboratory parameters. (A) The fraction of true positive results (sensitivity) and the fraction of false positive results (1-specificity) for LDH, HGB, SCr, PLT, THBD and ADAMTS13 activity were developed in 220 patients (all P≤0.001), and the levels of platelet and LDH showed acceptable discrimination, with AUC 0.739 and 0.756, respectively. (B) The levels of platelet and LDH could discriminate patients with TMA from those with no TMA in the validation cohort (n = 46), with AUC 0.747 and 0.741, respectively.

with renal biopsy-proven TMA presented with a poor outcome in the kidney and the patients with TMA had a 2.24-fold higher risk of renal failure than those without TMA.

The renal biopsy represents the gold standard in the management of patients with TMA, but a noninvasive diagnostic method for detection of TMA would be a valuable clinical application. Few studies have focused on the prediction of the histopathologic lesions, although abnormalities in the urinalysis and an increase in serum creatinine have been observed in patients with TMA lesions [25]. In addition, reports have demonstrated that laboratory variables were involved in clinical conditions associated with TMA [26–28], including hemolytic uremic syndrome and thrombotic thrombocytopenic purpura. Increased levels of LDH are associated with the severity of hemolysis and tissue ischemia, which might increase the risk of tissue lesions [29]. A deficiency of ADAMTS13 was related to thrombus formation and was subsequently noted in patients with thrombocytopenic purpura, who often suffered from TMA lesions in the kidney [30,31].

This study is the first to demonstrate the potential of routine laboratory parameters to be used in the detection of TMA without renal biopsy. Six parameters - serum creatinine, platelets, hemoglobin, THBD, ADAMTS13 activity and LDH - had

moderate diagnostic value for TMA. The strengths of this study are that we developed a diagnostic panel based on 4 laboratory variables (levels of serum creatinine, LDH, platelets and ADAMTS13 activity). This panel can noninvasively and accurately predict histological TMA. This is supported by the high AUC values of 0.800 derived from patients with and without TMA (sensitivity 81.6%; specificity 66.9%). Similar effects were noted when the predictive panel was validated using an independent population. The cross-validation further revealed that the 4-variable model tended to have high sensitivity, but a relatively low specificity. To the best of our knowledge, this is the first noninvasive biomarker that can detect TMA in the kidney. In addition, each individual parameter of the 5 or 6 variable model could not reach statistical significance (P<0.05, data not shown). The model of fewer variables could discriminate patients with TMA in derivation cohort, including the levels of LDH and platelets, but this effect was not proven by all different validation cohorts.

The 3 markers, LDH, platelets and the 4-variable panel, were further evaluated in a group of patients with SLE and expanded sets of patients. SLE is often reported with TMA lesions in the kidney [6,22], and there were 157 patients diagnosed with SLE

Table 2. Results of logistic regression analysis (n = 220).

Variable	B	S.E	Sig.	Exp (B)	95% CI
					Lower-Upper
Serum creatinine	0.140	0.060	0.020	1.150	1.022–1.295
LDH	0.004	0.001	0.002	1.004	1.001–1.006
Platelet	−0.010	0.004	0.021	0.990	0.981–0.998
ADAMTS 13 Activity	−0.002	0.001	0.014	0.998	0.996–1.000

Abbreviations: B: coefficient of regression; S.E.: Standard Error; Sig: P value; Exp (B): odds ratio; CI: confidence interval. LDH: L-lactate dehydrogenase; ADAMTS 13: a disintegrin and metalloprotease with thrombospondin type 1 repeats 13.

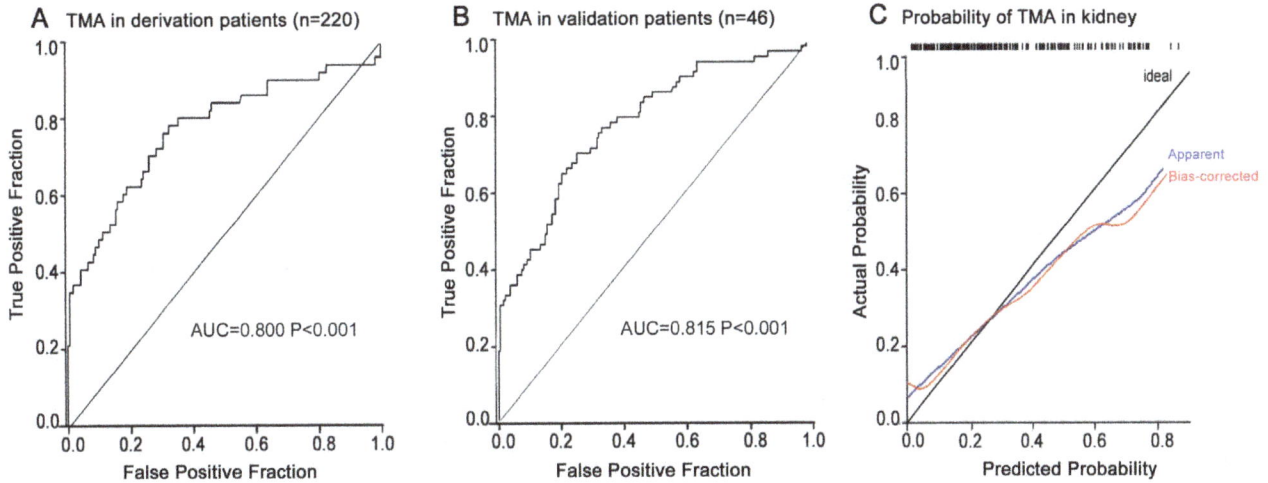

Figure 3. Receiver operating characteristic curves and calibration curve for a diagnostic panel. (A) The diagnostic panel was developed in the derivation group of 220 suspected patients, with AUC 0.800, P<0.001. (B) This marker was validated in 46 independent patients, with AUC 0.815, P<0.001. (C) Bootstrap validation shows the calibration curve of the diagnostic panel. Cross-validated estimates of the AUC, calibration-curve intercept and slope were 0.777, 0.07 and 0.64, respectively. The loess-smoothed estimates of the cross-validated and unadjusted calibration curves are overlaid on a diagonal reference line representing good model calibration.

among the suspected patients investigated. Focusing on one particular disease, all 3 markers showed discrimination values for patients with TMA. Because some patients with TMA exhibit little or no signs of clinical manifestations [31–33], we expanded the application of these markers. LDH levels and the 4-variable panel still demonstrated good discrimination, while platelets did not. Thus, LDH levels and the 4-variable panel might have wide usage in different cohorts of patients. In addition, data from patients with a repeat biopsy confirmed the association of increased LDH levels and the 4-variable signature with TMA status.

Another important finding of our study was that the 4-variable panel also serves as a prognostic biomarker for renal patients. The increased signature of the 4-variable panel was an independent prognostic parameter. The prognostic value of the 4-variable panel was similar with the histological diagnosis of TMA. As a noninvasive biomarker, the 4-variable panel showed an advantage in clinical application. However, LDH levels did not exhibit a prognostic value for renal outcome. Therefore, the 4-variable panel might not only diagnose TMA but also help predict renal

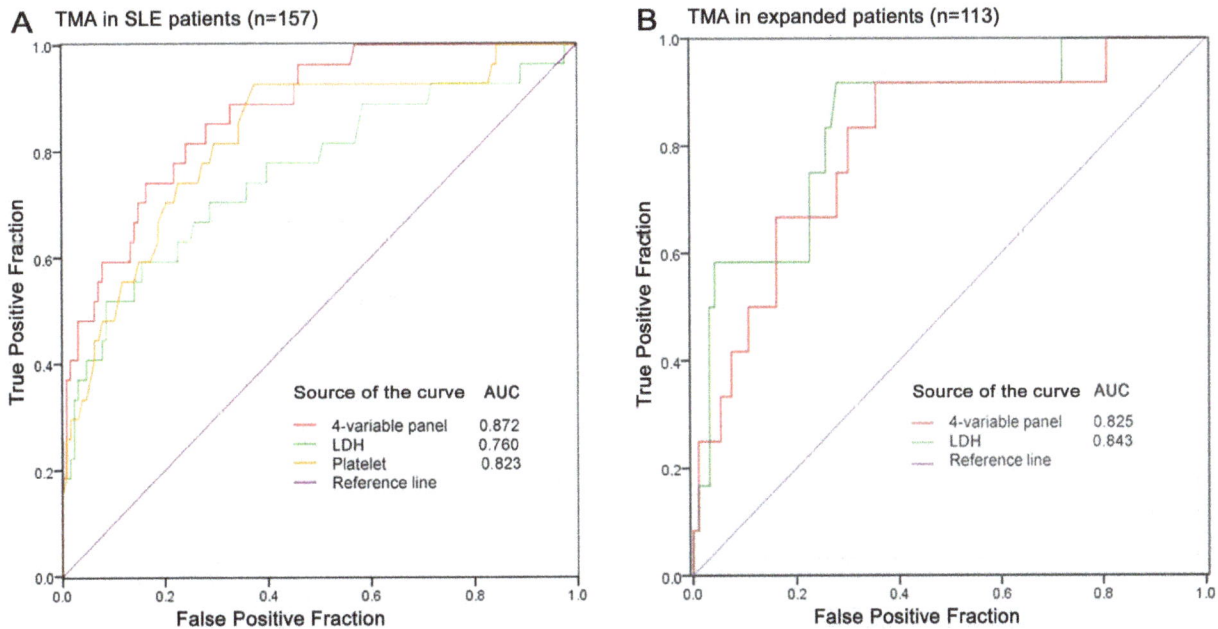

Figure 4. Evaluation of LDH, platelet and 4-variable panel in extra cohorts. (A) All levels of platelet, LDH and the 4-variable panel were evaluated in 157 suspected patients diagnosed with SLE and could discriminate patients with TMA, with an AUC of 0.823, 0.76 and 0.872, respectively. (B) To further validate in another independent group of 113 patients and ROC curve analysis showed that the levels of LDH and the 4-variable panel yielded an AUC of 0.843 and 0.825, showing an good discrimination of TMA (both P<0.001).

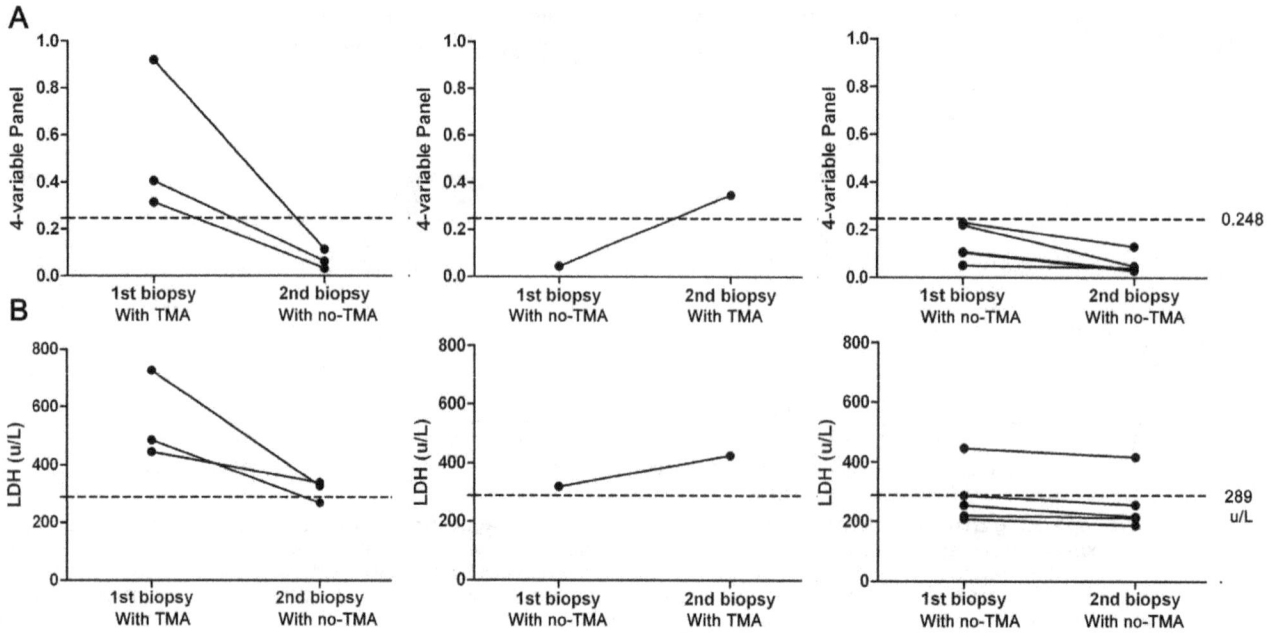

Figure 5. Evaluation of LDH and 4-variable panel in patients with repeat biopsy. (A)We analyzed paired first and second levels of LDH and 4-variable panel in a subset of 9 patients, who underwent repeat renal biopsy. The first figure shows 4-variable panel signature plummeted from 0.248 or greater in the same subset of patients, when three patients presented TMA at first biopsy but no TMA at second biopsy. In the second figure, only one patient had no TMA at first biopsy and TMA at second biopsy and 4-variable panel dramatically increased to 0.348. For other 5 patients, 4-variable signature was significantly decreased after treatment, although they consistently presented without TMA at two biopsies and the signature was 0.248 or less. (B) Similar pattern of LDH changes was observed in the patients with repeat biopsy, and increased LDH levels were associated with TMA status.

outcome with a higher accuracy than other single laboratory parameter.

Although our current assay may become a promising diagnostic tool for TMA, we acknowledge three potential limitations of this study. It is retrospective and will need to be validated with a prospective cohort of patients. Furthermore, the evaluation of prognosis was rendered difficult because of the variable nature of the treatments received. In addition, the number of patients with certain diseases was small and some validations were calculated using non-independent data, which prevented an in-depth

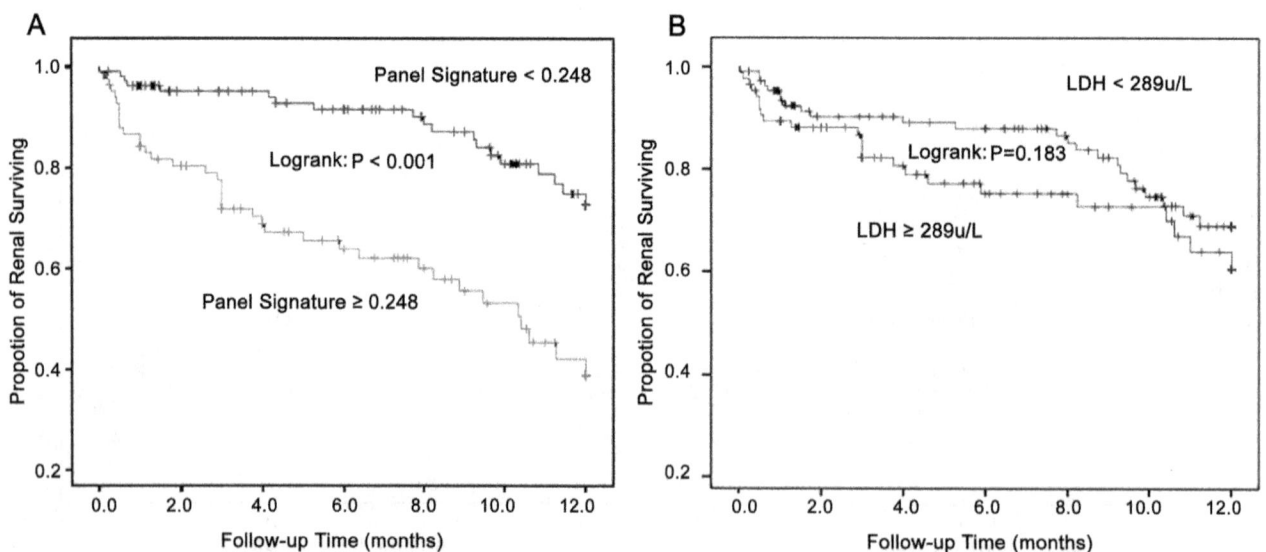

Figure 6. Association of LDH levels and 4-variable panel with renal survival. (A) Using the cutoff value of 0.248, suspected patients were divided into two groups by more or less than the value and the renal survival of two groups followed up 12 months was significantly different (P< 0.001). (B) The pattern of increased LDH concentrations (more than the cutoff point of 289 u/L) associated statistically poorer renal outcome was not observed (P = 0.183).

evaluation of the usefulness of the diagnostic panel for specifically predicting TMA in the kidney.

Conclusions

In conclusion, our results provide compelling evidence for the potential use of laboratory parameters as a noninvasive diagnostic and prognostic tool for TMA in the kidney. The 4-variable panel showed an advantage for the early detection of renal TMA lesions without renal biopsy and in directly predicting renal prognosis. In order for this concept to be incorporated into routine clinical practice in the near-future, validation is needed in large-scale prospective trials.

Supporting Information

File S1 Includes table S1–S5. **Table S1,** Diagnosis of TMA in kidney among patients (n = 220). **Table S2,** Laboratory variables in the validation group of internal patients (n = 46). **Table S3,** Clinical laboratory data for suspected patients with SLE (n = 157). **Table S4,** Clinical laboratory data for patients in expanded group (n = 113). **Table S5,** The laboratory feature of patients with/without TMA in the kidney at first renal biopsy and repeat biopsy.

Acknowledgments

We thank all the patients and their families who participated in this study.

Author Contributions

Conceived and designed the experiments: TZ HC ZL. Performed the experiments: TZ HC DC CZ SL CZ. Analyzed the data: TZ HC ZL. Contributed reagents/materials/analysis tools: DC SL HZ. Contributed to the writing of the manuscript: TZ HC ZL.

References

1. Moake JL (2002) Thrombotic microangiopathies. N Engl J Med 347: 589–600.
2. El Karoui K, Hill GS, Karras A, Jacquot C, Moulonguet L, et al. (2012) A clinicopathologic study of thrombotic microangiopathy in IgA nephropathy. J Am Soc Nephrol 23: 137–148.
3. Goldberg RJ, Nakagawa T, Johnson RJ, Thurman JM (2010) The role of endothelial cell injury in thrombotic microangiopathy. Am J Kidney Dis 56: 1168–1174.
4. van den Born BJ, van der Hoeven NV, Groot E, Lenting PJ, Meijers JC, et al. (2008) Association between thrombotic microangiopathy and reduced ADAMTS13 activity in malignant hypertension. Hypertension 51: 862–866.
5. Laurence J (2000) Pathological and therapeutic distinctions in HUS/TTP. Lancet 355: 497; author reply 497–498.
6. Hughson MD, Nadasdy T, McCarty GA, Sholer C, Min KW, et al. (1992) Renal thrombotic microangiopathy in patients with systemic lupus erythematosus and the antiphospholipid syndrome. Am J Kidney Dis 20: 150–158.
7. Eremina V, Jefferson JA, Kowalewska J, Hochster H, Haas M, et al. (2008) VEGF inhibition and renal thrombotic microangiopathy. N Engl J Med 358: 1129–1136.
8. Garg AX, Suri RS, Barrowman N, Rehman F, Matsell D, et al. (2003) Long-term renal prognosis of diarrhea-associated hemolytic uremic syndrome: a systematic review, meta-analysis, and meta-regression. JAMA 290: 1360–1370.
9. Reynolds JC, Agodoa LY, Yuan CM, Abbott KC (2003) Thrombotic microangiopathy after renal transplantation in the United States. Am J Kidney Dis 42: 1058–1068.
10. Clark WF (2012) Thrombotic microangiopathy: current knowledge and outcomes with plasma exchange. Semin Dial 25: 214–219.
11. Stiles KP, Yuan CM, Chung EM, Lyon RD, Lane JD, et al. (2000) Renal biopsy in high-risk patients with medical diseases of the kidney. Am J Kidney Dis 36: 419–433.
12. Symmers WS (1952) Thrombotic microangiopathic haemolytic anaemia (thrombotic microangiopathy). Br Med J 2: 897–903.
13. George JN, Vesely SK, James JA (2007) Overlapping features of thrombotic thrombocytopenic purpura and systemic lupus erythematosus. South Med J 100: 512–514.
14. D'Angelo WA, Fries JF, Masi AT, Shulman LE (1969) Pathologic observations in systemic sclerosis (scleroderma). A study of fifty-eight autopsy cases and fifty-eight matched controls. Am J Med 46: 428–440.
15. Cataland SR, Yang SB, Witkoff L, Kraut EH, Lin S, et al. (2009) Demographic and ADAMTS13 biomarker data as predictors of early recurrences of idiopathic thrombotic thrombocytopenic purpura. Eur J Haematol 83: 559–564.
16. Hochberg MC (1997) Updating the American College of Rheumatology revised criteria for the classification of systemic lupus erythematosus. Arthritis Rheum 40: 1725.
17. Peng J, Gong L, Si K, Bai X, Du G (2011) Fluorescence resonance energy transfer assay for high-throughput screening of ADAMTS1 inhibitors. Molecules 16: 10709–10721.
18. White LE, Cui Y, Shelak CM, Lie ML, Hassoun HT (2012) Lung endothelial cell apoptosis during ischemic acute kidney injury. Shock 38: 320–327.
19. Austin PC, Tu JV (2004) Bootstrap methods for developing predictive models. Am Stat 58: 131–137.
20. Baliga RS, Wingo CS (2003) Quinine induced HUS-TTP: an unusual presentation. Am J Med Sci 326: 378–380.
21. Noris M, Remuzzi G (2010) Thrombotic microangiopathy after kidney transplantation. Am J Transplant 10: 1517–1523.
22. Hu WX, Liu ZZ, Chen HP, Zhang HT, Li LS, et al. (2010) Clinical characteristics and prognosis of diffuse proliferative lupus nephritis with thrombotic microangiopathy. Lupus 19: 1591–1598.
23. Kaplan B, Meier-Kriesche HU (2002) Death after graft loss: an important late study endpoint in kidney transplantation. Am J Transplant 2: 970–974.
24. Michael M, Elliott EJ, Craig JC, Ridley G, Hodson EM (2009) Interventions for hemolytic uremic syndrome and thrombotic thrombocytopenic purpura: a systematic review of randomized controlled trials. Am J Kidney Dis 53: 259–272.
25. Droz D, Nochy D, Noel LH, Heudes D, Nabarra B, et al. (2000) Thrombotic microangiopathies: renal and extrarenal lesions. Adv Nephrol Necker Hosp 30: 235–259.
26. Vesely SK, George JN, Lammle B, Studt JD, Alberio L, et al. (2003) ADAMTS13 activity in thrombotic thrombocytopenic purpura-hemolytic uremic syndrome: relation to presenting features and clinical outcomes in a prospective cohort of 142 patients. Blood 102: 60–68.
27. Park YA, Waldrum MR, Marques MB (2010) Platelet count and prothrombin time help distinguish thrombotic thrombocytopenic purpura-hemolytic uremic syndrome from disseminated intravascular coagulation in adults. Am J Clin Pathol 133: 460–465.
28. Cataland SR, Yang S, Wu HM (2012) The use of ADAMTS13 activity, platelet count, and serum creatinine to differentiate acquired thrombotic thrombocytopenic purpura from other thrombotic microangiopathies. Br J Haematol 157: 501–503.
29. Cohen JA, Brecher ME, Bandarenko N (1998) Cellular source of serum lactate dehydrogenase elevation in patients with thrombotic thrombocytopenic purpura. J Clin Apher 13: 16–19.
30. Furlan M, Robles R, Solenthaler M, Wassmer M, Sandoz P, et al. (1997) Deficient activity of von Willebrand factor-cleaving protease in chronic relapsing thrombotic thrombocytopenic purpura. Blood 89: 3097–3103.
31. Galbusera M, Noris M, Rossi C, Orisio S, Caprioli J, et al. (1999) Increased fragmentation of von Willebrand factor, due to abnormal cleavage of the subunit, parallels disease activity in recurrent hemolytic uremic syndrome and thrombotic thrombocytopenic purpura and discloses predisposition in families. The Italian Registry of Familial and Recurrent HUS/TTP. Blood 94: 610–620.
32. George JN (2006) Clinical practice. Thrombotic thrombocytopenic purpura. N Engl J Med 354: 1927–1935.
33. Hastings MC, Wyatt RJ, Ault BH, Jones DP, Lau KK, et al. (2007) Diagnosis of de novo localized thrombotic microangiopathy by surveillance biopsy. Pediatr Nephrol 22: 742–746.

11

Average Values and Racial Differences of Neutrophil Lymphocyte Ratio among a Nationally Representative Sample of United States Subjects

Basem Azab[1], Marlene Camacho-Rivera[2], Emanuela Taioli[2]*

1 Department of Surgery, Staten Island University Hospital, Staten Island, New York, United States of America, 2 Department of Population Health, North Shore LIJ-Hofstra School of Medicine, Great Neck, New York, United States of America

Abstract

Introduction: Several studies reported the negative impact of elevated neutrophil/lymphocyte ratio (NLR) on outcomes in many surgical and medical conditions. Previous studies used arbitrary NLR cut-off points according to the average of the populations under study. There is no data on the average NLR in the general population. The aim of this study is to explore the average values of NLR and according to race in adult non-institutional United States individuals by using national data.

Methods: The National Health and Nutrition Examination Survey (NHANES) of aggregated cross-sectional data collected from 2007 to 2010 was analyzed; data extracted included markers of systemic inflammation (neutrophil count, lymphocyte count, and NLR), demographic variables and other comorbidities. Subjects who were prescribed steroids, chemotherapy, immunomodulators and antibiotics were excluded. Adjusted linear regression models were used to examine the association between demographic and clinical characteristics and neutrophil counts, lymphocyte counts, and NLR.

Results: Overall 9427 subjects are included in this study. The average value of neutrophils is 4.3k cells/mL, of lymphocytes 2.1k cells/mL; the average NLR is 2.15. Non-Hispanic Black and Hispanic participants have significantly lower mean NLR values (1.76, 95% CI 1.71–1.81 and 2.08, 95% CI 2.04–2.12 respectively) when compared to non-Hispanic Whites (2.24, 95% CI 2.19–2.28–p<0.0001). Subjects who reported diabetes, cardiovascular disease, and smoking had significantly higher NLR than subjects who did not. Racial differences regarding the association of smoking and BMI with NLR were observed.

Conclusions: This study is providing preliminary data on racial disparities in a marker of inflammation, NLR, that has been associated with several chronic diseases outcome, suggesting that different cut-off points should be set according to race. It also suggests that racial differences exist in the inflammatory response to environmental and behavioral risk factors.

Editor: Jian Zhang, The Ohio State University, United States of America

Funding: The authors have no support or funding to report.

Competing Interests: The authors have declared that no competing interests exist.

* Email: etaioli@nshs.edu

Introduction

Inflammation plays a major role in the pathophysiology of commonly considered non-inflammatory diseases, such as cancer and atherosclerosis [1–4]. Among many inflammatory markers, several studies demonstrated that elevated neutrophil/lymphocyte ratio (NLR) is a significant predictor of adverse outcomes for patients with cardiovascular disease or cancer [5–8]. NLR is believed to reflect the balance between innate (neutrophils) and adaptive (lymphocytes) immune responses. Previous research has shown that elevated NLR is associated with increased concentration of various pro-inflammatory cytokines [8–10] which may cause cellular DNA damage.

These studies corroborate the negative impact of elevated NLR, however they differ in their NLR cutoff points. While some studies categorized their patients according to NLR intervals (e.g. tertiles, quartiles, quintiles) [11–13], other studies used definite NLR cutoff points (e.g. NLR≥2.5 [14], NLR≥2.7 [15], NLR≥3 [16], NLR≥4 [17], and others used NLR≥5 [18–20]. Of note, the studies from western countries often used higher NLR cutoff points compared to other ethnicity (e.g. Asian and African), which reflect well known racial difference in the normal range of neutrophil and lymphocyte counts [21,22]. It is not known, however, if differences observed in NLR reflect real variation among healthy human subjects, or are related to the lack of standardization in the measurement of this biomarker. In fact, studies report differ timing for the collection of blood used to calculate NLR; some collect the

Table 1. Sample characteristics among NHANES 2007–2010 participants (n = 9427).

Variable	Categories	Subjects tested (N)	Weighted Prevalence (95% CI)
Race	Hispanic	2904	14.72 (10.92–18.53)
	Non-Hispanic White	4270	67.11 (61.77–72.44)
	Non-Hispanic Black	1756	11.03 8.92–13.14)
	Other Non-Hispanic	497	07.14 (5.46–8.82)
Sex	Male	4625	49.03 (47.95–50.11)
	Female	4802	50.97 (49.89–52.04)
Age (years)		9427	47.56 (46.92–48.21)
Education	< high school	2842	19.96 (18.15–21.77)
	High school or equiv	2246	24.09 (22.31–25.88)
	> high school	4325	55.84 (53.12–58.57)
Income/poverty ratio		8548	2.97 (2.88–3.07)
Health insurance	Insured	6871	78.33 (76.56–80.10)
Diabetes	Yes	1044	7.64 (6.69–8.60)
	Borderline	162	1.6 (1.25–1.86)
Heart condition	Yes	517	4.06 (3.57–4.55)
BMI (kg/m^2)	<18.5	140	1.64 (1.20–2.10)
	18.5–24.9	2469	29.20 (27.60–30.79)
	25.0–29.9	3167	33.82 (32.37–35.27)
	≥30.0	3562	35.34 (33.78–36.90)
Ever Smoker	Yes	4322	44.85 (42.37–47.34)
Current Drinker	Yes	6213	76.64 (74.43–78.55)
			Mean (95% CI)
Segmented Neutrophils (1000 cells/µL)		9427	4.27 (4.20–4.34)
Lymphocytes (1000 cells/µL)		9427	2.14 (2.11–2.16)
Neutrophil/lymphocyte ratio (NLR)		9427	2.15 (2.11–2.19)

blood sample on admission [23], others use preoperative NLR [24], maximum NLR during hospitalization [13], or average NLR of three readings during hospitalization [25]. Nevertheless, there is no study to our knowledge exploring the normal range and variability of NLR in a healthy population. Aim of this study was to investigate the normal range of NLR and its relationship with other demographic, risk factor and comorbidity variables in a well-known maintained national database of non-institutional individuals (NHANES).

Methods

Study design and participants

The National Health and Nutrition Examination Survey (NHANES) is a population-based survey designed to assess the health and nutritional status of non-institutionalized children and adults in the United States. NHANES uses a complex, multistage, probability sampling design to produce a nationally representative sample of non-institutionalized US children and adults. In this study, we aggregated cross-sectional data collected from 2007 to 2010; data extracted included markers of systemic inflammation (neutrophil count, lymphocyte count, and NLR), demographic

(age, sex, race, Body Mass Index) and clinical (history of diabetes, heart disease or heart attack) characteristics.

In the 2007–2008 NHANES survey, there were 8249 subjects of both sexes, aged ≥18 years, who had complete data on neutrophil or lymphocyte counts; 3,427 participants were excluded for reporting a history of cancer or malignancy or missing data on cancer or malignancy. An additional 279 participants were excluded for self-report of taking any of the following medications: steroids, chemotherapy, immunomodulators, antibiotics, leaving 4,548 subjects (55% of the original sample). In the 2009–2010 survey, the same exclusion criteria were applied; from the initial 8,786 men and women who had neutrophil and lymphocyte data, a total of 4,884 participants (approximately 56% of the original sample) were included in the present analysis. The final sample consisted of 9,427 subjects across both survey waves.

NHANES Data collection and laboratory analysis

Data collected regarding demographic information (age, race, education, health insurance status, and income to poverty ratio), current medication use, diagnosis of medical conditions (both previous and current), and lifestyle behaviors (smoking and alcohol use) were collected by trained interviewers. Body Mass Index

Table 2. Neutrophil, Lymphocyte, and NLR according to demographic and clinical characteristics (n = 9427).

Variable	Categories	Neutrophil Mean (95% CI)	Lymphocyte Mean (95% CI)	NLR Mean (95% CI)
Race	Hispanic	4.39 (4.31–4.48)	2.26 (2.23–2.29)	2.08 (2.04–2.12)
	Non-Hispanic White	4.35 (4.27–4.44)	2.09 (2.06–2.12)	2.24 (2.19–2.28)
	Non-Hispanic Black	3.65 (3.56–3.73)	2.24 (2.21–2.28)	1.76 (1.71–1.81)
	Other Non-Hispanic	4.18 (4.00–4.37)	2.11 (2.05–2.17)	2.10 (2.01–2.19)
Sex	Male	4.26 (4.18–4.33)	2.11 (2.08–2.13)	2.19 (2.14–2.25)
	Female	4.28 (4.20–4.36)	2.16 (2.14–2.19)	2.11 (2.07–2.16)
Education	< high school	4.44 (4.32–4.56)	2.22 (2.19–2.26)	2.16 (2.09–2.24)
	High school or equiv	4.45 (4.34–4.56)	2.19 (2.15–2.23)	2.20 (2.14–2.26)
	> high school	4.13 (4.07–4.20)	2.08 (2.06–2.10)	2.13 (2.08–2.17)
Health insurance	Insured	4.21 (4.14–4.28)	2.10 (2.08–2.12)	2.16 (2.11–2.21)
	Uninsured	4.48 (4.37–4.60)	2.26 (2.21–2.30)	2.12 (2.06–2.18)
Diabetes	Yes	4.66 (4.50–4.83)	2.21 (2.15–2.27)	2.34 (2.23–2.45)
	No	4.24 (4.17–4.30)	2.13 (2.11–2.15)	2.13 (2.09–2.17)
	Borderline	4.27 (3.88–4.67)	2.06 (1.97–2.15)	2.21 (2.01–2.41)
Heart condition	Yes	4.26 (4.19–4.33)	2.14 (2.12–2.16)	2.44 (2.30–2.58)
	No	4.45 (4.28–4.61)	2.03 (1.93–2.12)	2.14 (2.10–2.18)
BMI (kg/m^2)	<18.5	3.99 (3.64–4.34)	2.10 (1.97–2.23)	2.06 (1.85–2.27)
	18.5–24.9	3.97 (3.88–4.07)	2.01 (1.98–2.05)	2.11 (2.06–2.17)
	25.0–29.9	4.18 (4.08–4.28)	2.11 (2.08–2.15)	2.13 (2.07–2.20)
	≥30.0	4.62 (4.54–4.71)[#]	2.26 (2.23–2.29)[#]	2.21 (2.15–2.27)*
Ever Smoker	Yes	4.55 (4.43–4.66)	2.21 (2.19–2.24)	2.22 (2.16–2.28)
	No	4.04 (4.00–4.09)	2.07 (2.04–2.10)	2.10 (2.05–2.14)
Drinker	Yes	4.28 (4.21–4.35)	2.13 (2.10–2.16)	2.16 (2.11–2.20)
	No	4.22 (4.11–4.33)	2.12 (2.08–2.16)	2.17 (2.09–2.25)

*P for trend: 0.002;
[#]p for trend<0.0001.

(BMI) (kg/m^2) was measured during the medical examination. Laboratory tests were performed on collected blood specimens to provide information on neutrophil count (1,000 cells/µl) and lymphocyte count (1,000 cells/µl). NLR was calculated as the ratio of neutrophil cell count to lymphocyte cell count. The Coulter method was used to determine neutrophil and lymphocyte counts (Coulter Gen.S Hematology Analyzer, Beckman Coulter Corp, Hialeah, Florida).

Data analysis

The distribution of continuous variables was reported as means ± standard deviation, of categorical variables as frequencies and percentages. The main outcome of interest, neutrophil, lymphocyte counts and the NLR was reported as mean along with 95% confidence intervals. To examine the influence of demographic and clinical characteristics on neutrophil counts, lymphocyte counts, and NLR, linear regression models for each outcome were performed, including all the variables found to be statistically significant at univariate analysis (p<0.05) as well as clinically meaningful. Multivariate linear regression models were also stratified by race. All data analyses used the appropriate survey sample weights to provide nationally representative estimates. Statistical significance was determined at alpha level of 0.05. Analyses were performed using Stata/SE version 12 (StataCorp.

2011. *Stata Statistical Software: Release 12*. College Station, TX: StataCorp LP).

Results

There are 9427 subjects in this study (Table 1), distributed equally between males and female. The majority of subjects is white (67%), has completed at least high school or more (55%), and is covered by some form of insurance (78%). The average age is 47 years; roughly one third of the subjects is overweight (BMI≥ 30 km/m^2). The rate of comorbidities varies from 4% (heart condition) to 7% (diabetes). Forty four percent of subjects are classified as ever smokers, while 76% indentified themselves ad current drinkers. The average value of neutrophils is 4.27×1000 cells/µL, of lymphocytes 2.14×1000 cells/µL; the average NLR is 2.15.

NLR was studied in relation to personal and demographic variables (Table 2). Non-Hispanic Black participants and Hispanic participants had significantly lower mean NLR values (1.76, 95% CI 1.71–1.81 and 2.08, 95% CI 2.04–2.12 respectively) when compared to non-Hispanic Whites (mean NLR = 2.24, 95% CI 2.19–2.28–p<0.0001). Similar results were observed in children (table S1). Subjects who reported diabetes or a history of heart condition had higher NLR than subjects who did not, but only results on hearth condition were statistically significant (p< 0.0001). Ever smokers had significantly higher NLR than non

Table 3. Adjusted Linear Regression Estimates of the association between demographic and clinical characteristics and Neutrophil and Lymphocyte Values (n = 7736).

Variable	Categories	Neutrophil			Lymphocyte			NLR		
		Coeff	95% CI	p-value	Coeff	95% CI	p-value	Coeff	95% CI	p-value
Race	Hispanic	−0.14	(−0.27−−0.01)	0.03	0.09	(0.05−0.13)	<0.0001	−0.18	(−0.26−−0.11)	<0.0001
	Non-Hispanic White	REF			REF			REF		
	Non-Hispanic Black	−0.92	(−1.03−−0.81)	<0.0001	0.10	(0.06−0.15)	<0.0001	−0.55	(−0.61−−0.49)	<0.0001
	Other Non-Hispanic	−0.02	(−0.21−0.24)	0.89	0.05	(−0.04−0.13)	0.24	−0.07	(−0.19−0.05)	0.24
Sex	Female vs Male	0.16	(0.06−0.26)	0.002	0.10	(0.07−0.14)	<0.0001	−0.06	(−0.13−0.006)	0.07
Age (years)	Continuous	−0.007	(−0.009−−0.004)	<0.0001	−0.006	(−0.007−−0.005)	<0.0001	0.004	(0.002−0.006)	<0.0001
Education	<high school	REF			REF			REF		
	High school or equiv	0.10	(−0.02−0.21)	0.09	−0.013	(−0.06−0.31)	0.55	0.05	(−0.04−0.14)	0.29
	>high school	−0.12	(−0.25−0.004)	0.06	−0.06	(−0.10−−0.03)	0.002	−0.01	(−0.09−0.06)	0.72
Income/poverty ratio	Continuous	−0.05	(−0.08−−0.02)	0.003	−0.01	(−0.02−0.003)	0.14	−0.03	(−0.05−−0.007)	0.01
Health insurance	Uninsured vs Insured	0.20	(0.02−0.38)	0.03	0.05	(−0.07−0.10)	0.09	0.02	(−0.06−0.10)	0.61
Diabetes	Yes	0.32	(0.15−0.48)	<0.0001	0.08	(0.02−0.14)	0.009	0.11	(−0.004−0.23)	0.06
	No	REF			REF			REF		
	Borderline	−0.16	(−0.56−0.23)	0.40	−0.12	(−0.24−−0.11)	0.03	−0.006	(−0.22−0.21)	0.95
Heart condition	Yes vs No	.06	(−.13−.24)	0.55	−0.09	(−0.21−0.03)	0.13	0.17	(0.05−0.30)	0.008
BMI (kg/m²)	<18.5	0.04	(−0.37−0.45)	0.85	0.04	(−0.10−0.17)	0.59	0.008	(−0.22−0.24)	0.94
	18.5-24.9	REF			REF			REF		
	25.0-29.9	0.24	(0.09−0.38)	0.003	0.12	(0.07−0.16)	<0.0001	−0.005	(−0.10−0.09)	0.91
	≥30.0	0.71	(0.57−0.85)	<0.0001	0.27	(0.23−0.31)	<0.0001	0.08	(0.001−0.15)	0.046
Ever Smoker	Yes vs No	0.46	(0.33−0.60)	<0.0001	0.15	(0.12−0.19)	<0.0001	0.09	(0.02−0.16)	0.015
Drinker	Yes vs No	−0.02	(−0.14−0.10)	0.73	0.005	(−0.04−0.05)	0.81	−0.03	(−0.13−0.07)	0.55

Table 4. Linear Regression Estimates (β coefficients and 95% CI) of the association between clinical and demographic characteristics and NLR according to racial subgroups.

Variable	Categories	Blacks (n = 1440)	Whites (n = 3684)	Hispanics (n = 2255)
Sex	Female vs Male	−0.09 (−0.19–0.007)	−0.10 (−0.19− −0.02)^	0.04 (−0.05–0.13)
Age (years)	Continuous	0.001 (−0.001–0.005)	0.005 (0.002–0.007) #	0.002 (−0.0001–0.006)
Education	<high school	REF	REF	REF
	High school	0.08 (−0.05–0.21)	− 0.001 (−0.13–0.13)	0.10 (−0.03–0.23)
	>high school	0.06 (−.08–0.19)	−0.06 (−0.18–0.05)	0.02 (−0.04–0.09)
Income/poverty ratio	Continuous	−0.02 (−0.05–0.02)	−0.03 (−0.06− −0.008) ^	−0.03 (−0.06–0.003)
Health insurance	Uninsured vs Insured	−0.05 (−0.16–0.05)	0.02 (−0.10–0.13)	−0.02 (−0.13–0.08)
Diabetes	Yes	0.16 (−0.04–0.37)	0.15 (−0.05–0.34)	−0.02 (−0.13–0.09)
	No	REF	REF	REF
	Borderline	0.33 (−0.01–0.66)	−0.05 (−0.33–0.24)	−0.10 (−0.28–0.09)
Heart condition	Yes vs no	0.11 (−0.11–0.33)	0.15 (−0.01–0.31)	0.21 (0.002–0.42)*
BMI (kg/m²)	<18.5	0.12 (−0.50–0.73)	−0.02 (−0.31–0.28)	−0.11 (−0.92–0.69)
	18.5–24.9	REF	REF	REF
	25.0–29.9	−0.001 (−0.19–0.19)	−0.01 (−0.13–0.11)	−0.01 (−.12–0.11)
	≥30.0	0.15 (0.0005–0.29)*	0.05 (−0.06–0.15)	0.07 (−.05–0.20)
Ever Smoker	Yes vs no	0.02 (−0.08–0.12)	0.09 (0.002–0.18)*	0.01 (−0.07–0.10)
Drinker	Yes vs no	0.06 (−0.03–0.15)	−0.06 (−0.20–0.08)	0.06 (−0.04–0.16)

*$p = 0.04$;
#$p < 0.0001$;
^$p = 0.01$.

smokers ($p = 0.001$). There were no significant differences in NLR with sex, education, insurance status, or drinking habits. There was a significant trend of increasing NLR with increasing BMI (p for trend: 0.002). The associations persisted after adjustment for confounding factors (table 3). In addition NLR was significantly associated with increasing age and inversely associated with income poverty ratio.

When the analysis was repeated according to race (Table 4), among black subjects a high NLR was significantly associated only with increasing BMI (β coefficient = 0.15, 95% CI 0.0005–0.29). Among non-Hispanic Whites, older age ($p < 0.0001$) and being a smoker ($p = 0.04$) were positively associated with increasing NLR values, while income to poverty ratio was negatively associated with NLR ($p = 0.01$); women had significantly lower NLR values compared to men (β coefficient = −0.10, 95% CI −0.19− −0.02; $p = 0.01$). Among Hispanics, only having a heart condition was significantly associated with an increased NLR (β coefficient = 0.21, 95% CI 0.002–0.42; $p = 0.04$).

Discussion

The present analysis of a large US data set including over 9000 subjects reports the average value for NLR in the general population, and indicates that such normal value significantly varies with race; NLR is particularly low in Non-Hispanic Black subjects, from 2.24 observed in Whites to 1.76 in Blacks. This finding has important clinical implications. Several publications demonstrated that an elevated NLR is a predictor of poor outcome in cancer [7] and cardiovascular disease [5]; these studies however used arbitrary NLR cut off points for risk stratification, which were based on the average NLR values of each study population. Such

populations were mostly small in size, without consideration of racial differences and racial composition.

Because of the lower NLR observed in black in comparison to white subjects, it is possible that commonly reported high prognostic NLR cut-off points be hardly reached by non-white populations, or be a much worst prognostic indicator than in white patients. All these speculations need to be tested in multi ethnic populations affected by chronic diseases such as cancer and cardiovascular disease.

Another result of this analysis is that NLR is associated with several self-reported chronic conditions, such as diabetes and heart disease, with being a smoker, with high BMI, and with increasing age, all conditions that are known to increase the body inflammatory milieu [26]. In addition this study shows that an index of socioeconomic status, the income to poverty ratio, is inversely associated with NLR. A low socio economic status may be a proxy for poor dietary habits, low in nutrients and anti-oxidants, or lack of physical exercise, or occupational exposures to chemicals and carcinogens. We are not able to test these hypotheses given the retrospective nature of the NHANES data base, and the limited information available from the questionnaire.

This analysis also shows that the association between personal and behavioral factors and NLR differs with race. For example, among black patients only BMI was significantly associated with elevated NLR, while among white patients several expected factors, such as age and smoking habits were associated with higher NLR. These differences may be due to chance, or to a different host response to pro-inflammatory factors, a hypothesis that needs to be tested in *ad hoc* studies.

Despite the fact that this analysis relies on a large sample of the US population, a larger sample size collected over longer periods of time would help better defining NLR normal ranges. In addition, the NLR was an occasional, single measure, and as such does not reflect individual variability. Another limitation is that all the exposure variables, including race were self-reported, thus their accuracy could not be objectively verified. However, it is unlikely that the answers to the questionnaire could differ according to the NLR, since the participants were not aware of the results of the test.

This study is providing preliminary data on racial disparities in a marker of inflammation (NLR) that has been associated with several chronic diseases outcome, suggesting that different cut-off points should be set according to race. It also shows how NLR is associated with personal and behavioral factors, some of which are modifiable such as smoking and BMI. It suggests that together with public health interventions of the factors amenable of being modified, chemopreventive trials should be considered in an attempt to modify NLR in ageing people, smokers and populations at risk for chronic diseases such as cardiovascular disease and cancer.

Conclusions

The study indicates racial differences of average NLR among non-Hispanic black, Hispanic and non-Hispanic white subjects, with average NLR of 1.76, 2.08 and 2.24, respectively. The results corroborate prior studies on inflammation in reporting the association between elevated NLR and risk factors such as smoking, obesity, and diabetes. Moreover, differences in the association between some of these risk factors and elevated NLR across different races were observed. This may illustrate racial differences in inflammatory response to different risk factors, some of which are modifiable.

Author Contributions

Conceived and designed the experiments: BA ET. Performed the experiments: MCR. Analyzed the data: MCR. Contributed reagents/materials/analysis tools: ET. Contributed to the writing of the manuscript: ET BA.

References

1. Rueda-Clausen CF, López-Jaramillo P, Luengas C, del Pilar Oubiña M, Cachofeiro V, et al. (2009) Inflammation but not endothelial dysfunction is associated with the severity of coronary artery disease in dyslipidemic subjects. Mediators Inflamm 2009: 469169. Epub 2009 Jun 23. PMID: 19584917.
2. Libby P (2001) What have we learned about the biology of atherosclerosis? The role of inflammation. Am J Cardiol 88(7B): 3J–6J.
3. Balkwill F, Mantovani A (2001) Inflammation and cancer: back to Virchow? Lancet 357(9255): 539–45.
4. Coussens LM, Werb Z (2002) Inflammation and cancer. Nature 420(6917): 860–7.
5. Wang X, Zhang G, Jiang X, Zhu H, Lu Z, et al. (2014) Neutrophil to lymphocyte ratio in relation to risk of all-cause mortality and cardiovascular events among patients undergoing angiography or cardiac revascularization: a meta-analysis of observational studies. Atherosclerosis 234(1): 206–13.
6. Bhat T, Teli S, Rijal J, Bhat H, Raza M, et al. (2013) Neutrophil to lymphocyte ratio and cardiovascular diseases: a review. Expert Rev Cardiovasc Ther 11(1): 55–9.
7. Templeton AJ, McNamara MG, Seruga B, Vera-Badillo FE, Aneja P, et al. (2014) Prognostic Role of Neutrophil-to-Lymphocyte Ratio in Solid Tumors: A Systematic Review and Meta-Analysis. J Natl Cancer Inst 106(6): dju124.
8. Guthrie GJ, Charles KA, Roxburgh CS, Horgan PG, McMillan DC, et al. (2013) The systemic inflammation-based neutrophil-lymphocyte ratio: experience in patients with cancer. Crit Rev Oncol Hematol 88(1): 218–30.
9. Motomura T, Shirabe K, Mano Y, Muto J, Toshima T, et al. (2013) Neutrophil-lymphocyte ratio reflects hepatocellular carcinoma recurrence after liver transplantation via inflammatory microenvironment. J Hepatol 58: 58–64.
10. Kantola T, Klintrup K, Vayrynen JP, Vornanen J, Bloigu R, et al. (2012) Stage-dependent alterations of the serum cytokine pattern in colorectal carcinoma. Br J Cancer 107: 1729–36.
11. Uthamalingam S, Patvardhan EA, Subramanian S, Ahmed W, Martin W, et al. (2011) Utility of the neutrophil to lymphocyte ratio in predicting long-term outcomes in acute decompensated heart failure. Am J Cardiol 107(3): 433–8.
12. Azab B, Bhatt VR, Phookan J, Murukutla S, Kohn N, et al. (2012) Usefulness of the neutrophil-to-lymphocyte ratio in predicting short- and long-term mortality in breast cancer patients. Ann Surg Oncol 19(1): 217–24.
13. Núñez J, Núñez E, Bodi V, Sanchis J, Miñana G, et al. (2008) Usefulness of the neutrophil to lymphocyte ratio in predicting long-term mortality in ST segment elevation myocardial infarction. Am J Cardiol 101(6): 747–52.
14. Yamanaka T, Matsumoto S, Teramukai S, Ishiwata R, Nagai Y, et al. (2007) The baseline ratio of neutrophils to lymphocytes is associated with patient prognosis in advanced gastric cancer. Oncology 73(3–4): 215–20.
15. Ohno Y, Nakashima J, Ohori M, Hatano T, Tachibana M (2010) Pretreatment neutrophil-to-lymphocyte ratio as an independent predictor of recurrence in patients with nonmetastatic renal cell carcinoma. J Urol 184(3): 873–8.
16. Bhatti I, Peacock O, Lloyd G, Larvin M, Hall RI (2010) Preoperative hematologic markers as independent predictors of prognosis in resected pancreatic ductal adenocarcinoma: neutrophil-lymphocyte versus platelet-lymphocyte ratio. Am J Surg 200(2): 197–203.
17. Ding PR, An X, Zhang RX, Fang YJ, Li LR, et al. (2010) Elevated preoperative neutrophil to lymphocyte ratio predicts risk of recurrence following curative resection for stage IIA colon cancer. Int J Colorectal Dis 25(12): 1427–33.
18. Kishi Y, Kopetz S, Chun YS, Palavecino M, Abdalla EK, et al. (2009) Blood neutrophil-to-lymphocyte ratio predicts survival in patients with colorectal liver metastases treated with systemic chemotherapy. Ann Surg Oncol 16(3): 614–22.
19. Halazun KJ, Hardy MA, Rana AA, Woodland DC 4th, Luyten EJ, et al. (2009) Negative impact of neutrophil-lymphocyte ratio on outcome after liver transplantation for hepatocellular carcinoma. Ann Surg 250(1): 141–51.
20. Aliustaoglu M, Bilici A, Seker M, Dane F, Gocun M, et al. (2010) The association of pre-treatment peripheral blood markers with survival in patients with pancreatic cancer. Hepatogastroenterology 57(99–100): 640–5.
21. Bain BJ (1996) Ethnic and sex differences in the total and differential white cell count and platelet count. J Clin Pathol 49: 664–6.
22. Lichtman MA (1970) Cellular deformability during maturation of the myeloblast. Possible role in marrow egress. N Engl J Med 283: 943–8.
23. Tamhane UU, Aneja S, Montgomery D, Rogers EK, Eagle KA, et al. (2008) Association between admission neutrophil to lymphocyte ratio and outcomes in patients with acute coronary syndrome. Am J Cardiol 102: 653–7.
24. Azab B, Shariff MA, Bachir R, Nabagiez JP, McGinn JT Jr (2013) Elevated preoperative neutrophil/lymphocyte ratio as a predictor of increased long-term survival in minimal invasive coronary artery bypass surgery compared to sternotomy. J Cardiothorac Surg 8: 193.
25. Azab B, Zaher M, Weiserbs KF, Torbey E, Lacossiere K, et al. (2010) Usefulness of neutrophil to lymphocyte ratio in predicting short- and long-term mortality after non-ST-elevation myocardial infarction. Am J Cardiol 106(4): 470–6.
26. Seals DR, Kaplon RE, Gioscia-Ryan RA, LaRocca TJ (2014) You're Only as Old as Your Arteries: Translational Strategies for Preserving Vascular Endothelial Function with Aging. Physiology (Bethesda) 29(4): 250–264.

12

Increased C-C Chemokine Receptor 2 Gene Expression in Monocytes of Severe Obstructive Sleep Apnea Patients and under Intermittent Hypoxia

Li-Pang Chuang[1,2], Ning-Hung Chen[2], Shih-Wei Lin[2], Ying-Ling Chang[3], Hsiang-Ruei Liao[4], Yu-Sheng Lin[5], I-Ju Chao[1], Yuling Lin[1], Jong-Hwei S. Pang[1]*

1 Graduate Institute of Clinical Medical Sciences, College of Medicine, Chang Gung University, Taoyuan, Taiwan, 2 Sleep Center, Department of Pulmonary and Critical Care Medicine, Chang Gung Memorial Hospital, Taoyuan, Taiwan, 3 Department of Chinese Medicine, College of Medicine, Chang Gung University, Taoyuan, Taiwan, 4 Graduate Institute of Natural Products, College of Medicine, Chang Gung University, Taoyuan, Taiwan, 5 Division of Cardiology, Department of Internal Medicine, Chang Gung Memorial Hospital, Taipei, Taiwan

Abstract

Background: Obstructive sleep apnea (OSA) is known to be a risk factor of coronary artery disease. The chemotaxis and adhesion of monocytes to the endothelium in the early atherosclerosis is important. This study aimed to investigate the effect of intermittent hypoxia, the hallmark of OSA, on the chemotaxis and adhesion of monocytes.

Methods: Peripheral blood was sampled from 54 adults enrolled for suspected OSA. RNA was prepared from the isolated monocytes for the analysis of C-C chemokine receptor 2 (CCR2). The effect of intermittent hypoxia on the regulation and function of CCR2 was investigated on THP-1 monocytic cells and monocytes. The mRNA and protein expression levels were investigated by RT/real-time PCR and western blot analysis, respectively. Transwell filter migration assay and cell adhesion assay were performed to study the chemotaxis and adhesion of monocytes.

Results: Monocytic CCR2 gene expression was found to be increased in severe OSA patients and higher levels were detected after sleep. Intermittent hypoxia increased the CCR2 expression in THP-1 monocytic cells even in the presence of TNF-α and CRP. Intermittent hypoxia also promoted the MCP-1-mediated chemotaxis and adhesion of monocytes to endothelial cells. Furthermore, inhibitor for p42/44 MAPK or p38 MAPK suppressed the activation of monocytic CCR2 expression by intermittent hypoxia.

Conclusions: This is the first study to demonstrate the increase of CCR2 gene expression in monocytes of severe OSA patients. Monocytic CCR2 gene expression can be induced under intermittent hypoxia which contributes to the chemotaxis and adhesion of monocytes.

Editor: Vladimir V. Kalinichenko, Cincinnati Children's Hospital Medical Center, United States of America

Funding: This study was supported by Grant CMRPG3A1311, CMRPD190341 and CMRPD190342 from Chang Gung Memorial Hospital, Taiwan. The sponsors had no role in the study design, data collection and analysis, decision to publish, or preparation of the manuscript.

Competing Interests: The authors have declared that no competing interests exist.

* Email: jonghwei@mail.cgu.edu.tw

Introduction

Obstructive sleep apnea (OSA), defined as repeated episodes of obstructive apnea and hypopnea during sleep, together with symptoms of daytime sleepiness or frequently altered cardiopulmonary function, affects at least 5% of the general population [1,2]. OSA results in intermittent hypoxia (IH) and sleep fragmentation with neurocognitive dysfunction and cardiovascular disease as the major sequelae [3]. Previous studies report that patients with sleep apnea have an increased risk of diurnal hypertension, nocturnal dysrhythmias, pulmonary hypertension, right and left ventricular failure, myocardial infarction and stroke, suggesting that sleep apnea may be one of the important risk factors of cardiovascular disorders [4,5].

Most literatures conclude that acute coronary syndrome (ACS) would worsen OSA and vice versa, OSA would impair left ventricular function [6,7]. Some studies further demonstrate that the morning peak distribution of ACS onset (AM 6:00~12:00) might potentially be contributed by sleep apnea [8,9]. Possible mechanisms responsible for the development of those cardiovascular sequelae from OSA include intermittent hypoxia and hypercapnia, exaggerated negative intrathoracic pressure and bursts of sympathetic activity, which provoke surges in blood pressure and result in endothelial cell dysfunction [10,11]. Animal and cell culture studies have demonstrated preferential activation of inflammatory pathways by intermittent hypoxia, which is one of the integral features of OSA [12,13].

The excessive recruitment of monocytes to the sub-endothelial space is central to the pathology of atherosclerosis. The adhesion of circulating monocytes and consequent transmigration through the vascular endothelial layer are initiated from being attracted by chemokines released from injured endothelial cells which is a crucial step in the early atherosclerosis [14]. Monocyte chemotactic protein-1 (MCP-1), abundantly present in macrophage-rich atherosclerotic plaques in human, is responsible for the recruitment, activation and differentiation of monocytes in the vascular intima space [15,16]. Chemokine (C-C motif) receptor 2 (CCR2), one of the β-chemokine receptors characterized by seven-transmembrane domains and coupled to a GTP-binding protein is the major receptor of MCP-1. The binding of MCP-1 to CCR2 results in not only the chemotaxis of monocytes, but also the following adhesion and spreading of monocytes [17,18]. CCR2(-/-) mice show defect in monocyte recruitment and decreased atherosclerotic lesions, indicating the important role of CCR2 in the development of atherosclerosis [19].

The plasma MCP-1 level has been found to be elevated in OSA patients that is possibly secreted not only by endothelial cells but also by monocytes from OSA patients [20–22]. However, there is no report regarding the CCR2 expression level or the possible regulation by intermittent hypoxia in monocytes from OSA patients. Therefore, the present study aimed to investigate the CCR2 gene expression in monocytes of OSA patients; to examine whether intermittent hypoxia can exert effect on monocytic CCR2 gene expression and its related mechanism.

Materials and Methods

Patients

This study was approved by the Institutional Review Board of Chang Gung Memorial Hospital (No. 100-3166B). Written informed consents were obtained from 72 patients who enrolled in this study. The inclusion criteria of participants included any adult patient (>20 years old) who was suffering from snore with the suspect of OSA diagnosis. The exclusion criteria of participants included: chronic or recent (<1 month) clinically significant infectious or inflammatory condition; asthma; trauma; invasive medical/surgical/dental procedure; recent use (<1 month) of anti-inflammatory or antibiotics drugs; coexistence of ischemic heart disease, hypertension, diabetes, hyperlipidemia, cerebrovascular disease or renal disease. After the exclusion of 18 patients (3 patients have upper airway infectious symptoms, 4 patients have high blood pressure, 2 patients have elevated blood sugar, 5 patients have hyperlipidemia and high blood pressure, 2 patients have hyperlipidemia and elevated blood sugar, 1 patient has abnormal EKG, and 1 patient has recent dental procedure within one month), 54 patients were included in this study.

Polysomnography (PSG)

We use standard overnight PSG with the Siesta Physiological Monitoring System (Compumedics, Abbotsford, Australia) in the sleep center of our hospital with electroencephalography, electro-oculography, electromyography, and electrocardiography checks simultaneously. Ventilatory flow at the nose and mouth was measured with thermistors. Ventilatory movements of the chest and abdomen were monitored by inductive plethysmography bands. The arterial oxygen saturation (SaO_2) was measured transcutaneously with fingertip pulse oximetry (Nonin Xpod Patient Cable Oximeter 3011). Apnea was defined as continuous cessation of airflow for more than 10 seconds and hypopnea was defined as decreasing airflow more than 30% with arousal or oxygen desaturation more than 4%. Apnea-hypopnea index (AHI)

was determined by dividing the number of the total apnea/hypopnea events by the estimated hours of sleep. Adult with AHI $\leqq 5$ was considered as control, $5 <$ AHI $\leqq 15$ as mild OSA, $15 <$ AHI $\leqq 30$ as moderate OSA, and AHI >30 as severe OSA. Oxygen desaturation index (ODI) was determined by the number of times per hour of sleep that the blood's oxygen level drops by 4% or more from baseline. Polysomnography was performed from 10 PM to 6 AM next morning, and all the score were based on the 2010 AASM criteria.

Blood Sampling and Monocyte Isolation

Peripheral venous blood was sampled at 6 AM after patients woke up after the performance of PSG in supine position under fasting condition. Samples were collected in heparin rinse tubes and centrifugation (3,000 rpm for 20 min) was performed within 30 min. Peripheral blood mononuclear cells isolated by Ficoll-Hypaque centrifugation were enriched for CD14+ monocytes using the autoMACS magnetic cell sorting system (Miltenyi Biotec, Bergisch Gladbach, Germany) as described previously [23]. Briefly, peripheral blood mononuclear cells were incubated with saturating concentrations of CD14 microbeads on ice for 15 min, washed, and suspended in PBS containing 2 mM EDTA and 0.5% bovine serum albumin. The cell suspension was then applied to the autoMACS separator using the positive selection program. The CD14-positive monocytes were eluted from the magnetic column and placed into 3-cm culture dishes (1×10^6 cells per dish) containing RPMI 1640 medium supplemented with 10% (v/v) fetal bovine serum and antibiotics.

Cell Cultures

The human monocytic leukemia cell line THP-1 was obtained from ATCC and grown in suspension culture of RPMI 1640 medium supplemented with 10% (v/v) fetal bovine serum and antibiotics. Cells were subcultured by diluting the medium with fresh growth medium in a 1:4 ratio, and grown at 37°C in a humidified atmosphere with 5% CO_2/95% air. Human vascular endothelial cells (HUVECs) were isolated from the vein of human umbilical cords and grown in EGM-2 provided by Clonetics (MD, USA). Cells were maintained in a humidified atmosphere with 5% CO_2/95% air at 37°C. HUVECs were passaged 3–5 times prior to use in experiments.

Conditions of Normoxia and Intermittent Hypoxia

Human monocytes or THP-1 cells (1×10^6 cells/ml) were resuspended in a 5 cm culture dish containing 5 ml RPMI 1640 medium. Condition of normoxia or intermittent hypoxia (IH) was performed in a customized gas flow chamber modified from Hypo-Hyper Oxygen System (NexBioxy Inc., Taiwan). THP-1 cells or monocytes were placed in condition of normoxia (21% O_2, 5% CO_2, and balance N_2) or intermittent hypoxia (6 cycles of 35 min of hypoxia [0.1% or 5% O_2, 5% CO_2 and balance N_2] followed by 25 min of normoxia [21% O_2, 5% CO_2 and balance N_2] for 6 hr) and returned to normal culture condition for 18 hr before following analysis. The condition of intermittent hypoxia has used in a previously published literature and confirmed by the change of actual % O_2 in the medium [24]. The chamber was maintained in a standard humidified incubator at 37°C. TNF-α 10 uL or CRP 10 uL are co-cultured with THP-1 cells one day before *in vivo* intermittent hypoxia study.

RNA Extraction and RT/real-time PCR

Total cellular RNA was isolated by lysis in a guanidinium isothiocyanate buffer, followed by a single step of phenol–

chloroform–isoamyl alcohol extraction. In brief, 5×10^6 cells were lysed in 0.5 ml solution D containing 4 M guanidinium isothiocyanate, 25 mM sodium citrate (pH 7.0), 0.5% sodium sarcosine, and 0.1 M β-mercaptoethanol, with vigorous vortexing. Sequentially, 50 μl of 2 M sodium acetate (pH 4.0), 0.5 ml phenol, and 100 μl chloroform–isoamyl alcohol (49:1, v:v) were added to the homogenate. After vortexing for 1 min, the solution was centrifuged at 12,000 rpm for 20 min at 4°C. The RNA was precipitated by the addition of 0.5 ml isopropanol and kept at − 80°C for 1 h. RNA was pelleted by centrifuging the solution at 12,000 rpm for 20 min at 4°C. After the RNA pellet was rinsed in ice-cold 75% ethanol, the dry RNA was dissolved in DEPC-treated ddH$_2$O. The cDNA was synthesized from total RNA using M-MLV reverse transcriptase (USB Corporation, OH, USA). Quantitative real time PCR was performed with universal cycling conditions (15 min at 95°C, followed by 40 cycles of 30 s at 95°C, 1 min at 55°C, and 30 s at 72°C). Cycle threshold (CT) values were determined by automated threshold analysis with Mx-Pro Mx3005P v4.00 software (Agilent Tech, CA, USA). PCR primers used were as follows: CCR2 forward primer, 5′-ATGCTGTC-CACATCTCGTTCTCG-3′ and reverse primer, 5′-TTA-TAAACCAGCCGAGACTTCCTGC-3′; and GAPDH forward primer, 5′-GACCTGACCTGCCGTCTA-3′ and reverse primer, 5′-AGGAGTGGGTGTCGCTGT-3′.

Western Blot Analysis

Cell extract was prepared by processing cells in lysis buffer containing Tris–HCl, pH 7.5, 150 mM NaCl, 1 mM EDTA, 2 mM DTT, 2 mM PMSF and 1% Triton X-100 with three times of freeze–thaw cycles and centrifugation. The 1st supernatant was used as cytosolic protein extract. The pellet was re-dissolved in lysis buffer, sonicated until the solution became clear and after centrifuging again, the 2nd supernatant was used as the membrane protein extract. The protein concentration of the cell extract was determined by Bradford assay (Bio-Rad Laboratories, CA, USA). Extracts with the same amount of proteins were separated by 10% SDS–PAGE either for coomassie blue stain or transferred onto a PVDF membrane. Membrane was incubated at 4°C in blocking solution containing 5% bovine serum albumin (BSA) in TBST for 1 h, followed by 2 h incubation in blocking solution containing appropriate dilution of primary antibody. After washing three times in TBST, the membrane was then incubated in TBST containing secondary antibody conjugated with horseradish peroxidase for 1 h. Membranes were washed three times in TBST and positive signals were developed with enhanced chemiluminescence (Amershan Pharmacia Biotech, Little Chalfont Buckinghamshire, England). The semi-quantitative measurement of the band density was calculated by using 1D Digital Analysis Software (Kodak Digital ScienceTM, Eastman Kodak, Rochester, NY). Monoclonal antibody against CCR2 was obtained from Epitomics Inc. (CA, USA). Rabbit anti-p44/p42, and goat anti-rabbit secondary antibodies conjugated with horseradish peroxidase were acquired from Cell Signaling Technology (Danvers, MA, USA).

Transwell Filter Migration Assay

Microporous membrane (pore size, 8 μm) transwell inserts (Costar, Cambridge, MA) were used for the migration assay. THP-1 cells after normoxia or IH treatment were washed once with PBS, and 2×10^5 cells in 200 μl RPMI were added to the upper chamber, with 400 μl RPMI containing 20 ng/ml MCP-1 in the lower chamber. Recombinant MCP-1 was purchased from R&D Systems Inc. (Minneapolis, Minnesota, USA). THP-1 cells were allowed to migrate for 1 h at 37°C in an atmosphere of 5% CO$_2$/

95% air and then the inserts were fixed and stained with Liu's stain. The non-migratory cells were removed before the membrane was mounted and the number of migratory cells was observed and counted under a microscope.

Cell Adhesion Assay

THP-1 cells after normoxia or IH treatment were further activated by 20 ng/ml MCP-1 for 24 h. Recombinant MCP-1 was purchased from R&D Systems Inc. (Minneapolis, Minnesota, USA). THP-1 cells (2×10^5) were added to the monolayer of confluent HUVECs and incubated at 37°C in a humidified 95% air/5% CO$_2$ incubator for 30 min and non-adhered cells were removed by gentle washing with medium 199 twice, and the number of adhered THP-1 cells was counted using a microscope.

Statistical Analysis

T-test was used to compare the mean value of two groups, and one-way analysis of variance (ANOVA) was used for comparing the difference of more than two groups. Correlations were examined using the Spearman rank correlation coefficient. All statistical tests were performed with the use of SPSS software (SPSS Institute, Chicago, USA). A p value of 0.05 or less is considered to indicate statistical significance, and all data was expressed as mean ± SEM.

Results

Increased CCR2 Gene Expression in Monocytes Isolated from Severe OSA Patients

Patients recruited in this study were divided into four groups according to the severity of OSA as indicated by apnea-hypopnea index (AHI), an index used to assess the severity of sleep apnea based on the total number of complete cessations (apnea) and partial obstructions (hypopnea) of breathing occurring per hour of sleep. Table 1 listed the demographic data of these patients in four different groups (AHI ≦5, 5< AHI ≦15, 15< AHI ≦30 and AHI >30). There was no statistic significance over age, body mass index (BMI), neck circumference and smoking status among four groups. Except sleep efficiency, the parameters of polysomnography (PSG), including AHI, ODI, mean SaO$_2$, lowest SaO$_2$ and time with SaO$_2$ <85% showed statistic significance among these groups. Monocytes were isolated from the peripheral blood of these patients after sleep and processed for the analysis of CCR2 mRNA expression by RT/real-time PCR (Figure 1A). The monocytic CCR2 mRNA expression was found to be gradually increased along the severity of these OSA patients particularly in the group with AHI >30 which was statistically significant when compared with three other groups. Results shown in figure 1B demonstrated the positive correlation between AHI and CCR2 mRNA expression levels in monocytes (p<0.01, r = 0.507). Also, the monocytic CCR2 mRNA expression level was negatively correlated with average oxygen saturation in OSA patients (p< 0.05, r = 0.335) (Figure 1C). The monocytic CCR2 mRNA expression level was positively correlated with time under condition of SaO$_2$ <85% in OSA patients (p<0.05, r = 0.328) (Figure 1D).

Intermittent Hypoxia Induced the CCR2 Gene Expression in Monocytes

Since intermittent hypoxia is the hallmark of obstructive sleep apnea, we further examined the effect of intermittent hypoxia on the CCR2 expression in monocytes both at the mRNA and protein levels. Human monocytic THP-1 cells were treated with

Table 1. Baseline characterise and polysomnography parameters.

	Severity				
	AHI ≦5	5< AHI ≦15	15< AHI ≦30	AHI >30	
No. of subjects; (female/male)	8 (0/8)	11 (1/10)	15 (1/14)	20 (2/18)	
Age, yr	43.4±3.5	42.2±3.2	40.1±2.5	45.6±2.7	P=0.505
BMI, kg/m^2	24.9±1.0	24.9±1.5	26.1±0.8	28.1±1.0	P=0.096
NC, cm	37.9±0.7	38.0±0.6	38.7±0.9	39.9±0.6	P=0.210
Cholesterol, mg/dL	203.1±13.1	210.7±21.2	188.2±10.5	189.3±16.2	P=0.568
Smoker/Non	3/5	4/7	6/9	9/11	P=0.968
AHI, events/h	1.9±0.6	10.2±0.8^a	20.1±1.1^{ab}	52.4±3.4^{abc}	P<0.001
ODI, events/h	2.7±1.4	10.0±1.2^a	17.8±1.6^{ab}	51.4±4.6^{abc}	P<0.001
Sleep efficiency, %	73.3±6.6	72.2±4.8	70.1±3.1	63.7±3.2	P=0.296
Mean SaO$_2$, %	93.9±1.0	94.2±0.6	93.6±0.6	89.1±0.9^{abc}	P<0.001
Lowest SaO$_2$, %	88.6±2.2	84.8±1.2	79.1±1.6^{ab}	74.0±2.1^{ab}	P<0.001
Time with SaO2 <85%, minutes	0.5±0.3	0.9±0.9	2.6±2.8^a	18.6±4.3^{abc}	P<0.001

Definition of abbreviations: AHI = apnea-hypopnea index; BMI = body mass index; SaO$_2$ = oxygen saturation; NC = neck circumference; ODI = 4% oxygen desaturation index. (mean ± SE, ^{a}: P<0.05 vs. AHI ≦ 5, ^{b}: P<0.05 vs. 5< AHI ≦ 15, ^{c}: P<0.05 vs. 15< AHI ≦30).

normoxia or intermittent hypoxia as described for 6 hours, and RT/real-time PCR analysis was carried out after cells were placed in incubator under normal culture condition for another 18 hours. The CCR2 mRNA expression in human monocytic THP-1 cells was significantly increased by intermittent hypoxia (Figure 2A). Result from western blot analysis comparing the membrane proteins isolated from THP-1 cells with or without intermittent hypoxia also revealed a significant increase of CCR2 protein expression induced by intermittent hypoxia (Figure 2B). Similar increase of CCR2 mRNA expression was observed when monocytes isolated from human peripheral blood were treated by intermittent hypoxia under the same condition (Figure 2C). By comparing the CCR2 mRNA expression level in monocytes under different oxygen concentration, results further demonstrated the effect of intermittent hypoxia (21%, 5% and 0.1% oxygen levels) on the CCR2 mRNA expression was dose-dependent with highest induction level in cells treated with 0.1% hypoxia (Figure 3A). In the presence of TNF-α or CRP, two inflammatory markers known to be increased in OSA patients, the CCR2 mRNA expression could be further enhanced by intermittent hypoxia, suggesting a different molecular mechanism used by intermittent hypoxia to induce the mRNA expression of CCR2 in monocytes (Figure 3B and 3C, respectively).

Intermittent Hypoxia Enhanced Chemotaxis of Monocytes toward MCP-1

Since the major function of CCR2 is to respond to MCP-1 and induce the chemotaxis of monocytes, we further investigated whether the increased CCR2 expression by intermittent hypoxia might affect the chemotaxis of monocytes toward MCP-1. Monocytic THP-1 cells were treated under condition of normoxia or intermittent hypoxia as described, and the chemotaxis of monocytes toward MCP-1 was analyzed by transwell migration assay for 1 hour. For the first time, we demonstrated that intermittent hypoxia could significantly enhance the chemotaxis of THP-1 cells that were attracted by MCP-1 and migrated through the transwell filter (Figure 4A and 4B).

Intermittent Hypoxia Increased MCP-1-induced Adhesion of Monocytes to Vascular Endothelial Cells

The activation of monocytes by MCP-1 includes the enhanced ability of adhesion to the vascular endothelial cells which also contributes to the early development of atherosclerosis [25]. We therefore examined the modulating effect of intermittent hypoxia on this MCP-1-induced adhesive activity of monocytes. THP-1 cells were pretreated with normoxia or intermittent hypoxia as described and processed for MCP-1-stimulated adhesion assay. Results demonstrated that treatment with MCP-1 or intermittent hypoxia alone enhanced the adhesion of monocytes to vascular endothelial layer and combined MCP-1 and intermittent hypoxia treatment synergistically promoted the adhesive activity of monocytes (Figure 5A and 5B).

Intermittent hypoxia increased the CCR2 expression in monocytes through the activation of ERK and p38 MAPK signal pathways

The induction of CCR2 gene expression in monocytes has been reported to be dependent on the activation of signal pathways including ERK and p38 MAPK [26]. To further investigate the signaling pathways that might be activated by intermittent hypoxia, we performed western blot analysis to determine the phosphorylated levels of p44/42 and p38 MAPK in monocytes after treatment with intermittent hypoxia. Results demonstrated the time-dependent activation of both p44/42 and p38 MAPK in monocytes after intermittent hypoxia treatment (Figure 6A and 6B, respectively). Maximum level of phosphorylated p44/42 and p38 MAPK was found at 6 hr and 1 hr after intermittent hypoxia, respectively. Pretreatment with PD98095 and MSB202190 to inhibit p44/42 and p38 MAPK respectively in monocytes decreased the CCR2 gene expression induced by intermittent hypoxia (Figure 6C and 6D). Results demonstrated the activation of p44/42 and p38 MAPK was required for the increased CCR2 gene expression in monocytes by intermittent hypoxia.

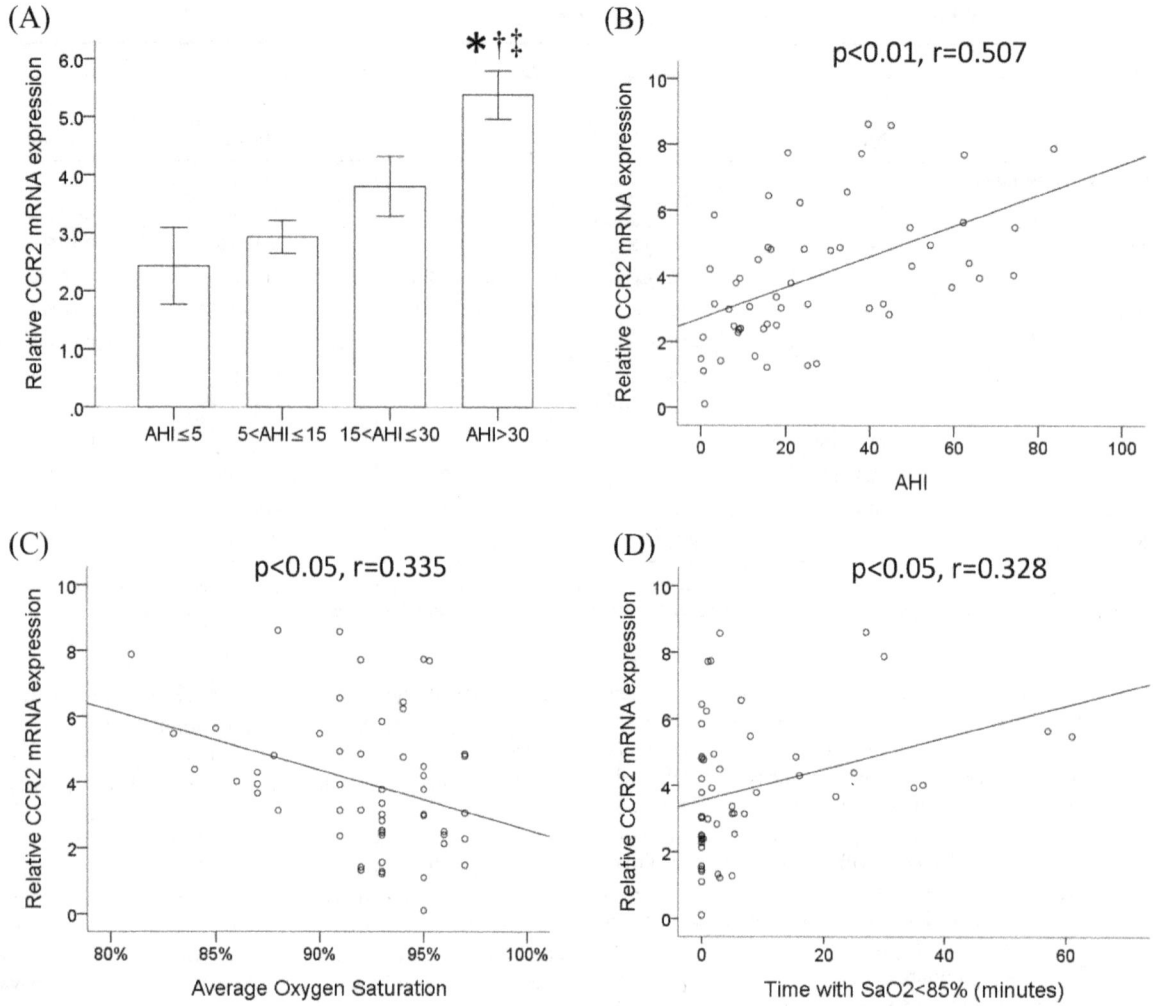

Figure 1. CCR2 mRNA expression significantly increased in monocytes of severe OSA patients. (A) The monocytic CCR2 mRNA expression of 54 patients from four different groups was analyzed by RT/real-time PCR. Data were means and standard errors. (mean ± SE, *: $P < 0.05$ vs. AHI ≤5, †: $P < 0.05$ vs $5 < $ AHI ≤15, ‡: $P < 0.05$ vs $15 < $ AHI ≤30) (B) Linear regression demonstrated the positive correlation between AHI and CCR2 mRNA expression levels in monocytes ($p < 0.01$, $r = 0.507$). (C) Linear regression demonstrated the negative correlation between average oxygen saturation in patients and CCR2 mRNA expression levels in monocytes ($p < 0.05$, $r = 0.335$). (D) Linear regression demonstrated the positive correlation between the monocytic CCR2 mRNA expression level and the time with $SaO_2 < 85\%$ in OSA patients ($p < 0.05$, $r = 0.328$).

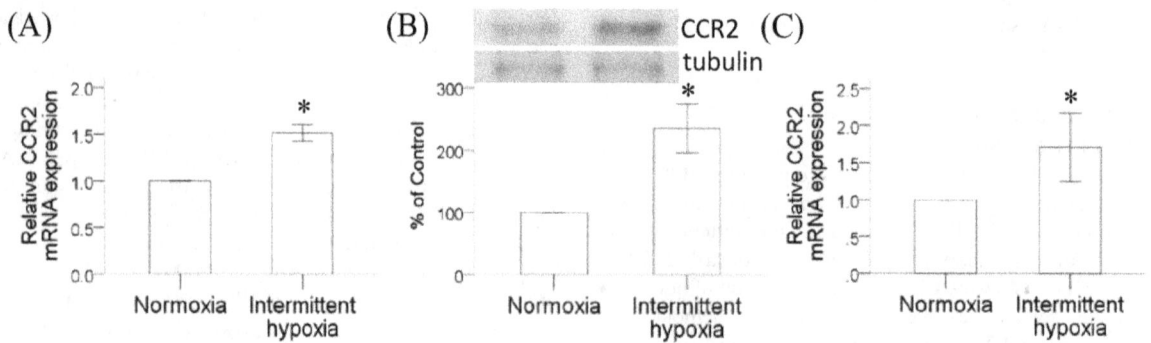

Figure 2. Intermittent hypoxia enhanced CCR2 gene expression in monocytes. THP-1 cells were treated with normoxia or intermittent hypoxia as described in methods. (A) RNA was isolated for the analysis of CCR2 gene expression by RT/real-time PCR. (B) Membrane proteins were prepared for western blot analysis. (C) Human peripheral monocytes were treated with the same conditions as in (A) and total RNA was isolated for the analysis of CCR2 gene expression by RT/real-time PCR. Data were present as means and standard errors from three independent experiments (mean ± SE, *: $P < 0.05$ vs. Normoxia).

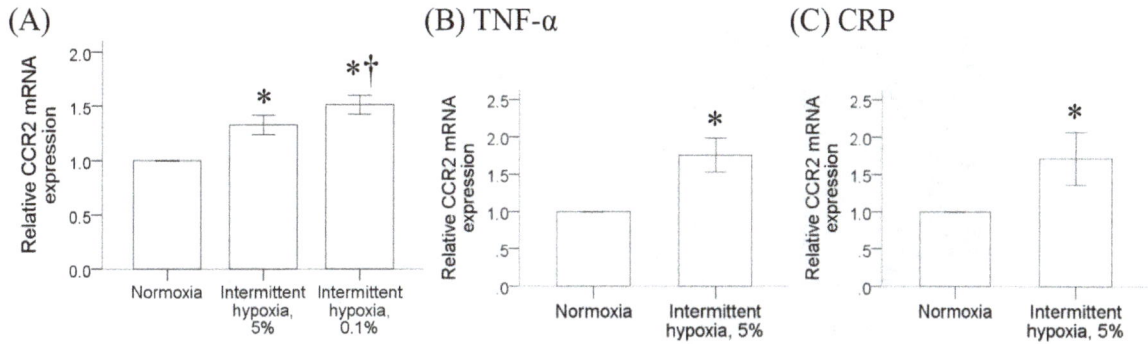

Figure 3. Up-regulation of monocytic CCR2 gene expression depended on the hypoxia level, but not TNF-α or CRP. (A) THP-1 cells were treated with normoxia or intermittent hypoxia with different hypoxia levels (lowest O_2 set-point at 5% or 0.1%) as described in methods. RNA was isolated for the analysis of CCR2 mRNA expression by RT/real-time PCR. In the presence of TNF-α (B) or CRP (C), THP-1 cells were treated with intermittent hypoxia as described in methods. RNA was isolated for the analysis of CCR2 mRNA expression by RT/real-time PCR. (mean ± SE, *: $P < 0.05$ vs. Normoxia, †: $P < 0.05$ vs Normoxia, three independent experiments).

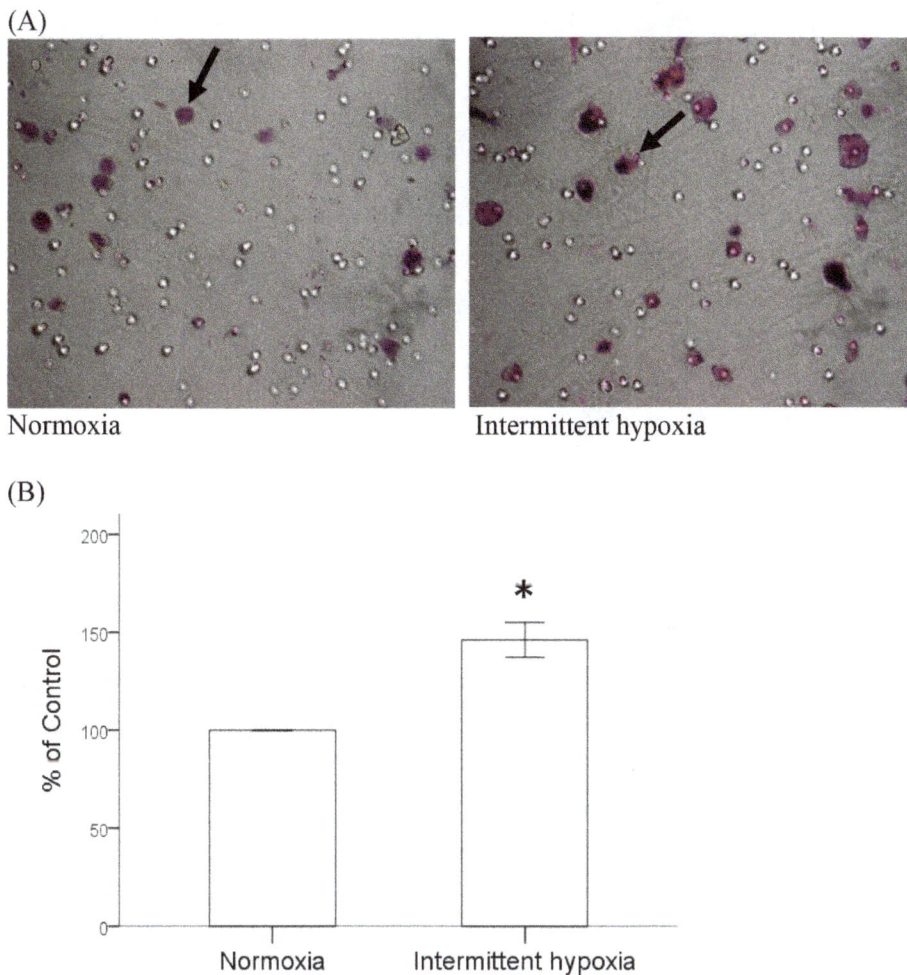

Figure 4. Intermittent hypoxia increased MCP-1-induced chemotaxis of monocytes. THP-1 cells were pretreated with normoxia or intermittent hypoxia as described in methods and then processed for the MCP-1-mediated chemotaxis assay. (A) Representative photos for normoxia- and intermittent hypoxia-treated THP-1 cells that migrated toward lower chamber indicated by black arrow. (B) Statistical results from three independent experiments were shown. Data were means and standard errors. (mean ± SE, *: $P < 0.05$ vs. Normoxia).

(A)

Normoxia   Normoxia + MCP-1

Intermittent hypoxia   Intermittent hypoxia + MCP-1

(B)

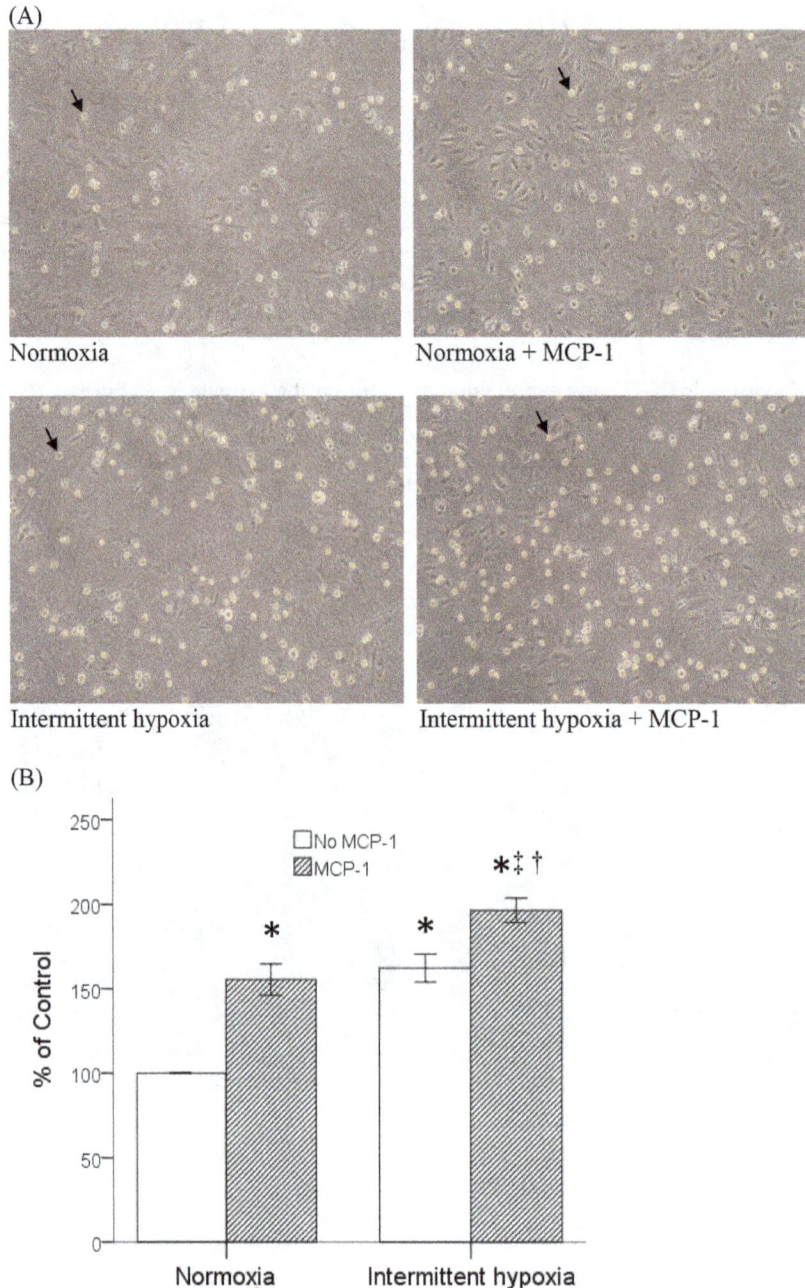

Figure 5. Intermittent hypoxia increased the MCP-1-enhanced adhesion of monocytes to vascular endothelial cells. THP-1 cells pretreated with normoxia or intermittent hypoxia were activated by 20 ng/ml MCP-1 for another 24 hours, and then processed for cell adhesion assay. (A) Representative photos for THP-1 cells after cell adhesion assay. Adhered cells were indicated by black arrow. (Normoxia: without any treatment, Normoxia + MCP-1: with MCP-1 stimulation only, Intermittent hypoxia: with intermittent hypoxia pretreatment only, Intermittent hypoxia + MCP-1: with intermittent hypoxia pretreatment and MCP-1 stimulation) (B) Statistical results from three independent experiments were shown. Data were means and standard errors. (mean ± SE, *: P<0.05 vs. Normoxia, †: P<0.05 vs. Normoxia + MCP-1, ‡: P<0.05 vs Intermittent hypoxia).

Discussion

Many chemokines and their receptors have been investigated and demonstrated to be responsible for the attraction, chemotaxis, adhesion and transendothelial migration of monocytes and involved in the early development of atherosclerosis [27]. Both CC and CXC chemokines are found to be expressed in human atherosclerotic plaques, and an increased expression of pro-inflammatory chemokines and their receptors correlates well with the progression of atherosclerosis within aortas of hyperlipidemic mice [28]. Studies in mice with chemokine or chemokine receptor deficient on the ApoE or LDL receptor knockout background have further confirmed their pathological roles in atherosclerosis [29]. Among the receptors, CCR2 is primarily expressed in almost all circulating monocytes, and mediates the chemotaxis of monocytes to the sites of inflammation that is involved in the

(A)

Phospho-p42/44 MAPK

p42/44 MAPK

Tubulin

Condition

N	IH	N	IH	N	IH
1 hour		3 hours		6 hours	

(N: normoxia; IH: intermittent hypoxia)

(B)

Phospho-p38 MAPK

P38 MAPK

Tubulin

Condition

N	IH	N	IH	N	IH
1 hour		3 hours		6 hours	

(N: normoxia; IH: intermittent hypoxia)

(C)

(D)

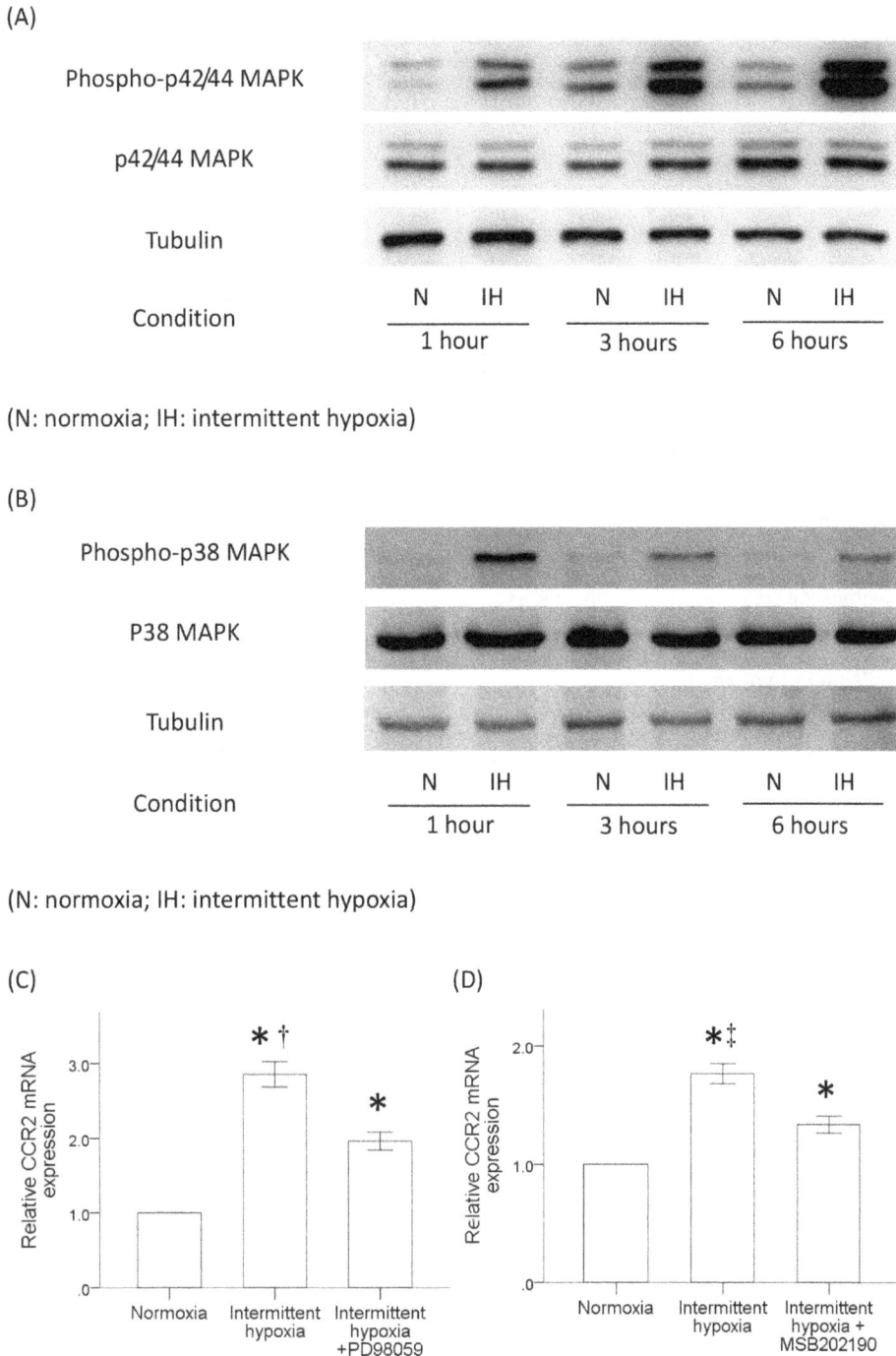

Figure 6. Intermittent hypoxia induced the activation of p44/42 and p38 MAPK signal pathways in THP-1 cells. THP-1 cells were treated with normoxia or intermittent hypoxia and cytosolic proteins were collected at 1, 3 and 6 hr for western blot analysis. The time-dependent activation of (A) p44/42 MAPK or (B) p38 MAPK through phosphorylation by intermittent hypoxia was investigated in THP-1 cells. Monocytes were pretreated with (C) PD98059 or (D) MSB202190 to inhibit p44/42 or p38 MAPK respectively for 1 hr and then the CCR2 mRNA expression was induced by intermittent hypoxia. (N: normoxia; IH: intermittent hypoxia) (mean ± SE, *: $P<0.05$ vs. Normoxia, †: $P<0.05$ vs Intermittent hypoxia + PD98059, ‡: $P<0.05$ vs Intermittent hypoxia + MSB202190).

pathogenesis of several inflammatory diseases [30]. Mice with deficiency of either CCL2 or CCR2 or with leukocyte CCR2-deficiency on an atherosclerotic background all showed decreased lesion formation and reduced macrophage number in the aortic root [31,32]. The number of circulating CCR2-positive inflam-matory monocytes in hypercholesterolemic animals is found to be increased [33]. In hemodialysis patients, the CCR2 expression of monocytes has been reported to positively correlate with the carotid intima-media thickness and cardio-ankle vascular index [34]. In addition to the chemotaxis of monocytes that can be induced by MCP-1 through CCR2 pathway, the activation of MCP-1-CCR2 axis in monocytes also enhances the adhesion of monocytes to vascular endothelial cells [25]. All these studies together with our novel findings that CCR2 gene expression in monocytes was up-regulated in severe OSA patients provide new evidence for the close association of OSA and cardiovascular diseases.

OSA is characterized by a cyclic occurrence of apneic events during sleep that is associated with intermittent hypoxemia and terminated by brief electroencephalographic and autonomic arousals [35]. Multiple cycles of hypoxia/reoxygenation can lead to the activation of inflammatory pathways, up-regulate the downstream expression of pro-inflammatory mediators including pro-inflammatory cytokines, chemokines and adhesion molecules, and result in the activation of various inflammatory cells, particularly lymphocytes and monocytes [36–38]. Except our study that demonstrated the increased CCR2 gene expression of monocytes in OSA patients and under in vitro condition of intermittent hypoxia, a recent study has reported the increase of CCR2 gene expression and macrophage infiltration in carotid body of rat treated with chronic intermittent hypoxia for 7 days [39]. Although the experimental conditions used in this study was different from ours, similar results all indicated that the CCR2 gene expression could be up-regulated by multiple cycles of hypoxia/reoxygenation both in vitro and in vivo. More interestingly, the monocytic CCR2 gene expression in patients of severe OSA group (AHI >30) was found to be further increased after sleep. It is likely that the condition of intermittent hypoxia during the sleep of severe OSA patients might play an important role on the increase of CCR2 expression in monocytes. As shown in our results, the increase of CCR2 expression in monocytes by intermittent hypoxia is demonstrated to be dose-dependent which might explain why the increase of CCR2 after sleep was observed only in severe OSA patients.

Growing evidence points out the importance of oxidative stress and activated inflammatory cells that play a role in the association between OSA and cardiovascular morbidity [40]. Monocytes, known to participate crucially in the entire pathological progression of atherosclerosis, have also been found to become active in OSA patients [22,41]. In the present study, we demonstrated the increase of monocytic CCR2 expression in monocytes of severe OSA patient. Together with the previous finding that MCP-1 level is significantly high in OSA patients, indicating the increase of monocytes could be more easily attracted and adhered to endothelial cells. In addition, the expression of adhesion molecules such as CD15 and CD11c, adhesion index and ROS in monocytes were also found to be up-regulated in OSA patients compared to control [42]. Indeed, monocytes isolated from OSA patients appeared to acquire increased adhesive activity to endothelial cells [43,44]. Circulating monocytes adhere to the endothelium, then transmigrate into the subendothelium, and subsequently invade the matrix of the intima during differentiation toward macrophages, which plays an important role in the early stage of atherosclerosis [45]. The number of macrophages is a lot more abundant in atherectomy materials from unstable angina and abdominal aortic aneurysm [46,47]. The activation and infiltration of monocytes not only directly participates in the formation of atherosclerotic plaque, but is also associated with the increased risk of plaque rupture [48,49].

It is interesting for our study to demonstrate the increase of CCR2 gene expression in monocytes of severe OSA patients, however, some limitations still need been to be discussed in this

study. Firstly, the small sample size was possibly due to the limited number of patients and stringent inclusion criteria. During patient recruitment, we have excluded the possible confounders that could influence the CCR2 expression such as ischemic heart disease, hypertension, diabetes, hyperlipidemia, cerebrovascular disease or renal disease. In addition, this study was carried out using the monocytes purified from each patient that made the study more difficult. Initially, 72 patients have enrolled in this study, but 18 patients were excluded to minimize the effects from other potential confounders. Based on our experience and also results published in previous studies comparing patients with normal control, BMI is often found to be a critical factor affecting OSA. In our study, both AHI and ODI in 54 patients were significantly different among four groups (AHI $\leqq$ 5, 5< AHI $\leqq$ 15, 15< AHI $\leqq$ 30, and AHI > 30). The potential influence by BMI was excluded because the BMI value among four groups did not differ significantly. Since this study aimed to understand the potential effect of intermittent hypoxia, patients with AHI $\leqq$ 5 were considered control in our study.

Instead of average total sleep time, we did measure the sleep efficiency as shown in Table 1 and the results had no statistical significance. As for the duration of OSA, since the record from each patient was considered not scientifically reliable, we did not add the data in our study. Results obtained from our in vitro cell study, though under the simplified condition, provided the first evidence that the CCR2 expression in monocytes was indeed up-regulated by intermittent hypoxia. Our results, for the first time, demonstrated that the induction level of CCR2 mRNA expression in monocytes was higher when cells treated with further hypoxia, providing a reason for the increase of CCR2 gene expression in severe OSA patient. Although we did not directly compare the response to intermittent hypoxia using monocytes from OSA patients with different severity, we tested the response of monocytes in vitro under condition that partially resembled the severe OSA. We found that in the presence of TNF-α or CRP, two inflammatory markers known to be increased in severe OSA patients, the CCR2 mRNA expression could be further enhanced at least 75% by intermittent hypoxia, suggesting the intermittent hypoxia-induced CCR2 mRNA expression in monocytes could further be up-regulated in the presence of other factors involved in severe OSA.

Finally, we divided recruited patients into 4 groups according to the standard OSA criteria, include the relative normal subjects who's AHI <5 as controls. It's not easy to find those patients with the same high body mass index but no any respiratory event during sleep. Thus, lack of normal controls is another limitation in our study.

In summary, this study, for the first time, demonstrated the increase of CCR2 gene expression in monocytes of severe OSA patients. Intermittent hypoxia, the hallmark of obstructive sleep apnea, was proved to increase the CCR2 gene expression and the chemotaxic ability of monocytes toward MCP-1. Intermittent hypoxia was also found to further enhance the adhesion of monocytes to vascular endothelial cells. Both ERK and p38 MAPK were confirmed to be involved in the signaling pathway for the induction of CCR2 in monocytes by intermittent hypoxia. These findings may shed some light on mechanisms involved in increased monocyte chemotaxis and adhesion under IH conditions that may lead to the development of atherosclerosis in patients with OSA. These results also strongly suggest an important role of CCR2, therefore, to reduce CCR2 expression or to block its function in monocytes by various antagonists could be a promising strategy to prevent atherosclerosis in patients with OSA.

Acknowledgments

The authors thank Dr. Samuel Chen from NexBiOxy Instruments Inc. for the technical help on the experimental setup of intermittent hypoxia chamber.

Author Contributions

Conceived and designed the experiments: LC JP. Performed the experiments: LC IC Yuling Lin JP. Analyzed the data: LC NC SL Yu-Sheng Lin JP. Contributed reagents/materials/analysis tools: YC HL. Wrote the paper: LC JP.

References

1. Young T, Peppard PE, Gottlieb DJ (2002) Epidemiology of obstructive sleep apnea: a population health perspective. American journal of respiratory and critical care medicine 165: 1217–1239.
2. (1994) Indications and standards for use of nasal continuous positive airway pressure (CPAP) in sleep apnea syndromes. American Thoracic Society. Official statement adopted March 1944. Am J Respir Crit Care Med 150: 1738–1745.
3. Malhotra A, White DP (2002) Obstructive sleep apnoea. Lancet 360: 237–245.
4. Newman AB, Nieto FJ, Guidry U, Lind BK, Redline S, et al. (2001) Relation of sleep-disordered breathing to cardiovascular disease risk factors: the Sleep Heart Health Study. Am J Epidemiol 154: 50–59.
5. Javaheri S, Parker TJ, Liming JD, Corbett WS, Nishiyama H, et al. (1998) Sleep apnea in 81 ambulatory male patients with stable heart failure. Types and their prevalences, consequences, and presentations. Circulation 97: 2154–2159.
6. Marin JM, Carrizo SJ, Vicente E, Agusti AG (2005) Long-term cardiovascular outcomes in men with obstructive sleep apnoea-hypopnoea with or without treatment with continuous positive airway pressure: an observational study. Lancet 365: 1046–1053.
7. Nakashima H, Katayama T, Takagi C, Amenomori K, Ishizaki M, et al. (2006) Obstructive sleep apnoea inhibits the recovery of left ventricular function in patients with acute myocardial infarction. Eur Heart J 27: 2317–2322.
8. Aboyans V, Cassat C, Lacroix P, Tapie P, Tabaraud F, et al. (2000) Is the morning peak of acute myocardial infarction's onset due to sleep-related breathing disorders? A prospective study. Cardiology 94: 188–192.
9. Gami AS, Howard DE, Olson EJ, Somers VK (2005) Day-night pattern of sudden death in obstructive sleep apnea. N Engl J Med 352: 1206–1214.
10. Parker JD, Brooks D, Kozar LF, Render-Teixeira CL, Horner RL, et al. (1999) Acute and chronic effects of airway obstruction on canine left ventricular performance. Am J Respir Crit Care Med 160: 1888–1896.
11. Tkacova R, Rankin F, Fitzgerald FS, Floras JS, Bradley TD (1998) Effects of continuous positive airway pressure on obstructive sleep apnea and left ventricular afterload in patients with heart failure. Circulation 98: 2269–2275.
12. Nacher M, Farre R, Montserrat JM, Torres M, Navajas D, et al. (2009) Biological consequences of oxygen desaturation and respiratory effort in an acute animal model of obstructive sleep apnea (OSA). Sleep medicine 10: 892–897.
13. Ryan S, McNicholas WT (2008) Intermittent hypoxia and activation of inflammatory molecular pathways in OSAS. Archives of physiology and biochemistry 114: 261–266.
14. Hansson GK (2009) Inflammatory mechanisms in atherosclerosis. Journal of thrombosis and haemostasis: JTH 7 Suppl 1: 328–331.
15. Amasyali B, Kose S, Kursaklioglu H, Barcin C, Kilic A (2009) Monocyte chemoattractant protein-1 in acute coronary syndromes: complex vicious interaction. International journal of cardiology 136: 356–357.
16. Tieu BC, Lee C, Sun H, Lejeune W, Recinos A 3rd, et al. (2009) An adventitial IL-6/MCP1 amplification loop accelerates macrophage-mediated vascular inflammation leading to aortic dissection in mice. The Journal of clinical investigation 119: 3637–3651.
17. Green SR, Han KH, Chen Y, Almazan F, Charo IF, et al. (2006) The CC chemokine MCP-1 stimulates surface expression of CX3CR1 and enhances the adhesion of monocytes to fractalkine/CX3CL1 via p38 MAPK. Journal of immunology 176: 7412–7420.
18. Hiraoka M, Nitta N, Nagai M, Shimokado K, Yoshida M (2004) MCP-1-induced enhancement of THP-1 adhesion to vascular endothelium was modulated by HMG-CoA reductase inhibitor through RhoA GTPase-, but not ERK1/2-dependent pathway. Life sciences 75: 1333–1341.
19. Kuziel WA, Morgan SJ, Dawson TC, Griffin S, Smithies O, et al. (1997) Severe reduction in leukocyte adhesion and monocyte extravasation in mice deficient in CC chemokine receptor 2. Proceedings of the National Academy of Sciences of the United States of America 94: 12053–12058.
20. Kaditis AG, Alexopoulos EI, Karathanasi A, Ntamagka G, Oikonomidi S, et al. (2010) Adiposity and low-grade systemic inflammation modulate matrix metalloproteinase-9 levels in Greek children with sleep apnea. Pediatr Pulmonol 45: 693–699.
21. Yamashita C, Hayashi T, Mori T, Matsumoto C, Kitada K, et al. (2010) Efficacy of olmesartan and nifedipine on recurrent hypoxia-induced left ventricular remodeling in diabetic mice. Life Sci 86: 322–330.
22. Tamaki S, Yamauchi M, Fukuoka A, Makinodan K, Koyama N, et al. (2009) Production of inflammatory mediators by monocytes in patients with obstructive sleep apnea syndrome. Intern Med 48: 1255–1262.
23. Chuang LP, Chen NH, Lin SW, Chang YL, Chao IJ, et al. (2013) Increased matrix metalloproteinases-9 after sleep in plasma and in monocytes of obstructive sleep apnea patients. Life Sci 93: 220–225.
24. Dyugovskaya L, Polyakov A, Lavie P, Lavie L (2008) Delayed neutrophil apoptosis in patients with sleep apnea. Am J Respir Crit Care Med 177: 544–554.
25. Chuang SY, Yang SH, Pang JH (2011) Cilostazol reduces MCP-1-induced chemotaxis and adhesion of THP-1 monocytes by inhibiting CCR2 gene expression. Biochem Biophys Res Commun 411: 402–408.
26. Ko J, Yun CY, Lee JS, Kim JH, Kim IS (2007) p38 MAPK and ERK activation by 9-cis-retinoic acid induces chemokine receptors CCR1 and CCR2 expression in human monocytic THP-1 cells. Exp Mol Med 39: 129–138.
27. Ono SJ, Nakamura T, Miyazaki D, Ohbayashi M, Dawson M, et al. (2003) Chemokines: roles in leukocyte development, trafficking, and effector function. J Allergy Clin Immunol 111: 1185–1199; quiz 1200.
28. Murphy N, Bruckdorfer KR, Grimsditch DC, Overend P, Vidgeon-Hart M, et al. (2003) Temporal relationships between circulating levels of CC and CXC chemokines and developing atherosclerosis in apolipoprotein E*3 Leiden mice. Arterioscler Thromb Vasc Biol 23: 1615–1620.
29. Boring L, Gosling J, Cleary M, Charo IF (1998) Decreased lesion formation in CCR2-/- mice reveals a role for chemokines in the initiation of atherosclerosis. Nature 394: 894–897.
30. Han KH, Tangirala RK, Green SR, Quehenberger O (1998) Chemokine receptor CCR2 expression and monocyte chemoattractant protein-1-mediated chemotaxis in human monocytes. A regulatory role for plasma LDL. Arterioscler Thromb Vasc Biol 18: 1983–1991.
31. Inoue S, Egashira K, Ni W, Kitamoto S, Usui M, et al. (2002) Anti-monocyte chemoattractant protein-1 gene therapy limits progression and destabilization of established atherosclerosis in apolipoprotein E-knockout mice. Circulation 106: 2700–2706.
32. Olzinski AR, Turner GH, Bernard RE, Karr H, Cornejo CA, et al. (2010) Pharmacological inhibition of C-C chemokine receptor 2 decreases macrophage infiltration in the aortic root of the human C-C chemokine receptor 2/apolipoprotein E-/- mouse: magnetic resonance imaging assessment. Arterioscler Thromb Vasc Biol 30: 253–259.
33. Ni W, Kitamoto S, Ishibashi M, Usui M, Inoue S, et al. (2004) Monocyte chemoattractant protein-1 is an essential inflammatory mediator in angiotensin II-induced progression of established atherosclerosis in hypercholesterolemic mice. Arterioscler Thromb Vasc Biol 24: 534–539.
34. Okumoto S, Taniguchi Y, Nakashima A, Masaki T, Ito T, et al. (2009) C-C chemokine receptor 2 expression by circulating monocytes influences atherosclerosis in patients on chronic hemodialysis. Ther Apher Dial 13: 205–212.
35. Kohler M, Stradling JR (2010) Mechanisms of vascular damage in obstructive sleep apnea. Nat Rev Cardiol 7: 677–685.
36. Nanduri J, Yuan G, Kumar GK, Semenza GL, Prabhakar NR (2008) Transcriptional responses to intermittent hypoxia. Respir Physiol Neurobiol 164: 277–281.
37. Morgan BJ (2007) Vascular consequences of intermittent hypoxia. Adv Exp Med Biol 618: 69–84.
38. Lavie L, Dyugovskaya L, Polyakov A (2008) Biology of peripheral blood cells in obstructive sleep apnea-the tip of the iceberg. Arch Physiol Biochem 114: 244–254.
39. Lam SY, Liu Y, Ng KM, Lau CF, Liong EC, et al. (2012) Chronic intermittent hypoxia induces local inflammation of the rat carotid body via functional upregulation of proinflammatory cytokine pathways. Histochem Cell Biol 137: 303–317.
40. Lavie L (2003) Obstructive sleep apnoea syndrome-an oxidative stress disorder. Sleep Med Rev 7: 35–51.
41. Minoguchi K, Tazaki T, Yokoe T, Minoguchi H, Watanabe Y, et al. (2004) Elevated production of tumor necrosis factor-alpha by monocytes in patients with obstructive sleep apnea syndrome. Chest 126: 1473–1479.
42. Lavie L, Dyugovskaya L, Lavie P (2005) Sleep-apnea-related intermittent hypoxia and atherogenesis: adhesion molecules and monocytes/endothelial cells interactions. Atherosclerosis 183: 183–184.
43. Dyugovskaya L, Lavie P, Lavie L (2002) Increased adhesion molecules expression and production of reactive oxygen species in leukocytes of sleep apnea patients. Am J Respir Crit Care Med 165: 934–939.
44. Lattimore JD, Wilcox I, Nakhla S, Langenfeld M, Jessup W, et al. (2005) Repetitive hypoxia increases lipid loading in human macrophages-a potentially atherogenic effect. Atherosclerosis 179: 255–259.

45. Glass CK, Witztum JL (2001) Atherosclerosis. the road ahead. Cell 104: 503–516.
46. Loftus IM, Naylor AR, Goodall S, Crowther M, Jones L, et al. (2000) Increased matrix metalloproteinase-9 activity in unstable carotid plaques. A potential role in acute plaque disruption. Stroke 31: 40–47.
47. Yamashita A, Ishida K, Aratake K, Wakamatsu H, Kawata R, et al. (2000) [Perioperative management of endovascular stent graft placement for abdominal aortic aneurysm]. Masui 49: 987–994.
48. Moreno PR, Falk E, Palacios IF, Newell JB, Fuster V, et al. (1994) Macrophage infiltration in acute coronary syndromes. Implications for plaque rupture. Circulation 90: 775–778.
49. Pasterkamp G, Schoneveld AH, Hijnen DJ, de Kleijn DP, Teepen H, et al. (2000) Atherosclerotic arterial remodeling and the localization of macrophages and matrix metalloproteases 1, 2 and 9 in the human coronary artery. Atherosclerosis 150: 245–253.

13

A New Recombinant BCG Vaccine Induces Specific Th17 and Th1 Effector Cells with Higher Protective Efficacy against Tuberculosis

Adeliane Castro da Costa[1], Abadio de Oliveira Costa-Júnior[1], Fábio Muniz de Oliveira[2], Sarah Veloso Nogueira[1], Joseane Damaceno Rosa[1], Danilo Pires Resende[1], André Kipnis[2], Ana Paula Junqueira-Kipnis[1]*

1 Laboratório de Imunopatologia das Doenças Infecciosas, Instituto de Patologia Tropical e Saúde Pública, Universidade Federal de Goiás, Goiânia, Goiás, Brazil, 2 Laboratório de Bacteriologia Molecular, Instituto de Patologia Tropical e Saúde Pública, Universidade Federal de Goiás, Goiânia, Goiás, Brazil

Abstract

Tuberculosis (TB) is an infectious disease caused by *Mycobacterium tuberculosis* (Mtb) that is a major public health problem. The vaccine used for TB prevention is *Mycobacterium bovis* bacillus Calmette-Guérin (BCG), which provides variable efficacy in protecting against pulmonary TB among adults. Consequently, several groups have pursued the development of a new vaccine with a superior protective capacity to that of BCG. Here we constructed a new recombinant BCG (rBCG) vaccine expressing a fusion protein (CMX) composed of immune dominant epitopes from Ag85C, MPT51, and HspX and evaluated its immunogenicity and protection in a murine model of infection. The stability of the vaccine *in vivo* was maintained for up to 20 days post-vaccination. rBCG-CMX was efficiently phagocytized by peritoneal macrophages and induced nitric oxide (NO) production. Following mouse immunization, this vaccine induced a specific immune response in cells from lungs and spleen to the fusion protein and to each of the component recombinant proteins by themselves. Vaccinated mice presented higher amounts of Th1, Th17, and polyfunctional specific T cells. rBCG-CMX vaccination reduced the extension of lung lesions caused by challenge with Mtb as well as the lung bacterial load. In addition, when this vaccine was used in a prime-boost strategy together with rCMX, the lung bacterial load was lower than the result observed by BCG vaccination. This study describes the creation of a new promising vaccine for TB that we hope will be used in further studies to address its safety before proceeding to clinical trials.

Editor: Delphi Chatterjee, Colorado State University, United States of America

Funding: This study was financed by the National Council for Scientific and Technological Development (CNPq, Project #301976/2011-2, 472906/2011-9, 301198/2009-8, 472909/2011-8) and by Fundação de Amparo a Pesquisa do Estado de Goiás (FAPEG-PRONEX). ACC received a PhD fellowship from CNPq. AOCJ, DPR, and FMO each received a MSc fellowship from CNPq. SVN received a Post Doc fellowship from CNPq. JDR received an undergraduate fellowship from PIBIC-CNPq. The funders had no role in study design, data collection and analysis, decision to publish, or preparation of the manuscript.

Competing Interests: The authors have declared that no competing interests exist.

* Email: apkipnis@gmail.com

Introduction

Tuberculosis (TB) is a public health problem causing 8.6 million new cases and 1.3 million deaths annually [1]. The causative agent of TB is *Mycobacterium tuberculosis* (Mtb), an intracellular pathogen that after infecting the host can either cause active disease or remain latent. In this context, it is estimated that one third of the world population is latently infected with Mtb, of which approximately 10% will develop active disease [2,1]. Currently, the vaccine used for TB prevention is Bacillus Calmette-Guérin (BCG), an attenuated *Mycobacterium bovis* strain used since 1921 [3]. Despite being the only approved vaccine for human use and conferring protection against tuberculous meningitis and miliary TB in children, its protective efficacy remains questionable, as it does not protect young adults against pulmonary TB [4,5,6].

The factors determining the variable protective mechanisms induced by BCG are not well understood. Some suppositions point towards the BCG sub-strain characteristics. It has acquired genotypic and phenotypic differences, such as residual virulence and epitope number variation, after the attenuation process and the several sub-culturing passages made through the years [7–8]. In addition, BCG has limited capacity to induce long lasting memory and, in humans, the vaccine induces an immune response with Th1 effector cells producing IFN-γ [9,10,11]. Although IFN-γ is crucial for the immune response to Mtb, studies have shown this cytokine is not a surrogate marker of the protection conferred by BCG [12,11]. To address this matter, several groups have been working on the development of protein subunit vaccines, new adjuvants, attenuated/auxotrophic Mtb strains, and recombinant BCG (rBCG) vaccines, among other approaches [13–14]. Different strategies are being used by the groups modifying BCG, such as the expression of immunodominant Mtb antigens [15], the association of re-introduction and super-expression of antigens lost during the process of BCG attenuation [16], the development of rBCG expressing cytokines and Mtb proteins [17], and the heterologous expression of proteins in rBCG to induce CD8[+] T lymphocytes [18].

While evaluating the rBCG vaccines produced in the last five years, it was observed that the selection of Mtb antigens used in the construction of the rBCG was more important for vaccine efficacy than the BCG subtypes used to make them [19]. However, comparing the BCG subtypes used to construct recombinant vaccines, sub strains BCG Tokyo and BCG Moreau presented more immune dominant epitopes than the other sub strains, and all rBCG produced using the Tokyo strain protected better than the wild type BCG [20]. Sequencing of the complete genome and an evaluation of the proteome profile of BCG Moreau were performed, but this strain was poorly used to build a TB recombinant vaccine [21–22]. Some studies have shown that BCG Moreau is a good carrier and efficiently induces a specific immune response to other diseases, such as pertussis, enteropathogenic *Escherichia coli*, or bladder cancer [23–25]. BCG Moreau has been used for more than 80 years in Brazil, attesting to its safety. This strain is currently being tested again as oral vaccine and is showing better performance than BCG Danish [26]. This prompted us to develop a recombinant TB vaccine using the BCG subtype Moreau.

Most of the time, the choice of the antigens used to develop an rBCG is based on the different phases of Mtb infection. Active and latent TB are distinct phases of the disease that can be characterized by their antigen expression, and these antigens are effective at inducing an immune response [27]. Our group and others have demonstrated that patients with active pulmonary TB and latently infected individuals respond differently to several Mtb antigens, such as antigen 85 complex proteins, MPT51 and HspX [28–31]. In our previous work, we developed a fusion protein (CMX) composed of the immunodominant antigens from Mtb: Ag85C, MPT51 and the entire HspX protein, [32] which are expressed in different stages of TB (active and latent phases of the disease). This construction retained the immunogenicity of the original proteins in vaccinated mice and was also specifically recognized by individuals with active TB [32]. To determine if this fusion protein could be expressed by a live vector, and consequently be used as a vaccine for TB, a recombinant *Mycobacterium smegmatis* (mc^2) was designed to express CMX (*mc^2-CMX*). This vaccine induced a specific immune response to CMX that culminated with protection similar to that observed following vaccination with BCG Moreau [33]. In this scenario, the fusion protein CMX was capable of adding important immunogenic properties to mycobacterium vaccine vectors, inducing an effective response to control Mtb infection in mice.

Based on the previous studies, both ours and others, we hypothesize that using BCG subtype Moreau to develop a new rBCG expressing CMX will add immunological characteristics that are missing in conventional BCG and therefore induce an specific immune response better able to control the infection by Mtb. Our data here show that the expression of CMX protein by the rBCG Moreau vaccine (rBCG-CMX) is a determining factor for inducing specific Th1 and Th17 responses, in addition to polyfunctional T cells. These responses may be responsible for the reduction in the inflammatory lung lesions induced by Mtb challenge in BALB/c mice and the reduction in the bacterial load. Moreover, prime vaccination with rBCG-CMX followed by boosting with rCMX further reduced the lung bacterial load as compared to the reduction caused by BCG Moreau.

Materials and Methods

Bacterial strains, growth conditions, and plasmid and vaccine preparations

The *M. bovis* BCG Moreau strain, kindly provided by the Butantan Institute, was grown in 7H9 media (Becton and Dickinson, Le pont de Claix- France) supplemented with 10 oleic acid, albumin, dextrose and catalase (OADC-Becton and Dickinson, Le pont de Claix- France), 0.5% glycerol and 0.05% Tween 80, at 37°C in a humid atmosphere and 5% CO_2 for approximately three weeks.

The recombinant BCG strains were obtained after electroporation of BCG Moreau with one of the three expression plasmids (pLA71, pLA72, and pMIP12). These plasmids have mycobacteria and *Escherichia coli* replication origins and use the gene for kanamycin resistance as a selection marker, as described by Varaldo et al. (2004) [34]. The gene coding for the fusion CMX protein (Ag85C, MPT51, and HspX) [32] was obtained from Mtb (H37Rv) DNA and inserted in the pLA71, pLA73 and pMIP12 mycobacteria expression vectors as described by Junqueira-Kipnis et al. (2013) [33]. The employed expression plasmids enable the recombinant gene to be expressed with either the signal peptide of the β-lactamase from *M. fortuitum* (pLA71) or the entire β-lactamase protein (pLA73), or, alternatively, the protein can be highly expressed intracellularly (pMIP12). Transformants with empty plasmids were used as controls. The recombinant vaccines obtained were cultured under the same conditions as the BCG Moreau described above, with the addition of 20 μg/mL of kanamycin.

The vaccines were grown in a single lot in 7H9 supplemented with OADC, and the concentration of the lots were determined by plating serial dilutions of each vaccine onto 7H11 agar plates with or without kanamycin (20 μg/mL).

Animals

BALB/c female mice, 4 to 8 weeks of age, from the Instituto de Patologia Tropical e Saúde Pública/UFG animal housing were maintained in micro-isolators equipped with HEPA filters for air intake and exhaustion, and provided with water and a chow diet *ad libitum*. The room temperature was kept at 20–24°C with a relative humidity of 40–70% and light/dark cycles of 12 hours. Mice were handled according to the Sociedade Brasileira de Ciência em Animais de Laboratório (SBCAL/COBEA) guidelines. The study was approved by the Ethical Committee for Animal use (CEUA: Comite de Ética no uso de animais; #229/11) of the Universidade Federal de Goiás.

PCR and Western blotting

To confirm the presence of the CMX fusion gene (~860 base pairs), a PCR reaction using Ag85C forward (5′ ggtctgcgggcccaggatg 3′) and HspX reverse (5′ tcagttggtggaccggatctgaatgtg 3′) primers (10 nmol of each) in the same conditions as described previously [32]. The expression of CMX (~35 kDa) by the different vectors was assessed by Western blot, as described previously [33].

Assessment of in vivo plasmid stability

BALB/c mice were immunized with 10^6 colony forming units (CFU) of rBCG-pLA71-CMX or rBCG-pLA71 subcutaneously in the dorsal region. Animals were euthanized at different time points (3 mice/group/time point) and the dorsal tissue at the injection site was cut out and macerated. The homogenized tissue was plated onto 7H11 agar supplemented with OADC, 0.5% glycerol and 20 μg/mL of kanamycin. After incubation at 37°C with 5%

CO_2 for approximately 30 days, the plates were analyzed for bacterial growth and the numbers of CFU were determined. The DNA from a representative colony was extracted by boiling the entire colony, and the supernatant was submitted to PCR for detection of the CMX gene. This experiment was repeated three times.

Mouse peritoneal macrophage preparation, culture, and infection

Peritoneal macrophages were obtained after injection of 1 mL of thioglycolate into the peritoneal cavity of BALB/c mice four days prior to macrophage collection. Mice were euthanized by cervical dislocation and 5 mL of ice cold phosphate buffered saline (PBS) was injected into the peritoneal cavity, followed by vigorous massage. The recovered cells were distributed in a 24 well plate at a concentration of 1×10^6 cells per mL and incubated with 5% CO_2 for 24 hours to allow for adherence. In some of the cultured wells, circular glass cover slides were introduced to allow for microscopic evaluation. Macrophages were infected with BCG or rBCG-CMX at a multiplicity of infection (MOI) = 10 or incubated with LPS (5 µg/mL), as a control. Infected macrophages were incubated at 37°C with 5% CO_2. After 3 hours, the supernatant was discarded, the cells were washed, and new media was added to the wells. After 18 hours, the supernatant was collected and plated on 7H11 agar plates to determine the number of bacteria that were not phagocytosed. Infected macrophages were washed three times with RPMI medium (HIMEDIA, Mumbai-India) and then lysed with water and plated on 7H11 agar to determine the level of CFU of the intracellular bacteria. Some of the infected macrophages were kept for an additional incubation of 48 hours and used for nitric oxide (NO) quantification of the supernatant by the Griess method, as described below. The cover slides from macrophages infected for 3 hours were washed three times with PBS at 37°C, fixed with methanol and stained with Ziehl Neelsen, for acid fast bacilli visualization, or Instant Prov (Newprov, Pinhais- Brazil), for cell visualization.

Nitric oxide determination

Supernatants (100 µL) from macrophage cultures that had been stimulated or not (control) with BCG, rBCG, or LPS were stored in a 96 well plate at −20°C until use. Fifty microliters of the supernatant was transferred to another 96 well plate and 50 µL Griess reagent (1% sulphanilamide, 2% phosphoric acid, and 0.1% naphthylethylene diamine dihydrochloride) was added, followed by 15 minutes of incubation at room temperature, protected from the light. A serial dilution of nitrite was included in additional wells to provide a standard curve for comparison. The absorbance was measured in a spectrophotometer (Thermo LabSystems Multiskan RC/MS/EX Microplate Reader) at 595 nm.

BCG and rBCG-CMX immunizations

BALB/c mice were separated into three groups: Control, BCG Moreau, and rBCG-CMX. Five to six animals were used in each group. Prior to use, the vaccines were thawed and the concentrations adjusted with PBS/0.05% Tween 80, so that each animal would receive 10^6 CFU in 100 µL by subcutaneous injection in the dorsal region. The vaccine concentrations were confirmed by plating the remaining inocula on 7H11 agar supplemented with OADC. An additional group of animals, previously vaccinated with rBCG-CMX (N = 5) was given a booster, 30 days later with 20 µg/mL of rCMX/CPG DNA prepared as described at de Souza et al, 2012 [32]. This

experiment was repeated two times in BALB/c mice and one time in C57BL/6 mice.

Cell preparation for immune response evaluation

Thirty days after immunization, six animals from each group of the BALB/c mice were euthanized and the spleens and left lung lobes were collected. Spleens were prepared into single cell suspensions using 70 µm cell strainers (BD Biosciences, Lincoln Park, NJ) and the cells were resuspended with RPMI medium. Erythrocytes were lysed with lysis solution (0.15 M NH_4Cl, 10 mM $KHCO_3$) and the cells were washed and resuspended with RPMI supplemented with 20% fetal calf serum, 0.15% sodium bicarbonate, 1% L-glutamine (200 mM; Sigma-Aldrich-Brazil, São Paulo), 1% non-essential amino acids (Sigma-Aldrich). Cells were counted in a Neubauer chamber and the concentration was adjusted to 1×10^6 cells/mL. Prior to collection, the lungs were perfused with ice-cold PBS containing 45 U/mL of heparin (Sigma-Aldrich-Brazil, São Paulo) and processed as described previously [33]. The lungs were digested with DNAse IV (30 µg/mL; Sigma-Aldrich) and collagenase III (0.7 mg/mL; Sigma-Aldrich-Brazil, São Paulo) for 30 min at 37°C. The digested lungs were prepared into single cell suspensions using 70 µm cell strainers and submitted to erythrocyte lysis. The cells were washed and resuspended with RPMI, and the concentrations were adjusted to 1×10^6 cells/mL.

Ag85 (Rv0129c), MPT51 (Rv3803c), HspX (Rv2031c) and CMX specific cytokine evaluation by lung and spleen lymphocytes

In a 96 well cell culture plate (CellWells TM), 200 µL of spleen or lung cell suspensions were cultivated without (media alone) or with recombinant CMX or with only one of the component recombinant proteins, Ag85, MPT51 or HspX (single proteins were used at a concentration of 10 µg/mL) or ConA (positive control) in a 5% CO_2 incubator at 37°C for 4 hours. Monensin (3 µM; eBioscience) was then added to the wells and the cultures were further incubated for 4 hours. Cells were treated with 0.1% sodium azide in PBS for 30 min at room temperature. After centrifuging, the cells were stained with anti-CD4 Percp (eBioscience, clone RM4-5) or anti-CD4 FITC (BD PharMingen, clone RM4-5) for 30 min. Cells were then, permeabilized with Perm Fix/Perm Wash (BD PharMingen), washed with 0.1% sodium azide in PBS, and then stained with the following antibodies to access the expressions of a panel of Th1 cytokines. anti-TNF-α FITC (BD PharMingen-MP6; clone: XT22), anti-IL-2 PE (eBioscience-JES6; clone: 5H4), and anti-IFN-γ APC (eBioscience; clone: XMG1.2). To access the expression of a panel of Th17 cytokines, cells were stained with: anti-IL-2 PE (eBioscience, clone: JES6-5H4), anti-IL-17A Percp (eBioscience, clone: eBio17B7), and anti-IFN-γ APC (eBioscience, clone: XMG1.2) for 30 min. Cell acquisition of 100,000 events per sample was performed in a BD FACS Verse (Universidade de Brasília-UNB) flow cytometer and the acquired data were analyzed using FlowJo 8.7 software. Lymphocytes were selected based on their size (Forward scatter, FSC) and granularity (side scatter, SSC). The specific immune responses were determined by subtracting the result of the media alone stimulation from the responses to each of the antigens.

Mycobacterium tuberculosis intravenous infection

The *Mycobaterium tuberculosis* (H37Rv) strain was maintained as described previously [33]. A vial from a constant lot was thawed and the inoculum was adjusted to the concentration of 10^6 CFU/

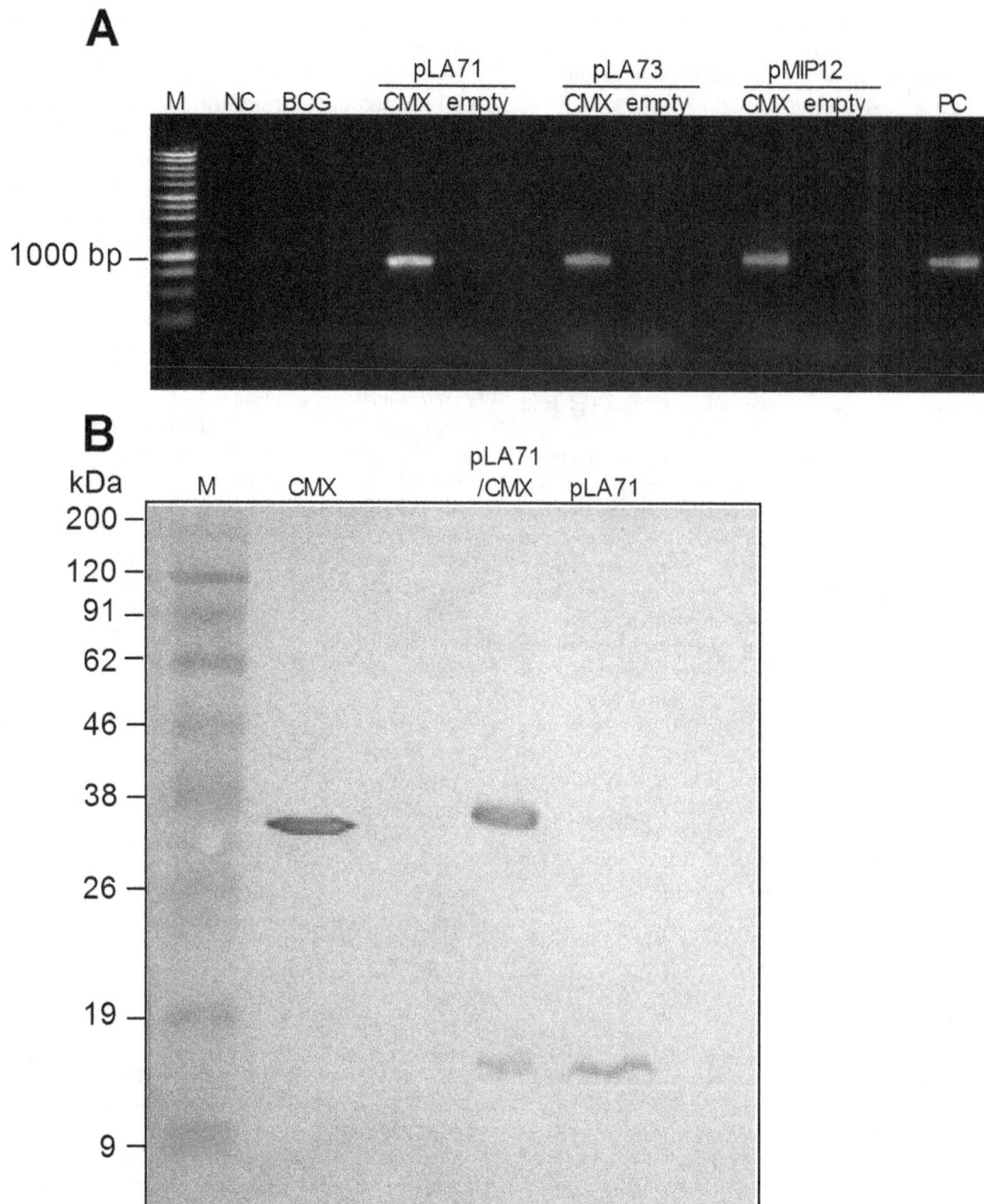

Figure 1. Plasmid construction and CMX expression for three different rBCG-CMX vaccines. (A) PCR products corresponding to the CMX fusion gene, CMX (~860 bp), from all three plasmid constructions and their respective empty controls: pLA71, pLA73 and pMIP12. M: molecular weight marker; NC: negative control reaction, using water; BCG: DNA from BCG-Moreau; rBCG transformed with pLA71, pLA73 and pMIP12, with (CMX) or without (empty) the fusion gene; PC: positive control reaction. (B) Analysis of CMX expression in rBCG-pLA71/CMX. Western blot of BCG transformants containing pLA71/CMX or empty vector using polyclonal antibody produced against rCMX. M: molecular mass marker; CMX: purified recombinant CMX; pLA71/CMX: rBCG with plasmid pLA71/CMX; pLA71: rBCG with plasmid pLA71.

mL by diluting with PBS containing 0.05% Tween 80. Ninety days after immunization with rBCG-CMX or BCG Moreau, 100 μL of the inoculum was injected into the retro-orbital plexus. The bacterial load of infection was determined by plating the lung homogenates from one mouse from each group on the day following infection on 7H11 agar supplemented with OADC. Forty-five days after infection, mice were euthanized and the anterior and mediastinal right lung lobes were collected, homogenized, and plated on 7H11 agar supplemented with OADC. The bacterial load was determined by counting the CFU after 21 days of incubation at 37°C.

Histopathology

The lungs of mice euthanized 45 days after the Mtb challenge were perfused with 0.05% heparin by injection in the heart right ventricle. The posterior right lobes were collected, conditioned in histological cassettes, and fixed with 10% buffered formaldehyde. Samples were sectioned into 5 μm thick slices and stained with

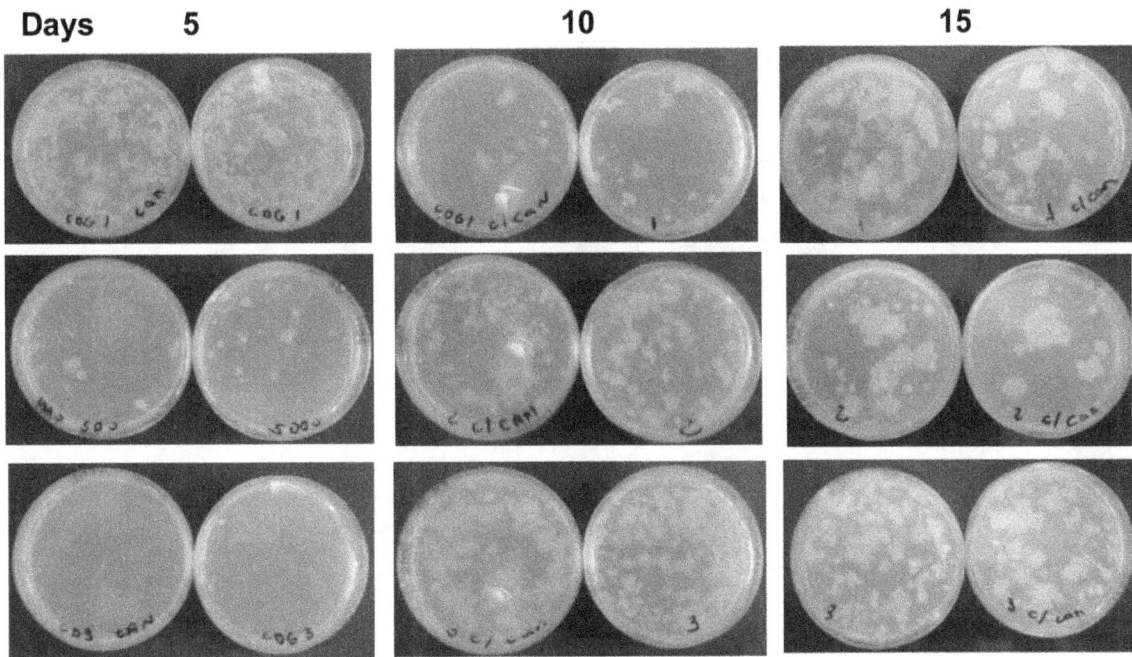

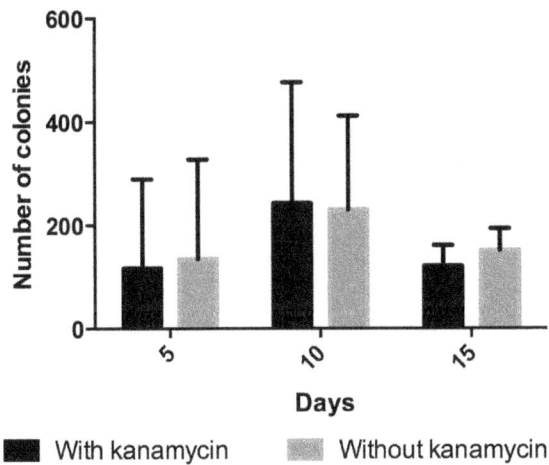

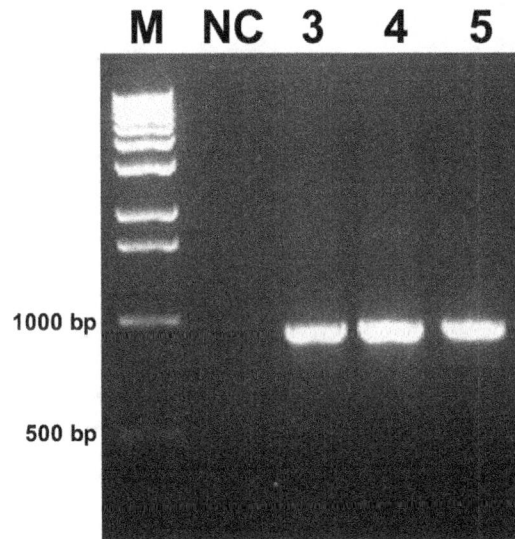

Figure 2. Stability of rBCG-CMX *in vivo*. (A) Images of plates showing the mycobacterial growth of rBCG-CMX recovered from the dorsal region of mice 5, 10 and 15 days after subcutaneous immunization, and plated on media with kanamycin (kan) or without (W/o). (B) CFU counts recovered at different time points from the dorsal region of mice after immunization. (C) CMX gene detection by PCR for three isolated colonies from plates W/o kanamycin (Lanes 3–5). Lanes 1: M: molecular weight marker; 2: Negative control: NC: water.

hematoxylin and eosin (HE) for analysis via microscopy (Axio scope.A1 - Carl Zeiss). Scores for the observed lesions were determined based on the area with lesions relative to the area of the total visual field. The results are presented as the percentage of area with lesions. Three different fields were evaluated per slide for each animal of each group.

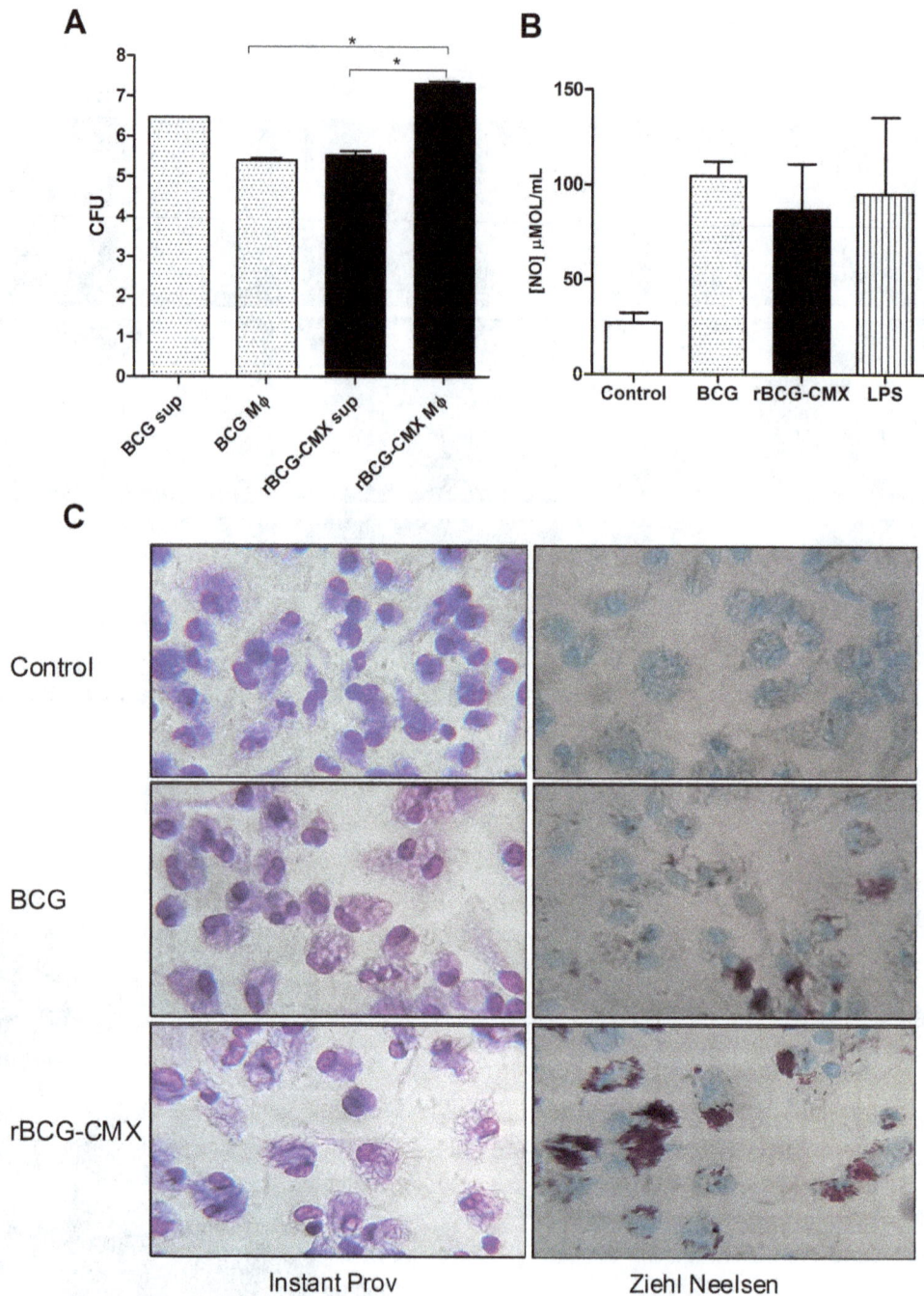

Figure 3. Levels of phagocytosis by peritoneal macrophages of BCG and rBCG-CMX after infection (MOI = 10). (A) Macrophages were infected with BCG or rBCG-CMX and the bacterial load in both the supernatant (sup) and inside the macrophages (Mφ) were determined. The amount of viable bacteria was determined by plating supernatant or cell lysates onto 7H11 agar supplemented with OADC and counting the CFU 28 days after incubation at 37°C. *(p<0.01) significant difference between the compared groups (log10 scale). (B) Nitric oxide (NO) production by macrophages infected with BCG or rBCG-CMX was determined. Uninfected media (Control) and LPS-stimulated (LPS) macrophages were included as controls. (C) Microscopic evaluation of peritoneal macrophages, 3 hours after infection with BCG or rBCG-CMX stained with Instant Prov or Ziehl Neelsen. Uninfected macrophages (Control) were included as a negative control. The results shown are representative of three different experiments.

Statistical analysis

The data were analyzed using Microsoft Office Excel 2011 and Prism (version 5.0c, GraphPad) software. The results represent the mean and standard deviation for each experimental group. The results from rBCG-CMX and BCG groups were compared using One-Way Anova followed by Dunnett's post-hoc test. Values of p<0.05 were considered statistically significant. All experiments repetition showed similar responses.

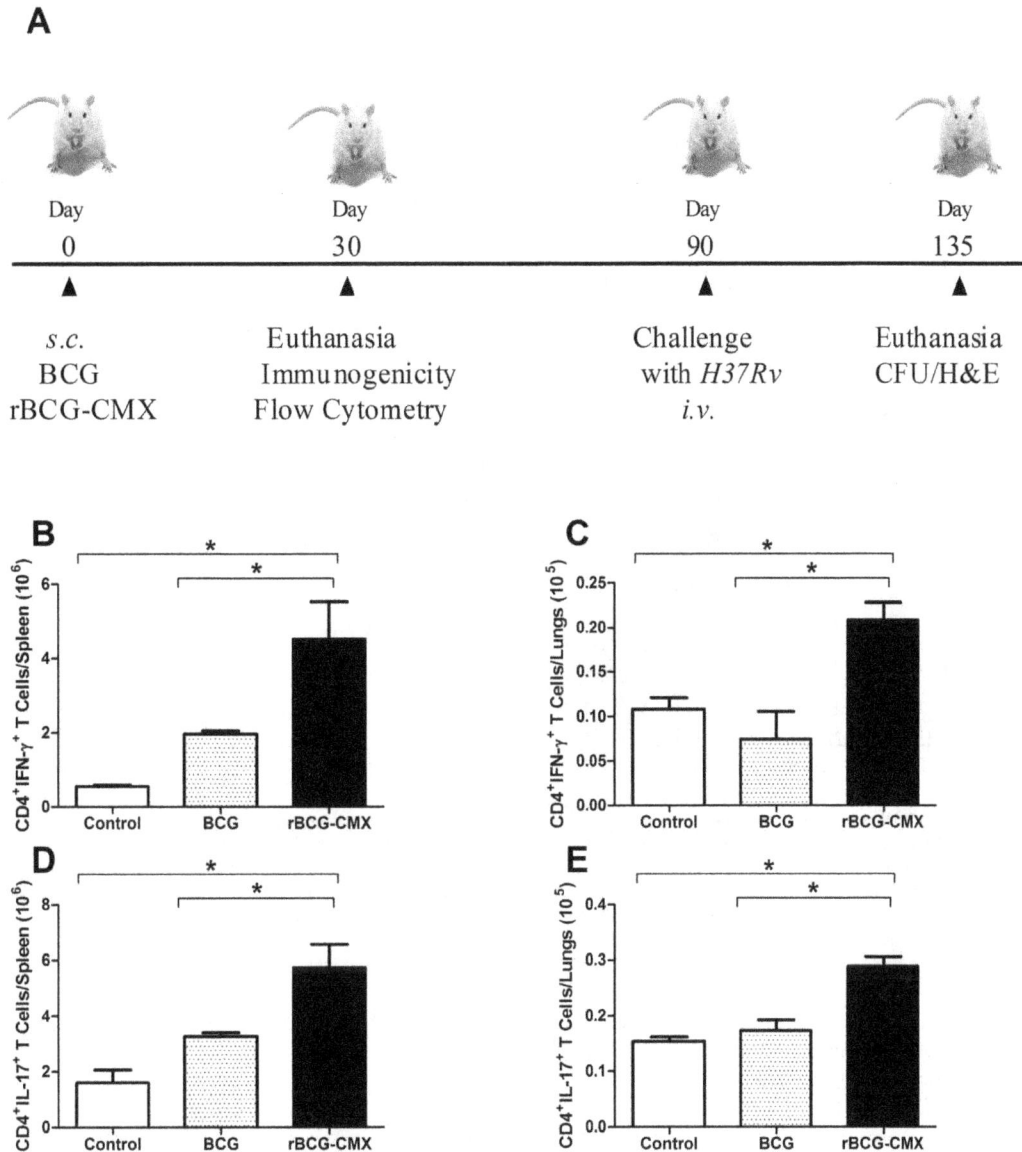

Figure 4. Immunogenicity of rBCG-CMX in BALB/c mice. (A) Experimental time line. BALB/c mice were immunized with rBCG-CMX or BCG Moreau. Thirty days later, 6 mice per group were euthanized for evaluation of vaccine-induced immunogenicity. Ninety days after immunization, mice were intravenously (*i.v.*) challenged with 10^5 CFU of H37Rv. Forty-five days after *i.v.* challenge, the lung bacterial load (CFU) and lesions (H&E) were assessed. (B–E) Specific cellular immune responses induced with rCMX stimulation *ex vivo*. Spleen (B and D) and lung (C and E) cell suspensions from vaccinated and unvaccinated (Control) mice were stimulated with rCMX. Cells positive for both CD4 and IFN-γ (B and C) or CD4 and IL-17 (D and E) were determined by flow cytometry. Lymphocytes were selected based on size and granularity. Flow cytometry gates were set to analyze CD4$^+$ T cells, and then the fluorescence of antibodies detecting IFN-γ$^+$ or IL-17$^+$ cells was recorded. These data are representative of two independent experiments (N = 6, *p<0.05).

Results

1. Recombinant vaccine construction, rCMX expression analysis and *in vivo* plasmid stability

The expression of heterologous proteins in mycobacteria can be influenced by several factors such as administration dose, cellular localization, and expression stability, among others [34–35]. To obtain the best possible expression, we tested three different plasmid constructions to express CMX: pLA71/CMX, pLA73/CMX, and pMIP12/CMX. As shown in Figure 1A, all three constructions contained the CMX fused gene and were successfully transformed into BCG Moreau. Western blot analysis of

recombinant BCG cultures revealed that only the plasmid pLA71/CMX was capable of inducing the expression of CMX protein (Fig. 1B, Figure S1). Thus we performed the following analysis only with the recombinant vaccine rBCG-pLA71/CMX, henceforward referred to as rBCG-CMX.

In order to verify the stability of the plasmid within the recombinant vaccine rBCG-CMX *in vivo* without antibiotic selective pressure, mice were vaccinated subcutaneously and the tissue of the site of infection was macerated at different time points and plated on media with or without the selective antibiotic kanamycin. As shown in Figure 2, the number of CFU recovered from media with or without antibiotic was similar, indicating that

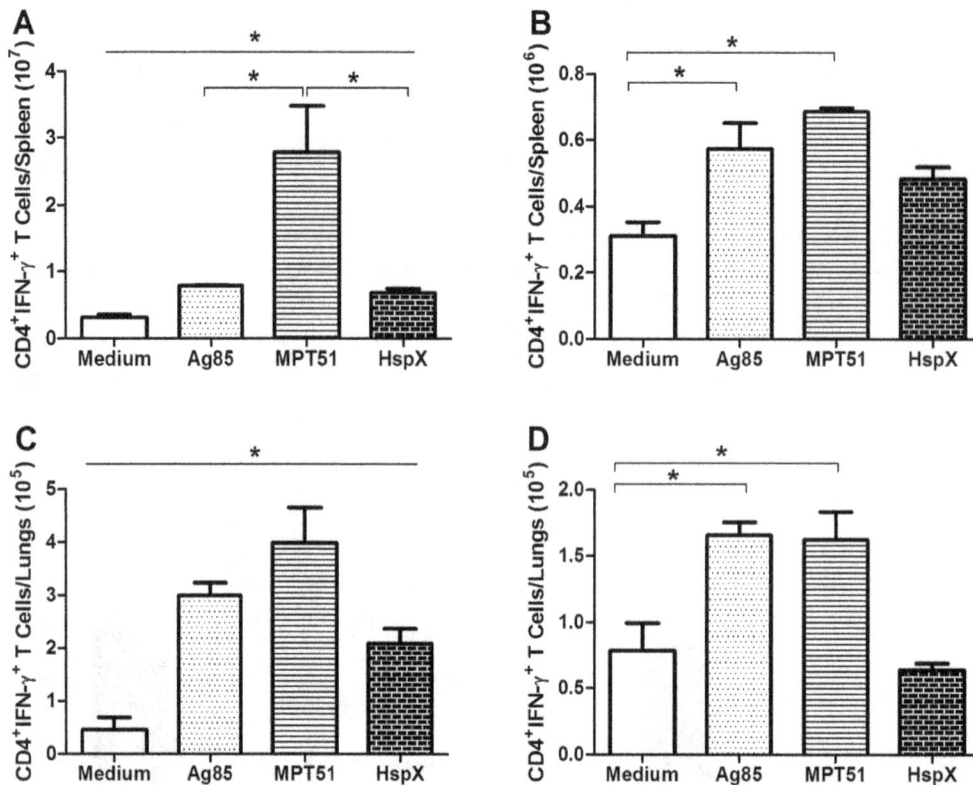

Figure 5. Levels of CD4⁺IFN-γ⁺ T cells induced by *ex vivo* stimulation with recombinant Ag85, MPT51, and HspX. Thirty days after vaccination, lung and spleen suspensions were stimulated *ex vivo* with Ag85, MPT51, HspX, or medium alone. The number of cells positive for CD4 and IFN-γ was determined by flow cytometry. Lymphocytes were selected based on size and granularity. Gates were set to analyze CD4⁺ T cells, and then the fluorescence of antibodies detecting IFN-γ⁺ cells was recorded. (A–B) Spleen cells from mice vaccinated with (A) rBCG-CMX or (B) BCG. (C–D) Lung cells from mice vaccinated with (C) rBCG-CMX or (D) BCG. In A and C, all results were different from the medium stimulation. These data are representative of two independent experiments (N = 6, *p<0.05).

the recombinant vaccine recovered from mice retained the plasmids up to 15 days after immunization (Figs. 2A and B). The presence of plasmid was further confirmed by performing PCR specific to the CMX gene (Fig. 2C).

2. rBCG-CMX is phagocytosed by peritoneal macrophages at higher levels than BCG Moreau but induces similar levels of NO

Vaccine phagocytosis and processing to present antigens has been shown to be an important factor responsible for the capacity to induce a protective immune response [36]. Thus the tendency of peritoneal macrophages to phagocytose rBCG-CMX was analyzed (Fig. 3). After 18 hours of infection, the recovered CFU from rBCG-CMX infected macrophages was higher than that from BCG Moreau infected macrophages (Fig. 3A, p<0.01). Acid fast staining of infected macrophage cultures confirmed that peritoneal macrophages had higher numbers of rBCG-CMX than of BCG (Fig. 3C). The analysis of CFU from culture supernatants confirmed that the groups were equally infected by the different vaccines (Fig. 3A).

Phagocytosis induces respiratory burst activation with its consequent production of NO. As another way to evaluate phagocytosis rates, the production of nitric oxide (NO) was evaluated in the culture supernatant of infected peritoneal macrophages. No difference in NO production was observed between the two vaccines evaluated (Fig. 3B). Despite the increased number of bacilli inside the peritoneal macrophages

infected with rBCG-CMX, similar levels of NO were induced by both vaccines.

3. rBCG-CMX vaccine induces a specific cellular immune response

Since rBCG-CMX was stable *in vivo* and phagocytosis of it induced macrophage activation (as measured by NO production), we questioned whether this vaccine would be able to induce a specific response to CMX and/or to the recombinant antigens alone (Fig. 4A). Immunization with rBCG-CMX vaccine induced higher numbers of CD4⁺ T lymphocytes positive for IFN-γ specific for CMX in cells from the spleen and lungs of BALB/c immunized mice 30 days after vaccination than did immunization with BCG Moreau (Figs. 4B and C, p<0.05; Th1 representative dot plots in Figure S2A). Similarly, rBCG-CMX induced higher levels of specific Th17 cells, an important group of cells for protection from Mtb and development of memory, in the cells from the spleen and lungs of immunized mice (Figs. 4D and E, p<0.05; Th17 representative dot plots in Fig. S2B).

We next questioned which protein(s) of the recombinant CMX fusion protein could contribute to the induction of IFN-γ (Fig. 5) and/or IL-17 (Fig. 6) by CD4⁺ T lymphocytes. As depicted in Figure 5, *ex vivo* stimulation of spleen and lung cells from rBCG-CMX vaccinated mice with Ag85, MPT51, or HspX all specifically induced CD4⁺IFN-γ⁺ cells (Figs. 5A and C, p<0.05). A significantly higher number of spleen cells were observed responding to MPT51 than to Ag85 or HspX. In mice vaccinated

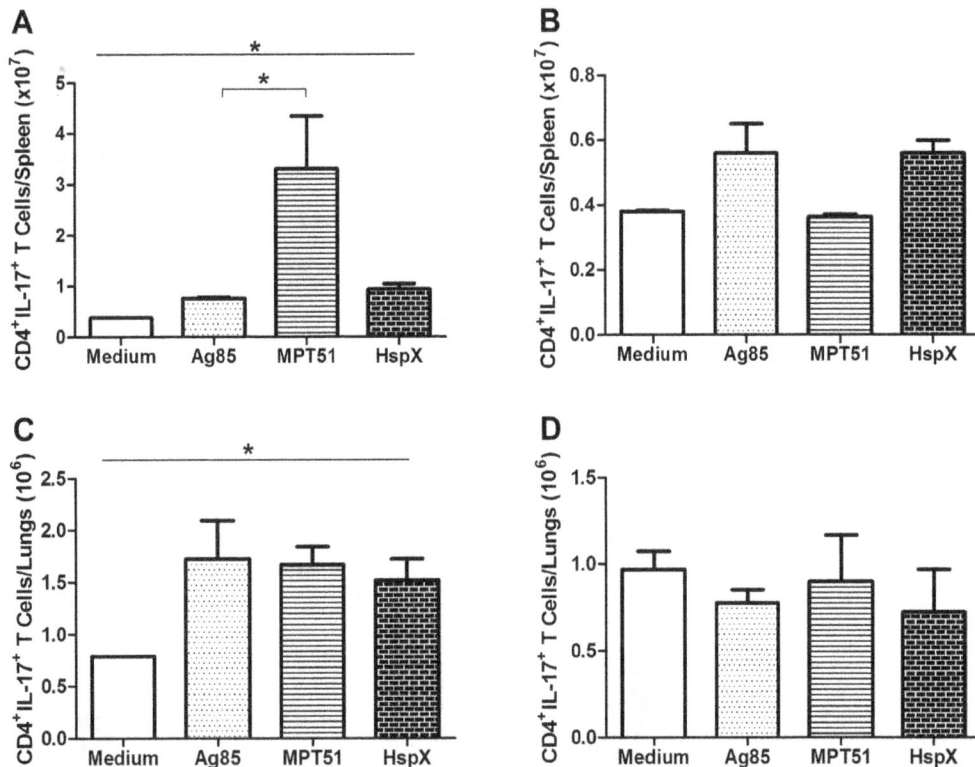

Figure 6. Levels of CD4$^+$IL-17$^+$ T cells induced by *ex vivo* stimulation with recombinant Ag85, MPT51, and HspX. Thirty days after vaccination, lung and spleen suspensions were stimulated *ex vivo* with Ag85, MPT51, HspX, or medium alone. The number of cells positive for CD4 and IL-17 was determined by flow cytometry. Lymphocytes were selected based on size and granularity. Gates were set to analyze CD4$^+$ T cells, and then the fluorescence of antibodies detecting IL-17$^+$ cells was recorded. (A–B) Spleen cells from mice vaccinated with (A) rBCG-CMX or (B) BCG. (C–D) Lung cells from mice vaccinated with (C) rBCG-CMX or (D) BCG. In A and C, all results were different from the medium stimulation. These data are representative of two independent experiments (N = 6, *p<0.05).

with BCG, cells that were CD4$^+$IFN-γ^+ were only induced in response to Ag85 and MPT51 stimulation, but not in response to HspX. Additionally, these CD4$^+$IFN-γ^+ cells were induced to a lesser extent than in the spleen or lung cells from mice vaccinated with rBCG-CMX (Figs. 5B and D, p<0.05).

Upon antigen stimulation in cells from rBCG-CMX-immunized mice, high numbers of Th17 lymphocytes were induced. In spleen cells, the highest response was to MPT51 (Fig. 6A), while in the lungs, all antigens stimulated the production of IL-17 to a similar degree (Fig. 6C). The number of CD4$^+$IL-17$^+$ spleen cells responding to MPT51 was significantly higher than the amount of cells responding to Ag85 antigen (Fig. 6A, p<0.05). Th17 expression was not induced in spleen or lung cells from mice vaccinated with BCG when stimulated with any of the recombinant proteins (Ag85, MPT51 and HspX) (Figs. 6B and D).

Although the above experiments determined that the rBCG-CMX vaccine generates Th1 (IFN-γ) and Th17 specific responses, it remained important to verify the induction of polyfunctional CD4$^+$ T cells, since several publications have associated these cells with protection against Mtb [33,37]. *Ex vivo* stimulation of spleen and lung cells with CMX increased the numbers of CD4$^+$ T cells positive for both IL-2 and IFN-γ (Figs. 7A and C) as well as for both TNF-α and IFN-γ (Figs. 7B and D) in cells from rBCG-CMX vaccinated mice as compared to the levels in cells from BCG Moreau vaccinated mice.

4. rBCG-CMX reduces the lung bacterial load

Although we found that immunization with rBCG-CMX was capable of inducing a specific immune response to CMX in BALB/c mice, this response alone is not sufficient to predict the protection properties of a vaccine. Thus, immunized mice were challenged with Mtb and the protective capacity was evaluated by assessing the bacterial load 45 days later. As observed in Figure 8, mice immunized with rBCG-CMX had a significantly lower bacterial load in the lungs than the unimmunized mice. To test if the protection could be improved in a prime-boost strategy, rBCG-CMX immunized mice were boosted 30 days later with rCMX/CPG DNA vaccine formulation and challenged with Mtb. Surprisingly, a boost with rCMX subunit vaccine showed the lowest lung bacterial load at 45 days post Mtb infection (Fig. 8).

5. The immune response induced by the rBCG-CMX vaccine reduces TB pulmonary lesions

Lung architecture preservation is yet another important aspect of a successful vaccine against TB. Histological analysis of the lungs of vaccinated mice challenged with Mtb showed that 45 days after challenge, unimmunized mice had intensive lymphocytic and neutrophilic infiltrates, significantly compromising the lung tissue architecture, together with the presence of a few hemorrhagic foci and foamy macrophages (Fig. 9A). BCG-vaccinated mice, instead, showed significantly fewer lung lesions, with a preservation of alveolar spaces and very limited lymphocytic infiltrate foci (Fig. 9B). The recombinant vaccine greatly preserved the lung

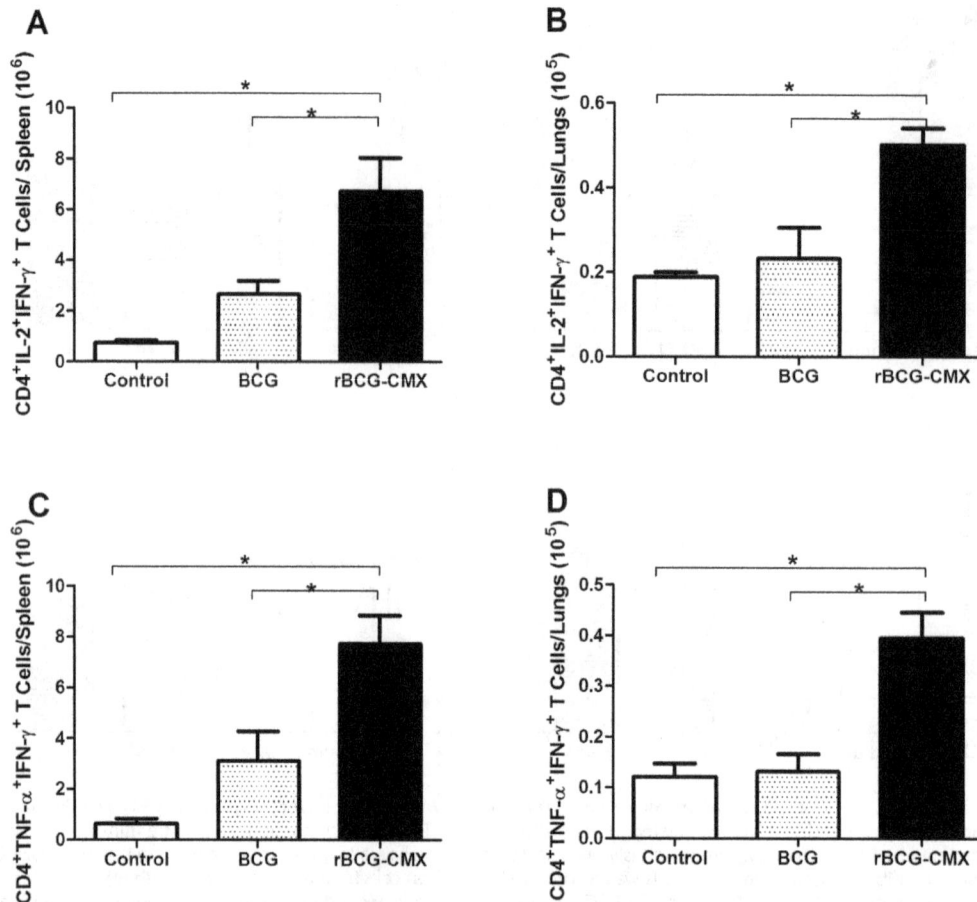

Figure 7. Levels of polyfunctional CD4⁺ T cells induced by BCG and rBCG-CMX vaccines. Spleen (A and C) and lung (B and D) cell suspensions from vaccinated and control mice stimulated with rCMX. (A–B) CD4⁺IL-2⁺IFN-γ⁺ cells or (C–D) CD4⁺TNF-α⁺IFN-γ⁺ cells were analyzed by flow cytometry. Lymphocytes were selected based on size and granularity. Gates were set to analyze CD4⁺ T cells, and then the fluorescence of antibodies detecting IL-2⁺ and IFN-γ⁺ or TNF-α⁺ and IFN-γ⁺ cells was recorded. These data are representative of two independent experiments (N = 6, *p<0.05).

architecture, showing very few inflammatory infiltrates (Fig. 9C). Similar results were obtained for animals immunized with rBCG-CMX and boosted with rCMX (Data not shown). The differences in inflammatory responses upon Mtb challenge between all three groups are summarized in the scores of their lung lesions, which are presented in Figure 9D.

Discussion

In this study, a recombinant vaccine expressing the fusion protein CMX (rBCG-CMX) was used to immunize BALB/c mice and was shown to be efficient in protecting mice against Mtb challenge. The recombinant vaccine induced higher levels of CD4⁺IFN-γ⁺ and CD4⁺IL-17⁺ T cells, as well as higher levels of CD4⁺TNF-α⁺IFN-γ⁺ and CD4⁺IL-2⁺IFN-γ⁺ polyfunctional T lymphocytes specific for CMX in BALB/c mice.

During the attenuation process of BCG, some antigens important for the induction of a protective immune response were lost [38]. This is thought to be one reason that BCG does not provide long lasting protection in humans. In the pursuit of a new TB vaccine, several groups have tried to insert heterologous genes into BCG and in doing so many different expression systems have been tested [35]. Our approach was to test three different plasmid constructions to express the fusion protein CMX. Of the systems

we tested, only the one that expressed the recombinant fusion protein together with the signal peptide β-lactamase (pLA71) was successful and stable in vivo. Other antigens have been expressed with the same three plasmids used in this study, but with different results. For example, the Schistosoma mansoni antigen Sm14 [34] and the pertussis toxin subunit S1 [39] were only successfully expressed in plasmid pLA73, which expresses the recombinant gene with the entire β-lactamase protein.

Macrophages infected with wild type BCG or rBCG produced similar amounts of NO. In the murine model, the production of NO has been shown to be critical for the control of mycobacterial growth [40]. Although NO production helps to control the progression of infection, its effects are concentration dependent. In low doses, NO acts as a signaling molecule to promote vascular integrity, mediate neurotransmission, and help regulate cellular respiration. In high concentrations, NO inhibits respiration and can cause protein and DNA damage [41–42]. In M. bovis BCG, NO seems to limit inflammatory responses, in part by down-regulating the accumulation of activated T cells [43]. We found that a significant amount of rBCG-CMX was phagocytosed, and that it can reside and survive within the macrophages (Fig. 3). Our data show that rBCG-CMX was phagocytosed in higher amounts than BCG Moreau (Figs. 3A and B). However, the induction of NO by the recombinant vaccine was similar to that induced by

A

B

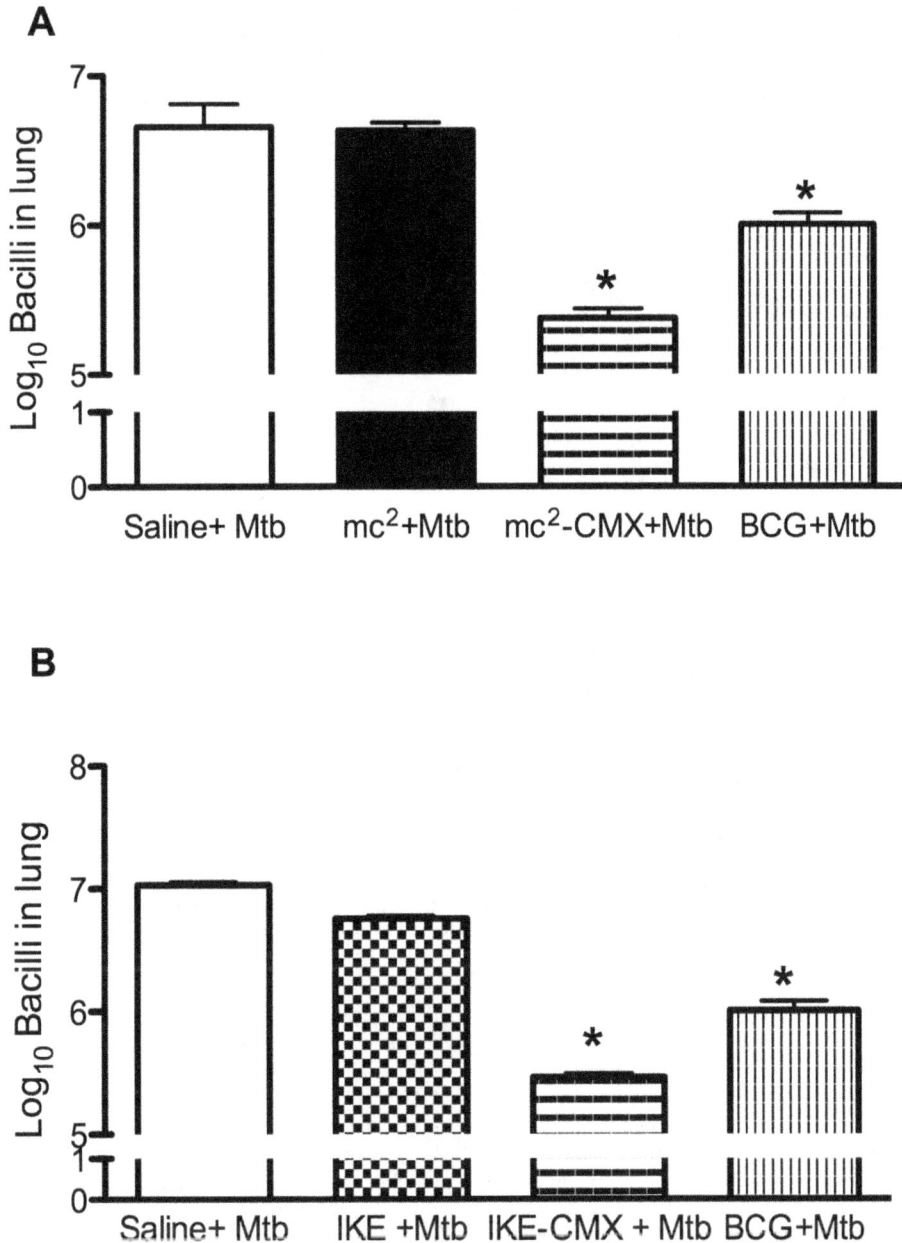

Figure 8. Bacterial load in the lungs of BALB/c mice 45 days after *Mycobacterium tuberculosis* challenge. Ninety days after immunization, three mice from each group (control, BCG and rBCG-CMX) were challenged with 10^5 CFU of *Mycobacterium tuberculosis* H37Rv intravenously into the orbital sinus plexus. One additional group of animals received a booster of rCMX/CPG DNA, 30 days after rBCG-CMX vaccination and challenged with Mtb 30 days post the immunization (rBCG-CMX+CMX). Forty-five days after challenge, mice were euthanized and the anterior and mediastinal right lung lobes were collected, homogenized, and plated on Middlebrook 7H11agar supplemented with OADC to determine the bacterial load by counting the number of CFU. * Significant differences between infected (control) and vaccinated groups. # Significant differences between rBCG-CMX and rBCG-CMX+CMX groups. | Significant differences between rBCG-CMX and BCG groups analyzed by *t* test (p<0.05).

BCG Moreau. These data suggest that our recombinant vaccine is viable, since it has not lost its ability to induce an immune response.

After finding that rBCG-CMX was efficiently phagocytosed, we anticipated that antigen processing and presentation to naive T lymphocytes *in vivo* would be favored, and data from our next experiment support this idea. In cells from the lungs and spleen of rBCG-CMX vaccinated mice, stimulation with CMX induced high levels of T cells that were $CD4^+IFN$-γ^+ (Figs. 4B and C). The importance of IFN-γ in protection against TB is well established,

as it induces an increase in phagocytosis and Mtb destruction, consequently reducing the bacterial load [44]. In spite of this, there is controversy about the role of IFN-γ in vaccine models. In high concentrations, IFN-γ induces apoptosis of $CD4^+$ effector T lymphocytes, lowering the potential to generate memory cells [11].

Th17 cells are thought to be responsible for TB protection, as they have an early memory cell signature [45]. Our recombinant vaccine was shown to induce CMX-specific $CD4^+IL$-17^+ T cells in the spleen and lungs (Figs. 4D and E). The expression of CMX by *Mycobacterium smegmatis* (mc^2-CMX) was also shown to induce

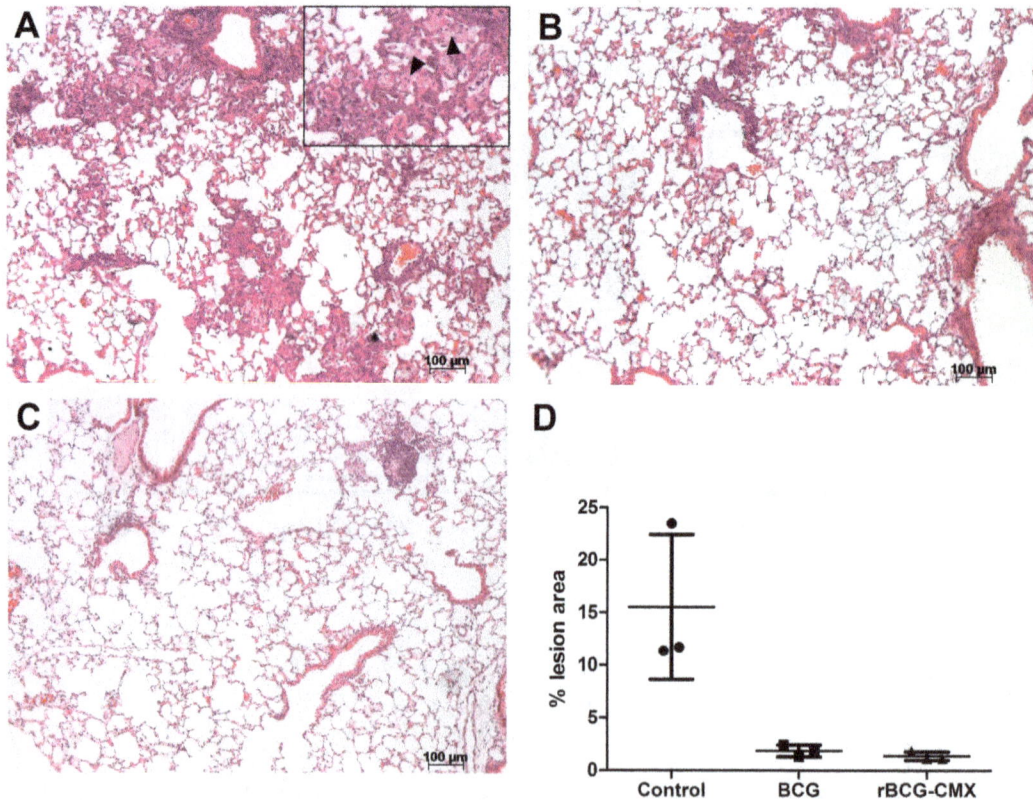

Figure 9. Representative lung pathology of Balb/c mice after challenge. Vaccinated mice were challenged *i.v.* with 10^5 CFU of virulent *M. tuberculosis* H37Rv strain. Forty-five days after infection, lung tissue sections from different vaccine groups were harvested. Images are representative of two distinct experiments. HE staining is shown with 20X magnification. (A) Unvaccinated group. Black arrowheads: Foamy macrophages. (B) BCG-vaccinated group. (C) rBCG-CMX vaccinated group. (D) Histological score of the lesion area from three representative fields obtained by AxioVision 4.9.1 software, through ratio of lesioned and total field area. Data are presented as percentages (%).

high levels of CD4$^+$IL-17$^+$ T lymphocytes in the spleen and lungs [33] that directly correlated to protection. The importance of Th17 in vaccine models and in TB is controversial, but it is known that in chronic infections, such as TB, constitutive or late IL-17 production is related to the degree of interstitial inflammatory involvement and tissue lesion [46]. Instead, when produced early as is the case for vaccination, IL-17 is important for the induction of protective memory cells for TB [47,45].

Our vaccine, rBCG-CMX, induced Th1 and Th17 immune responses that were specific to CMX. Furthermore, we demonstrated that this recombinant vaccine induced Th1 and Th17 immune responses to each of the CMX component proteins, rAg85, rMPT51, and rHspX, alone (Figs. 5A and C; Figs. 6A and C). The induction of immune responses to these proteins suggests that the construction of the CMX protein retained the immunodominant characteristics of its components. It is important to note that the use of recombinant BCG vaccines described in the literature, most of the times did not test the specific immune response to the heterologous antigens [48–49]. Most studies only evaluated the specific response to PPD (Purified Protein derivative) as a stimulus, and here we showed that an immune response was generated to the heterologous protein [49].

It has already been shown that rBCG expressing HspX or Ag85 complex proteins (Ag85A, Ag85B, Ag85C) induce superior protection to wild type BCG [50–52]. Interestingly, we found a pronounced response to stimulation with MPT51. This protein belongs to new family of non-catalytic alfa/beta hydrolases (*Fbpc*1) which act in binding the fibronectin extracellular matrix [53]. As

demonstrated by another study, MPT51 effectively induces Th1 immune responses, promoting protection in mice challenged with Mtb [54]. The characteristics of these proteins were retained in CMX, which contributed to the ability of rBCG-CMX to promote important immune responses and protection.

In spleen and lung cells from mice immunized with the BCG vaccine, stimulation with rAg85 and rMPT51 induced a Th1 response, but not stimulation with HspX or CMX (Figs. 5A and B). This may be related to the poor ability of BCG to induce specific responses to certain proteins, such as HspX which is expressed in low levels by BCG [55,50,56]. Interestingly, despite containing the same original proteins as those composing the CMX protein, immunization with BCG Moreau did not induce a specific response against CMX. Additionally, BCG was not able to induce a Th17 immune response to any of the component recombinant proteins (Figs. 6A and B). Although it has previously been shown that Th17 responses generated by BCG vaccination induce TB infection control in non-human primates [47], we did not observe similar results with our recombinant proteins.

We found an increased number of CD4$^+$ polyfunctional T cells among mice immunized with rBCG-CMX relative to the number in those who received the BCG Moreau vaccine. The recombinant vaccine induced high levels of polyfunctional T cells expressing both IL-2 and IFN-γ (Figs. 7A and B) and high levels of these cells expressing both TNF-α and IFN-γ (Figs. 7C and D). It has been demonstrated that polyfunctional cells are important for protection against intracellular bacteria, as well as viral, parasitic, and chronic bacterial infections, such as TB [57,37]. Additionally, it has been shown that polyfunctional cells are involved in providing protection against TB [37]. Consequently, we believe that the cellular profile induced by rBCG-CMX is likely the result of our addition of CMX to BCG [32].

The ability of rBCG-CMX to induce protection against Mtb challenge showed a tendency to improve the protection conferred by BCG Moreau. Vaccination with rBCG-CMX significantly reduced the lung bacterial load of BALB/c mice (Fig. 8). Because the only difference between the vaccines were the presence of CMX, we decided to address if using a booster with rCMX would increase the immune response to CMX, and consequently the protection to Mtb. The improved protection observed (rBCG-CMX + rCMX) must be due to the extra presence of the recombinant fusion protein CMX, as only the recombinant vaccine induced a significant increase in the proliferation and migration of specific CD4+ T cells in the spleen and lungs (Figs. 4 and 5) of immunized mice. Like in here, not all recombinant BCG vaccines expressing fusion proteins that have been tested were able to induce superior protection when compared with BCG [58]. Thus we believe that the recombinant CMX protein, composed of Mtb immunodominant antigens (Ag85C, MPT-51, and HspX) that relate to different infection phases, added significant immunogenic properties to BCG which were crucial to the observed protection. This is the first study using limited number of animals (3–6) to demonstrate the efficacy of the fusion protein CMX. We are now setting up collaborations to test the CMX in a more appropriate guinea pig model. Other studies from our group have characterized those properties by investigating rCMX in the context of *M. smegmatis* mc^2 155 (mc^2-CMX). Additionally, we observed this phenomenon with the IKE vaccine (IKE-CMX), which also induced a significant reduction in bacterial load in comparison to vaccination with IKE lacking the recombinant antigen [33]. Taken together, the data demonstrate that CMX can play an important role in the enhancement of protective immune responses induced by vaccines against Mtb [32–33].

Achieving the correct balance between the induction of Th1 and Th17 cells is an important goal for an effective vaccine against Mtb. While the induced IFN-γ will act on the activation of infected cells, IL-17 will regulate the resulting inflammatory response by inducing protective cells [49]. As shown in Figure 9, the lungs of mice vaccinated with rBCG-CMX had a larger preserved area of the lungs compared to the lungs of BCG Moreau immunized mice. In addition the group receiving the recombinant vaccine showed little inflammatory infiltration and very few necrotic foci and coalescent alveoli, all of which are known for being favorable areas for bacilli replication [59–60]. The reduced bacterial load of the lungs found in rBCG-CMX challenged mice corroborates those observations (Fig. 8). In addition, no foamy macrophages were found in the lungs of mice vaccinated with the recombinant

vaccine (Fig. 9), which is important as those cells are known to be bacilli reservoirs [61–62].

In conclusion, the addition of the recombinant fusion protein CMX to BCG Moreau generated a recombinant vaccine with superior immunological properties. This vaccine induced a balanced IFN-γ and IL17 cytokine response from CD4+ T cells and was able to protect mice from Mtb.

Supporting Information

Figure S1 CMX expression analysis from rBCG transformed with recombinant plasmids pLA73/CMX and pMIP12/CMX. Western blot analysis of whole cell lysates from rBCG transformants using polyclonal antibodies raised against rCMX. (A) rBCG containing pLA73/CMX or empty vector. M: molecular mass marker; CMX: purified recombinant CMX; pLA73/CMX: rBCG with plasmid pLA73/CMX; pLA73: rBCG with plasmid pLA73. (B) rBCG containing pMIP12/CMX or empty vector. M: molecular mass marker; CMX: purified recombinant CMX; pMIP12/CMX: rBCG with plasmid pMIP12/CMX; pMIP12: rBCG with plasmid pMIP12.

Figure S2 Representative dot plots of TCD4+IFN-γ+ and TCD4+IL-17+ cells. Splenic cells from non-immunized mice (Control) or mice immunized with BCG or with rBCG-CMX were stimulated with medium or one of the following recombinant proteins: rAg85, rMPT51, rHspX or rCMX. Lymphocytes were selected based on their size and granulocity and antigen specific TCD4+IFN-γ+ (A) and TCD4+IL-17+ (B) cells were analyzed based on their fluorescence.

Acknowledgments

We are thankful to Associação de Combate ao Câncer de Goiás and Universidade de Brasília (UnB) for allowing access to their flow cytometry core facilities, to Dr. Aline Carvalho Batista, from Faculdade de Odontologia – UFG, for collaborating in the processing and analysis of histological preparations, and to Drs. Alexander Augusto da Silveira and Lorena Cristina Santos for technical assistance in constructing the recombinant vaccines.

Author Contributions

Conceived and designed the experiments: APJK AK. Performed the experiments. APJK AK ACC AOCJ FMO SVN JDR DPR. Analyzed the data: APJK AK ACC AOCJ FMO SVN JDR DPR. Contributed reagents/materials/analysis tools: APJK AK. Contributed to the writing of the manuscript: APJK AK ACC AOCJ FMO SVN JDR DPR. Cytometry experiments and analysis: ACC.

References

1. World Health Organization (WHO) (2013) Global tuberculosis control-epidemiology, strategy, financing.
2. Kamath AT, Fruth U, Brennan MJ, Dobbelaer R, Hubrechts P, et al. (2005) New live mycobacterial vaccines: the Geneva consensus on essential steps towards clinical development. Vaccine 23: 3753–3761.
3. Calmette A (1929) Sur la vaccination preventive des enfants nouveau-nes contre tuberculose par le BCG. Ann Inst Pasteur 41: 201–232.
4. World Health Organization (WHO) (1998) Global tuberculosis control.
5. Partnership WST (2010) The Global Plan to Stop TB 2011–2015: Transforming the Fight- Towards Elimination of Tuberculosis.
6. Lienhardt C, Zumla A (2005) BCG: the story continues. Lancet 366: 1414–1416.
7. Behr MA, Small PM (1997) Has BCG attenuated to impotence? Nature 389: 133–134.
8. Zhang W, Zhang Y, Zheng H, Pan Y, Liu H, et al. (2013) Genome sequencing and analysis of BCG vaccine strains. PLoS One 8: e71243.
9. Soares AP, Scriba TJ, Joseph S, Harbacheuski R, Murray RA, et al. (2008) Bacille Calmette–Guérin vaccination of human newborns induces T cells with complex cytokine and phenotype profiles. J Immunol 180: 3569–77.
10. Stenger S, Hansen DA, Teitelbaum R, Dewan P, Niazi KR, et al. (1998) An antimicrobial activity of cytolytic T cells mediated by granulysin. Science 282: 121–5.
11. Abebe F (2012) Is interferon-gamma the right marker for bacilli Calmette-Guérin-induced immune protection? The missing link in our understanding of tuberculosis immunology. Clin Exp Immunol 169: 213–219.
12. Mittrucker HW, Stenhoof U, Kohler A, Krause M, Lazar D, et al. (2007) Poor correlation between BCG vaccination-induced T cell response and protection against tuberculosis. Proc Natl Acad A Sci USA 104: 12434–124.
13. Junqueira-Kipnis AP, Marques Neto LM, Kipnis A (2014) Role of Fused *Mycobacterium tuberculosis* Immunogens and Adjuvants in Modern Tuberculosis Vaccines. Front Immunol 5: 188.

14. Kaufmann SH, Lange C, Rao M, Balaji KN, Lotze M, et al. (2014) Progress in tuberculosis vaccine development and host- directed therapies – a state of the art review. Lancet Respir Med 4: 301–321.

15. Hoft DF, Blazevic A, Abate G, Hanekom WA, Kaplan G, et al. (2008) A new recombinant bacille Calmette-Guérin vaccine safely induces significantly enhanced tuberculosis-specific immunity in human volunteers. J Infect Dis 198: 1491–1501.

16. Deng YH, He HY, Zhang BS (2012) Evaluation of protective efficacy conferred by a recombinant Mycobacterium bovis BCG expressing a fusion protein of Ag85A-ESAT-6. J Microbiol Immunol Infect 25: S1684–1182.

17. Tang C, Yamada H, Shibata K, Maeda N, Yoshida S, et al. (2008) Efficacy of Recombinant Bacille Calmette-Guérin Vaccine Secreting Interleukin-15/ Antigen 85B Fusion Protein in Providing Protection against Mycobacterium tuberculosis. J Infect Dis 197: 1263–1274.

18. Farinacci M, Weber S, Kaufmann SH (2012) The recombinant tuberculosis vaccine rBCGΔureC::hly+ induces apoptotic vesicles for improved priming of CD4+ and CD8+ T cells. Vaccine 30: 7608–7614.

19. da_Costa AC, Nogueira SV, Kipnis A, Junqueira-Kipnis AP (2014) Recombinant BCG: innovations on an old vaccine. Scope of BCG strains and strategies to improve long-lasting memory. Front Immunol 5: 152.

20. Lin CW, Su IJ, Chang JR, Chen YY, Lu JJ, et al. (2011). Recombinant BCG coexpressing Ag85B, CFP10, and interleukin-12 induces multifunctional Th1 and memory T cells in mice. APMIS 120: 72–82.

21. Gomes LH, Otto TD, Vasconcellos EA, Ferrão PM, Maia RM, et al. (2011) Genome sequence of Mycobacterium bovis BCG Moreau, the Brazilian vaccine strain against tuberculosis. J Bacteriol 193: 5600–1.

22. Berrêdo-Pinho M, Kalume DE, Correa PR, Gomes LH, Pereira MP, et al. (2011) Proteomic profile of culture filtrate from the Brazilian vaccine strain Mycobacterium bovis BCG Moreau compared to M. bovis BCG Pasteur. BMC Microbiol 11: 80.

23. Nascimento IP, Dias WO, Quintilio W, Hsu T, Jacobs WR Jr, et al. (2009) Construction of an unmarked recombinant BCG expressing a pertussis antigen by auxotrophic complementation: protection against Bordetella pertussis challenge in neonates. Vaccine 27: 7346–51.

24. Andrade PM, Chade DC, Borra RC, Nascimento IP, Villanova Fe, et al. (2010) The therapeutic potential of recombinant BCG expressing the antigen S1PT in the intravesical treatment of bladder cancer. Urol Oncol 28: 520–525.

25. Vasconcellos HL, Scaramuzzi K, Nascimento IP, Da Costa Ferreira JM Jr, Abe CM, et al. (2012) Generation of recombinant bacillus Calmette-Guérin and Mycobacterium smegmatis expressing BfpA and intimin as vaccine vectors against enteropathogenic Escherichia coli. Vaccine 30: 5999–6005.

26. Clark SO, Kelly DL, Badell E, Castello-Branco LR, Aldwell F, et al. (2010) Oral delivery of BCG Moreau Rio de Janeiro gives equivalent protection against tuberculosis but with reduced pathology compared to parenteral BCG Danish vaccination. Vaccine 28(43): 7109–16.

27. Yuk JM, Jo EK (2014) Host immune responses to mycobacterial antigens and their implications for the development of a vaccine to control tuberculosis. Clin Exp Vaccine Res 3: 155–167.

28. Achkar JM, Jenny-Avital E, Yu X, Burger S, Leibert E, et al. (2010) Antibodies against immunodominant antigens of Mycobacterium tuberculosis in subjects with suspected tuberculosis in the United States compared by HIV status. Clin Vaccine Immunol 17: 384–392.

29. Rabahi MF, Junqueira-Kipnis AP, Dos Reis MC, Oelemann W, Conde MB (2007) Humoral response to HspX and GlcB to previous and recent infection by Mycobacterium tuberculosis. BMC Infect Dis 7: 148.

30. de Araujo-Filho JA, Vasconcelos AC Jr, Martins de Sousa E, Kipnis A, Ribeiro E, et al. (2008) Cellular responses to MPT-51, GlcB and ESAT-6 among MDR-TB and active tuberculosis patients in Brazil. Tuberculosis 88: 474–481. doi:10.1016/j.tube.2008.06.002.

31. Kashyap RS, Shekhawat SD, Nayak AR, Purohit HJ, Taori GM, et al. (2013) Diagnosis of tuberculosis infection based on synthetic peptides from Mycobacterium tuberculosis antigen 85 complex. Clin Neurol Neurosurg 115: 678–683.

32. de Sousa EM, da Costa AC, Trentini MM, de Araujo Filho JA, Kipnis A, et al. (2012) Immunogenicity of a fusion protein containing immunodominant epitopes of Ag85C, MPT51, and HspX from Mycobacterium tuberculosis in mice and active TB infection. PLoS One 7: e47781.

33. Junqueira-Kipnis AP, de Oliveira FM, Trentini MM, Tiwari S, Chen B, et al. (2013) Prime-Boost with Mycobacterium smegmatis Recombinant Vaccine Improves Protection in Mice Infected with Mycobacterium tuberculosis. PLoS One 8: e78639.

34. Varaldo PB, Leite CC, Dias WO, Miyaji EN, Torres FIG, et al. (2004) Recombinant Mycobacterium bovis BCG Expressing the Sm14 Antigen of Schistosoma mansoni Protects Mice from Cercarial Challenge. Infect Immun 72: 3336–3343.

35. Bastos RG, Borsuk S, Seixas FK, Dellagostin OA (2009) Recombinant Mycobacterium bovis BCG. Vaccine 27: 6495–6503.

36. Jagannath C, Lindsey DR, Dhandayuthapani S, Xu Y, Hunter RL Jr, et al. (2011) Autophagy enhances the efficacy of BCG vaccine by increasing peptide presentation in mouse dendritic cells. Nat Med 15: 267–276.

37. Forbes EK, Sander C, Ronan EO, McShane H, Hill AV, et al. (2008) Multifunctional, High-level cytokine-producing Th1 cells in the lung, but not spleen, correlate with protection against Mycobacterium tuberculosis aerosol challeng in mice.J Immunol 181: 4955–64.

38. Brosch R, Gordon SV, Pym A, Eiglmeier K, Garnier T, et al. (2000) Comparative genomics of the mycobacteria. Int J Med Microbiol. 290: 143–152.

39. Nascimento IP, Dias WO, Mazzantini RP, Miyaji EN, Gamberini M, et al. (2000) Recombinant Mycobacterium bovis BCG expressing pertussis toxin subunit S1 induces protection against an intracerebral challenge with live Bordetella pertussis in mice. Infect Immun 68: 4877–4883.

40. Chan J, Xing Y, Magliozzo RS, Bloom BR (1992) Killing of virulent Mycobacterium tuberculosis by reactive nitrogen intermediates produced by activates murine macrophages. J Exp Med 175: 1111–1122.

41. Xu W, Charles IG, Moncada S (2005) Nitric Oxide: orchestrating hypoxia regulation through mitochondrial respiration and the endoplasmic reticulum stress response. Cell Res 15: 63–65.

42. Pearl JE, Torrado E, Tighe M, Fountain JJ, Solache A, et al. (2012) Nitric oxide inhibits the accumulation of CD4+CD44hiTbet+CD69lo T cells in mycobacterial infection. Eur J Immunol 42: 3267–3279.

43. Cooper AM, Adams LB, Dalton DK, Appelberg R, Ehlers S (2002) IFN-γ and NO in mycobacterial disease: new jobs for hands. Trends Microbiol 10: 221–226.

44. North RJ, Jung YJ (2004) Immunity to tuberculosis. Annu Rev Immunol 22: 599–623.

45. Muranski P, Borman ZA, Kerkar SP, Klebanoff CA, Ji Y, et al. (2011) Th17 Cells Are Long Lived and Retain a Stem Cell-like Molecular Signature. Immunity 35: 972–985.

46. Cruz A, Fraga AG, Fountains JJ, Rangel-Moreno J, Torrado E, et al. (2010) Pathological role of interleukin 17 in mice subjected to repeated BCG vaccination after infection with Mycobacterium tuberculosis. J Exp Med 207: 1609–1616.

47. Wareham AS, Tree JA, Marsh PD, Butcher PD, Dennis M, et al. (2014) Evidence for a role for interleukin-17, Th17 cells and homeostasis in protective immunity against tuberculosis in cynomolgus macaques. PloS One 9: e88149.

48. Tullius MV, Harth G, Maslesa-Galic S, Dillon BJ, Horwitz MA (2008) A replication-limited recombinant Mycobacterium bovis BCG vaccine against tuberculosis designed for human immuno deficiency virus-positive persons is safer and more efficacious than BCG. Infect Immun 76: 5200–14.

49. Desel C, Dorhoi A, Bandermann S, Grode L, Eisele B, et al. (2011) Recombinant BCGΔureC::hly Induces Superior Protection over Parental BCG by Stimulating a Balanced Combination of Type 1 and Type 17 Cytokine Responses. J Infect Dis 204: 1573–1584.

50. Shi C, Chen L, Chen Z, Zhang Y, Zhou Z, et al. (2010) Enhanced protection against tuberculosis by vaccination with recombinant BCG over-expressing HspX protein. Vaccine 28: 5237–5244.

51. Wang C, Fu R, Chen Z, Tan K, Chen L, et al. (2012) Immunogenicity and protective efficacy of a novel recombinant BCG strain over expressing antigens Ag85A e Ag85B. Clin. Dev. Immunol. 2012: 1–9.

52. Jain R, Dey B, Dhar N, Rao V, Singh R, et al. (2008) Enhanced and enduring protection against tuberculosis by recombinant BCG-Ag85C and its association with modulation of cytokine profile in lung. PLoS One 3: e3869.

53. Wilson RA, Maughan WN, Kremer L, Besra GS, Fütterer K (2004) The structure of Mycobacterium tuberculosis MPT51 (FbpC1) defines a new family of non-catalytic alpha/beta hydrolases. J Mol Biol 9: 519–530.

54. Silva BD, da Silva EB, do Nascimento IP, Dos Reis MC, Kipnis A, et al. (2009) MPT-51/CpG DNA vaccine protects mice against Mycobacterium tuberculosis. Vaccine 27: 4402–4407.

55. Geluk A, Lin MY, van Meijgaarden KE, Leyten EM, Franken KL, et al. (2007) T-cell recognition of the HspX protein of Mycobacterium tuberculosis correlates with latent M. tuberculosis infection but not with M. bovis BCG vaccination. Infect Immun 75: 2914–2921.

56. Spratt JM, Britton WJ, Triccas JA (2010) In vivo persistence and protective efficacy of the bacille Calmette Guerin vaccine overexpressing the HspX latency antigen. Bioeng Bugs 1: 61–65.

57. Maroof A, Yorgensen YM, Li Y, Evans JT (2014) Intranasal vaccination promotes detrimental Th17-mediated immunity against influenza infection. PLoS Pathog 10: e1003875.

58. Deng YH, He HY, Zang BS (2014) Evaluation of protective efficacy conferred by a recombinant Mycobacterium bovis BCG expressing a fusion protein Of Ag85A-ESAT-6. J Microbiol Immunol Infect 47: 48–56.

59. Ulrichs T, Kosmiadi GA, Jorg S, Pradl L, Titukhina M, et al. (2005) Differential organization of the local immune response in patients with active cavitary tuberculosis or with nonprogressive tuberculoma. J Infect Dis192: 89–97.

60. Lenaerts AJ, Hoff D, Aly S, Ehlers S, Andries K, et al. (2007) Mycobacteria in a guinea pig model of tuberculosis revealed by r207910. Antimicrob Agents Chemother 51: 3338–3345.

61. Russell DG, Cardona PJ, Kim MJ, Allain S, Altare F (2009) Foamy macrophages and the progression of the human tuberculous granuloma. Nature Immunol 10: 943–948.

62. Huynh KK, Joshi SA, Brown EJ (2011) A delicate dance: host response to mycobacteria. Current Opinion in Immunology 23: 464–472.

14

Differential Control of Interleukin-6 mRNA Levels by Cellular Distribution of YB-1

Sujin Kang, Taeyun A. Lee, Eun A. Ra, Eunhye Lee, Hyun jin Choi, Sungwook Lee*, Boyoun Park*

Department of Systems biology, College of Life Science and Biotechnology, Yonsei University, Seoul, South Korea

Abstract

Cytokine production is essential for innate and adaptive immunity against microbial invaders and must be tightly controlled. Cytokine messenger RNA (mRNA) is in constant flux between the nucleus and the cytoplasm and in transcription, splicing, or decay; such processes must be tightly controlled. Here, we report a novel function of Y-box-binding protein 1 (YB-1) in modulating interleukin-6 (IL-6) mRNA levels in a cell type-specific manner. In lipopolysaccharide (LPS)-stimulated macrophages, YB-1 interacts with IL-6 mRNA and actively transports it to the extracellular space by YB-1-enriched vesicles, resulting in the proper maintenance of intracellular IL-6 mRNA levels. YB-1 secretion occurs in a cell type-specific manner. Whereas macrophages actively secret YB-1, dendritic cells maintain it predominantly in the cytoplasm even in response to LPS. Intracellular YB-1 has the distinct function of regulating IL-6 mRNA stability in dendritic cells. Moreover, because LPS differentially regulates the expression of histone deacetylase 6 (HDAC6) in macrophages and dendritic cells, this stimulus might control YB-1 acetylation differentially in both cell types. Taken together, these results suggest a unique feature of YB-1 in controlling intracellular IL-6 mRNA levels in a cell type-specific manner, thereby leading to functions that are dependent on the extracellular and intracellular distribution of YB-1.

Editor: Georg Stoecklin, German Cancer Research Center, Germany

Funding: This study was supported by grants from Basic Science Research Program through the National Research Foundation of Korea (NRF) funded by the Ministry of Education, Science and Technology (2011-0015372, 2010-0009203) and from the National R&D Program for Cancer Control, Ministry of Health & Welfare, Republic of Korea. SL was supported by the Yonsei University Research Fund of 2014 (2014-12-0135). SK, TAL, and EAR were supported by BK21 PLUS (Brain Korea 21 Program for Leading University & Students). HJC was supported by NRF (National Research Foundation of Korea) grant funded by the Korean Government (NRF-2013- Global Ph.D. Fellowship Program). The funders had no role in study design, data collection and analysis, decision to publish, or preparation of the manuscript.

Competing Interests: The authors have declared that no competing interests exist.

* Email: bypark@yonsei.ac.kr (BP); swlee1905@yonsei.ac.kr (SL)

Introduction

The immune response comprises a variety of processes in response to infection or tissue damage; immune cells and soluble mediators, such as cytokines of the innate and adaptive immune system, play important roles in the host defense mechanism. The inflammatory response is generally a protective reaction and maintains tissue homeostasis [1]. Although an uncontrolled response causes chronic inflammation, scarring, and fibrosis, inflammation in a normal context results in a complete resolution of the response and return to the local homeostatic state after pathogen elimination or tissue repair [2].

YB-1 is a member of a large family of cold shock domain-containing proteins and is involved in inflammatory processes [3,4]. YB-1 consists of the alanine/proline-rich N-terminal domain (A/P domain), the cold shock domain (CSD), and the large C-terminal domain (CTD) with alternating clusters of positively and negatively charged amino acids. The consensus sequences of the CSD mediate YB-1 interactions with DNA and RNA, and the CTD of YB-1 is associated with the majority of its protein partners [5]. The N-terminal A/P domain binds to actin microfilaments, which contribute to mRNA localization [3]. YB-1 has been identified as a pleiotropic protein that participates in DNA repair, pre-mRNA splicing, the regulation of transcription and transla-

tion, and mRNA packing and stability [6]. It can be secreted from the cell to perform extracellular functions, acting as an extracellular mitogen [7]. The multiple activities of YB-1 are exemplified by its involvement in cell proliferation and differentiation, the stress response, and inflammatory responses [4].

The importance of the balance between stabilization and degradation of cytokine mRNA is illustrated by the differences between inflammatory diseases and immune homeostasis [8,9]. Cytokine mRNA decay is tightly regulated at the post-transcriptional level through cis- or trans-acting elements [10], where cytokine transcripts are transiently stabilized and then undergo regulated degradation. However, the precise mechanisms controlling cytokine mRNA metabolism remain to be elucidated.

In this study, we demonstrate a distinct role of YB-1 in the tight regulation of intracellular IL-6 mRNA levels in a cell type-specific manner. YB-1 is secreted from macrophages but not dendritic cells after inflammatory stimuli and interacts with IL-6 mRNA. YB-1-depleted macrophages exhibit increased intracellular IL-6 mRNA levels, whereas dendritic cells exhibit decreased IL-6 mRNA expression after YB-1 depletion. In macrophages, the amount of intracellular IL-6 mRNA is controlled by YB-1 secretion, which enables cytosolic IL-6 mRNA to be exported into the extracellular fluid. In contrast, intracellular YB-1 enhances IL-6 mRNA stability in dendritic cells. These findings illustrate the distinct function of YB-1 as a critical regulator in controlling intracellular IL-6 mRNA levels differentially in a cell type-specific manner.

Results

YB-1 is secreted in a cell type-dependent manner

Studies have shown that YB-1 exhibits various subcellular localization patterns depending on the stimulus [7,11]. In particular, human monocytes stimulated with LPS secrete YB-1 from micro-vesicles [7]. We began examining the role(s) of YB-1 in the immune response by reproducing documented observations of YB-1 secretion in response to LPS, which promotes robust cytokine production to induce innate and adaptive immunity [7]. First, we assessed YB-1 subcellular localization in LPS-stimulated macrophages and dendritic cells. As shown previously, we observed intracellular secretory vesicle formation with enriched levels of endogenous YB-1 in LPS-treated macrophages, but not in unstimulated cells (**Figure 1A**). To explore TLR-agonist specificity in YB-1 secretion, we measured the pattern of intracellular vesicles in macrophages exposed to CpG-DNA, which activates the TLR9 signaling cascade. In CpG-DNA-stimulated macrophages, YB-1 secretory vesicles were clearly detected to an extent similar to LPS (**Figure 1A**). Interestingly, unlike macrophages, YB-1 was distributed throughout the cytoplasm, with one or two speckles close to the nuclear membrane in LPS- or CpG-DNA-stimulated bone marrow-derived dendritic cells (BMDCs) (**Figure 1B**). Therefore, YB-1 exhibits differential subcellular distribution that varies according to cell type, resulting in the regulation of distinct biological functions in macrophages and dendritic cells.

To confirm these findings, we examined YB-1 secretion from macrophages and dendritic cells following LPS stimulation. Equal numbers of macrophages and dendritic cells were exposed to LPS or CpG-DNA for 24 h and then the supernatants were immunoblotted with anti-YB-1 antibody. Macrophages showed secretion of YB-1, whereas no release of cytosolic protein was observed from dendritic cells (**Figure 1C, upper left panels**). The actual molecular weight of YB-1 is 35.9 kDa; however, this intracellular protein exhibits an electrophoretic mobility of ~50 kDa. Interestingly, the molecular mass of intracellular YB-1 was detectable at 50 kDa but the majority of extracellular YB-1 exhibited the ~37 kDa size along with several other molecular weight species, indicating that YB-1 may undergo fragmentation processing at different sites in LPS-stimulated macrophages (**Figure 1C, asterisks**). Because YB-1 knockdown resulted in no detectable protein bands in the immunoblot assay, it was confirmed that the protein bands observed were not due to non-specific proteins (**Figure 1C, bottom panel, asterisk**). Therefore, we conclude that YB-1 is secreted in a cell type-specific manner.

The localization of YB-1 affects IL-6 production

Because YB-1 serves as a regulator in both pro- and anti-inflammatory responses [4,12] and its cellular distribution was quite different between macrophages and dendritic cells, we investigated whether this differential localization of YB-1 affects its ability to induce cytokine production in response to LPS. YB-1 was depleted in macrophages or BMDCs using YB-1-specific RNA interference (RNAi). Unexpectedly, depletion of YB-1 enhanced LPS-induced production of IL-6 but not TNF-α in macrophages (**Figure 2A**). Likewise, CpG-DNA-stimulated macrophages expressing YB-1-specific RNAi exhibited increased production of IL-6 but not TNF-α (**Figure 2B**). In contrast to macrophages, LPS-exposed dendritic cells expressing YB-1 RNAi reduced IL-6

production but not TNF-α (**Figure 2C**). To confirm these findings, we examined the effect of YB-1 depletion on IL-6 mRNA production by quantitative RT-PCR (qRT-PCR) in macrophages and dendritic cells. The quantity of IL-6 mRNA produced upon LPS stimulation was increased in YB-1-depleted macrophages (**Figure 2D**) and was decreased in dendritic cells under the same conditions (**Figure 2E**). Similarly, RT-PCR confirmed that YB-1 affected IL-6 mRNA production in macrophages and dendritic cells in opposite ways (**Figure 2F and 2G**). Therefore, we conclude that YB-1-mediated IL-6 mRNA production is dependent upon cell type and tightly co-regulated with differential localization patterns of YB-1.

YB-1 negatively regulates intracellular IL-6 mRNA levels in macrophages

YB-1 binds near the cap structure of mRNA and also interacts with granulocyte monocyte colony stimulating factor (GM-CSF) mRNA [13,14]. YB-1 consists of three major domains: a glycine-rich N-terminal domain, a C-terminal domain containing alternating charged amino acids, and a highly conserved cold shock domain [4,5,15]. The glycine-rich and cold shock domains of YB-1 are thought to bind nucleic acid, based on previous reports and our results. Therefore, we determined whether YB-1 could bind IL-6 mRNA by conducting IL-6 mRNA pull-down analysis with the indicated primers using LPS-stimulated macrophages. We demonstrated that YB-1 interacts with IL-6 mRNA but not TNF-α mRNA (**Figure 3A**). Because YB-1 depletion increased IL-6 production, the ability of YB-1 to bind IL-6 mRNA suggested a possible role of YB-1 in regulating IL-6 mRNA stability. To investigate this possibility, we treated LPS-stimulated macrophages with the transcriptional inhibitor actinomycin D (Act.D) and then examined IL-6 mRNA stability by RT-PCR. We found that the amount of IL-6 mRNA during ActD exposure was much higher than in control macrophages, but the half-life of IL-6 mRNA in YB-1-depleted macrophages was similar to that of control macrophages. YB-1 depletion did not affect TNF-α mRNA expression or stability (**Figure 3B**). Calculation of mRNA band intensities also indicated that in YB-1-depleted macrophages, the relative amount of IL-6 mRNA increased more than two fold compared to control cells (**Figure 3C, upper graphs**); however, we found that the half-life of IL-6 mRNA or TNF-α mRNA was unaffected (**Figure 3C, bottom graphs**). These results suggest that YB-1 negatively regulates intracellular IL-6 mRNA expression levels, but it is not due to an increase in RNA turnover.

YB-1 actively exports cytosolic IL-6 mRNA to the extracellular space to control intracellular IL-6 mRNA levels in macrophages

Previous studies have shown that YB-1 associates with GM-CSF mRNA and thereby protects it from degradation, resulting in the development of allergic asthma by accumulating eosinophils in the lung parenchyma and airways [13,16]. However, our results showed that YB-1 depletion clearly increases IL-6 mRNA levels by a mechanism other than enhancing its stability in macrophages (**Figure 2**). Therefore, we hypothesized that in macrophages, YB-1 may facilitate IL-6 mRNA export to the extracellular space by YB-1 secretory micro-vesicles, resulting in a reduction of total cytosolic IL-6 mRNA levels. It is known that extracellular RNA (exRNA) species present outside the cells from which were transcribed, but their biological function is not fully understood [17,18]. To explore this possibility, we determined whether IL-6 mRNA exists extracellularly and whether or not secretory YB-1 functions in exporting IL-6 mRNA from cytosol to the extracel-

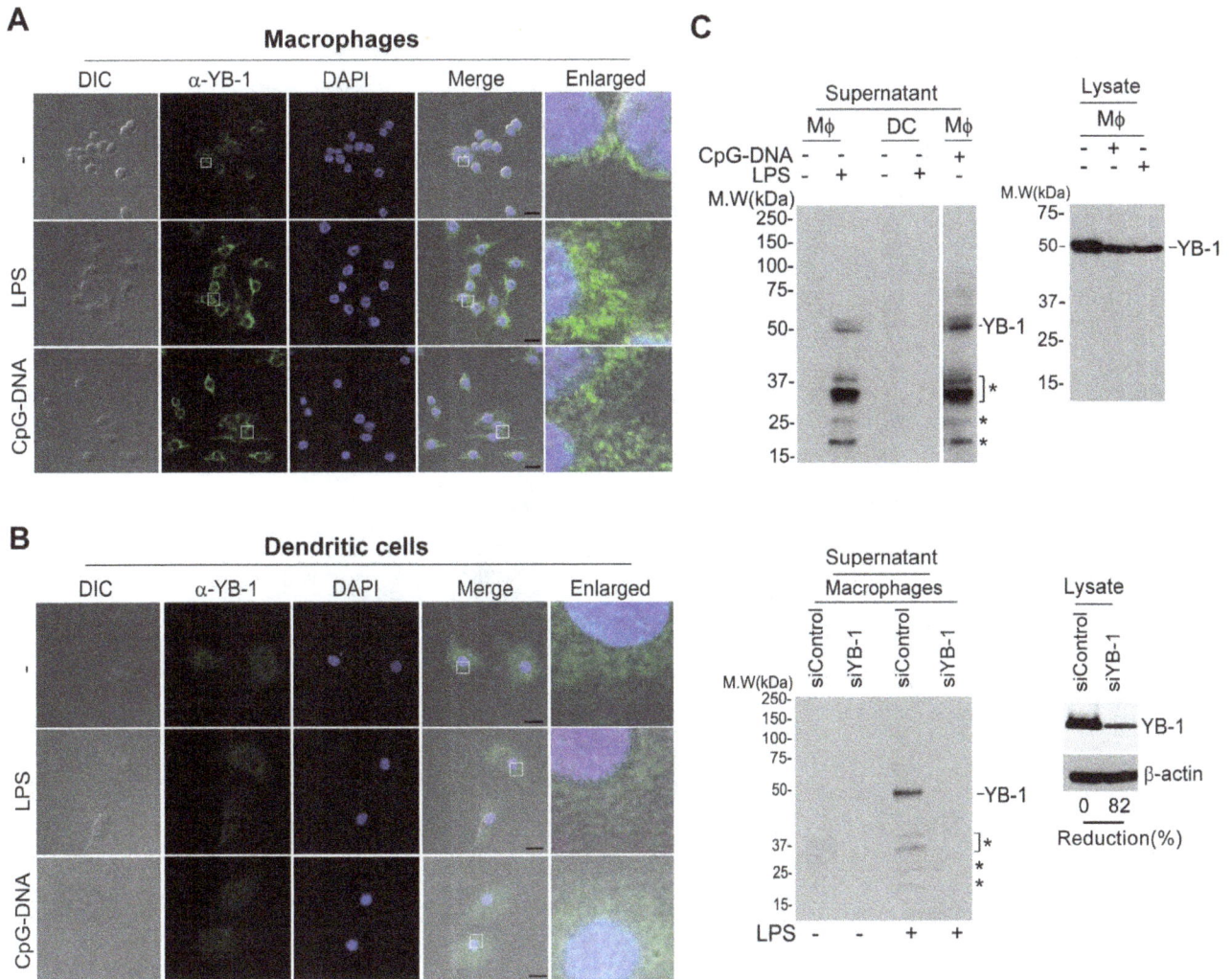

Figure 1. Inflammatory stimuli induce YB-1 secretion in a cell type-specific manner. (**A**) Immunofluorescence microscopy assay (IFA) of YB-1 in RAW macrophages following exposure to LPS (80 ng/ml) or CpG-DNA (1 μM). LPS or CPG-DNA-stimulated macrophages exhibited YB-1-enriched exporting vesicles. 6.5× digital enlargement of main image, Scale bars, 10 μm. (**B**) Bone marrow-derived Dendritic cells (BMDC) were stimulated with LPS (80 ng/ml) or CpG-DNA (1 μM). Anti-YB-1 antibody with Alexa 488-conjugated secondary antibody and DAPI were used. YB-1-enriched vesicles were not detected in BMDC. 6.5× digital enlargement of main image, Scale bars, 10 μm. (**C**) Western blot analyses of YB-1 in macrophages and dendritic cells with anti-YB-1antibody. TCA-precipitated extracellular supernatant from macrophages contained secreted YB-1, which was confirmed by depletion of YB-1. Lineage markers were used to characterize macrophages or dendritic cells (Fig. S1). Asterisk indicates the molecular weight species of extracellular YB-1. Data are representative of three (**A–B**), or two (**C**) experiments.

lular space. Macrophages expressing either control or YB-1 RNAi were incubated in serum-free medium in the absence or presence of LPS for 24 h. Culture medium was collected from the macrophages and then assayed for IL-6 mRNA by RT-PCR. Surprisingly, we found that IL-6 mRNA was secreted to the extracellular space from macrophages (**Figure 4A, lane 7 of left panel**); in contrast, we did not observe any secreted TNF-α mRNA (**Figure 4A, lane 5 of right panel**). Furthermore, intracellular and extracellular IL-6 mRNA levels correlated with YB-1 expression levels in macrophages. YB-1 depletion increased the amount of intracellular IL-6 mRNA and decreased levels of extracellular IL-6 mRNA (**Figure 4A, comparing lane 3 with 4 and lane 7 with 8 of left panel**). TNF-α mRNA levels were unaffected, as shown previously (**Figure 4A, right panel**). We quantified the IL-6 mRNA band intensities from RT-PCR and showed that IL-6 mRNA increased in the intracellular space by

51% in YB-1-depleted macrophages and extracellular IL-6 mRNA levels decreased by 58% (**Figure 4B**).

Because YB-1 binds to single-stranded cisplatin-modified Y box DNA sequences and degrades DNA by its exonuclease activity [19], we investigated whether YB-1 could also degrade RNA. We purified YB-1 by immunoprecipitation and then incubated the protein with oligonucleotides or poly-A tail RNAs. An *in vitro* degradation assay showed that YB-1 degraded oligonucleotides but not RNA (**Figure 4C, comparing lane 2 with 3 and lane 5 with 6**), indicating that YB-1 does not have an exoribonuclease activity. Taken together, we demonstrate that YB-1 tightly controls intracellular IL-6 mRNA levels by binding and exporting cytosolic IL-6 mRNA to the extracellular fluid, but does not act as an exoribonuclease.

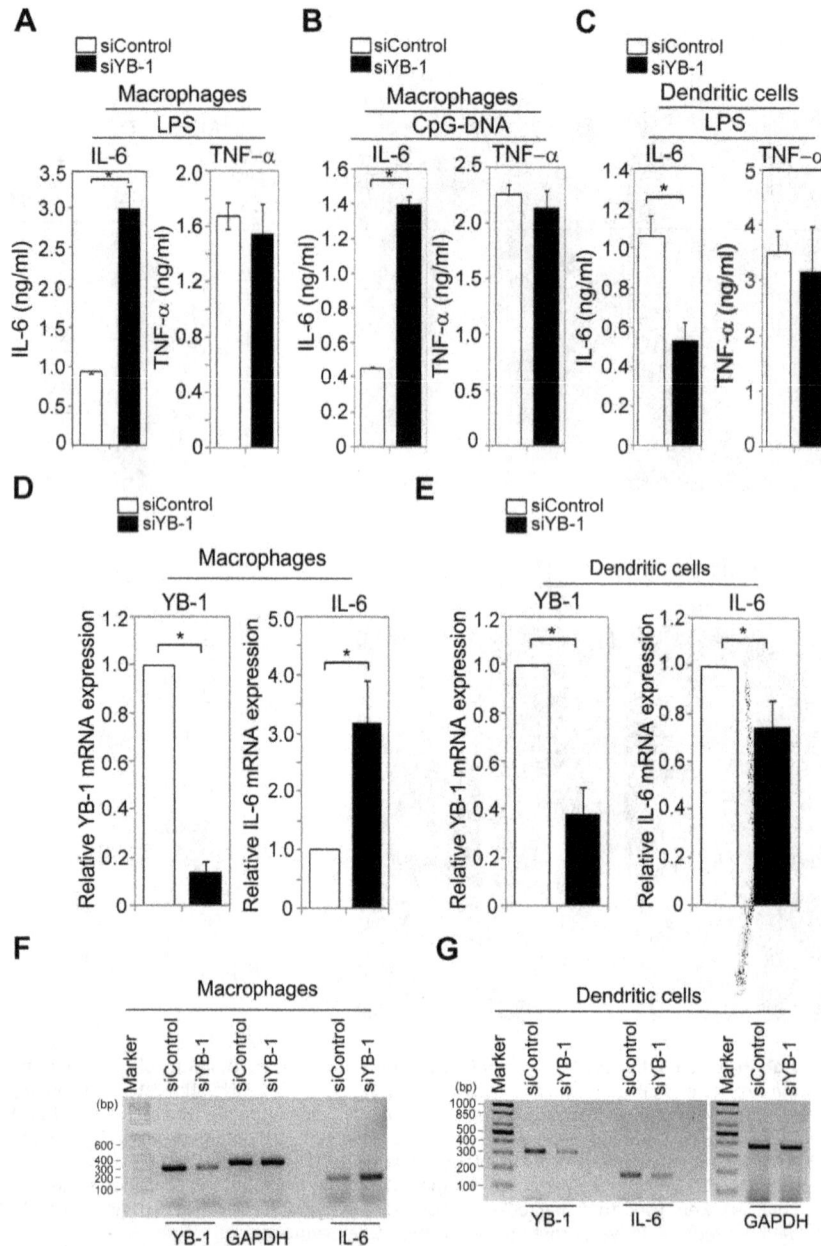

Figure 2. Depletion of YB-1 affects IL-6 mRNA production in a cell type-specific manner. (A–C) The increased production of IL-6 was observed in YB-1-depleted macrophages but not BMDC. After depletion of YB-1, macrophages were stimulated with LPS (80 ng/ml) or CpG-DNA (1 μM). ELISA was performed to measure IL-6 and TNF-α levels in RAW macrophages (**A** and **B**) and BMDC (**C**). *$P<0.001$ (student's t-test) (**D–G**) YB-1 knockdown led to increased IL-6 mRNA levels in macrophages, but reduced in BMDC. IL-6 mRNA levels were assessed by qRT-PCR (**D–E**, primer pairs: P2, P3, and P5 in **Table S1**) or RT-PCR (**F–G**, primer pairs: P1, P3, and P5) in YB-1-depleted macrophages (**D** and **F**) or BMDC (**E** and **G**), stimulated with LPS (80 ng/ml). *$P<0.001$ (student's t-test). Data are representative of at least three independent experiments.

Intracellular YB-1 is essential for IL-6 mRNA stability in dendritic cells

Because YB-1 is involved in regulating transcription, RNA processing, and mRNA stabilization [14,20,21], we next investigated whether intracellular YB-1 controls IL-6 mRNA metabolism in dendritic cells. To examine the effects of YB-1 on IL-6 mRNA transcription and splicing, dendritic cells expressing YB-1 RNAi were stimulated with LPS and then IL-6 mRNA production was measured. YB-1 depletion in dendritic cells resulted in reduced IL-6 mRNA production following LPS stimulation. In contrast, TNF-

α mRNA levels were unaffected. In addition, IL-6 pre-mRNA accumulation was not observed, suggesting that YB-1 is not involved in IL-6 pre-mRNA processing (**Figure 5A**). To explore whether YB-1 activates IL-6 gene expression, we examined luciferase activity in YB-1-expressing macrophages or dendritic cells using an *IL-6* promoter luciferase reporter. The luciferase assay showed no significant effect by YB-1 on *IL-6* promoter activity (**Figure 5B**), indicating that YB-1 may not be involved in regulating IL-6 mRNA transcription but rather its stability. Indeed, we found that the half-life of IL-6 mRNA in YB-1-

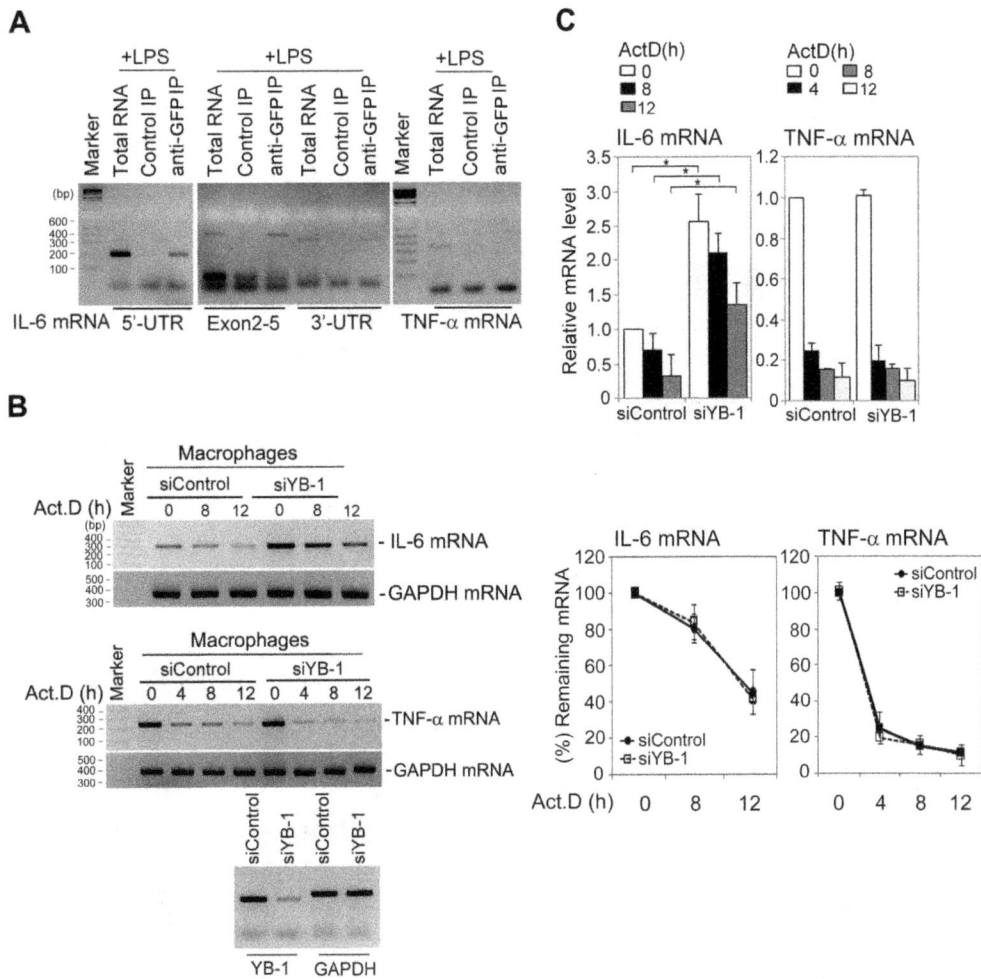

Figure 3. YB-1 interacts with IL-6 mRNA but does not affect IL-6 mRNA stability. (**A**) Macrophages were exposed to LPS (80 ng/ml) and then subjected to RIP assay using appropriate primer pairs (P4, P6, P8, and P9 in **Table S1**). YB-1 bound IL-6 mRNA, but not TNF-α mRNA. (**B**) The effect of YB-1 depletion on IL-6 or TNF-α mRNA stability in LPS-stimulated macrophages. Total mRNA was isolated at different time points after actinomycin D (6 µg/ml) treatment and each RT-PCR was analyzed by the indicated primer pairs (P4, P5, and P8). (**C**) Each graph represents densitometric analysis of RT-PCR data. Relative densitometric values for each mRNA were corrected by dividing each value by that for the GAPDH mRNA in each blot. *P<0.001 (student's t-test). Data are representative of at least three independent experiments.

depleted dendritic cells was less than in control dendritic cells (**Figure 5C**). Taken together, we conclude that cytosolic YB-1 controls IL-6 production by regulating IL-6 mRNA stability in dendritic cells.

LPS induces YB-1 acetylation, which differentially regulates HDAC6 expression between macrophages and dendritic cells

Based on previous observations that YB-1 acetylation is essential for its secretion [7], we examined this post-translational modification of YB-1 in LPS-stimulated macrophages or dendritic cells. Immunoprecipitation of intracellular YB-1 using anti-YB-1 antibody followed by immunoblotting with anti-Pan-acetyl antibody revealed weak but detectable YB-1 acetylation in macrophages but not in dendritic cells (**Figure 6A**).

Studies have demonstrated that LPS regulates the expression of several members of the HDAC family in macrophages in a time-dependent manner [22]. In particular, the expression of HDAC6 was highly expressed in non-stimulated macrophages, but its

expression was significantly reduced after 2 hours of LPS stimulation in macrophages. Therefore, we hypothesized that LPS blocks the activity of HDAC6, allowing intracellular YB-1 to be efficiently acetylated for its secretion. We performed RT-PCR or qRT-PCR assays to examine HDAC6 expression in LPS-stimulated macrophages and dendritic cells over time. Indeed, the levels of HDAC6 decreased in LPS-treated macrophages (**Figure 6B**). Interestingly, in contrast to macrophages, the expression of HDAC6 during LPS stimulation was highly increased in dendritic cells (**Figure 6B**). Similarly, qRT-PCR confirmed that LPS affected HDAC6 mRNA production in macrophages and dendritic cells in opposite ways (**Figure 6C**). These results demonstrate that LPS negatively regulates the expression of HDAC6 in macrophages; in contrast, it positively regulates the expression of both HDACs in dendritic cells, indicating that different expression patterns of HDAC6 may differentially control YB-1 acetylation and secretion in a cell type-dependent manner.

A

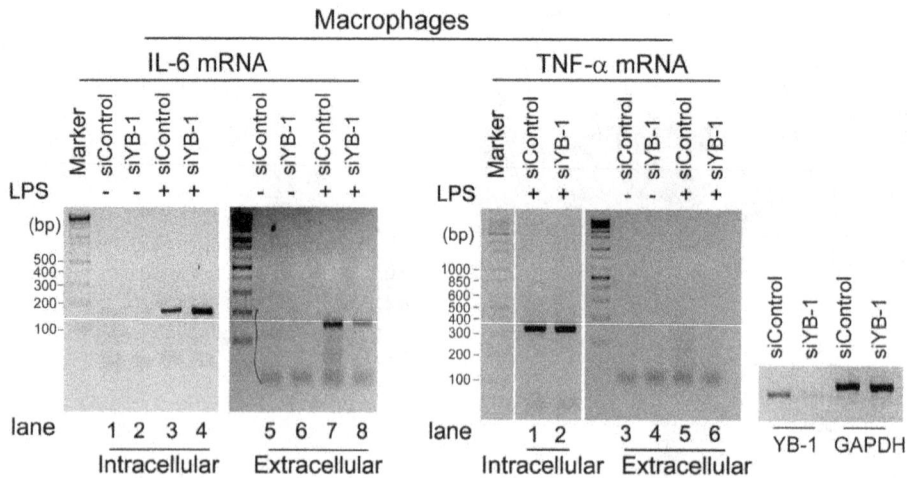

B

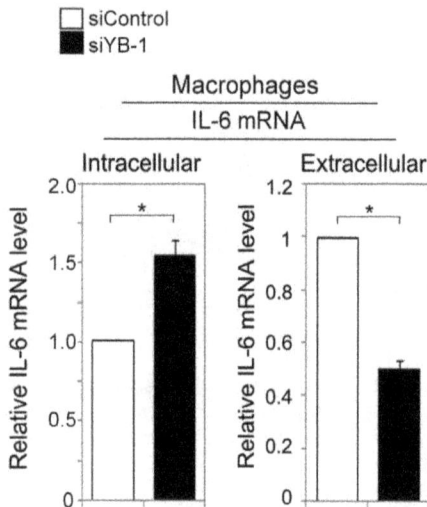

C

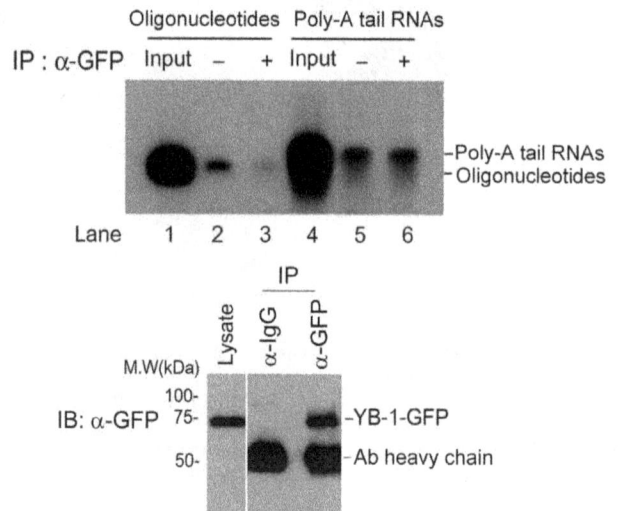

Figure 4. YB-1 is essential for maintaining intracellular IL-6 mRNAs levels by secreting mRNA to the extracellular space in macrophages. (**A**) After LPS stimulation for 24 h, total RNAs were purified separately from medium or cell lysates and the presence of IL-6 or TNF-α mRNAs was examined by RT-PCR. (**B**) The ratio of IL-6 mRNA between intracellular and extracellular fluid was correlated to YB-1 expression level. *$P <$ 0.005 (student's t-test). (**C**) YB-1 does not act as an exoribonuclease enzyme. Cell lysates from macrophages stably expressing YB-1-GFP were immunoprecipitated with anti-GFP antibody. YB-1-GFP proteins were then purified and incubated with the P^{32}-labeled single-stranded 21mer oligonucleotides or 12mer Poly-A tail RNAs. Exonuclease or exoribonuclease assay was performed at 37°C for 2 h and terminated by adding 2× sample buffer and reaction products were separated on a 15% polyacrylamide 7 M urea gel. YB-1-GFP proteins were probed by anti-GFP-antibody. Data are representative of three (**A, B**), or two (**C**) experiments.

Discussion

These studies describe a critical role of YB-1 in controlling intracellular IL-6 mRNA levels in a cell type-specific manner. In macrophages responding to inflammatory stimuli, YB-1 is actively secreted, allowing it to bind IL-6 mRNA and promote the export of intracellular IL-6 mRNA to the extracellular fluid, thereby maintaining immune homeostasis by reducing excess IL-6 mRNA within the cell. However, the function of YB-1 in dendritic cells is distinct from that in macrophages. Dendritic cells do not exhibit YB-1 secretion in response to LPS. Instead, cytosolic YB-1 is

essential for IL-6 mRNA stability as a positive regulator. Therefore, YB-1 is needed for IL-6 mRNA production to protect against microbial infection. Moreover, YB-1 is involved in maintaining intracellular IL-6 mRNA levels to prevent a hyperactive immune response. These distinct functions are dependent on the subcellular distribution of YB-1 (**Figure 6D**). Depending on the context of cell type-dependent YB-1 function, our data imply that there may be potential relevance to the differences in YB-1 function between the inflammatory infiltrating macrophages and tissue-resident macrophages during various immune responses.

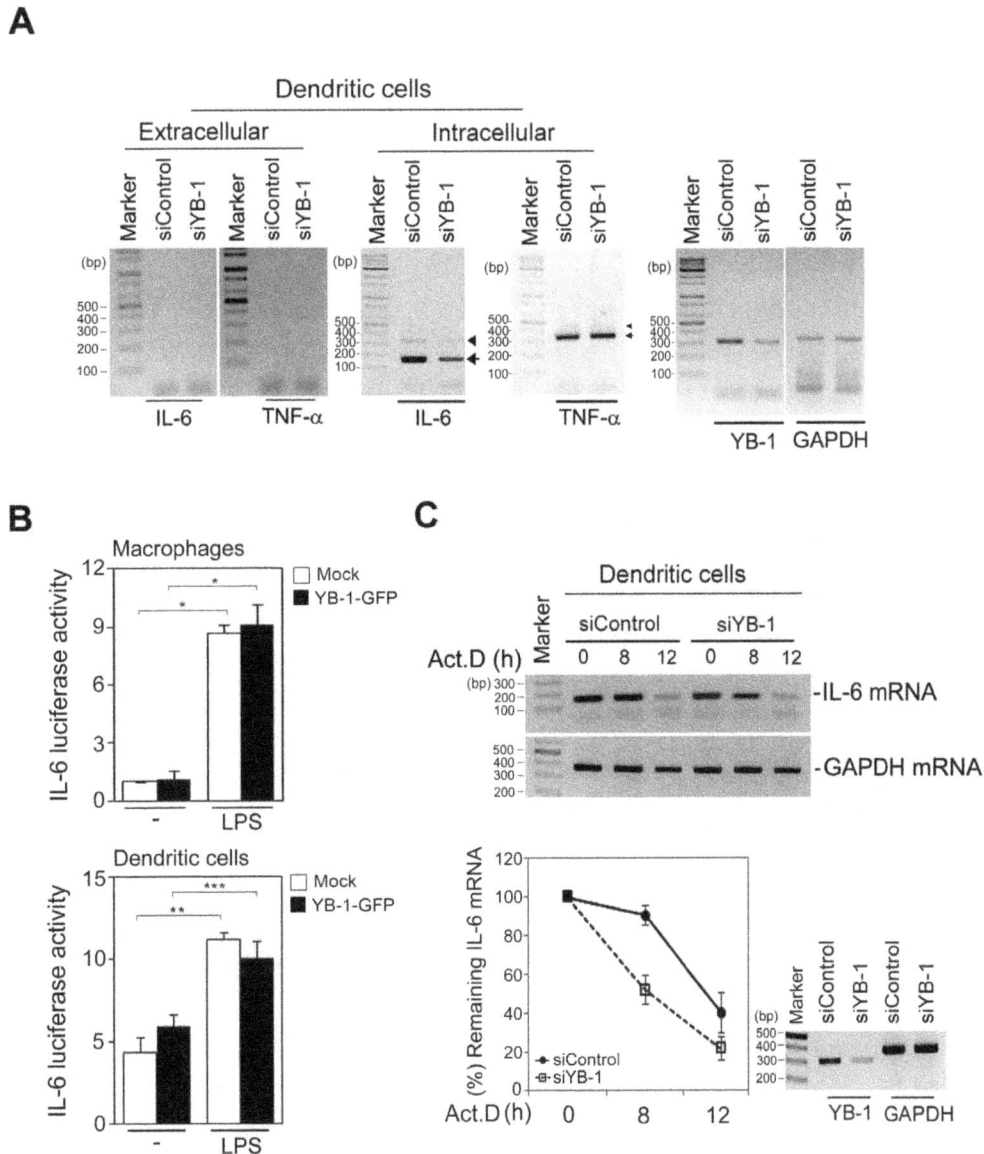

Figure 5. YB-1 has a distinct role in dendritic cells, capable of enhancing IL-6 RNA stability. (A) Total RNAs were purified from culture medium or cell lysates from LPS-stimulated BMDCs expressing either control or YB-1 RNAi. The extracellular or intracellular IL-6 mRNA or TNF-α mRNA was examined by RT-PCR (primer pairs: P4 and P7 in Table S1). YB-1 knockdown and RNA quantitation were determined by RT-PCR using the indicated primers (primer pairs: P3 and P5). Arrowheads and arrows indicate pre-mRNA and mRNA, respectively. (B) Macrophages or dendritic cells were cotransfected with empty vector or YB-1-GFP together with IL-6 and a *Renilla* luciferase reporter gene and then stimulated with LPS for 12 h. Cell lysates were prepared and then measured by *Renilla*-Firefly luciferase dual assay. Luciferase activity was determined using a luminometer. All luciferase assays were performed in triplicate for each reporter construct. (C) The effect of YB-1 depletion on IL-6 mRNA stability in LPS-stimulated dendritic cells was assessed by RT-PCR analysis of IL-6 mRNA levels (primer pairs: P1 and P5). Total mRNA was isolated at different time points after ActD treatment. Each graph represents densitometric analysis of RT-PCR data. Relative densitometric values for each mRNA were corrected by dividing each value by that for the GAPDH mRNA in each blot. *$P < 0.0005$, ** $P < 0.001$, *** $P < 0.005$ (Student's t-test). Data are representative of three independent experiments.

Several reports have documented different post-translational modifications for YB-1, including fragmentation, acetylation, and phosphorylation. Interestingly, we show that secretion of YB-1 is dependent on cell type, and that the molecular mass of intracellular and extracellular YB-1 is quite different. The molecular mass of intracellular YB-1 is mostly detectable at ~50 kDa, whereas the majority of extracellular YB-1 exhibits a size of approximately 37 kDa, along with several other molecular weight species. Previous reports have shown that YB-1 is cleaved by the 20S proteasome, which allows its truncated form to

translocate to the nucleus, resulting in more efficient protection of cells from DNA damage [23–25]. In particular, the 18-kDa fragment of secreted YB-1 was detected in the plasma of cancer patients [26] and we also show the 18 kDa fragment in TCA-precipitated extracellular supernatant from LPS-stimulated macrophages. Therefore, it is possible that the various YB-1 fragments that form in response to LPS may result in altered subcellular localization and immunological function.

Furthermore, YB-1 acetylation is required for its secretion [7]. Our results show that YB-1 is acetylated in LPS-stimulated

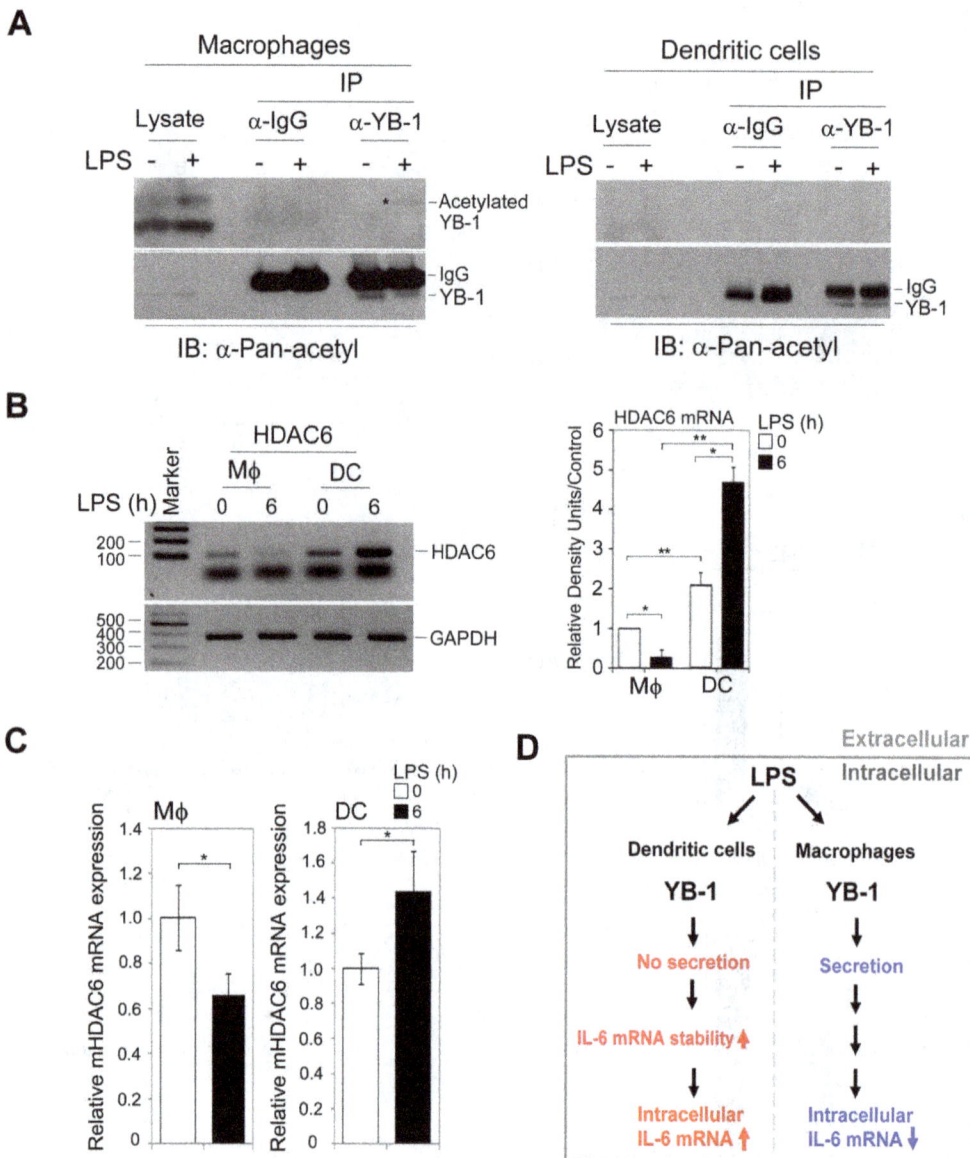

Figure 6. YB-1 acetylation leads to differential regulation of HDAC6 between macrophages and dendritic cells. (**A**) Equal numbers of macrophages and dendritic cells were exposed to LPS for 12 h and then lysed. The lysates were immunoprecipitated with anti-YB-1 antibody and then immunoblotted with anti-Pan-acetyl or anti-YB-1 antibody. (**B and C**) Macrophages or dendritic cells were stimulated with LPS for 0 h or 6 h before total RNA was purified. The expression level of HDAC6 was examined by RT-PCR or qRT-PCR (primer pairs: P10 and P5). *$P<0.001$, **$P<0.005$ (Student's t-test). Data are representative of two (**A**) or three (**B, C**) experiments. (**D**) Schematic model of YB-1 controlling intracellular IL-6 mRNA levels in a cell type-specific manner. The proper maintenance of intracellular IL-6 mRNA expression is dependent on the extracellular and intracellular distribution of YB-1.

macrophages, but not in dendritic cells. In addition, we demonstrate that HDAC6 expressions differ in a cell type-dependent manner, indicating that differences in YB-1 secretion between macrophages and dendritic cells may be correlated with differential HDAC6 expression. In addition, during the early phase of inflammation, YB-1 is phosphorylated at Ser102, a site located in the highly conserved cold-shock domain [12]. In addition, calcineurin-mediated YB-1 dephosphorylation regulates CCL5 expression during monocyte differentiation [27]. Because YB-1 contains several possible sites for phosphorylation, it may be possible that LPS regulates YB-1 phosphorylation, leading to changes in its subcellular localization.

YB-1 can function as a negative or positive regulator on RNA metabolism [20,28]. For example, heterozygous YB-1 knockout mice show increased basal expression levels of CXCL1 in the kidney and liver, whereas LPS stimulation results in decreased CXCL1 expression in these organs. Interestingly, the peritoneal lavage fluid of these mice treated with LPS contains elevated CXCL1 levels as compared with wild-type mice. Our study also shows that YB-1 exhibits different functions depending on the cell type, capable of controlling intracellular IL-6 mRNA levels through export or enhancement of stability.

Several types of extracellular RNAs have been described. Recent studies have shown that microRNAs (miRNAs) are released and that secretory miRNAs are transferable by packaged vesicles and functional in recipient cells [29,30]. It is possible that secreted IL-6 mRNA may be packaged with YB-1-containing exosomal vesicles and transferred to neighboring cells, resulting in IL-6 production in these cells without LPS stimulation. In particular, our results imply that YB-1 could also regulate the secretion or stability of other mRNA species.

Because misregulation of IL-6 mRNA expression levels contributes to autoimmune and chronic inflammatory diseases, an understanding of the regulatory proteins involved in controlling cytokine mRNA levels is essential for the development of new classes of immunomodulatory therapies.

Materials and Methods

Cell lines

Murine RAW 264.7 macrophages (ATCC TIB-71) were cultured in DMEM supplemented with 10% heat inactivated fetal bovine serum (HyClone, Logan, UT) and penicillin/streptomycin (Hyclone). Cells were grown at 37°C in humidified air with 5% CO_2.

Generation of BMDC

Bone marrow-derived dendritic cells (BMDC) were generated from wild-type C57BL/6 mice (Orient Bio, Gyeonggi-do, South Korea), in medium containing 5 ng/ml GM-CSF (BioLegend, San Diego, CA). Briefly, femurs and tibiae were collected from 4-week-old mice. After removing bone-adjacent muscles, marrow cells were extracted by flushing with a 25-gauge needle. Bone marrow cells were then resuspended in DMEM (10% FBS and 1% antibiotics) with GM-CSF (5 ng/ml). Fresh medium was replenished on Days 2 and 4. BMDC were generated after 6–8 days of culture. Mice were maintained under pathogen-free conditions according to guidelines set by the committee for animal care at the Yonsei University.

Reagents

LPS (E. coli 026:B6) and 1826-CpG DNA (5′-TsCsCsAsTsgsAsCsgsTsTsCsCsTsgsAsCsgsTsT-3′) were purchased from Sigma (St. Louis, MO) and TIB Molbiol (Berlin, Germany), respectively. YB-1 antibodies were obtained from Cell Signaling Technology (Danvers, MA) and Santa Cruz Biotechnology (Santa Cruz, CA). Actinomycin D (Act. D) and Trichloroacetic acid (TCA) were purchased from Sigma.

Retroviral transduction and RNAi production

HEK 293T cells were transfected with plasmids encoding VSV-G and Gag-Pol, as well as either shRNA for YB-1 or shRNA for GFP (Control). Thirty-six to forty-eight hours post-transfection, media containing viral particles were collected, filtered through a 0.45 μm membrane and incubated with RAW macrophages for 24 h. Cells were selected with puromycin. The shRNA sequence against YB-1 was annealed and subcloned into the pSUPER retroviral vector (Oligoengine, Seattle, WA) using the following primers: 5′-GATCCGGTCATCGCAACGAAGGTTTTCTCGAGAAAACCTTCGTTGCGATGACCTTTTTTGGAAA-3′ and 5′-AGCTTTTCCAAAAAA GGTCATCGCAACGAAGGTTTTCTCGAGAAAACCTTCGTTGCGATGACC-3′. The siRNA sequence against GFP, which was used as a negative control, was cloned using the following primers: 5′-GATCCGCAAGCTGACCCTGAAGTTCCTCGAGGAACTTCAGGGTCAGCTTGCTTTTTTGGAAA-3′ and 5′-AGCTTTTCCAAAAAAGCAAGCTGACCCTGAAGTTCCTCGAGGAACTTCAGGGTCAGCTTGCGG-3′.

ELISA and siRNA transfection

Cells were treated with 80 ng/ml LPS or 1 μM CpG-DNA for 12 h. The media were collected and mouse IL-6 and TNF-α levels were analyzed by ELISA according to the manufacturer's recommendations (BD Biosciences, San Jose, CA). BMDC were transfected (DharmaFECT; Thermo scientific, Rockford, IL) with either scrambled siRNA (Control) or YB-1 siRNA for 48 h. The siRNA sequences were as follows: YB-1 (5′- UCAUCGCAACGAAGGUUUUTT-3′, 5′- AAAACCUUCGUUGCGAUGATT-3′) and negative control (5′-UUCUCCGAACGUGUCACGUTT-3′, 5′-ACGUGACACGUUCGGAGAATT-3′).

Immunofluorescence assay (IFA)

For immunofluorescent staining, cells were fixed in 3.7% formaldehyde and permeabilized with 0.1% Triton X-100 prior to incubation with anti-YB-1 antibody and Alexa Fluor 488-conjugated secondary antibody (Life technologies, Carlsbad, CA). DAPI (4′, 6-diamidino-2-phenylindole) (Sigma) was used as a nuclear counterstain. Cells were imaged using a fluorescence microscope.

RNA Immunoprecipitation (RIP assay)

Cytosolic fractions were isolated from macrophages expressing YB-1-GFP using a hypotonic buffer containing 10 mM HEPES, pH 7.9, 15 mM $MgCl_2$, 10 mM KCl, 0.05% NP-40, protease inhibitor cocktail (Roche, Mannheim, Germany), and 100 units of RNase inhibitor (TaKaRa, Otsu, Japan). After incubation with anti-GFP antibody and protein G-Sepharose beads (Sigma), samples were washed with ice-cold RIP buffer (150 mM KCl, 25 mM Tris-Cl, pH 7.4, and 0.5% NP-40) and RNA was extracted using an RNA purification kit (GeneAll, Seoul, South Korea) according to the manufacturer's instructions.

Purification of YB-1 protein

Macrophages stably expressing YB-1-GFP were lysed with 1% NP-40 with protease inhibitor cocktail (Roche) for 30 min. Lysates were incubated with anti-GFP antibody (Roche) at 4°C overnight. After incubation with protein G-Sepharose beads (Sigma) for 1 h, samples were washed twice with ice-cold 0.1% NP-40. Then beads containing YB-1-GFP were incubated with 10 μl reaction buffer at 37°C for 2 h and purified.

Exonuclease or Exoribonuclease activity assay

The single-stranded oligonucleotides (21mer; Cosmo Genetech, Seoul, South Korea) and Poly-A tail RNA (12 mer; Bioneer, Seoul, South Korea) were end-labeled with [α-^{32}P] ATP (Perkin Elmer, Waltham, MA) using T4 polynucleotide kinase (Thermo Scientific) at 37°C for 1 h and then heat inactivated at 75°C for 10 min. Purified YB-1 proteins were incubated with labeled oligonucleotides (30 pmol) or poly-A tail RNA (30 pmol) in a reaction mixture containing 10 mM Tris-HCl pH 8.0, 5 mM $MgCl_2$, 50 mM KCl, 10 mM DTT, and 40 units of recombinant RNase inhibitor (TaKaRa) at 37°C for 2 h. The reactions were terminated by adding 2× loading buffer (90% formamide, 10 mM EDTA, 0.1% Xylene cyanol, 0.1% bromophenol blue) and boiling at 95°C for 1 min. After vortex and gentle centrifugation, samples were separated on a 15% polyacrylamide 7 M urea gel in TBE buffer at 70 V for 90 min and dried at 60°C for 1 h. Dried gels were exposed to film.

TCA precipitation

Samples were precipitated with TCA(10% v/v), collected by centrifugation at 20,000 g for 45 min at 4°C, washed twice with ice-cold 70% ethanol, and then dried completely. Air-dried pellet were resuspended in distilled water.

Flow cytometry

The surface expression of F4/80 or CD11c, which are lineage markers on macrophages or dendritic cells, was determined by flow cytometry (FACScalibur, Becton Dickinson Biosciences). Cells (1×10^6) were washed twice with cold PBS containing 1% bovine serum albumin (BSA) and incubated for 1 h at 4°C with a saturating concentration of mAb F4/80 or CD11c (R&D Systems, Minneapolis, MN). Normal mouse IgG was used as a negative control for each test. The cells were washed twice with cold PBS containing 1% BSA and then stained with FITC-conjugated goat anti-mouse IgG for 50 min. A total of 10,000 gated events were collected by the FACScalibur cytometer and analyzed with CellQuest software (BD Biosciences).

Real time PCR and RT-PCR assays

Total cellular RNA was prepared using an RNA prep kit (GeneAll, Seoul, South Korea) and RNA (0.5 µg) was reverse transcribed for 1 h with random hexamers at 42°C using M-MLV (Moloney Murine Leukemia Virus) reverse transcriptase (Enzynomic, Seoul, South Korea). PCR was then performed and PCR products were visualized on ethidium bromide-stained gels. Real time PCR was performed using TOPreal qPCR premix (SYBR Green, Enzymonics) and an Applied Biosystems 7300 Real-Time PCR System (Life technologies). Results were normalized to expression of the gene encoding GAPDH and were quantified by the change-in-threshold method ($\Delta\Delta$CT). All primer sequences are listed in **Table S1**.

Luciferase assay

Macrophages or dendritic cells were dispensed into each well of 24 well plates and were transfected with YB-1, renilla reporter gene, or IL-6 reporter plasmid. After 24 h, the transfected cells were stimulated by LPS for 12 h and lysed with luciferase buffer. The luciferase assays were performed with the Dual-luciferase Reporter Assay System (Pierce) and measured with a luminometer. All the luciferase assays were performed in triplicate for each luciferase reporter construct.

Ethics statement

All animal experiments were performed in accordance with the Korean Food and Drug Administration (KFDA) guidelines. Protocols were reviewed and approved by the Institutional Animal Care and Use Committee (IACUC) of the Yonsei Laboratory Animal Research Center (YLARC). All mice were maintained in the specific pathogen-free facility of the YLARC.

Author Contributions

Conceived and designed the experiments: BP SL. Performed the experiments: SK TAL EAR EL HJC. Analyzed the data: BP SL SK. Contributed reagents/materials/analysis tools: BP SL. Wrote the paper: BP SL.

References

1. Medzhitov R (2008) Origin and physiological roles of inflammation. Nature 454: 428–435.
2. Norling LV, Serhan CN (2010) Profiling in resolving inflammatory exudates identifies novel anti-inflammatory and pro-resolving mediators and signals for termination. J Intern Med 268: 15–24.
3. Ruzanov PV, Evdokimova VM, Korneeva NL, Hershey JW, Ovchinnikov LP (1999) Interaction of the universal mRNA-binding protein, p50, with actin: a possible link between mRNA and microfilaments. J Cell Sci 112 (Pt 20): 3487–3496.
4. Raffetseder U, Liehn EA, Weber C, Mertens PR (2012) Role of cold shock Y-box protein-1 in inflammation, atherosclerosis and organ transplant rejection. Eur J Cell Biol 91: 567–575.
5. Wolffe AP (1994) Structural and functional properties of the evolutionarily ancient Y-box family of nucleic acid binding proteins. Bioessays 16: 245–251.
6. Lyabin DN, Eliseeva IA, Ovchinnikov LP (2014) YB-1 protein: functions and regulation. Wiley Interdiscip Rev RNA 5: 95–110.
7. Frye BC, Halfter S, Djudjaj S, Muehlenberg P, Weber S, et al. (2009) Y-box protein-1 is actively secreted through a non-classical pathway and acts as an extracellular mitogen. EMBO Rep 10: 783–789.
8. Anderson P (2008) Post-transcriptional control of cytokine production. Nat Immunol 9: 353–359.
9. Seko Y, Cole S, Kasprzak W, Shapiro BA, Ragheb JA (2006) The role of cytokine mRNA stability in the pathogenesis of autoimmune disease. Autoimmun Rev 5: 299–305.
10. Ivanov P, Anderson P (2013) Post-transcriptional regulatory networks in immunity. Immunol Rev 253: 253–272.
11. Cohen SB, Ma W, Valova VA, Algie M, Harfoot R, et al. (2010) Genotoxic stress-induced nuclear localization of oncoprotein YB-1 in the absence of proteolytic processing. Oncogene 29: 403–410.
12. Hanssen L, Alidousty C, Djudjaj S, Frye BC, Rauen T, et al. (2013) YB-1 is an early and central mediator of bacterial and sterile inflammation in vivo. J Immunol 191: 2604–2613.
13. Bousquet J, Chanez P, Lacoste JY, Barneon G, Ghavanian N, et al. (1990) Eosinophilic inflammation in asthma. N Engl J Med 323: 1033–1039.
14. Evdokimova V, Ruzanov P, Imataka H, Raught B, Svitkin Y, et al. (2001) The major mRNA-associated protein YB-1 is a potent 5′ cap-dependent mRNA stabilizer. EMBO J 20: 5491–5502.
15. Wolffe AP, Tafuri S, Ranjan M, Familari M (1992) The Y-box factors: a family of nucleic acid binding proteins conserved from Escherichia coli to man. New Biol 4: 290–298.
16. Capowski EE, Esnault S, Bhattacharya S, Malter JS (2001) Y box-binding factor promotes eosinophil survival by stabilizing granulocyte-macrophage colony-stimulating factor mRNA. J Immunol 167: 5970–5976.
17. Valadi H, Ekstrom K, Bossios A, Sjostrand M, Lee JJ, et al. (2007) Exosome-mediated transfer of mRNAs and microRNAs is a novel mechanism of genetic exchange between cells. Nat Cell Biol 9: 654–659.
18. Hunter MP, Ismail N, Zhang X, Aguda BD, Lee EJ, et al. (2008) Detection of microRNA expression in human peripheral blood microvesicles. PLoS One 3: e3694.
19. Izumi H, Imamura T, Nagatani G, Ise T, Murakami T, et al. (2001) Y box-binding protein-1 binds preferentially to single-stranded nucleic acids and exhibits 3′−>5′ exonuclease activity. Nucleic Acids Res 29: 1200–1207.
20. Diamond P, Shannon MF, Vadas MA, Coles LS (2001) Cold shock domain factors activate the granulocyte-macrophage colony-stimulating factor promoter in stimulated Jurkat T cells. J Biol Chem 276: 7943–7951.
21. Raffetseder U, Frye B, Rauen T, Jurchott K, Royer HD, et al. (2003) Splicing factor SRp30c interaction with Y-box protein-1 confers nuclear YB-1 shuttling and alternative splice site selection. J Biol Chem 278: 18241–18248.
22. Aung HT, Schroder K, Himes SR, Brion K, van Zuylen W, et al. (2006) LPS regulates proinflammatory gene expression in macrophages by altering histone deacetylase expression. FASEB J 20: 1315–1327.
23. Sorokin AV, Selyutina AA, Skabkin MA, Guryanov SG, Nazimov IV, et al. (2005) Proteasome-mediated cleavage of the Y-box-binding protein 1 is linked to DNA-damage stress response. EMBO J 24: 3602–3612.
24. Kim ER, Selyutina AA, Buldakov IA, Evdokimova V, Ovchinnikov LP, et al. (2013) The proteolytic YB-1 fragment interacts with DNA repair machinery and enhances survival during DNA damaging stress. Cell Cycle 12: 3791–3803.
25. van Roeyen CR, Scurt FG, Brandt S, Kuhl VA, Martinkus S, et al. Cold shock Y-box protein-1 proteolysis autoregulates its transcriptional activities. Cell Commun Signal 11: 63.
26. Tacke F, Kanig N, En-Nia A, Kaehne T, Eberhardt CS, et al. (2011) Y-box protein-1/p18 fragment identifies malignancies in patients with chronic liver disease. BMC Cancer 11: 185.
27. Alidousty C, Rauen T, Hanssen L, Wang Q, Alampour-Rajabi S, et al. (2014) Calcineurin-mediated YB-1 dephosphorylation regulates CCL5 expression during monocyte differentiation. J Biol Chem.

28. Raffetseder U, Rauen T, Djudjaj S, Kretzler M, En-Nia A, et al. (2009) Differential regulation of chemokine CCL5 expression in monocytes/macrophages and renal cells by Y-box protein-1. Kidney Int 75: 185–196.

29. Kosaka N, Iguchi H, Yoshioka Y, Takeshita F, Matsuki Y, et al. (2010) Secretory mechanisms and intercellular transfer of microRNAs in living cells. J Biol Chem 285: 17442–17452.

30. Kosaka N, Iguchi H, Hagiwara K, Yoshioka Y, Takeshita F, et al. (2013) Neutral sphingomyelinase 2 (nSMase2)-dependent exosomal transfer of angiogenic microRNAs regulate cancer cell metastasis. J Biol Chem 288: 10849–10859.

15

Host Genetic Factors Associated with Symptomatic Primary HIV Infection and Disease Progression among Argentinean Seroconverters

Romina Soledad Coloccini[1], **Dario Dilernia**[1], **Yanina Ghiglione**[1], **Gabriela Turk**[1], **Natalia Laufer**[1,2], **Andrea Rubio**[1], **María Eugenia Socías**[2,3], **María Inés Figueroa**[2,3], **Omar Sued**[2,3], **Pedro Cahn**[2,3], **Horacio Salomón**[1], **Andrea Mangano**[4], **María Ángeles Pando**[1]*

1 Instituto de Investigaciones Biomédicas en Retrovirus y SIDA (INBIRS), Universidad de Buenos Aires-CONICET, Buenos Aires, Argentina, 2 Hospital Juan A. Fernandez, Buenos Aires, Argentina, 3 Fundación Huésped, Buenos Aires, Argentina, 4 Laboratorio de Biología Celular y Retrovirus, CONICET, Hospital de Pediatría "Prof. Dr. Juan P. Garrahan", Buenos Aires, Argentina

Abstract

Background: Variants in HIV-coreceptor C-C chemokine receptor type 5 (CCR5) and Human leukocyte antigen (HLA) genes are the most important host genetic factors associated with HIV infection and disease progression. Our aim was to analyze the association of these genetic factors in the presence of clinical symptoms during Primary HIV Infection (PHI) and disease progression within the first year.

Methods: Seventy subjects diagnosed during PHI were studied (55 symptomatic and 15 asymptomatic). Viral load (VL) and CD4 T-cell count were evaluated. HIV progression was defined by presence of B or C events and/or CD4 T-cell counts < 350 cell/mm^3. CCR5 haplotypes were characterized by polymerase chain reaction and SDM-PCR-RFLP. HLA-I characterization was performed by Sequencing.

Results: Symptoms during PHI were significantly associated with lower frequency of CCR5-CF1 (1.8% vs. 26.7%, p = 0.006). Rapid progression was significantly associated with higher frequency of CCR5-CF2 (16.7% vs. 0%, p = 0.024) and HLA-A*11 (16.7% vs. 1.2%, p = 0.003) and lower frequency of HLA-C*3 (2.8% vs. 17.5%, p = 0.035). Higher baseline VL was significantly associated with presence of HLA-A*11, HLA-A*24, and absence of HLA-A*31 and HLA-B*57. Higher 6-month VL was significantly associated with presence of CCR5-HHE, HLA-A*24, HLA-B*53, and absence of HLA-A*31 and CCR5-CF1. Lower baseline CD4 T-cell count was significantly associated with presence of HLA-A*24/*33, HLA-B*53, CCR5-CF2 and absence of HLA-A*01/*23 and CCR5-HHA. Lower 6-month CD4 T-cell count was associated with presence of HLA-A*24 and HLA-B*53, and absence of HLA-A*01 and HLA-B*07/*39. Moreover, lower 12-month CD4 T-cell count was significantly associated with presence of HLA-A*33, HLA-B*14, HLA-C*08, CCR5-CF2, and absence of HLA-B*07 and HLA-C*07.

Conclusion: Several host factors were significantly associated with disease progression in PHI subjects. Most results agree with previous studies performed in other groups. However, some genetic factor associations are being described for the first time, highlighting the importance of genetic studies at a local level.

Editor: Srinivas Mummidi, South Texas Veterans Health Care System and University of Texas Health Science Center at San Antonio, United States of America

Funding: This research was funded by grants from: Agencia Nacional de Promoción Científica y Tecnológica (grant number 2008-0559), "Fundación Florencio Fiorini" (period: 2009–2010), UBACYT (period: 2010–2012) and CONICET (PIP 2011–2013). The funders had no role in study design, data collection and analysis, decision to publish, or preparation of the manuscript.

* Email: mpando@fmed.uba.ar

Introduction

Research studies on primary HIV infection (PHI) are increasing worldwide to better understand the natural history of HIV infection and to identify the most important disease prognostic markers. As most of these studies were performed in other countries and due to genetic differences in the circulating virus and in the host, local studies are needed to better understand the particular characteristics of HIV infection dynamics [1].

In Argentina, an estimated 110,000 persons live with HIV (approximately 5,000 new cases per year) [2]. The first multicenter follow-up study of PHI (*Grupo Argentino de Seroconversión*) started in 2008. Retrospective and prospective data analyses allowed identifying factors associated with disease progression among untreated subjects. Symptomatic PHI, high VL (≥100,000

RNA copies/ml) or low CD4 T-cell count (≤ 350 cell/mm^3) at baseline were identified as relevant factors for faster progression during the first year follow-up [3]. Data comparisons with other PHI cohorts revealed that VL at baseline in the Argentinean cohort was higher than those found in developed countries [4–5], closer to African and Asian levels [6–7]. Globally, 50–90% of subjects diagnosed during PHI are symptomatic [8–10], reaching 74% in the mentioned Argentinean cohort [3].

Previous studies demonstrated extensive variability in host susceptibility to HIV infection and disease progression [11–13]. Several host genetic factors affecting HIV infection and pathogenesis were identified, like chemokine receptors and HLA alleles [14–17]. Multiple variations were described in the CCR5 gene, in particular the 32 base-pair deletion (CCR5-Δ32). This deletion provides protection against HIV-1 infection with CCR5 tropic viruses in homozygotes and delays progression in heterozygous subjects [16,18–19]. Seven Single Nucleotide Polymorphisms (SNPs) were defined in the cis-regulatory region between −2761 and −1835 of the CCR5 gene: −2733, −2554, −2459, −2135, −2132, −2086 and −1835 (GenBank accession number AF031236 and AF031237) [20]. Based on these variations and on the CCR2-V64I polymorphism, nine polymorphisms, called CCR5 Human Haplotypes (HH)-A, -B, -C, -D, -E, -F (F*1 and F*2), and –G (G*1 and G*2) were defined [15,20–21]. One of the largest studies in the subject demonstrated that the frequency and effect of CCR5-HH differ among different ethnic groups. CCR5-HHA was associated with disease retardation among African-Americans, whereas CCR5-HHC did so among European-Americans. In the same study, specific sequences of CCR5-HHE were associated with higher transcriptional activity, surface expression and HIV/AIDS susceptibility [21]. Another factor associated with disease progression is the dose of the gene encoding CCL3L1 (MIP-1α), a natural ligand of CCR5. A previous study found an association between lower gene dose and disease progression, and this susceptibility is even greater in individuals with CCR5 genotypes associated with disease progression [22].

The HLA system has an impact on several aspects of HIV infection such as transmission, progression and therapeutic response [23–24]. HLA class I molecules are involved in peptide presentation to CD8 cytotoxic T lymphocytes (CTLs), which play a key role in reducing viral replication. HIV specific CD8 T-cell response emerges along with the control of viremia and resolution of clinical symptoms, which varies from person to person and constitutes a strong predictor of disease progression [25–26]. Heterozygosis at HLA class I region is considered to be a selective advantage because those individuals are able to present a greater range of antigenic peptides to CTLs than homozygotes, deferring the emergence of escape mutants and prolonging the period before the development of AIDS [18]. Even when several HLA alleles were associated with disease progression, HLA-B*27 and HLA-B*57 alleles showed a particularly strong association with delayed progression [27] and HLA-B*35 and HLA-B*53 with acceleration to AIDS [28].

Based on the effects of host genetic variations described on HIV disease progression, our aim was to analyze the association of CCR5/CCL3L1 system and HLA in the presence of clinical symptoms during PHI and disease progression within the first year post-infection.

Materials and Methods

Study population

A group of 70 individuals recruited through 2008–2012 was studied. Inclusion criteria for enrolment in the cohort were: >16 years old at first evaluation, PHI confirmed diagnosis, and first medical and laboratory evaluation (i.e., CD4 T-cell count and plasma HIV RNA) within six months of the probable date of infection. Primary HIV infection is defined as: (1) detection of HIV RNA or p24 antigen with a simultaneous negative or indeterminate Western blot assay [12]; or (2) positive Western blot with a negative test within the previous six months. Hence, it includes both acute and recently infected patients [3].

In this study, PHI was defined as symptomatic if one or more of the following symptoms, associated with acute retroviral syndrome, were present: fever, rash, lymphadenopathy, headache, oral ulcers, dysphagia or pharyngitis. Disease progression was defined by clinical B or C events (according to the Centers for Disease Control and Prevention 1993 classification [29]) and/or CD4 T-cell count <350 cells/mm^3 within the first year of infection [3].

Ethics Statement

International and national ethical guidelines for biomedical research involving human subjects were followed. This research study was reviewed and approved by a local Institutional Review Board (IRB), "Fundación Huésped" and was conducted in compliance with all federal regulations governing the protection of human subjects. All potential participants signed an informed consent prior to entering the study.

Study Procedure

Once subjects were identified as PHI, they were included in the cohort. Subjects were evaluated at the time of diagnosis (baseline), at 6 months and at one year. On each visit, HIV plasma VL (branched-DNA, Versant HIV-1 RNA 3.0 assay, Siemmens Healthcare, USA), CD4 T-cell count (flow cytometry double platform, BD FACSCanto, BD Biosciences, USA), and clinical information were updated.

Study samples

Peripheral blood samples were obtained on each visit. Whole blood samples or peripheral blood mononuclear cells (PBMC) were used for DNA extraction using QIAmp DNA Blood Mini Kit (QIAGEN GmbH, Hilden, Germany). Plasma samples from the first visit after HIV diagnosis were used for lipopolysaccharide (LPS) quantification (Limulus Amebocyte Lysate test, LAL assay, QCL-1000, Lonza, DK). HIV tropism was determined by sequencing a region of V3 loop from env gene (HXB2) [30]. Viral DNA was amplified in duplicate by nested PCR and amplicons were sequenced by Big Dye Terminator Kit (Amersham, Sweden). Viral tropism was inferred from Geno2Pheno algorithm (http://coreceptor.bioinf.mpi-inf.mpg.de/index.php) using a false positive rate of 10%.

CCR5 and CCL3L1 characterization

CCR5-Δ32 deletion was identified by differences in PCR products size. CCR2 genotypes and Single Nucleotide Polymorphisms (SNPs) of the CCR5 gene corresponding to positions 29, 208, 627, 630, 676 and 927 (Genbank accession number: AF031236 and AF031237) [31] were determined with Site Directed Mutagenesis-PCR-Restriction Fragment Length Polymorphism (SDM-PCR-RFLP) assay. Primers used in each determination, PCR cycling condition and RFLP assay were reported previously [15,21,32–33]. Haplotype classification (HHA, HHB, HHC, HHD, HHE, HHF*1, HHF*2, HHG*1 and HHG*2) was determined as reported previously [15,20–21]. CCL3L1 Copy Number (CN) was determined by Taqman real-time PCR [22].

HLA characterization

HLA class I characterization was performed by sequencing-based typing (SBT). HLA-A exons 2 and 3 were amplified together. HLA-B and HLA-C exons 2 and 3 were amplified separately as reported in Table S1 and Figure S1 [34–36]. Amplicons were sequenced using the Big Dye Terminator sequencing kit (Amersham, Sweden) [36]. Sequence interpretation was performed using the NCBI SBT Interpretation software (http://www.ncbi.nlm.nih.gov/gv/mhc/sbt.cgi?cmd=main).

Genetic score

Additive genetic score was used to compile host genetic information [37]. In our model, alleles with a previous reported protective effect were added, and risk alleles were subtracted. For CCR5 polymorphisms, Δ32 and CCR2-64I alleles were considered as protective (1) [21]. Regarding CCR5 genotypes, HHC/HHF*2 and HHC/HHG*2 were considered as protective (1), HHC/HHE, HHE/HHE and HHE/HHG*2 as deleterious (–1), and the others as neutral (0) [21,32]. Two CCL3L1 cpg (mean in the Argentinean population) were considered as neutral (0). Lower CCL3L1 CN than the mean was considered as deleterious (–1) and higher CN as protective (1) [22]. HLA-A*02, HLA-A*32, HLA-A*68, HLA-B*15, HLA-B*13, HLA-B*27, HLA-B*32, HLA-B*39, HLA-B*44, HLA-B*51 and HLA-B*57 were considered as protective (1). HLA-A*11, HLA-A*23, HLA-A*24, HLA-B*08, HLA-B*35, HLA-B*53, HLA-C*04 and HLA-C*07 were considered as deleterious (–1). Other HLA alleles were considered as neutral (0) [11–13,23–24,27–28,37–39]. Heterozygosis for HLA was considered as protective (1) and homozygosis as deleterious (–1) [18].

Statistical analysis

Baseline characteristics were described using mean or medians and standard deviation or interquartile ranges [IQRs] for continuous variables respectively, and counts and percentages for categorical data. Chi-square test or Fisher's exact test were used to compare proportions. Differences among continuous variables were analyzed using Student's t-test or Wilcoxon test. Spearman correlation was calculated for genetic score and HIV viral load and CD4 T-cell count (baseline and follow up). All p values were two-sided; p values<0.05 were considered to be statistically significant. Lack of complete data values in table is expressed in numbers. Data analysis was performed using SPSS 15.0, 2007 (Chicago, Illinois).

Results

Characteristics of the study population

We studied 70 HIV-infected adults diagnosed during primary HIV infection (PHI) (49 men and 21 women), 55 were symptomatic and 15 asymptomatic. Sixty of them were also classified according to disease progression within the first year post diagnosis, 18 progressed and 42 did not. Most PHI subjects were recruited during Fiebig stages V and VI [40]. Sexual transmission was reported as the main route: all the women reported heterosexual transmission whereas 82.2% of men reported sexual relationship with other men as the probably route of acquisition of the virus. All subjects were from Buenos Aires City and surrounding areas. The population of this area is mostly descendent from South Europe [41]. Median HIV VL at diagnosis was 61862 RNA copies/ml, whit significantly higher VL in those who presented symptoms and those who progressed (Table 1). The same trend was observed for VL at 6 months. Baseline CD4 T-cell count was 514 cells/mm^3 without statistical differences between symptomatic and asymptomatic subjects. Significantly higher CD4 T-cell counts (baseline, 6 and 12 months) were observed among subjects who did not progress to disease during the first year (Table 1).

Frequency of CCR5 haplotypes/genotypes and CCL3L1

Similar to the results found in Argentinean children exposed perinatally to HIV (including both HIV infected and not infected) [42] and blood donors [43], the most frequent CCR5 haplotypes in the PHI group were HHE (36.4%) and HHC (30.7%). Frequencies of all the other haplotypes were lower than 10% (Figure 1; Table S2). Regarding CCR5 genotypes, HHC/HHE (21.4%) and HHE/HHE (12.9%) were the most commonly found. Other genotypes were present with frequencies lower than 10% (Table 2 and Table S3). The CCL3L1 gene copy number, one of the main ligands of CCR5, was evaluated in 50 PHI subjects with a median of two copies (IQR25-75, 1–4), as reported in persons of European origin [22].

Frequency of HLA variants

Given the essential role of CTL responses during PHI as well as the description of a strong association among certain HLA-I alleles with virus control, HLA-I frequencies were studied in this cohort finding 17 HLA-A, 27 HLA-B and 14 HLA-C different alleles. The HLA-A alleles most frequently found were HLA-A*02 (27.2%) and HLA-A*24 (12.5%). In HLA-B locus, HLA-B*35 (15.6%) and HLA-B*44 (12.9%) were the most frequent. In HLA-C, HLA-C*07 (27.9%), HLA-C*04 (16.2%) and HLA-C*03 (11.8%) were the most frequent. Other HLA-A, B and C alleles showed frequencies lower than 10% (Table S4). HLA class I alleles were found in homozygosis in the following frequencies: 32.4% for HLA-A, 3.0% for HLA-B and 17.6% for HLA-C (Table S5). The most common combinations for HLA-A were A*02-A*02 (11.8%) and A*02-A*68 (8.8%), for HLA-B were B*15-B*35 (4.5%) and B*35-B*44 (4.5%), and for HLA-C, C*04-C*07 (8.8%), C*07-C*07 (8.8%) and C*03-C*07 (7.4%) (data not shown).

Influence of CCR5 haplotypes/genotypes, CCL3L1 copy number, and HLA variants on symptoms present during acute HIV infection

In order to identify individual host genetic determinants of early HIV disease progression, the PHI cohort was stratified according to the presence/absence of symptoms during the seroconversion period. Regarding the CCR5 coreceptor, HHC was overrepresented (40% vs. 28.2%) and HHE (23.3% vs. 40%) was less frequent in asymptomatic as compared to symptomatic subjects, however without statistical significance (Figure 1). Concerning CCR5 genotypes, HHC/HHF*1 was detected in a significantly higher percentage among asymptomatic subjects (26.7% vs. 1.8%, p = 0.006). Even when it was not statistically significant, genotype HHE/HHF*1 was only found among symptomatic subjects (10.9%) (Table 2 and Table S3). No significant differences were found in the CCL3L1 copy number, even when a higher copy number was detected among asymptomatic (median (IQR25-75); 3 (2–3) and 2 (1–4), respectively). No influence of HLA-A, -B and -C alleles was detected in the presence of symptoms during PHI (Table S4). Likewise, no influence of HLA homozygosis was

Table 1. HIV viral load and CD4 T-cell count of the study population diagnosed during primary HIV infection [PHI] (N = 70).

		Symptomatic PHI		p	Progressor at one year		p	All (N = 70)
		Yes (N = 55)	No (N = 15)		Yes (N = 18)	No (N = 42)		
HIV RNA median copies/ml (IQR)	Baseline	77,080	7,024	**0.003**	193,601	41,402	**0.003**	61,862
		(30,449–386,715)	(2,699–76,466)		(80,545–500,000)	(10,409–154,476)		(17,050–257,524)
	6 month	66,002	9,018	**0.004**	166,812	33,508	**0.001**	40,231
		(17,959–178,030)	(3,820–34,624)		(47,167–321,018)	(8,578–73,231)		(117,17–165,238)
CD4 T-cell count median cells/mm³ (IQR)	Baseline	502	587	0.322	306	602	**<0.001**	514
		(356–649)	(416–876)		(237–346)	(500–741)		(387–671)
	6 month	499	555	0.694	323	602	**<0.001**	503
		(356–665)	(424–665)		(172–386)	(488–690)		(404–65)
	12 month	491	534	0.296	330	534	**0.001**	501
		(389–615)	(436–672)		(289–504)	(435–643)		(400–619)

PHI: primary HIV infection. IQR: interquartile range. Statistically significant p values are in bold.

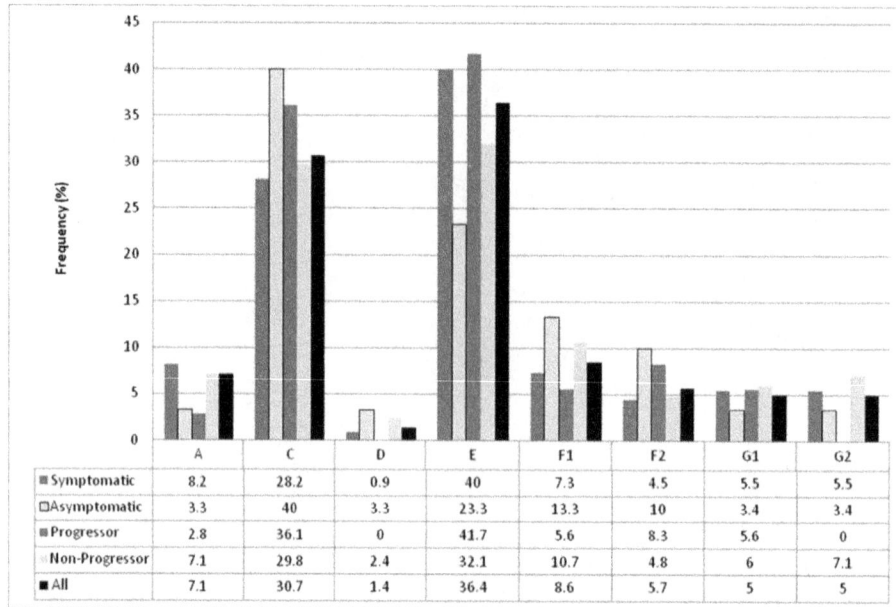

Figure 1. Frequency of CCR5 haplotypes of the study population diagnosed during primary HIV infection [PHI] (N = 70). Full information is available on supplementary material (Table S1).

observed in the presence of symptoms during seroconversion (Table S5). When HLA pairs were compared, HLA-B*35-B*44 was found in a significantly higher frequency among asymptomatic subjects (21.4% vs. 0%, p = 0.007) (data not shown).

Only CCR5 genotypes with a frequency higher than 10% in some of the study groups were included in the table. No significant differences were observed among CCR5 genotypes with frequencies lower than 10%. Full information is on supplementary material (Table S2).

Influence of CCR5 haplotypes/genotypes, CCL3L1 and HLA variants on disease progression within the first year

Additionally, the PHI group was analyzed in order to identify possible genetic factors that might influence the rate of progression within the first year. Several CCR5 haplotypes were most frequently detected in individuals who did not progress (e.g. HHA, HHF*1 and HHG*2) and HHF*2 was most represented in subjects who progressed to disease (Table S2), without statistical differences. Regarding CCR5 genotypes, HHC/HHF*2 was significantly associated with progression (p = 0.024) and a higher, but not significant proportion of subject who progress had HHE/HHE also as compared with those who do not progress (22.2% vs. 7.1%) (Table S3). Regarding HLA alleles, a strong association was found between disease progression and higher frequency of HLA-A*11 (16.7% vs. 1.2%, p = 0.003) and lower frequency of HLA-C*03 (17.5% vs. 2.8%, p = 0.035) (Table S4). No influence of HLA homozygosis was observed in disease progression (Table S5).

Influence of CCR5 haplotypes/genotypes, CCL3L1 and HLA variants on plasma HIV viral load and CD4 T-cell count

As the CD4 T-cell count and HIV plasma VL are good predictors of disease progression [3], the association of these parameters with host genetic factors was also analyzed. Subjects with CCR5 HHE haplotype had higher VL after 6 months

(66,001 copies/ml vs. 31,718 copies/ml, p = 0.039) and also higher baseline VL (98,684 copies/ml vs. 41,402 copies/ml, p = 0.082). On the other hand, HHA was found to be associated with higher baseline CD4 T-cell levels (656 cells/mm^3 vs. 499 cells/mm^3, p = 0.044). Regarding CCR5 genotypes, HHC/HHF*1 was associated with lower VL (6,243 copies/ml vs. 53,997 copies/ml, p = 0.027) and HHC/HHF*2 with lower CD4 T-cell levels at baseline (379 cells/mm^3 vs. 545 cells/mm^3, p = 0.046), at 6 months (355 cells/mm^3 vs. 531 cells/mm^3, p = 0.024) and at 12 months (290 cells/mm^3 vs. 510 cells/mm^3, p = 0.034).

Concerning the HLA influence on CD4 T-cell count and HIV plasma VL, the presence of several alleles was found to be beneficial for HIV subjects, with an association with higher CD4 T-cell count (HLA-A*01, HLA-A*23, HLA-B*07, HLA-B*39 and HLA-C*07) or lower HIV plasma VL (HLA-A*31 and HLA-B*57). Conversely, some alleles were found to be detrimental for subjects, with an association with higher HIV plasma VL (HLA-A*11, HLA-A*24 and HLA-B*53) or lower CD4 T-cell count (HLA-A*24, HLA-A*33, HLA-B*14, HLA-B*53 and HLA-C*08) (Table 3).

Additive genetic score

Additive genetic score was calculated for each subject and average values were calculated considering symptoms during PHI (2.6 for asymptomatic and 1.4 for symptomatic subjects) and disease progression within the first year (1.8 for those who did not progress and 0.6 for those who progressed). Subjects were grouped according to both characteristics: Group 1: Asymptomatic/Non-progressors, Group 2: Asymptomatic/Progressors and Symptomatic/Non-progressors, and Group 3: Symptomatic/Progressors. Mean genetic score was: 2.8, 1.6 and 0.5 for groups 1, 2 and 3, respectively. Correlation analyses revealed a significant negative correlation between genetic score and HIV viral load at baseline (p = 0.008) (Figure 2). No significant association was observed between genetic score and CD4 T-cells count.

Table 2. Frequency of CCR5 human genotypes of the study population diagnosed during primary HIV infection [PHI] (N = 70).

Genotype	Symptomatic PHI			Progressor at one year			All (N = 70)
	Yes (N = 55)*	No (N = 15)*	p	Yes (N = 18)*	No (N = 42)*	p	
HHC/HHC	2 (3.6)	1 (6.7)	0.521	2 (11.1)	1 (2.4)	0.212	3 (4.3)
HHC/HHE	12 (21.8)	3 (20)	1.000	4 (22.2)	9 (21.4)	1.000	15 (21.4)
HHC/HHF*1	1 (1.8)	4 (26.7)	0.006	1 (5.6)	4 (9.5)	1.000	5 (7.1)
HHC/HHF*2	3 (5.5)	1 (6.7)	1.000	3 (16.7)	0	0.024	4 (5.7)
HHC/HHG*1	5 (9.1)	1 (6.7)	1.000	1 (5.6)	5 (11.9)	0.658	6 (8.6)
HHE/HHE	8 (14.5)	1 (6.7)	0.672	4 (22.2)	3 (7.1)	0.220	9 (12.9)
HHE/HHF*1	6 (10.9)	0	0.329	1 (5.6)	4 (9.5)	1.000	6 (8.6)

*Data are no. (%) of CCR5 haplotypes.

Complementary studies

HIV infection has been associated with disruption of mucosal barrier and CD4 T-cell depletion in the gastrointestinal tract. This damage is caused, at least in part, by increased translocation of microbial products, mainly lipopolysaccharides (LPS), a major component of gram-negative bacterial cell walls [44–46]. Since immune activation is a good predictor of disease progression, plasma LPS levels were determined in the baseline sample of 65 individuals finding a median of 39.0 pg/ml (IQR25-75, 26.7–56.8) with significantly higher levels in the symptomatic than the asymptomatic group (43.5 pg/ml vs. 29.0 pg/ml, p = 0.040). No association was found among LPS levels, disease progression, CD4 T-cell count, HIV VL or host genetic factors. HIV tropism was determined given that the presence of X4 tropic viruses was associated with a more rapid disease progression (data not shown). Fourteen out of 59 (23.7%) PHI subjects presented X4 tropic HIV variants. Even when no statistically significant differences were observed, X4 tropic HIV variants were overrepresented among symptomatic subjects (26.1% vs. 15.4%, p = 0.713). No differences were observed among HIV tropism, disease progression, CD4 T-cell count or HIV VL.

Discussion

Other countries reported associations between human genes and HIV susceptibility. However, local studies are needed considering differences in genetic background [14,17,19]. In line with this, for the first time in Argentina, this study reports several human genes associated with early HIV disease progression among adults.

Buenos Aires population is mainly descendant of Southern Europe. The frequency of CCR5 haplotypes reported here correlates with reports in Hispanic and other Argentinean groups [21,43], with HHE and HHC being the most common haplotypes. Regarding CCR5 genotypes, the most common were HHC/HHE and HHE/HHE, with other genotypes having frequencies lower than 10%. In comparison with blood donors, PHI individuals were found to have a higher but not significant frequency of HHE/HHE genotype (5.9% vs. 12.9% respectively). This result is consistent with previous reports evidencing an association between presence of HHE/HHE genotype and enhancement of HIV infection [21,42]. Even when the HHE haplotype and the HHE/HHE genotype were overrepresented among symptomatic subjects and those who progressed, no significant associations were observed, maybe due to sample size. Data on HIV VL also supports the same trend with significantly higher VL at 6 months among subjects carrying HHE. This trend is in line with previous studies that associated disease progression with HHE [21,42]. However, this disease-modified effect was not observed among other ethnic groups (i.e., Africans) where the frequency of HHE haplotype was much lower (~10%) [21]. As HHE is the most frequent CCR5 haplotype in our cohort, the potential adverse effect of this haplotype deserves special attention.

HHC/HHF*1 genotype was associated with asymptomatic PHI and HHC/HHF*2 with disease progression. In line with these results, we found that the HHC/HHF*1 genotype was associated with lower levels of VL and HHC/HHF*2, with lower CD4 T-cell levels at baseline and during one-year follow-up. Only few studies support these findings, maybe due to the fact that these genotypes were found in low frequency in most cohorts [21,42]. One of the most important studies in the subject found a disease accelerating effect for HHC/HHF*1 among African Americans [21]. However, this study also reports that the effect of HHC haplotypes on HIV disease differed among ethnic groups. While the HHC

Table 3. HIV viral load and CD4 T-cell count of the study population diagnosed during primary HIV infection [PHI] according to HLA alleles (N = 70).

Alleles		CD4 T-cell count			HIV RNA	
		median cells/mm^3			median copies/ml	
		Baseline	6 months	12 months	Baseline	6 months
HLA-A*01	Yes	902	810	716	5160	4298
	No	500	499	491	64045	40083
	p	**0.022**	**0.019**	0.112	0.241	0.317
HLA-A*11	Yes	347	344	475	477708	166930
	No	525	517	492	52352	38270
	p	0.070	0.071	0.447	**0.020**	0.059
HLA-A*23	Yes	736	637	534	36101	24322
	No	499	497	475	61862	40232
	p	**0.038**	0.072	0.195	0.374	0.290
HLA-A*24	Yes	393	403	483	500000	89517
	No	576	545	500	41402	30591
	p	**0.049**	**0.048**	0.371	**0.001**	**0.004**
HLA-A*31	Yes	602	563	612	24654	19603
	No	502	502	491	67397	56594
	p	0.494	0.616	0.883	**0.032**	**0.038**
HLA-A*33	Yes	387	387	347	67660	67660
	No	535	528	515	55276	39484
	p	**0.046**	0.100	**0.021**	0.818	1.00
HLA-B*07	Yes	535	818	679	378025	133268
	No	525	499	474	52352	38720
	p	0.972	**0.015**	**0.005**	0.177	0.280
HLA-B*14	Yes	466	485	410	213099	117061
	No	575	542	534	52352	37506
	p	0.167	0.135	**0.002**	0.229	0.260
HLA-B*39	Yes	644	780	573	4383	18062
	No	509	497	483	62679	42753
	p	0.098	**0.027**	0.175	0.073	0.085
HLA-B*53	Yes	288	248	286	500000	349244
	No	545	531	509	54286	39033
	p	**0.046**	**0.036**	0.117	0.058	**0.028**
HLA-B*57	Yes	525	495	654	16926	12971
	No	529	528	492	66821	47077
	p	0.819	0.865	0.272	**0.046**	0.058
HLA-C*07	Yes	525	527	534	66821	60546
	No	497	491	449	62679	40083
	p	0.738	0.527	**0.038**	0.584	0.563
HLA-C*08	Yes	437	499	409	184000	163664
	No	519	499	533	61045	40083
	p	0.290	0.200	**0.001**	0.443	0.286

haplotype in African Americans was associated with disease acceleration, in Caucasians and Hispanics it was associated with disease retardation. Regarding the HHF*2 haplotype, a previous report found similar results in individuals carrying the allele with lower CD4 T-cell counts during follow-up [47]. However, these results disagree with previous studies that observed a protective effect against disease progression among subjects carrying the CCR2-64I allele [33]. HHC/HHF*2 genotype was also associated with disease retardation among Argentinean children [42]. Even when no statistically significant association was established, the

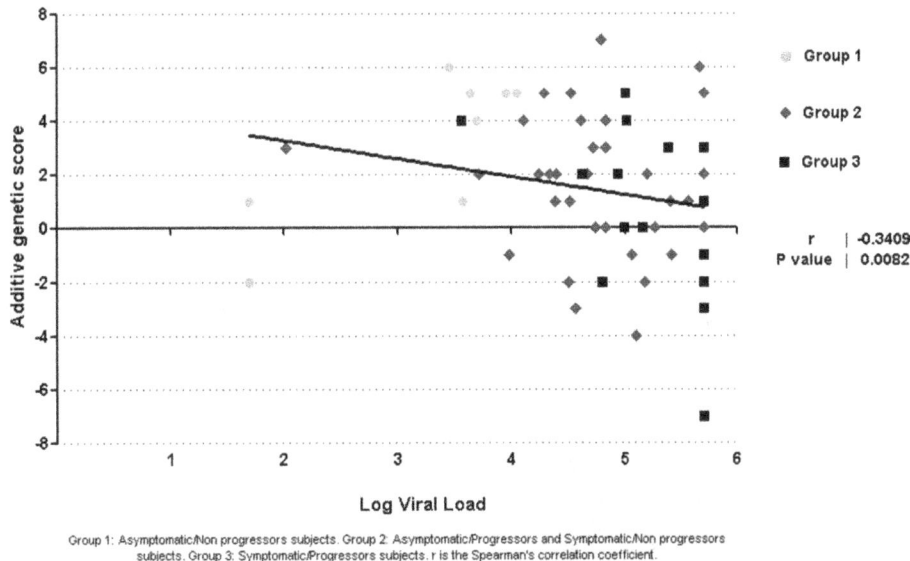

Group 1: Asymptomatic/Non progressors subjects. Group 2: Asymptomatic/Progressors and Symptomatic/Non progressors subjects. Group 3: Symptomatic/Progressors subjects. r is the Spearman's correlation coefficient.

Figure 2. Correlation between baseline HIV viral load and additive genetic score on the study population diagnosed during primary HIV infection [PHI] (N = 70).

CCR5 genotype HHE/HHF*1 was only detected among symptomatic subjects in more than 10% of the group. CCL3L1 copy number distribution in PHI population was similar to that observed in the European population [22] with a median of two copies. Even when no significant differences were observed, asymptomatic individuals had a higher copy number, maybe suggesting that CCL3L1 would have an impact since the HIV infection onset.

Identifying HLA alleles associations with HIV disease progression is complex due to the extreme variability of the loci. In fact, this study identifies 17, 27 and 14 HLA-A, B and C alleles, respectively. Coincident with previous reports, including our blood donors group, the alleles most frequently reported here were HLA-A*02 and HLA-*24, HLA-B*35 and HLA-B*44, and HLA-C*07, HLA-C*04 and HLA-C*03 [41]. Even when it was proposed that heterozygosis on HLA confers advantages on disease progression revealing a greater variety of the immune response [18,48–49], no significant differences in disease progression were detected between heterozygotes and homozygotes at any individual HLA locus or homozygosis at one, two, or all three class I loci.

Several HLA alleles identified in our study were associated with disease progression. Our results adds more evidence to the protective effect of HLA-B*57 allele on disease progression [23], with significantly lower VL at baseline and also lower, but not significant, VL at 6 months. Moreover, the allele was only found among those who did not progress. Even when HLA-B*57 was previously associated with the absence of symptoms during seroconversion, our study failed to confirm these findings [50]. Regarding HLA-B*27, reported as a protective allele [50], we did not observe this trend or evidence, likely due to the low frequency found (1.5% among HIV positive and 2.0% among blood donors). Another HLA allele, several times associated with disease progression is HLA-B*35 [18,23]. However, our study did not find any statistical association or trend even when the frequency of the allele was around 15% in the overall group.

HLA-A*11 was associated with disease progression during the first year and with higher VL at baseline. We also found a trend in the presence of the allele and higher HIV VL at 6 months and

lower CD4 T-cell counts at baseline and during follow-up. These results agree with a previous study that found a higher frequency of HLA-A*1101 among subjects with AIDS compared with other HIV subjects who did not progress [51]. Even when this study performed high resolution HLA-typing, in contrast to our low resolution data, it is important to mention that typing studies reported that most of the typed HLA-A*11 are HLA-A*1101 [41,52].

HLA-B*53 was associated with lower CD4 T-cell counts and higher HIV VL levels, even when only two subjects carried that allele. Elevated VL levels among subjects with HLA-B*53 were previously observed among African seroconverters [53]. Although only few subjects carried the HLA-B*53, the potential impact of this allele on disease progression may deserve more investigation. Another interesting allele is HLA-A*24, associated with lower CD4 T-cell counts and higher VL levels at baseline and during follow-up. This allele frequency was also higher (but not significant) among subjects who presented symptoms during seroconversion as compared with those without them. Previous studies also found a deleterious effect of this allele, enhancing HIV infection [54], showing rapid decline in CD4 T-cells [27] and favouring disease progression [55]. HLA-B*39 confers a beneficial effect on disease evolution yielding high CD4 T-cell counts and low VL levels [16,55]. We also observed a trend in higher frequency of HLA-B*39 among asymptomatic vs. symptomatic (10.7% vs. 2.9%) subjects. Controversial results were found in other alleles. While our study suggests that subjects with HLA-B*14 (with significantly lower CD4 T-cell counts at 12 months and a trend of lower levels of CD4 T-cells at baseline and at 6 months and higher VL) progressed faster to disease, others found significant associations between allele and low disease progression [56] and that the allele had enhanced HIV infection [57].

Previous studies showed that plasma LPS levels among subjects with acute HIV infection were similar to non-infected subjects [58]. In fact, our study found similar levels in the PHI group (39.0 pg/ml) and a group of HIV-negative subjects (37.4 pg/ml, data not shown). However, we found that higher plasma LPS levels are significantly associated with presence of symptoms during PHI.

These results suggest higher immune activation in symptomatic subjects since the establishment of infection.

An important limitation of the current research was the low frequency of asymptomatic subjects included due to the difficulty in identifying them during the seroconversion period. The lack of progression data in a group of patients also influenced the possibility of finding significant associations. It is also important to note the difficulty in finding associations when genetic variants are in low frequency. Given these limitations, a score was constructed in order to combine some of the most important human genetic factors previously associated with HIV/AIDS and to look for associations with presence of symptoms, disease progression and other progression markers like HIV viral load and CD4 T-cell count. Results reveal a higher score in asymptomatic and those who did not progress, revealing the presence of more protective genetic factors in these groups. Even more, when data were analysed considering both variables (symptoms and progression) a higher score was observed for those who did not present symptoms during PHI and did not progress at one year. As described by other authors, the genetic score was a useful tool to evaluate the additive influence of human genetic factors with high variability on small groups [37].

Conclusions

This study reveals that some host genetic variants identified previously as disease-modifying factors influence disease progression from the very beginning of the HIV infection. However, here we also described some associations for the first time. Variability of host genetic factors as well as their association with HIV infection and/or disease progression relies strongly on the ethnic population background. Therefore, the population ethnicities are growing it is becoming increasingly difficult to extrapolate results from one study to other populations. In this context, it is important to highlight the need to perform studies at a in this setting not only these genetic differences in the population but also the environmental variance and the circulating virus.

Acknowledgments

We thank all the physicians of the "Grupo Argentino de Seroconversión" Study Group: Lorena Abusamra, Marcela Acosta, Carolina Acuipil, Viviana Alonso, Liliana Amante, Graciela Ben, M. Belén Bouzas, Ariel Braverman, Mercedes Cabrini, Pedro Cahn, Osvaldo Cando, Cecilia Cánepa, Daniel Cangelosi, Juan Castelli, Mariana Ceriotto, Carina Cesar, María Collins, Fabio Crudo, Darío Dilernia, Andrea Duarte, Gustavo Echenique, María I. Figueroa, Valeria Fink, Claudia Galloso, Palmira Garda, Manuel Gómez Carrillo, Ana Gun, Alejandro Krolewiecki, Natalia Laufer, María E. Lázaro, Alberto Leoni, Eliana Loiza, Patricia Maldonado, Horacio Mingrone, Marcela Ortiz, Patricia Patterson, Héctor Pérez, Norma Porteiro, Daniel Pryluka, Carlos Remondegui, Raúl Román, Horacio Salomón, M. Eugenia Socías, Omar Sued, J. Gonzalo Tomás, Gabriela Turk, Javier Yave, Carlos Zala, Inés Zapiola. Authors also thank Sergio Mazzini for assistance during manuscript preparation.

Author Contributions

Conceived and designed the experiments: RSC AM HS MAP. Performed the experiments: RSC DD YG GT AR. Analyzed the data: MAP RSC. Contributed to the writing of the manuscript: MAP AM RSC. Participants' recruitment: NL MES MIF OS PC.

References

1. Pilcher CD, Eron JJ Jr, Galvin S, Gay C, Cohen MS (2004) Acute HIV revisited: new opportunities for treatment and prevention. J Clin Invest 113: 937–945.
2. Boletín N°30 sobre VIH-sida e ITS en la Argentina (2013) Ministerio de Salud. Presidencia de la Nación. Available: http://www.msal.gov.ar/sida. Accessed 2014 July 3.
3. Socías ME, Sued O, Laufer N, Lázaro ME, Mingrone H, et al. (2011) Acute retroviral syndrome and high baseline VL are predictors of rapid HIV progression among untreated Argentinean seroconverters. J Int AIDS Soc: 14–40.
4. Hubert JB, Burgard M, Dussaix E, Tamalet C, Deveau C, et al. (2000) Natural history of serum HIV-1 RNA levels in 330 patients with a known date of infection. The SEROCO Study Group. AIDS 14: 123–131.
5. Lyles RH, Muñoz A, Yamashita TE, Bazmi H, Detels R, et al. (2000) Natural history of human immunodeficiency virus type 1 viremia after seroconversion and proximal to AIDS in a large cohort of homosexual men. Multicenter AIDS Cohort Study. J Infect Dis 181: 872–880.
6. Salamon R, Marimoutou C, Ekra D, Minga A, Nerrienet E, et al. (2002) Clinical and biological evolution of HIV-1 seroconverters in Abidjan, Côte d'Ivoire, 1997–2000. J Acquir Immune Defic Syndr 29: 149–157.
7. Buchacz K, Hu DJ, Vanichseni S, Mock PA, Chaowanachan T, et al. (2004) Early markers of HIV-1 disease progression in a prospective cohort of seroconverters in Bangkok, Thailand: implications for vaccine trials. J Acquir Immune Defic Syndr 36: 853–860.
8. Lavreys L, Thompson ML, Martin HL Jr, Mandaliya K, Ndinya-Achola JO, et al. (2000) Primary human immunodeficiency virus type 1 infection: clinical manifestations among women in Mombasa, Kenya. Clin Infect Dis 30: 486–490.
9. Hightow-Weidman LB, Golin CE, Green K, Shaw EN, MacDonald PD, et al. (2009) Identifying people with acute HIV infection: demographic features, risk factors, and use of health care among individuals with AHI in North Carolina. AIDS Behav 13: 1075–1083.
10. Richey LE, Halperin J (2013) Acute human immunodeficiency virus infection. Am J Med Sci 345: 136–142.
11. O'Brien SJ, Nelson GW (2004) Human genes that limit AIDS. Nat Genet 36: 565–574.
12. Smith MZ, Kent SJ (2005) Genetic influences on HIV infection: implications for vaccine development. Sex Health 2: 53–62.
13. Telenti A, Goldstein DB (2006) Genomics meets HIV-1. Nat Rev Microbiol 4: 865–873.
14. Marmor M, Hertzmark K, Thomas SM, Halkitis PN, Vogler M (2006) Resistance to HIV Infection. J Urban Health 83: 5–17.
15. Mummidi S, Ahuja SS, Gonzalez E, Anderson SA, Santiago EN, et al. (1998) Genealogy of the CCR5 locus and chemokine system gene variants associated with altered rates of HIV-1 disease progression. Nat Med 4: 786–793.
16. Tang J, Shelton B, Makhatadze NJ, Zhang Y, Schaen M, et al. (2002) Distribution of Chemokine Receptor CCR2 and CCR5 Genotypes and Their Relative Contribution to Human Immunodeficiency Virus Type 1 (HIV-1) Seroconversion, Early HIV-1 RNA Concentration in Plasma, and Later Disease Progression. J Virol 76: 662–672.

17. Telenti A, Bleiber G (2006) Host genetics of HIV-1 susceptibility. Future Virology 1: 55–70.
18. Carrington M, Dean M, Martin MP, O'Brien SJ (1999) Genetics of HIV-1 infection: chemokine receptor CCR5 polymorphism and its consequences. Human Molecular Genetics 8: 1939–1945.
19. Smith MZ, Kent SJ (2005) Genetic influence on HIV infection: implications for vaccine development. Sexual Health 2: 53–62.
20. Mummidi S, Bamshad M, Ahuja SS, Gonzalez E, Feuillet PM, et al. (2000) Evolution of human and nonhuman primate CC chemokine receptor 5 gene and mRNA. Potential roles for haplotype and mRNA diversity, differential haplotype-specific transcriptional activity and altered transcription factor binding to polymorphic nucleotides in the pathogenesis of HIV-1 and SIV. J Biol Chem 275: 18946–18961.
21. Gonzalez E, Bamshad M, Sato N, Mummidi S, Dhanda R, et al. (1999) Race-specific HIV-1 disease-modifying effects associated with CCR5 haplotypes. Proc Natl Acad Sci U S A 96: 12004–12009.
22. Gonzalez E, Kulkarni H, Bolivar H, Mangano A, Sanchez R, et al. (2005) The influence of CCL3L1 gene-containing segmental duplications on HIV-1/AIDS susceptibility. Science 307: 1434–1440.
23. Carrington M, O'Brien SJ (2003) The influence of HLA genotype on AIDS. Annu Rev Med 54: 535–551.
24. Goulder PJ, Walker BD (2012) HIV and HLA class I: an evolving relationship. Immunity 37: 426–440.
25. Borrow P, Lewicki H, Hahn BH, Shaw GM, Oldstone MB (1994) Virus-specific CD8+ cytotoxic T-lymphocyte activity associated with control of viremia in primary human immunodeficiency virus type 1 infection. J Virol 68: 6103–6110.
26. Koup RA, Safrit JT, Cao Y, Andrews CA, McLeod G, et al. (1994) Temporal association of cellular immune responses with the initial control of viremia in primary human immunodeficiency virus type 1 syndrome. J Virol 68: 4650–4655.
27. Kaslow RA, Carrington M, Apple R, Park L, Muñoz A, et al. (1996) Influence of combinations of human major histocompatibility complex genes on the course of HIV-1 infection. Nat Med 2: 405–411.
28. Gao X, Nelson GW, Karacki P, Martin MP, Phair J, et al. (2001) Effect of a single amino acid change in MHC class I molecules on the rate of progression to AIDS. N Engl J Med 344: 1668–1675.
29. 1993 revised classification system for HIV infection and expanded surveillance case definition for AIDS among adolescents and adults (1992) MMWR Recomm Rep 14: 1–19.
30. McGovern RA, Harrigan PR, Swenson LC (2010) Genotypic inference of HIV-1 tropism using population-based sequencing of V3. J Vis Exp 46: 2531.
31. Mummidi S, Ahuja SS, McDaniel BL, Ahuja SK (1997) The human CC chemokine receptor 5 (CCR5) gene. Multiple transcripts with 5'-end heterogeneity, dual promoter usage, and evidence for polymorphisms within the regulatory regions and noncoding exons. J Biol Chem 272: 30662–30671.
32. Mangano A, Kopka J, Batalla M, Bologna R, Sen L (2000) Protective Effect of CCR2-64I and Not of CCR5-Δ32 and SDF-1-3' in Pediatric HIV-1 infection. JAIDS 23: 52–57.
33. Smith MW, Dean M, Carrington M, Winkler C, Huttley GA, et al. (1997) Contrasting Genetic Influence of CCR2 and CCR5 Variants on HIV-1 Infection and Disease Progression. Science 277: 959–965.
34. Cereb N, Maye P, Lee S, Kong Y, Yang SY (1995) Locus-specific amplification of HLA class I genes from genomic DNA: locus-specific sequences in the first and third introns of HLA-A, -B, and -C alleles. Tissue Antigens 45: 1–11.
35. Hurley CK, Fernandez-Vina M, Hildebrand WH, Noreen HJ, Trachtenberg E, et al. (2007) A high degree of HLA disparity arises from limited allelic diversity: analysis of 1775 unrelated bone marrow transplant donor-recipient pairs. Hum Immunol 68: 30–40.
36. Dun PPJ, Day S (2001) Sequencing-Based Typing for HLA-A, B and C. International Histocompatibility Working Group (IHWG). Chapter 30 A, 1–5.
37. Casado C, Colombo S, Rauch A, Martínez R, Günthard HF, et al (2010) Host and viral genetic correlates of clinical definitions of HIV-1 disease progression. PLoS One 5: e11079.
38. Fellay J, Shianna KV, Ge D, Colombo S, Ledgerber B, et al. (2007) A whole-genome association study of major determinants for host control of HIV-1. Science 317: 944–947.
39. Fellay J, Ge D, Shianna KV, Colombo S, Ledgerber B, et al. (2009) Common genetic variation and the control of HIV-1 in humans. PLoS Genet 5: e1000791.
40. Fiebig EW, Wright DJ, Rawal BD, Garrett PE, Schumacher RT, et al. (2003) Dynamics of HIV viremia and antibody seroconversion in plasma donors: implications for diagnosis and staging of primary HIV infection. AIDS 17: 1871–1879.
41. Gonzalez-Galarza FF, Christmas S, Middleton D, Jones AR (2011) Allele frequency net: a database and online repository for immune gene frequencies in worldwide populations. Nucleic Acid Research 39: D913–D919.
42. Mangano A, Gonzalez E, Dhanda R, Catano G, Bamshad M, et al. (2001) Concordance between the CC chemokine Receptor 5 Genetic Determinants That Alter Risks of Transmission and Disease Progression in Children Exposed Perinatally to Human Immunodeficiency Virus. J Infect Dis 183: 1574–1585.
43. Rocco CA, Mangano A, del Pozo A, Sen L (2003) Distribution of CCR5-CCR2 haplotypes in an Argentinean population. AIDS Res Hum Retroviruses 19: 943–945.
44. Brenchley JM, Price DA, Schacker TW, Asher TE, Silvestri G, et al. (2006) Microbial translocation is a cause of systemic immune activation in chronic HIV infection. Nat Med 12: 1365–1371.
45. Hunt PW, Brenchley J, Sinclair E, McCune JM, Roland M, et al. (2008) Relationship between T cell activation and CD4+ T cell count in HIV-seropositive individuals with undetectable plasma HIV RNA levels in the absence of therapy. J Infect Dis 197: 126–133.
46. Tincati C, Bellistrì GM, Ancona G, Merlini E, d'Arminio Monforte A, et al. (2012) Role of in vitro stimulation with lipopolysaccharide on T-cell activation in HIV-infected antiretroviral-treated patients. Clin Dev Immunol 2012: 935425.
47. Nguyen L, Chaowanachan T, Vanichseni S, McNicholl JM, Mock PA, et al. (2004) Frequent human leukocyte antigen class I alleles are associated with higher viral load among HIV type 1 seroconverters in Thailand. J Acquir Immune Defic Syndr 37: 1318–1323.
48. Tang J, Rivers C, Karita E, Costello C, Allen S, et al. (1999) Allelic variants of human beta-chemokine receptor 5 (CCR5) promoter: evolutionary relationships and predictable associations with HIV-1 disease progression. Genes Immun 1: 20–27.
49. Naruto T, Gatanaga H, Nelson G, Sakai K, Carrington M, et al. (2012) HLA class I-mediated control of HIV-1 in the Japanese population, in which the protective HLA-B*57 and HLA-B*27 alleles are absent. J Virol 86: 10870–10872.
50. Altfeld M, Addo MM, Rosenberg ES, Hecht FM, Lee PK, et al. (2003) Influence of HLA-B57 on clinical presentation and viral control during acute HIV-1 infection. AIDS 17: 2581–2591.
51. Huang X, Ling H, Mao W, Ding X, Zhou Q, et al. (2009) Association of HLA-A, B, DRB1 alleles and haplotypes with HIV-1 infection in Chongqing, China. BMC Infect Dis 9: 201.
52. Li L, Chen W, Bouvier M (2005) A biochemical and structural analysis of genetic diversity within the HLA-A*11 subtype. Immunogenetics 57: 315–325.
53. Prentice HA, Price MA, Porter TR, Cormier E, Mugavero MJ, et al. (2014) Dynamics of viremia in primary HIV-1 infection in Africans: insights from analyses of host and viral correlates. Virology 449: 254–262.
54. de Sorrentino AH, Marinic K, Motta P, Sorrentino A, López R, et al. (2000) HLA class I alleles associated with susceptibility or resistance to human immunodeficiency virus type 1 infection among a population in Chaco Province, Argentina. J Infect Dis 182: 1523–1526.
55. Leslie A, Matthews PC, Listgarten J, Carlson JM, Kadie C, et al. (2010) Additive contribution of HLA class I alleles in the immune control of HIV-1 infection. J Virol 84: 9879–9888.
56. Magierowska M, Theodorou I, Debré P, Sanson F, Autran B, et al. (1999) Combined genotypes of CCR5, CCR2, SDF1, and HLA genes can predict the long-term nonprogressor status in human immunodeficiency virus-1-infected individuals. Blood 93: 936–941.
57. Li S, Jiao H, Yu X, Strong AJ, Shao Y, et al. (2007) Human leukocyte antigen class I and class II allele frequencies and HIV-1 infection associations in a Chinese cohort. J Acquir Immune Defic Syndr 44: 121–131.
58. Douek D (2007) HIV disease progression: immune activation, microbes, and a leaky gut. Top HIV Med 15: 114–117.

16

Identification and Characterization of HTLV-1 HBZ Post-Translational Modifications

Nathan Dissinger[1,2], Nikoloz Shkriabai[1,5], Sonja Hess[6], Jacob Al-Saleem[1,2], Mamuka Kvaratskhelia[1,5], Patrick L. Green[1,2,3,4]*

1 Center for Retrovirus Research, The Ohio State University, Columbus, Ohio, United States of America, **2** Department of Veterinary Biosciences, The Ohio State University, Columbus, Ohio, United States of America, **3** Comprehensive Cancer Center and Solove Research Institute, Columbus, Ohio, United States of America, **4** Department of Molecular Virology, Immunology, and Medical Genetics, The Ohio State University, Columbus, Ohio, United States of America, **5** College of Pharmacy, The Ohio State University, Columbus Ohio, United States of America, **6** Proteome Exploration Laboratory, Beckman Institute, California Institute of Technology, Pasadena, California, United States of America

Abstract

Human T-cell leukemia virus type-1 (HTLV-1) is estimated to infect 15–25 million people worldwide, with several areas including southern Japan and the Caribbean basin being endemic. The virus is the etiological agent of debilitating and fatal diseases, for which there is currently no long-term cure. In the majority of cases of leukemia caused by HTLV-1, only a single viral gene, *hbz*, and its cognate protein, HBZ, are expressed and their importance is increasingly being recognized in the development of HTLV-1-associated disease. We hypothesized that HBZ, like other HTLV-1 proteins, has properties and functions regulated by post-translational modifications (PTMs) that affect specific signaling pathways important for disease development. To date, PTM of HBZ has not been described. We used an affinity-tagged protein and mass spectrometry method to identify seven modifications of HBZ for the first time. We examined how these PTMs affected the ability of HBZ to modulate several pathways, as measured using luciferase reporter assays. Herein, we report that none of the identified PTMs affected HBZ stability or its regulation of tested pathways.

Editor: Dong-Yan Jin, University of Hong Kong, Hong Kong

Funding: National Cancer Institute National Institutes of Health CA100730 to PLG (http://www.cancer.gov/). The funders had no role in study design, data collection and analysis, decision to publish, or preparation of the manuscript.

Competing Interests: The authors have declared that no competing interests exist.

* Email: green.466@osu.edu

Introduction

Human T-cell leukemia virus type 1 (HTLV-1) was the first human retrovirus discovered to be associated with diseases [1,2] including the aggressive CD4[+] T-cell malignancy, adult T-cell leukemia (ATL) [3], as well as the neurodegenerative disease HTLV-1-associated myelopathy/tropical spastic paraparesis, and other inflammatory diseases [4]. HTLV-1 encodes the structural and enzymatic proteins, Gag, Pol, and Env, as well as the regulatory proteins, Tax and Rex. The virus also encodes accessory proteins that are required for efficient infection and persistence *in vivo*, but are dispensable for T-cell immortalization *in vitro* [5]. The accessory/regulatory protein HBZ is unique in that it is the only viral protein encoded by the minus strand of the proviral genome while the rest of the viral proteins are encoded by the plus strand [6–8]. HBZ is expressed in all HTLV-1 cell lines and cases of ATL; in fact, in 60% of those ATL cases, *hbz* is typically the only viral gene expressed (eg. no Tax) [9]. This finding is attributed to deletion or hyper-methylation-silencing of the promoter in the 5′ LTR or a non-functional mutation in the Tax transactivator, which significantly disrupts plus-strand transcription [9,10].

When HBZ was discovered, it was first shown to repress Tax transactivation of the viral promoter [7,11,12]. Since then, other functions have been reported such as modulation of the AP-1 [13–17] and the classical NF-κB signaling pathways [18,19]. More recent studies have shown that HBZ may regulate the cell-mediated immune response to the virus infection [20,21]. There also is growing evidence that HBZ is important in the oncogenic process since it plays a role in driving infected cell proliferation [22–24], increasing hTERT transcription [25,26], and inhibiting apoptosis [20,27].

Post-translational modifications (PTMs) are chemical modifications added to proteins that can alter many aspects of a protein, including conformation, localization, and activity. This common mechanism of cellular regulation is utilized by several pathogens, including HTLV-1, to alter the expression of their own proteins. Tax contains several PTMs, for example, phosphorylation of Tax both stabilizes the protein [28] and inhibits its activity [29]. In addition, a phosphorylation site is required for the addition of an acetyl group that activates Tax to enhance NF-κB and induce transformation [30,31]. Furthermore, our lab has shown phosphorylation to be vital for the regulation of Rex function [32].

There currently are no published data about whether HBZ is post-translationally modified; however, it is known that HBZ interacts with acetyl-transferases [12,33]. Therefore, we hypothesized that HBZ, like Tax and Rex, would contain PTMs that regulate important functions. In this study, we purified an affinity-tagged-HBZ protein and analyzed this protein by LC-MS/MS. A high percentage of the protein, including the majority of the key leucine-zipper domain at the C-terminus, was covered in this analysis. This approach identified 7 modifications, which were further characterized by mutational analysis to determine if they regulated known HBZ functions.

Materials and Methods

Cells

293T cells were maintained in Dulbecco's modified Eagle's medium and Jurkat T-cells were maintained in RPMI medium at 37°C in a humidified atmosphere of 5% CO_2 and air. Media was supplemented with 10% fetal bovine serum (FBS), 2 mM glutamine, penicillin (100 U/ml), and streptomycin (100 μg/ml). Cells were originally obtained from ATCC.

Plasmids

To generate the Flag-6xHis-HBZ construct, the HBZ cDNA was inserted downstream of an N-terminal Flag-6xHis affinity tag and expression was driven by a CMV promoter. Amino acid exchanges were made using the QuickChange site-directed mutagenesis kit (Stratagene, La Jolla, CA). All mutations were confirmed by DNA sequencing and expression was verified by transfection and Western blot analysis. The pCMV-c-Jun and pLG4-10-6xAP-1-Luc plasmids were graciously provided by Dr. John C. McDermott of York University. The p65 expression plasmid and κB-Luc plasmid were a kind gift from Dr. Dean Ballard of Vanderbilt University. The IRF-1 expression plasmid and IRF-1 luciferase reporter plasmid were graciously provided by Dr. John Yim of the Beckman Research Institute.

Protein Purification

293T cells were plated in six 100 mm dishes, three per condition, and each plate was transfected with 10 μg of empty vector or Flag-6xHis-HBZ plasmid using lipofectamine (Invitrogen, Carlsbad, CA). Twenty-four hours post-transfection, cells were collected, combined, washed in cold 1x PBS, and lysed following the FLAG fusion protein immunoprecipitation and SDS-PAGE buffer elution protocols of the FLAG M Purification Kit (Sigma Aldrich, St. Louis, MO). Samples were loaded on a large 12% SDS-PA gel and electrophoresed for 3 hours at 55 mA. The gel was washed with Millipore water and stained using GelCode Blue Stain (Thermo Scientific, Rockford, IL). The HBZ band was excised from the gel for further proteomic analysis.

Mass Spectrometry and Proteomic Analysis

LC-MS/MS analysis was performed as described previously [34] with following modifications. HBZ excised gel slices were cut into small pieces (2–3 mm cubes) and incubated on a shaker overnight in 50% acetonitrile to distain gel pieces from Coomassie dye. Samples were reduced with 7.5 mM DTT in 75 mM ammonium bicarbonate solution at 50°C for 30 min, after which DTT was removed and the protein was alkylated with 40 mM iodoacetamide in 75 mM ammonium bicarbonate solution for 20 min at room temperature in dark. The gel pieces were washed with acetonitrile, desiccated in a speed-vac. Aliquots were, subjected to in-gel proteolysis using the following endoproteinases (5 ng/μl): i) sequencing grade modified trypsin (Promega); ii) sequencing grade chymotrypsin (Roche); iii) sequencing grade endoproteinase Asp-N, (Roche) and iv) Trypsin/Asp-N combination. The resulting peptides were extracted in 100 μl of acetonitrile by vortexing for 10 min. The solution was transferred to new small microcentrifuge tubes and desiccated in a speed-vac. Dried

samples were resuspended in 6 μl buffer A (2% acetonitrile, 0.2% formic acid,) and 5 μl were separated on a 15 cm×0.075 mm fused silica capillary column packed with reversed phase 3 μm ReproSil-Pur C_{18AQ} resin (Dr. Maisch GmbH, Ammerbuch-Entringen, Germany) using a nano EASY HPLC. Peptides were eluted over 50 min by applying a 0–30% linear gradient of buffer B (80% acetonitrile, 19.8% water and 0.2% formic acid) at a flow rate of 350 nL/min. The Orbitrap (Thermo Fischer Scientific, San Jose, CA) was run in data dependent mode with 10 data-dependent scan events for each full MS scan. Normalized collision energy was set at 35, activation Q was 0.250. AGC target for MS was 1×10^6 and AGC target for MS/MS was 5×10^4. Dynamic exclusion was set to 60 s and early expiration was disabled. Sequence analysis was performed with MASCOT (Matrix Sciences, London GB) software using an indexed human subset database of Swissprot, supplemented with HTLV, 263 contaminants and 114960 decoy sequences.

Reporter Assays

Each functional reporter assay had its own set of conditions for plasmid concentrations. In brief, 293 T cells were seeded in 6-well plates at 2×10^5 cells per well. Twenty-four hours post-plating, cells were transfected with 10 or 20 ng of renilla-TK, a luciferase reporter, an expression plasmid of a specific transcription factor, and an HBZ expression plasmid at one of two concentrations (1:5 or 1:10 ratio). Empty vector was added to make the total DNA concentration equal among all transfections. Transfections were performed using Lipofectamine (Invitrogen, Carlsbad, CA). Twenty-four hours post-transfection, cells were collected and analyzed using a dual luciferase assay kit (Promega, Madison, WI). Levels of firefly luciferase and renillia luciferase were measured using a Packard LumiCount luminometer. Each experiment was performed three independent times in duplicates. Jurkat T-cells were plated in 6-well dishes at 3.5×10^5 cells per well. Twenty-four hours post-plating, cells were transfected using TransFectin lipid reagent (Bio-Rad Laboratories, Hercules, CA) by following the manufacturer's guidelines. Forty hours post-transfection, cells lysates were collected and analyzed as described above.

Western Blot Analysis

Transfected cells were lysed in 1x Passive Lysis Buffer (Promega, Madison, WI) with protease inhibitor cocktail (Roche, Mannheim, Germany). Protein concentrations were measured using a Nano-drop spectrophotometer (Thermo Fisher Scientific, Waltham, MA). SDS dye (6x solution) was added to the lysates and samples were boiled for 10 min. Twenty micrograms of protein were resolved by SDS-PAGE and transferred to nitrocellulose membranes. Blots were probed with a rabbit polyclonal anti-HBZ antiserum (1:1000), a mouse anti-Flag M2 antibody (1:5000) (Sigma Aldrich, St. Louis, MO), or mouse anti-Actin (1:10000) according to standard procedures. Secondary antibodies used included goat anti-rabbit and goat anti-mouse conjugated with horseradish peroxidase (Santa Cruz Biotechnology, Santa Cruz, CA) at a dilution of 1:2000. Blots were developed using Immunocruz luminol reagent (Santa Cruz Biotechnology) and imaged using the Fuji LAS 4000 imaging system (GE Healthcare Life Sciences, Piscataway, NJ). Densitometry was measured using Multi Gauge version 3.0 software (Fujifilm, Tokyo, Japan).

Results

Prediction of HBZ PTMs

There are currently no reports on whether HBZ is post-translationally modified, but it is well known that PTMs can play a

Table 1. Predicted and Identified Phosphorylation Sites of HBZ.

Predicted Phosphorylation Site	Score	Threshold	Times Modified/Times Detected	% Modified
S29	0.974	0.5	0/5	0.00%
S49	0.975	0.5	1/27	3.70%
S54	0.965	0.5	0/15	0.00%
T73	0.991	0.5	0/5	0.00%
S150	0.993	0.5	N.D.	N/A
S174	0.929	0.5	0/87	0.00%

N.D. means Not Detected. N/A means Not Applicable.

major role in the properties and functions of proteins. Two major types of modification are phosphorylation and acetylation. These modifications are reversible and are used to modify the activity of many transcription factors [35]. Using the online phosphorylation prediction tool, NetPhos 2.0 Server [36], we found 6 potential phosphorylation sites on HBZ (Table 1). We also used the online tool PAIL [37] for acetylation prediction (Table 2) that predicted 16 acetylated lysines. These data suggested that HBZ was likely modified by the cell. Instead of mutating all predicted modified residues, we first set out to identify modified residues by performing mass spectrometry (MS). This approach would allow us to identify both phosphorylation and acetylation added to HBZ within a eukaryotic cell in a single assay. This analysis was dependent on the production and purification of substantial quantities of HBZ protein.

Function and purification of Flag-6xHis-HBZ

Varying amounts of the Flag-6xHis-HBZ construct were transfected into 293T cells along with a Tax expression plasmid and the HTLV-1-LTR-Luciferase reporter plasmid (Figure 1A). As expected, Flag-6xHis-HBZ was able to repress Tax transactiva-

tion in a dose-dependent manner similarly to untagged, wild-type HBZ. We next verified that we would be able to adequately purify HBZ for mass spectrometry analysis. Using components of Sigma's FLAG M Purification kit, lysates from HBZ-transfected 293T cells were collected and HBZ was purified using agarose beads conjugated with mouse anti-Flag antibody. SDS-PAGE and GelCode Blue visualization revealed a specific band correlating to tagged HBZ that could be processed for mass spectrometry (Figure 1B).

Identification of PTMs

Multiple runs of LC-MS/MS were performed with protein digestion schemes described in the Materials and Methods section. Overall, we were able to obtain 68% coverage of the amino acid sequence, including the majority of the key leucine-zipper functional domain and identified several PTMs (Figure 2). We detected phosphorylation on S49, acetylation on K66 and K155, and methylation on K35, K37, K181 and K186 (Figure 2 and Tables 1–3). The majority of these modifications occur in the important protein-protein interaction domains of HBZ. Of the predicted phosphorylation sites, we covered 5 of the 6 predicted

Table 2. Predicted and Identified Acetylation Sites of HBZ.

Predicted Acetylation Site	Score	Threshold	Times Modified/Times Detected	% Modified
K66	2.09	0.5	39/39	100.00%
K84	2.64	0.5	N.D.	N/A
K86	1.65	0.5	N.D.	N/A
K88	2.42	0.5	N.D.	N/A
K89	1.96	0.5	N.D.	N/A
K93	1.47	0.5	0/2	0.00%
K106	0.79	0.5	N.D.	N/A
K110	1.37	0.5	N.D.	N/A
K119	1.51	0.5	N.D.	N/A
K120	2.43	0.5	0/1	0.00%
K128	0.75	0.5	N.D.	N/A
K145	1.6	0.5	N.D.	N/A
K147	1.89	0.5	N.D.	N/A
K153	1.26	0.5	N.D.	N/A
K155	1.13	0.5	2/71	2.82%
K181	0.67	0.5	0/73	0.00%

N.D. means Not Detected. N/A means Not Applicable.

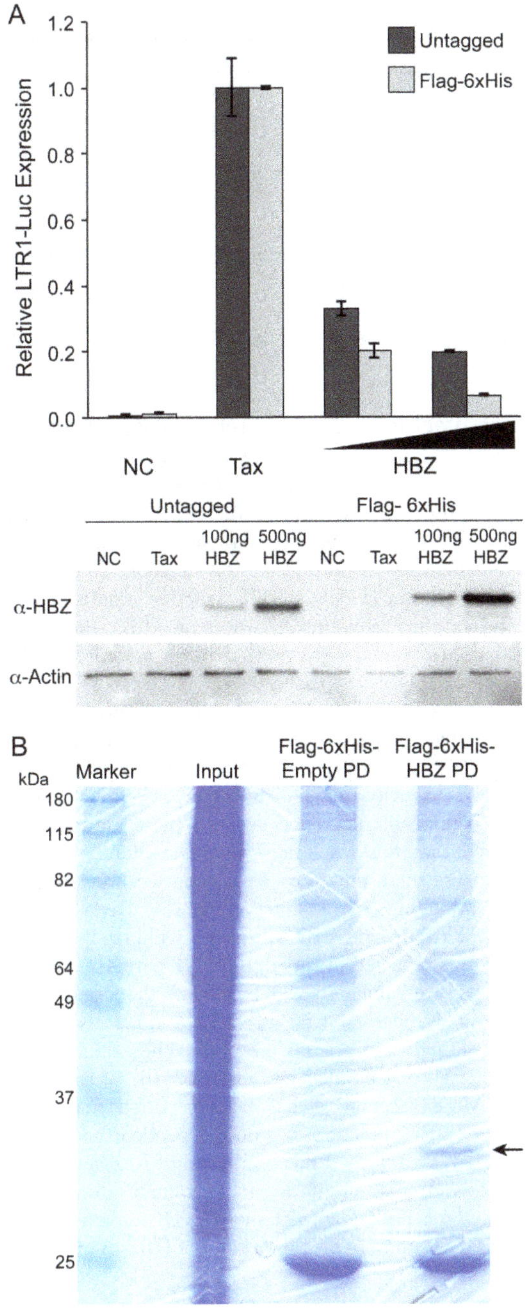

Figure 1. Flag-6xHis-tagged HBZ represses Tax transactivation and can be purified. (A) The functional activity of Flag-6xHis-HBZ was determined by measuring its ability to repress Tax trans-activation of a LTR1-luc reporter in 293T cells. Cells were transfected with S-tag Tax (200 ng), LTR-1 luciferase reporter (100 ng) renilla-TK (20 ng) and a titration of HBZ constructs (100 and 500 ng.) Values represent mean measurements relative to Tax expression alone. Error bars represent standard deviation. Western blots were performed on 20 ug total cell lysate and probed with rabbit HBZ-specific antisera. Actin was used as a loading control. (B) Flag-6xHis-HBZ was purified from lysates of transfected 293T cells using agarose beads conjugated with anti-Flag antibody. Bands were resolved by SDS-PAGE and the gel was stained with GelCode Blue.

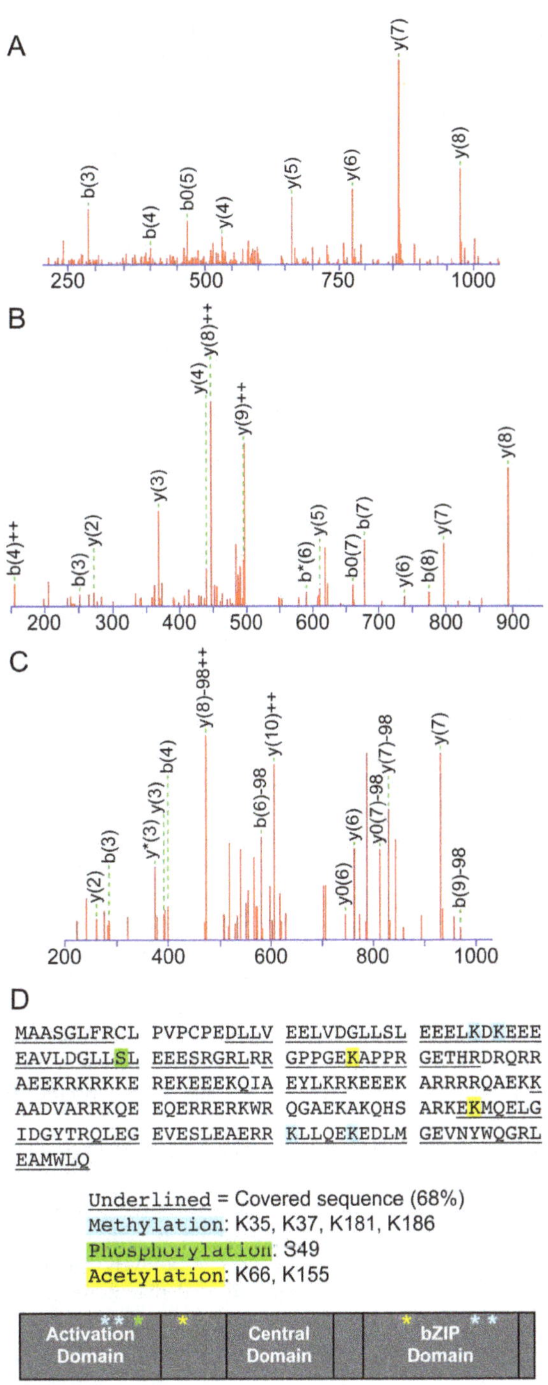

Figure 2. MS based analysis of PTMs in HBZ. (A) MS/MS fragmentation of HBZ peptide DGLLSLEEELK*, where Lys is methylated. (B) MS/MS Fragmentation of HBZ peptide GPPGEK*APPR, where Lys is acetylated. (C) MS/MS Fragmentation of HBZ peptide DGLLS*LEEESR, where Ser is phosphorylated. (D) Summary of MS results. The HBZ sequence is provided, with covered sequences underlined. PTMs found are highlighted in the sequence and marked relative to the three domains of HBZ in a cartoon.

sites (Table 1), and 5 of the 16 predicted acetylation sites (Table 2). We compared MS spectrum counts for modified peptides with their unmodified counterparts, which allowed semiquantitative analysis for the frequency of modifications (Tables 1–3). Our data suggest that the phosphorylation of HBZ is an infrequent occurrence since S49 showed limited phosphorylation. The addition of an acetyl group to K155 also seems to be a rare event, being detected approximately 3% of the time. Of the

Table 3. Detected Methylation Sites of HBZ.

Methylated Residue	Times Modified/Times Detected	% Modified
K35	3/10	30.00%
K37	1/6	16.67%
K181	3/73	4.11%
K186	1/80	1.25%

discovered methylations, our data indicate that only K35 is methylated with some consistency. Furthermore, we provide evidence that K66 is constitutively acetylated, neutralizing the positive charge of this amino acid. All these identified modifications are novel and, we hypothesized, could regulate the properties and/or functions of HBZ.

PTMs do not affect HBZ steady-state levels

In the current study, we decided to examine the roles of phosphorylation and acetylation individually by mutating modified amino acids to mimetic (S→D and K→Q, respectively) and inhibitory (S→A and K→R, respectively) residues for each PTM. We also created a phospho-, acetyl-mimetic mutant (PhAc-mim: S49D-K66Q-K155Q), and a phospho-, acetyl-inhibitory mutant (PhAc-inh: S49A-K66R-K155R) for the discovered modified sites to investigate if they act in concert. The approach of having mimetic and inhibitory mutants allowed us to compare each mutant to the wild-type protein and the paired residue mutation. It also is important to examine both the mimetic and inhibitory mutations as both phosphorylation and acetylation can positively or negatively regulate the functions of proteins. We decided not to focus on the discovered methylation sites currently since all methylated states were found in less than half the cases of detected peptides and we cannot create a methylated lysine mimetic mutation. If future studies identify methyltransferases that interact with HBZ, it would be interesting to see if over-expression of these enzymes modifies these residues of HBZ and are important for HBZ function.

After the creation of the mutant forms of HBZ in the Flag-6xHis vector, Western blot analysis was performed to examine if any of the modifications affected the steady-state levels of the protein. We hypothesized that acetylation of K66 would be important for protein stability as it was found to be constitutively modified. However, probing for the affinity-tag showed that none of the

modifications affected the steady state level of the protein (Figure 3).

PTMs do not affect inhibition of viral regulatory proteins

HBZ inhibits Tax-transactivation of the LTR promoter by binding to the co-activators CREB and p300 [11,12] and by up-regulating the ubiquitin E3 ligase PDLIM2, which targets Tax for degradation [38]. To examine if the phosphorylation and acetylation of HBZ were important for this function, 293 T cells were transfected with an HTLV-1 LTR-luciferase reporter along with Tax and titrating amounts of wild-type HBZ, the PTM mutants, and a ΔLZ mutant (previously shown to repress Tax-transactivation to a lesser extent than wild-type) [11,12] (Figure 4A). As expected, wild-type HBZ and, to a lesser degree, HBZΔLZ, were able to repress Tax trans-activation of the HTLV-1 LTR promoter. We observed that all PTM mutants tested were able to inhibit Tax activity to a similar degree as wild-type HBZ and found no significant difference between paired mutants. It should be noted that this result for the S49 mutants was not unexpected because these mutations were reported previously to bind to p300, inhibiting it from interacting with Tax [12]. To examine if the PTMs affected HBZ's functions within a T-cell, the luciferase assay was repeated in Jurkat T-cells (Figure 4B). Results in Jurkat T-cells were similar to 293 T cells; all the tested PTM mutants functioned similarly to wild-type HBZ and repressed Tax-transactivation of the HTLV-1 LTR promoter. These data suggest that the tested PTMs do not affect the ability of HBZ to modulate Tax activity. More recently, it has been reported that HBZ modestly repressed Rex function in a dose-dependent manner in HeLa cells [39]. We confirmed this repression of Rex activity by wild-type HBZ and that all of the PTM mutants functioned similarly to wild-type HBZ (data not shown). These data suggest that the tested PTMs do not affect the ability of HBZ to modulate Rex activity.

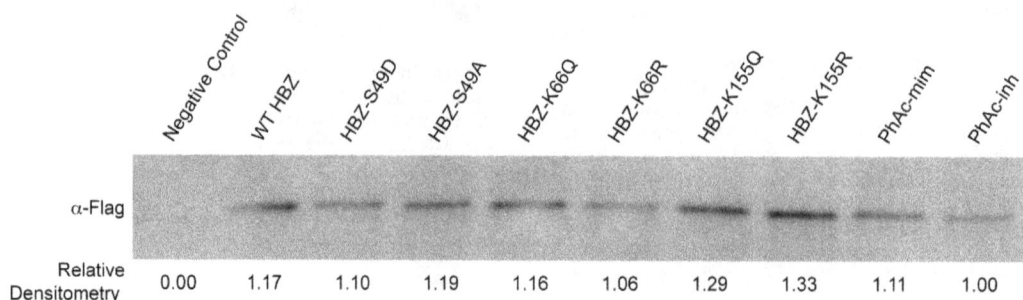

Figure 3. Steady-state levels of HBZ protein is not altered by identified PTMs. Lysates were collected from transfected 293 T cells and were resolved by SDS-PAGE. The amount of lysate loaded was normalized to measured renilla-TK values. The blot was probed with mouse anti-Flag M2 (1:5000). Densitometries were measured and the ratios are reported under the blot.

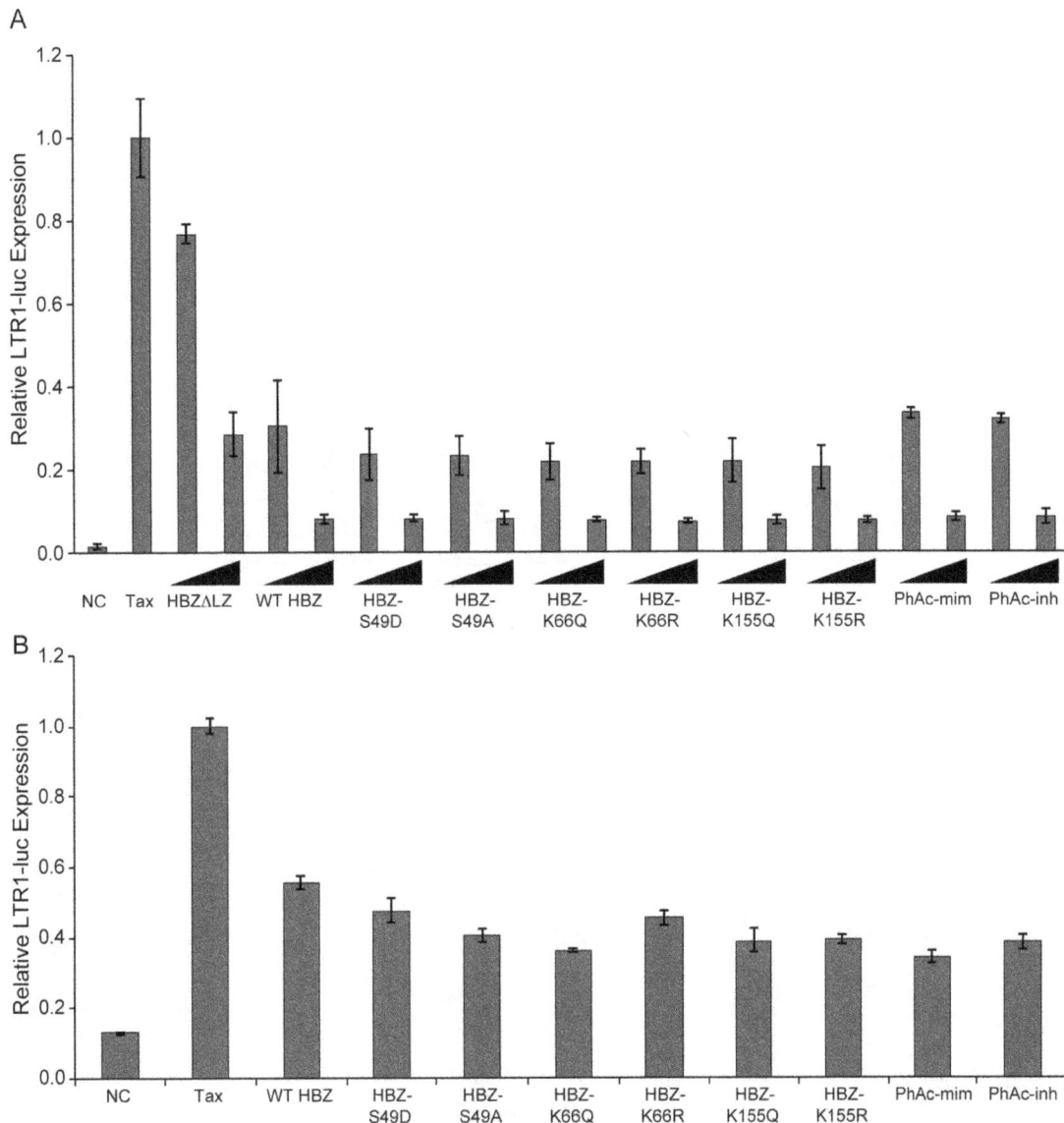

Figure 4. Phosphorylation and acetylation do not alter the ability of HBZ to repress Tax transactivation of the LTR promoter. (A) 293 T cells were transfected with LTR-1-luc reporter (100 ng), renilla-TK (20 ng), S-tagged Tax (200 ng) and a titration of HBZ mutants (100 ng and 500 ng). DNA amounts were normalized with empty Flag-6xHis plasmid. Twenty-four hours post-transfection, lysates were collected and luciferase levels were measured. (B) Jurkat T-cells were transfected with LTR-1-luc reporter (300 ng), renilla-TK (100 ng), S-tagged Tax (600 ng) and HBZ mutants (1500 ng). Forty hours post-transfection, lysates were collected and luciferase levels were measured. Error bars represent standard deviations.

PTMs of HBZ do not affect p65 or c-Jun transcriptional activity

It previously was reported that HBZ represses the classical NF-κB pathway by inhibiting the DNA-binding of p65 and inducing p65 degradation [18]. This finding was important because this binding stopped cells from entering Tax-induced senescence [19]. We used a reporter assay to examine if the discovered PTMs affected the ability of HBZ to repress p65 in both 293 T cells and Jurkat T-cells (Figure 5A and 5B). These data demonstrated that the PTMs of HBZ, individually and in combination with each other, did not affect HBZ's ability to repress p65 transcriptional activity in either cell type.

We next examined how the PTMs affect the ability of HBZ to repress c-Jun transcriptional activity because HBZ and APH-2, the

HBZ counterpart in non-pathogenic HTLV-2, differentially regulate this cellular pathway [13,40]. 293 T cells were transfected with a 6xAP-1-luciferase construct along with pCMV-c-Jun and titrating amounts of HBZ. Because HBZ interacts with c-Jun through its leucine zipper domain [13], we also included the HBZΔLZ mutant (Figure 6). Our results show WT HBZ was able to repress c-Jun-mediated transcription and the HBZΔLZ mutant was unable to repress c-Jun. All PTM mutants acted in a manner similar to WT HBZ, indicating none of the PTMs affected the interaction of HBZ with c-Jun. Taken together, our data indicate that the phosphorylation and acetylation state at these residues are not important for the ability of HBZ to modulate the classical NF-κB and AP-1 pathways.

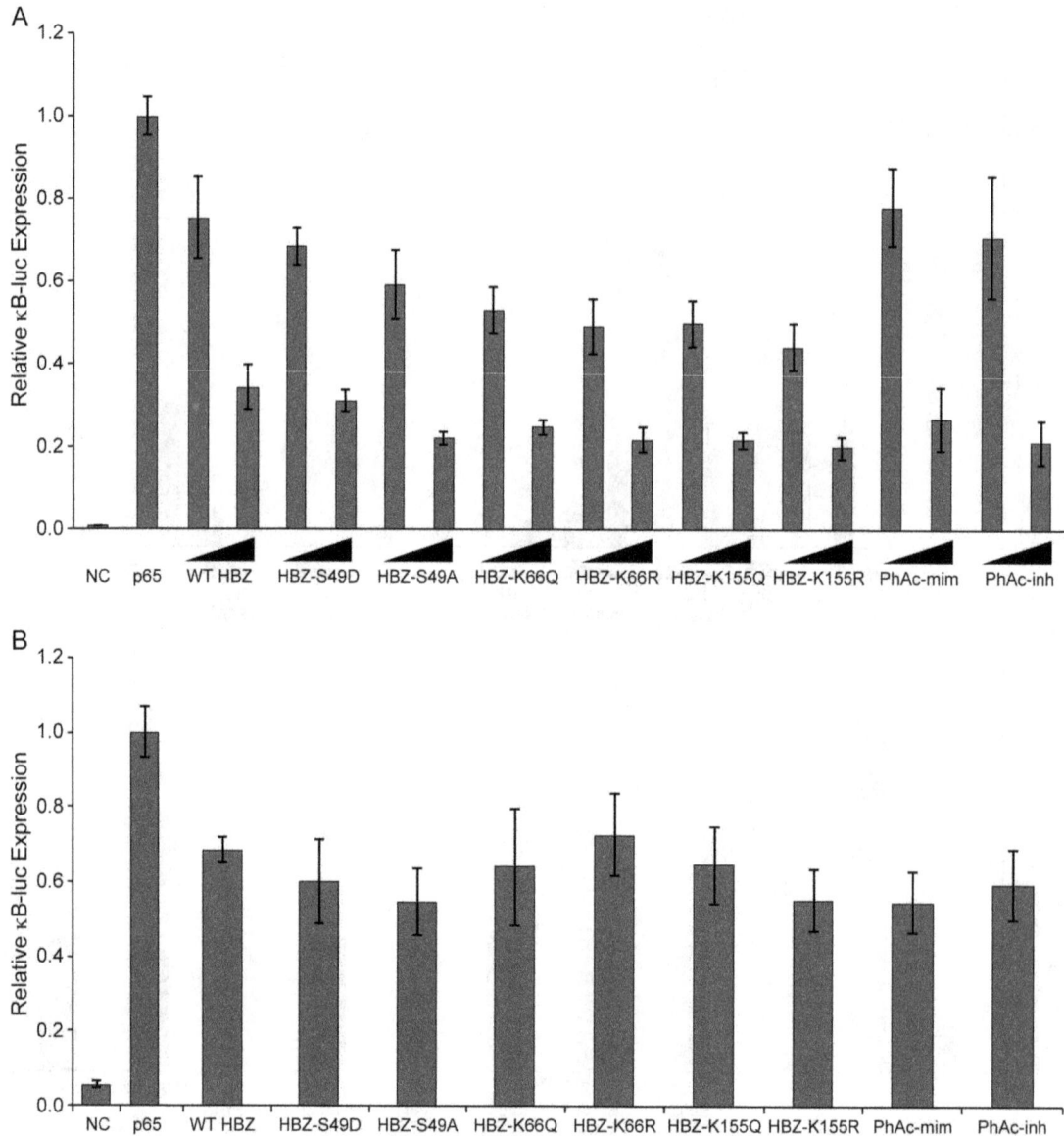

Figure 5. Phosphorylation and acetylation do not affect the ability of HBZ to repress p65-mediated transcription. (A) 293 T cells were transfected with κB-luc reporter (100 ng), renilla-TK (20 ng), p65 expression plasmid (50 ng) and a titration of HBZ constructs (100 ng and 500 ng). DNA amounts were normalized with empty Flag-6xHis plasmid. Lysates were collected 24 hours post-transfection and luciferase levels were measured. (B) Jurkat T-cells were transfected with κB-luc reporter (200 ng), renilla-TK (100 ng), p65 expression plasmid (100 ng) and HBZ mutants (1000 ng). Lysates were collected 40 hours post-transfection and luciferase levels were measured. Error bars represent standard deviations.

Repression of IRF-1 is not dependent on HBZ PTMs

After testing whether PTMs regulate the ability of HBZ to repress viral expression and growth pathways, we next turned our attention to a component of the innate immune system. Interferon (IFN) regulatory factors (IRFs) are key components of the immune system as they control interferon production and development of immune cells, but they also play a role in regulating oncogenesis [41]. IRF-1 induces the expression of type-I IFN and acts as a tumor suppressor by inducing apoptosis [42]. Clinical data have shown that IRF-1 expression is lost in many cases of leukemia [43]. Since HBZ is typically the only HTLV-1 protein expressed in cases of ATL, Mukai et al investigated if HBZ and IRF-1 interacted [20]. They discovered that the N-terminus of HBZ was important for binding IRF-1 and repressing its activity. We

performed a reporter assay to assess whether the PTMs of HBZ regulated the repression of IRF-1 transcriptional activity (Figure 7). All PTM mutants were able to repress IRF-1 in a dose-dependent manner and there were no significant differences between paired mutations. These data suggest that PTMs are not involved in the regulation of IRF-1 activity by HBZ.

Discussion

Our present research is the first to report PTMs of HBZ and to define the potential role of these PTMs in the known functions of HBZ. Using online prediction tools, we found 6 potential sites of phosphorylation and 16 sites of acetylation. Our MS data covered 68% of the amino acids of HBZ, including 5 of the 6 potential phosphorylation sites and 5 of the 16 acetylation sites. In total, 7

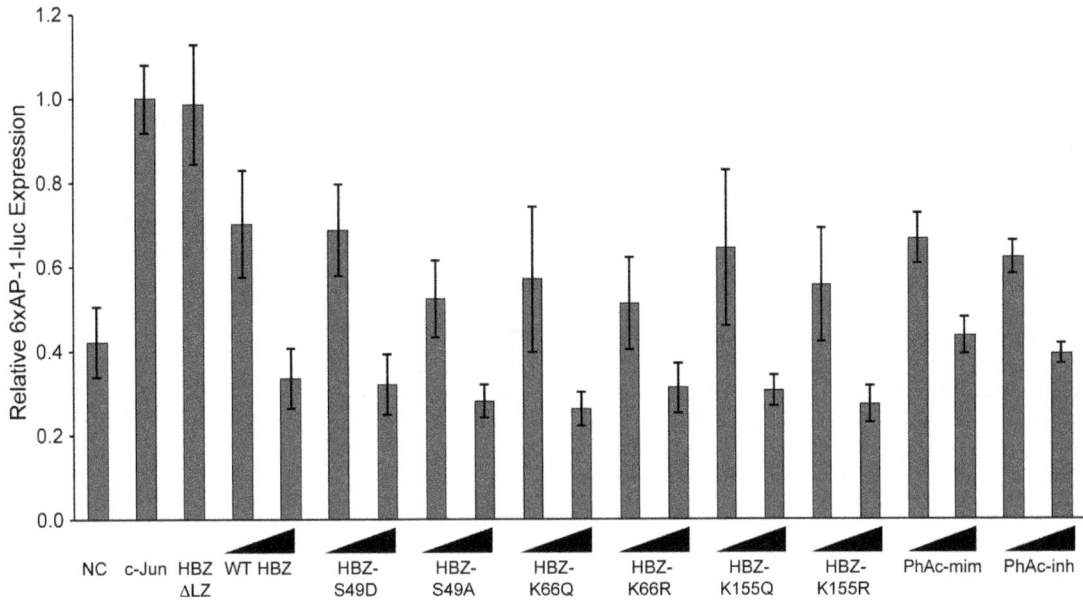

Figure 6. Phosphorylation and acetylation do not affect the ability of HBZ to inhibit c-Jun-mediated transcription. 293 T cells were transfected with a 6xAP-1-luc reporter (50 ng), renilla-TK (10 ng), pCMV-c-Jun (25 ng) and a titration of HBZ constructs (10 ng and 100 ng). DNA amounts were normalized with empty Flag-6xHis plasmid. Lysates were collected 24 hours post-transfection and luciferase levels were measured. Error bars represent standard deviations.

modifications were identified: 1 phosphorylation, 2 acetylations, and 4 methylations. Three of these modifications occur in the N-terminal activation domain, one in between the activation domain and central domain, and the final three occur in the leucine zipper domain. Only acetylation of K66 occurred at a high frequency, with the 6 other modifications occurring at low frequency. The negative predicted sites that were covered cannot be fully ruled out as being modified, but we are confident that the modifications do not occur at a high frequency. Of the uncovered predicted sites, it would seem likely that acetylation would occur more frequently than phosphorylation because there are more sites available and HBZ is known to interact with acetyl-transferases.

We first examined the effect that these PTMs had on the steady state levels of the protein, but found no difference between samples and controls. We next tested how PTMs affect the ability of HBZ to repress Tax transactivation. Because none of the mutants acted

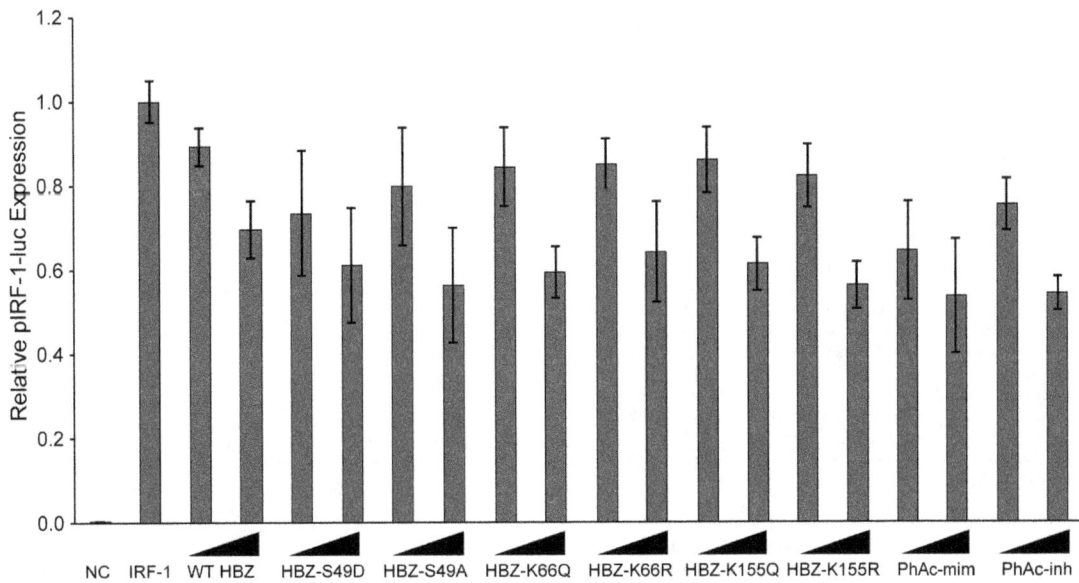

Figure 7. The ability of HBZ to repress IRF-1 activity is not affected by the identified PTMs. 293 T cells were transfected with pIRF-1-luc (50 ng), renilla-TK (20 ng), IRF-1 expression plasmid (100 ng) and a titration of HBZ constructs (50 ng and 500 ng). DNA amounts were normalized with empty Flag-6xHis plasmid. Lysates were collected 24 hours post-transfection and luciferase levels were measured. Error bars represent standard deviations.

differently than the wild-type at a low or high concentration, we are able to infer two aspects of the identified phosphorylation and acetylation: 1) they do not affect the interaction of HBZ with p300, and 2) they do not affect the interaction of HBZ with CREB. The cellular signaling pathways AP-1 and NF-κB, along with IRF-1-mediated transcription were examined. Although the modifications found were in domains that modulate the activity of the tested transcription factors, they did not play any role in the ability of HBZ to repress these selected pathways.

HBZ is known to interact with several proteins and affect various cellular pathways. While we could not identify any role for PTMs in the pathways examined, it remains possible that these PTMs have a function. Although the enzymes that add PTMs to their cognate proteins within the cell are not 100% specific for functionality, their promiscuity is still expected to be limited due to the importance of strict regulation and localization. The possibility that a combination of identified and unidentified PTMs may be necessary cannot be ruled out at this point. Furthermore, it is important to note that there could be unknown functions of HBZ that are regulated by these three PTMs. Future studies should focus on modifications that cannot be readily detected by MS such as SUMOylation [44,45] as these have also been shown to be important for regulating protein functions.

Acknowledgments

We thank Kate Hayes-Ozello for editorial comments on the manuscript and Tim Vojt for figure preparation. We thank the Proteome Exploration Laboratory members for technical assistance.

Author Contributions

Conceived and designed the experiments: PLG MK. Performed the experiments: ND JA NS. Analyzed the data: ND JA SH MK PLG. Contributed reagents/materials/analysis tools: ND SH MK PLG. Wrote the paper: ND MK PLG.

References

1. Poiesz BJ, Ruscetti FW, Gazdar AF, Bunn PA, Minna JD, et al. (1980) Detection and isolation of type C retrovirus particles from fresh and cultured lymphocytes of a patient with cutaneous T-cell lymphoma. Proc Natl Acad Sci USA 77: 7415–7419.

2. Yoshida M, Miyoshi I, Hinuma Y (1982) Isolation and characterization of retrovirus from cell lines of human adult T-cell leukemia and its implication in the disease. Proc Natl Acad Sci USA 79: 2031–2035.

3. Takatsuki K (2005) Discovery of adult T-cell leukemia. Retrovirology 2: 16. doi:10.1186/1742-4690-2-16.

4. Bangham CRM, Osame M (2005) Cellular immune response to HTLV-1. Oncogene 24: 6035–6046. doi:10.1038/sj.onc.1208970.

5. Nicot C, Harrod RL, Ciminale V, Franchini G (2005) Human T-cell leukemia/lymphoma virus type 1 nonstructural genes and their functions. Oncogene 24: 6026–6034. doi:10.1038/sj.onc.1208977.

6. Larocca D, Chao LA, Seto MH (1989) HUMAN T-CELL LEUKEMIA VIRUS MINUS STRAND TRANSCRIPTION IN INFECTED T-CELLS. Biochemical and Biophysical Research Communications 163: 1006–1013.

7. Gaudray G, Gachon F, Basbous J, Biard-Piechaczyk M, Devaux C, et al. (2002) The Complementary Strand of the Human T-Cell Leukemia Virus Type 1 RNA Genome Encodes a bZIP Transcription Factor That Down-Regulates Viral Transcription. Journal of Virology 76: 12813–12822. doi:10.1128/JVI.76.24.12813–12822.2002.

8. Cavanagh M-H, Landry S, Audet B, Arpin-André C, Hivin P, et al. (2006) HTLV-I antisense transcripts initiating in the 3′LTR are alternatively spliced and polyadenylated. Retrovirology 3: 15. doi:10.1186/1742-4690-3-15.

9. Matsuoka M, Jeang K-T (2007) Human T-cell leukaemia virus type 1 (HTLV-1) infectivity and cellular transformation. Nat Rev Cancer 7: 270–280. doi:10.1038/nrc2111.

10. Miyazaki M, Yasunaga JI, Taniguchi Y, Tamiya S, Nakahata T, et al. (2007) Preferential Selection of Human T-Cell Leukemia Virus Type 1 Provirus Lacking the 5′ Long Terminal Repeat during Oncogenesis. Journal of Virology 81: 5714–5723. doi:10.1128/JVI.02511-06.

11. Lemasson I, Lewis MR, Polakowski N, Hivin P, Cavanagh MH, et al. (2007) Human T-Cell Leukemia Virus Type 1 (HTLV-1) bZIP Protein Interacts with the Cellular Transcription Factor CREB To Inhibit HTLV-1 Transcription. Journal of Virology 81: 1543–1553. doi:10.1128/JVI.00480-06.

12. Clerc I, Polakowski N, Andre-Arpin C, Cook P, Barbeau B, et al. (2008) An Interaction between the Human T Cell Leukemia Virus Type 1 Basic Leucine Zipper Factor (HBZ) and the KIX Domain of p300/CBP Contributes to the Down-regulation of Tax-dependent Viral Transcription by HBZ. Journal of Biological Chemistry 283: 23903–23913. doi:10.1074/jbc.M803116200.

13. Basbous J, Arpin C, Gaudray G, Piechaczyk M, Devaux C, et al. (2003) The HBZ Factor of Human T-cell Leukemia Virus Type I Dimerizes with Transcription Factors JunB and c-Jun and Modulates Their Transcriptional Activity. Journal of Biological Chemistry 278: 43620–43627. doi:10.1074/jbc.M307275200.

14. Matsumoto J, Ohshima T, Isono O, Shimotohno K (2004) HTLV-1 HBZ suppresses AP-1 activity by impairing both the DNA-binding ability and the stability of c-Jun protein. Oncogene 24: 1001–1010. doi:10.1038/sj.onc.1208297.

15. Clerc I, Hivin P, Rubbo P-A, Lemasson I, Barbeau B, et al. (2009) Propensity for HBZ-SP1 isoform of HTLV-I to inhibit c-Jun activity correlates with sequestration of c-Jun into nuclear bodies rather than inhibition of its DNA-binding activity. Virology 391: 195–202. doi:10.1016/j.virol.2009.06.027.

16. Hivin P, Basbous J, Raymond F, Henaff D, Arpin-André C, et al. (2007) The HBZ-SP I isoform of human T-cell leukemia virus type I represses JunB activity by sequestration into nuclear bodies. Retrovirology 4: 14. doi:10.1186/1742-4690-4-14.

17. Thebault S, Basbous J, Hivin P, Devaux C, Mesnard J (2004) HBZ interacts with JunD and stimulates its transcriptional activity. FEBS Letters 562: 165–170. doi:10.1016/S0014-5793(04)00225-X.

18. Zhao T, Yasunaga J-I, Satou Y, Nakao M, Takahashi M, et al. (2009) Human T-cell leukemia virus type 1 bZIP factor selectively suppresses the classical pathway of NF-kB. Blood: 1–10. doi:10.1181/blood-2008-06-161729.

19. Zhi H, Yang L, Kuo Y-L, Ho Y-K, Shih H-M, et al. (2011) NF-κB Hyper-Activation by HTLV-1 Tax Induces Cellular Senescence, but Can Be Alleviated by the Viral Anti-Sense Protein HBZ. PLoS Pathog 7: e1002025. doi:10.1371/journal.ppat.1002025.g007.

20. Mukai R, Ohshima T (2011) Dual effects of HTLV-1 bZIP factor in suppression of interferon regulatory factor 1. Biochemical and Biophysical Research Communications 409: 328–332. doi:10.1016/j.bbrc.2011.05.014.

21. Sugata K, Satou Y, Yasunaga JI, Hara H, Ohshima K, et al. (2012) HTLV-1 bZIP factor impairs cell-mediated immunity by suppressing production of Th1 cytokines. Blood 119: 434–444. doi:10.1182/blood-2011-05-357459.

22. Arnold J, Zimmerman B, Li M, Lairmore MD, Green PL (2008) Human T-cell leukemia virus type-1 antisense-encoded gene, Hbz, promotes T-lymphocyte proliferation. Blood 112: 3788–3797. doi:10.1182/blood-2008.

23. Hagiya K, Yasunaga J-I, Satou Y, Ohshima K, Matsuoka M (2011) ATF3, an HTLV-1 bZip factor binding protein, promotes proliferation of adult T-cell leukemia cells. Retrovirology 8: 19. doi:10.1186/1742-4690-8-19.

24. Ma G, Yasunaga J, Fan J, Yanagawa S, Matsuoka M (2012) HTLV-1 bZIP factor dysregulates the Wnt pathways to support proliferation and migration of adult T-cell leukemia cells. Oncogene: 1–9. doi:10.1038/onc.2012.450.

25. Kuhlmann A-S, Villaudy J, Gazzolo L, Castellazzi M, Mesnard J-M, et al. (2007) HTLV-1 HBZ cooperates with JunD to enhance transcription of the human telomerase reverse transcriptase gene (hTERT). Retrovirology 4: 92. doi:10.1186/1742-4690-4-92.

26. Borowiak M, Kuhlmann A-S, Girard S, Gazzolo L, Mesnard JM, et al. (2013) HTLV-1 bZIP factor impedes the menin tumor suppressor and upregulates JunD-mediated transcription of the hTERT gene. Carcinogenesis 34: 2664–2672. doi:10.1093/carcin/bgt221.

27. Tanaka-Nakanishi A, Yasunaga JI, Takai K, Matsuoka M (2014) HTLV-1 bZIP Factor Suppresses Apoptosis by Attenuating the Function of FoxO3a and Altering Its Localization. Cancer Research 74: 188–200. doi:10.1158/0008-5472.CAN-13-0436.

28. Jeong S-J, Ryo A, Yamamoto N (2009) The prolyl isomerase Pin1 stabilizes the human T-cell leukemia virus type 1 (HTLV-1) Tax oncoprotein and promotes malignant transformation. Biochemical and Biophysical Research Communications 381: 294–299. doi:10.1016/j.bbrc.2009.02.024.

29. Durkin SS, Ward MD, Fryrear KA, Semmes OJ (2006) Site-specific Phosphorylation Differentiates Active from Inactive Forms of the Human T-cell Leukemia Virus Type 1 Tax Oncoprotein. Journal of Biological Chemistry 281: 31705–31712. doi:10.1074/jbc.M607011200.

30. Lodewick J, Lamsoul I, Polania A, Lebrun S, Burny A, et al. (2009) Acetylation of the human T-cell leukemia virus type 1 Tax oncoprotein by p300 promotes activation of the NF-κB pathway. Virology 386: 68–78. doi:10.1016/j.virol.2008.12.043.

31. Lodewick J, Sampaio C, Boxus M, Rinaldi A-S, Coulonval K, et al. (2013) Acetylation at lysine 346 controls thetransforming activity of the HTLV-1 Taxoncoprotein in the Rat-1 fibroblast model. Retrovirology 10: 1–1. doi:10.1186/1742-4690-10-75.

32. Kesic M, Doueiri R, Ward M, Semmes OJ, Green PL (2009) Phosphorylation regulates human T-cell leukemia virus type 1 Rex function. Retrovirology 6: 105. doi:10.1186/1742-4690-6-105.

33. Simonis N, Rual J-F, Lemmens I, Boxus M, Hirozane-Kishikawa T, et al. (2012) Host-pathogen interactome mapping for HTLV-1 and -2 retroviruses. Retrovirology 9: 26. doi:10.1186/1742-4690-9-26.

34. Kalli A, Hess S (2012) Effect of mass spectrometric parameters on peptide and protein identification rates for shotgun proteomic experiments on an LTQ-orbitrap mass analyzer. Proteomics 12: 21–31. doi:10.1002/pmic.201100464.

35. Tootle TL, Rebay I (2005) Post-translational modifications influence transcription factor activity: A view from the ETS superfamily. Bioessays 27: 285–298. doi:10.1002/bies.20198.

36. Blom N, Gammeltoft S, Brunak S (1999) Sequence and structure-based prediction of eukaryotic protein phosphorylation sites. J Mol Biol 294: 1351–1362. doi:10.1006/jmbi.1999.3310.

37. Li A, Xue Y, Jin C, Wang M, Yao X (2006) Prediction of Nε-acetylation on internal lysines implemented in Bayesian Discriminant Method. Biochemical and Biophysical Research Communications 350: 818–824. doi:10.1016/j.bbrc.2006.08.199.

38. Kannian P, Green PL (2010) Human T Lymphotropic Virus Type 1 (HTLV-1): Molecular Biology and Oncogenesis. Viruses 2: 2037–2077. doi:10.3390/v2092037.

39. Philip S, Zahoor MA, Zhi H, Ho Y-K, Giam C-Z (2014) Regulation of human T-lymphotropic virus type I latency and reactivation by HBZ and Rex. PLoS Pathog 10: e1004040. doi:10.1371/journal.ppat.1004040.

40. Marban CL, McCabe I, Bukong TN, Hall WW, Sheehy N (2012) Interplay between the HTLV-2 Tax and APH-2 proteins in the regulation of the AP-1 pathway. Retrovirology 9: 1–1. doi:10.1186/1742-4690-9-98.

41. Tamura T, Yanai H, Savitsky D, Taniguchi T (2008) The IRF Family Transcription Factors in Immunity and Oncogenesis. Annu Rev Immunol 26: 535–584. doi:10.1146/annurev.immunol.26.021607.090400.

42. Tanaka N, Ishihara M, Kitagawa M, Harada H, Kimura T, et al. (1994) Cellular Commitment to Oncogene-Induced Transformation or Apoptosis Is Dependent on the Transcription Factor IRF-1. Cell 77: 829–839.

43. Willman CL, Sever CE, Pallavicini MG, Harada H, Tanaka N, et al. (1993) Deletion of IRF-1, mapping to chromosome 5q31.1, in human leukemia and preleukemic myelodysplasia. Science 259: 968–971. Available: http://eutils.ncbi.nlm.nih.gov/entrez/eutils/elink.fcgi?dbfrom=pubmed&id=8438156&retmode=ref&cmd=prlinks.

44. Lamoliatte F, Bonneil E, Durette C, Caron-Lizotte O, Wildemann D, et al. (2013) Targeted identification of SUMOylation sites in human proteins using affinity enrichment and paralog-specific reporter ions. Mol Cell Proteomics 12: 2536–2550. doi:10.1074/mcp.M112.025569.

45. Griffiths JR, Chicooree N, Connolly Y, Neffling M, Lane CS, et al. (2014) Mass Spectral Enhanced Detection of Ubls Using SWATH Acquisition: MEDUSA-Simultaneous Quantification of SUMO and Ubiquitin-Derived Isopeptides. J Am Soc Mass Spectrom. doi:10.1007/s13361-014-0835-x.

17

Mean Platelet Volume (MPV) Predicts Middle Distance Running Performance

Giuseppe Lippi[1]*, Gian Luca Salvagno[2], Elisa Danese[2], Spyros Skafidas[3], Cantor Tarperi[4], Gian Cesare Guidi[2], Federico Schena[4]

1 Laboratory of Clinical Chemistry and Hematology, Academic Hospital of Parma, Parma, Italy, **2** Laboratory of Clinical Biochemistry, Department of Life and Reproduction Sciences, University of Verona, Verona, Italy, **3** CeRiSM (Centre for Mountain Sport and Health), Rovereto (TN), Italy, **4** Department of Neurological, Neuropsychological, Morphological and Movement Sciences, University of Verona, Verona, Italy

Abstract

Background: Running economy and performance in middle distance running depend on several physiological factors, which include anthropometric variables, functional characteristics, training volume and intensity. Since little information is available about hematological predictors of middle distance running time, we investigated whether some hematological parameters may be associated with middle distance running performance in a large sample of recreational runners.

Methods: The study population consisted in 43 amateur runners (15 females, 28 males; median age 47 years), who successfully concluded a 21.1 km half-marathon at 75–85% of their maximal aerobic power (VO_2max). Whole blood was collected 10 min before the run started and immediately thereafter, and hematological testing was completed within 2 hours after sample collection.

Results: The values of lymphocytes and eosinophils exhibited a significant decrease compared to pre-run values, whereas those of mean corpuscular volume (MCV), platelets, mean platelet volume (MPV), white blood cells (WBCs), neutrophils and monocytes were significantly increased after the run. In univariate analysis, significant associations with running time were found for pre-run values of hematocrit, hemoglobin, mean corpuscular hemoglobin (MCH), red blood cell distribution width (RDW), MPV, reticulocyte hemoglobin concentration (RetCHR), and post-run values of MCH, RDW, MPV, monocytes and RetCHR. In multivariate analysis, in which running time was entered as dependent variable whereas age, sex, blood lactate, body mass index, VO_2max, mean training regimen and the hematological parameters significantly associated with running performance in univariate analysis were entered as independent variables, only MPV values before and after the trial remained significantly associated with running time. After adjustment for platelet count, the MPV value before the run (p = 0.042), but not thereafter (p = 0.247), remained significantly associated with running performance.

Conclusion: The significant association between baseline MPV and running time suggest that hyperactive platelets may exert some pleiotropic effects on endurance performance.

Editor: Pedro Tauler, University of the Balearic Islands, Spain

Funding: The authors have no support or funding to report.

Competing Interests: The authors have declared that no competing interests exist.

* Email: glippi@ao.pr.it

Introduction

According to a recent on-line survey, recreational running is the most popular leisure sport activity, followed by lifting weights, biking, hiking and other outdoor activities [1]. More specifically, 75% of adults aged 24 to 44 years are engaged in outdoor running activities at least once a week in the US [2]. The typical middle distance runner is a "normal" trained adult subject, with few previous experiences in competitive sport and without special functional characteristics. The broad popularity of middle distance is mostly attributable to a variety of reasons, which include no need of special talent or highly-specialized and expensive equipment, and the remarkable benefits on health, fitness, stress reduction and weight control [2]. It is also noteworthy that the practice of habitual running has been associated with a significantly reduced risk of obesity, hypertension, diabetes, cardiovascular disease, cancer, osteoporosis, depression and several other chronic conditions, thus resulting in an overall 20% to 40% lower risk of mortality [3].

Both running economy and overall performance in middle distance running depend on a number of physiological factors, which are partially different from those required for short and long distance running [4,5]. The published research on half-marathon runners has mainly focused on a number of specific anthropometric variables (i.e., midaxillary skinfold, body mass index, percent body fat), functional characteristics (i.e., maximal aerobic power [VO_2max]), body core temperature), volume and intensity in training [6–8]. Despite the well-established relationship existing between packed cell volume, VO₂max, aerobic performance and maximal exercise capacity [9–11], a fact that has also contributed to the increase use of blood doping in sports during the past decades [12], there is little information about the association between hematological variables and middle distance running performance. As such, the aim of this study was to investigate whether some hematological parameters may predict half-marathon running time in a large sample of recreational runners.

Materials and Methods

The study was performed during a specific event called "Run For Science", held in Verona (Italy) in April 2014, with the purpose of analyzing the normal response of adult person to middle distance running. Forty three amateur runners were recruited (15 females and 28 males; median age 47 years and IQR 42–50 years; median body mass index 23 kg/m² and IQR, 22–25 kg/m²), who successfully concluded a 21.1 km half-marathon at 75–85% of their VO₂max. All athletes were members of a non professional team, were habitually involved in recreational running (mean training regimen 222 min/week and IQR 191–253 min/week; maximal oxygen uptake 50 mL/kg/min and IQR 46–55 mL/kg/min), and had rested for not less than 36 hours before the trial. Maximal aerobic capacity was individually measured in the last two weeks before the event by a running test on a treadmill using a breath by breath ergospirometric system (Quark B2, Cosmed Italy). After appropriate familiarization, each runner underwent a progressive incremental test, starting from habitual running pace and increasing speed of 0.5 km/h every min till reaching the volitional exhaustion. None of the subjects were taking medications known to alter erythrocyte or platelet metabolism, including antiplatelet or antihypertensive drugs and erythropoiesis stimulating substances. The trial started at 9.30 AM and the 21.1 km distance was covered on a relatively flat route near Verona (35 m vertical gain, with maximal slope of 1.8%), in a partially sunny day with temperatures between 12–19°C and humidity between 55–75%. Participants were free to drink *ad libitum* during the run. Blood was drawn in primary blood tubes containing K₂EDTA (Terumo Europe N.V., Leuven, Belgium) 10 min before the start of the run and immediately thereafter (i.e., within 15 min after conclusion). The whole blood samples were immediately transported to the local laboratory under controlled conditions of temperature and humidity, where a complete blood cell count (CBC) was performed on Advia 2120 (Siemens Healthcare Diagnostics, Tarrytown NY, USA), which included measurement of hematocrit, hemoglobin, red blood cell (RBC) count, mean corpuscular volume (MCV), mean corpuscular hemoglobin (MCH), mean corpuscular hemoglobin concentration (MCHC), RBC distribution width (RDW), platelet count, mean platelet volume (MPV), white blood cell (WBC) count and differential, reticulocyte count and reticulocyte hemoglobin concentration (RetCHR). The analysis of blood specimens was concluded within 2 hours after sample collection and all results were finally expressed as median and interquartile range (IQR). Differences of pre-run and post-run values were analyzed with Wilcoxon's test for paired samples. Univariate (i.e., Spearman's correlation) and multivariate analysis (with adjustment for age, sex, blood lactate, body mass index, VO₂max, mean training regimen and CBC parameters significantly associated with running time in univariate correlation) were performed, in order to identify potential predictors of running performance. The statistical analysis was performed with Analyse-it (Analyse-it Software Ltd, Leeds, UK) for Microsoft Excel (Microsoft Corporation, Redmond, WA, USA). All subjects gave a written consent for being enrolled in this investigation. The study was approved by the local ethical committee (Department of Neurological, Neuropsychological, Morphological and Movement Sciences, University of Verona) and performed in accord with the Helsinki Declaration of 1975 (additional information can be downloaded from the institutional Website: http://www.dsnm.univr.it/?ent=iniziativa&id=5382, Last accessed, 10 October 2014).

Results

The 43 amateur runners completed the run in a median time of 113 min (IQR, 105–121 min). As predictable, the median running performance of the 28 male athletes (100 min and IQR 101–118 min) was significantly better than that of the 15 females athletes (120 min and IQR 113–123 min; p<0.001). The median body weight decreased by 2.2% after the run (from 73.1 to 71.5 kg; p<0.001). The median lactate value measured in capillary blood at the end of the run was 4.0 mmol/L (IQR, 3.0–4.9 mmol/L). The variation of the CBC parameters after the run is shown in table 1. The values of lymphocytes and eosinophils exhibited a significant decrease compared to pre-run values, whereas those of MCV, platelets, MPV, WBC, neutrophils and monocytes were found to be significantly increased after the run. In univariate analysis, significant predictors of finishing time were the pre-run values of hematocrit, hemoglobin, MCH, RDW, MPV, RetCHR, whereas the post-run values of MCH, RDW, MPV, monocytes and RetCHR were also associated with running performance (Table 2). The VO₂max was the best overall predictor of running time (r = −0.601; p<0.001), whereas neither body mass index or blood lactate at the end of the half-marathon were significantly associated with running performance (Table 2). In multivariate analysis, in which running time was entered as dependent variable whereas age, sex, blood lactate, body mass index, VO₂max, mean training regimen and the CBC parameters significantly associated with running performance in univariate analysis were entered as independent variables, only MPV values before and after the trial remained significantly associated with running time (Table 3). After adjustment for the platelet count, the MPV value before the run (p = 0.042), but not thereafter (p = 0.247), remained significantly associated with running performance (Fig. 1). Neither the platelet count (r = −0.210; p = 0.303) or the MPV (r = 0.039; p = 0.851) were significantly associated with VO₂max in univariate analysis.

Discussion

Due to the increasing popularity of recreational running as a form of leisure activity and health-promoting behavior, a large number of studies have been performed over the past decades to identify the most reliable predictors of running economy and performance. The large majority of these investigations focused on anthropometric variables, functional characteristics, as well as volume and intensity of training [13]. With the notable exception of hemoglobin and packed cell volume, little information is available on other hematological parameters that may predict middle distance running performance [14]. This investigation was hence specifically planned to establish whether some hematological parameters comprised within the CBC may be significantly associated with half-marathon running time.

The leukocytes variations recorded in this study are not new, since an increase of total leukocyte, neutrophil and monocyte counts along with a decrease of lymphocyte and eosinophils values have already been reported in a number of previous investigations, and are prevalently attributable to the well-documented release of catecholamines and cortisol during exercise [8,15,16].

The significant increase of both platelet count (median increase, 17%; IQR, 10–34%) and MPV (median increase, 6%; IQR, 1–9%) recorded immediately after the half-marathon run substantially exceeded the inter-individual biological variation of these parameters (platelet count, 9.1%; MPV, 4.3%) [17], and is also consistent with the well established evidence that aerobic physical activity is effective to enhance circulating activated platelets, as well as platelet-platelet and platelet-leukocyte aggregates [18–22]. More specifically, it has been recently demonstrated that the hyperactive platelets generated during exercise are rapidly cleared by the spleen, which is also a dynamic reservoir of younger and larger platelets (i.e., the human spleen retains one-third of total body platelets, with MPV approximately 20% greater than that of circulating platelets) [23]. The younger platelets are then released into the circulation, thus explaining the significant increase of platelet count and MPV observed after endurance exercise in this and other previous studies [18–22]. Another putative mechanism that may contribute to increase the MPV has been reported by Hilberg et al. [24], who observed that moderate exercise increased both platelet reactivity and platelet-leukocyte conjugate formation, which both contribute to increase the measured value of MPV. Regardless of the underlying mechanism(s), the significant increase of MPV recorded after exercise in this and other studies [18–22] has meaningful clinical implications, suggesting that the enhanced risk of cardiovascular events that is occasionally observed in athletes may be at least in part mediated by platelet hyper-reactivity [20]. Indeed, further studies are advisable to define whether an improvement of physical fitness is also accompanied with an increased MPV.

Interestingly, although the pre-run values of hematocrit, hemoglobin, MCH, RDW, MPV, RetCHR, along with the post-run values of MCH, RDW, MPV, monocytes and RetCHR were significantly associated with running time in univariate analysis, only the MPV values before and after the half-marathon remained significantly correlated with running performance in the fully-adjusted model. As predictable, both hemoglobin and hematocrit values were found to be positively correlated with running performance in univariate analysis, but the significance of these associations was lost in the fully adjusted model, especially when VO_2max was entered as covariate. This is plausible, since VO_2max and both hemoglobin and hematocrit clearly interplay in increasing sport performance, and VO_2max is in fact enhanced by approximately 1% for each 3 g/L increase of hemoglobin [25].

As such, this is the first study demonstrating a direct correlation between platelet size and endurance performance to the best of our knowledge. It is noteworthy that the inverse association between pre-run MPV value and half-marathon running time remained significant after adjustment for a number of factors such as age, sex, blood lactate, body mass index, VO_2max, mean training regimen and platelet count, thus confirming the existence of an effective interplay between platelet metabolism and aerobic performance. In univariate analysis, the correlation between running time and pre-run MPV value was the second highest overall, only preceded by that between running time and VO_2max (Table 2). In agreement with a previous study [26], neither the platelet count or the MPV at baseline were significantly associated with VO_2max, thus confirming that the influence of MPV on running performance may be virtually independent from the baseline cardiorespiratory fitness level.

An increased platelet volume is a well established surrogate marker of platelet activation, wherein large platelets are reportedly more active than small platelets [27–29]. The association of this evidence with our data would imply that platelet hyperactivity may be a significant determinant of performance in medium distance running. The use of platelets in sports medicine has risen sharply in recent times. The platelet-rich plasma (PRP), an autologous blood fraction rich in platelets and associated cytokines and growth factors, is mainly used for treatment of sports related

Table 1. Variation of the complete blood cell count after a 21.1 km half-marathon run in 43 amateur runners.

	Pre-run	Post-run	P
Hematocrit	0.45 (0.44–0.47)	0.45 (0.43–0.47)	0.420
Hemoglobin (g/L)	148 (140–155)	148 (138–155)	0.137
RBC (10^{12}/L)	4.8 (4.6–5.0)	4.8 (4.5–5.1)	0.162
MCV (fL)	94 (91–96)	95 (92–97)	**0.004**
MCH (pg)	31 (30–32)	31 (30–32)	0.400
MCHC (g/dL)	32.7 (32.4–33.2)	32.5 (3.19–3.32)	0.068
RDW (%)	13.4 (13.1–13.5)	13.5 (13.1–13.6)	**0.001**
Platelets (10^9/L)	260 (218–299)	321 (287–361)	**<0.001**
MPV (fL)	9.2 (8.6–9.8)	9.5 (8.9–10.1)	**<0.001**
WBC (10^9/L)	5.6 (4.9–6.4)	12.4 (9.8–13.9)	**<0.001**
Neutrophils (10^9/L)	3.1 (2.5–3.6)	9.3 (7.4–11.5)	**<0.001**
Lymphocytes (10^9/L)	2.0 (1.7–2.3)	1.8 (1.5–2.2)	**0.037**
Monocytes (10^9/L)	0.3 (0.2–0.4)	0.5 (0.4–0.6)	**<0.001**
Eosinophils (10^9/L)	0.2 (0.1–0.2)	0.1 (0.0–0.01)	**<0.001**
Basophils (10^9/L)	0.1 (0.1–0.1)	0.1 (0.0–0.1)	0.052
LUC (10^9/L)	0.01 (0.1–0.1)	0.01 (0.1–0.1)	0.063
Reticulocytes (10^9/L)	62 (54–74)	60 (52–73)	0.138
RetCHR (pg)	31 (31–32)	31 (31–32)	0.243

RBC, red blood cell; MCV, mean corpuscular volume; MCH, mean corpuscular hemoglobin (MCH); MCHC, mean corpuscular hemoglobin concentration; (MCHC); RDW, red blood cell distribution width; MPV, mean platelet volume (MPV); WBC, white blood cell; LUC, large unstained cells; RetCHR, reticulocyte hemoglobin concentration.

Table 2. Univariate correlation (r) analysis between running performance and parameters of the complete blood cell count in 43 amateur athletes who completed a 21.1 km half-marathon run.

	Pre-run value		Post-run value	
	r	**p**	**r**	**p**
Hematocrit	−0.329	**0.031**	−0.298	0.052
Hemoglobin	−0.388	**0.010**	−0.291	0.059
RBC	−0.074	0.635	−0.086	0.584
MCV	−0.234	0.131	−0.257	0.097
MCH	−0.306	**0.046**	−0.341	**0.025**
MCHC	−0.240	0.122	−0.199	0.200
RDW	0.316	**0.039**	0.336	**0.027**
Platelets	0.300	0.052	0.256	0.097
MPV	−0.450	**0.002**	−0.476	**0.001**
WBC	−0.208	0.181	0.248	0.109
Neutrophils	−0.142	0.365	0.262	0.090
Lymphocytes	−0.072	0.647	−0.028	0.861
Monocytes	−0.262	0.090	0.361	**0.017**
Eosinophils	−0.143	0.360	−0.258	0.095
Basophils	−0.096	0.538	−0.197	0.207
LUC	−0.039	0.805	0.185	0.234
Ret	0.290	0.059	0.208	0.181
RetCHR	−0.390	**0.001**	−0.379	**0.012**
Blood lactate	–	–	−0.069	0.663
Body mass index	0.092	0.555	-	-
VO2max (mL/min/Kg)	−0.601	**0.001**	-	-

RBC, red blood cell; MCV, mean corpuscular volume; MCH, mean corpuscular hemoglobin (MCH); MCHC, mean corpuscular hemoglobin concentration; (MCHC); RDW, red blood cell distribution width; MPV, mean platelet volume (MPV); WBC, white blood cell; LUC, large unstained cells; RetCHR, reticulocyte hemoglobin concentration; VO2max, maximal aerobic power.

injuries [30–32]. It was recently proven that injection of PRP may also exert some ergogenic effects. In particular, Wasterlain et al. studied the effect of PRP injection on variation of performance-enhancing systemic growth factors in 25 patients [33], and observed that the administration of PRP increased the concentration of insulin-like growth factor-1 (IGF-1), basic fibroblast growth factor (bFGF) and VEGF. Interestingly, Kasuya et al. also showed that a symptom-limited treadmill exercise test was effective to enhance the platelet release of nitric oxide (NO) [34], which would then contribute to raise exercise tolerance and performance [35].

Another mechanism by which platelets may contribute to enhance sport performance is the attenuation of neuropathic pain and/or fatigue during exercise [36]. Kennedy et al. studied platelet activation and function in 17 patients with chronic fatigue

Table 3. Multivariate correlation analysis between running performance and parameters of the complete blood cell count in 43 amateur athletes who completed a 21.1 km half-marathon run.

	Pre-run value	Post-run value
	p	**p**
Hematocrit	0.338	-
Hemoglobin	0.216	-
MCH	0.512	0.567
RDW	0.272	0.216
MPV	**0.042**	**0.026**
Monocytes	-	0.080
RetCHR	0.967	0.925

Results were also adjusted for age, sex, body mass index, post-run blood lactate, maximal aerobic power (VO$_2$max) and training regimen.
MCH, mean corpuscular hemoglobin (MCH); RDW, red blood cell distribution width; MPV, mean platelet volume (MPV); RetCHR, reticulocyte hemoglobin concentration.

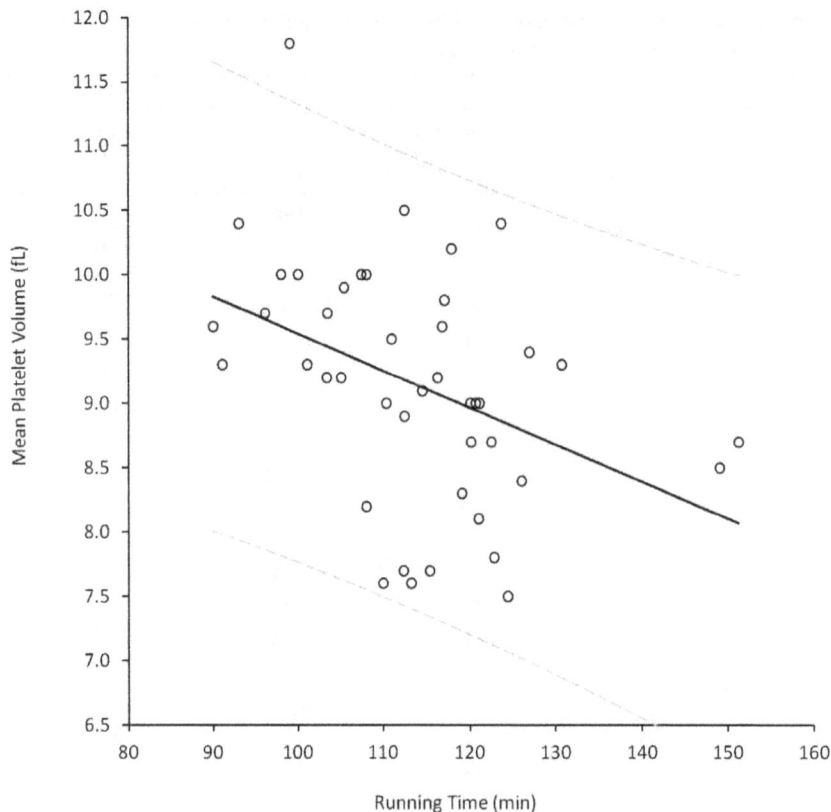

Figure 1. Correlation (and 95% prediction interval, 95% PI) between running performance and baseline value of mean platelet volume (MPV) in 43 amateur athletes completing a 21.1 km half-marathon run.

syndrome and 16 healthy controls [37], reporting that patients displayed lower platelet aggregability and reduced MPV. This would be consistent with the fact that smaller and less active platelets may somehow increase the fatigue threshold, thus conditioning exercise output. A series of studies also demonstrated that platelet gel or autologous platelet tissue graft are effective to lower pain after surgery and are associated with less pain medications and broader range of motion prior to discharge [38–40]. As specifically regards sports, the use of PRP was proven to be effective in reducing pain and promoting function improvement in tennis elbow [41] and other painful tendinopathies [42], as well as for accelerating muscle recovery after acute injury [43].

According to these evidences, it seems hence plausible that hyperactive platelets may exert some pleiotropic effects on endurance sport performance, by both releasing ergogenic mediators as well as by triggering an increase in performance-enhancing substances such as NO into the circulation. Further studies, involving also different running distances, sports and different categories of athletes are needed to confirm these findings and to elucidate the potential underlining mechanisms linking platelet volume and aerobic performance.

Author Contributions

Conceived and designed the experiments: GL CT FS. Performed the experiments: GLS ED SS. Analyzed the data: GL GLS GCG FS. Wrote the paper: GL GCG FS.

References

1. Reuters Press. Americans say they're creatures of simple, solo exercise habits. Available at: http://www.reuters.com/article/2013/09/23/us-fitness-habits-idUSBRE98M0KN20130923. Accessed: 16 August 2014.
2. Knechtle B, Barandun U, Knechtle P, Zingg MA, Rosemann T, et al. (2014) Prediction of half-marathon race time in recreational female and male runners. Springerplus 3:248.
3. Kokkinos P, Myers J (2010) Exercise and physical activity: clinical outcomes and applications. Circulation 122:1637–1648.
4. Brandon LJ (1995) Physiological factors associated with middle distance running performance. Sports Med 19:268–277.
5. Saunders PU, Pyne DB, Telford RD, Hawley JA (2004) Factors affecting running economy in trained distance runners. Sports Med 34:465–485.
6. Williams C, Nute ML (1983) Some physiological demands of a half-marathon race on recreational runners. Br J Sports Med 1983;17:152–161.
7. Knechtle B, Knechtle P, Barandun U, Rosemann T (2011) Anthropometric and training variables related to half-marathon running performance in recreational female runners. Phys Sportsmed 39:158–166.
8. Del Coso J, Fernández D, Abián-Vicen J, Salinero JJ, González-Millán C, et al. (2013) Running pace decrease during a marathon is positively related to blood markers of muscle damage. PLoS One 8:e57602.
9. Kanstrup IL, Ekblom B (1984) Blood volume and hemoglobin concentration as determinants of maximal aerobic power. Med Sci Sports Exerc 16:256–262.
10. Joyner MJ (2003) VO2MAX, blood doping, and erythropoietin. Br J Sports Med 37:190–191.
11. Calbet JA, Lundby C, Koskolou M, Boushel R (2006) Importance of hemoglobin concentration to exercise: acute manipulations. Respir Physiol Neurobiol 151:132–140.
12. Lippi G, Franchini M, Salvagno GL, Guidi GC (2006) Biochemistry, physiology, and complications of blood doping: facts and speculation. Crit Rev Clin Lab Sci 43:349–391.

13. Midgley AW, McNaughton LR, Jones AM (2007) Training to enhance the physiological determinants of long-distance running performance: can valid recommendations be given to runners and coaches based on current scientific knowledge? Sports Med 37:857–880.

14. Joyner MJ, Coyle EF (2008) Endurance exercise performance: the physiology of champions. J Physiol 586:35–44.

15. Lippi G, Schena F, Salvagno GL, Aloe R, Banfi G, et al. (2010) Foot-strike haemolysis after a 60-km ultramarathon. Blood Transfus 10:377–383.

16. Lippi G, Salvagno GL, Danese E, Tarperi C, Guidi GC, et al. (2014) Variation of Red Blood Cell Distribution Width and Mean Platelet Volume after Moderate Endurance Exercise. Adv Hematol 2014:192173. doi:10.1155/2014/192173.

17. Ricós C, Alvarez V, Cava F, García-Lario JV, Hernández A, et al. (1999) Current databases on biological variation: pros, cons and progress. Scand J Clin Lab Invest 59:491–500.

18. Knudsen JB, Brodthagen U, Gormsen J, Jordal R, Nørregaard-Hansen K, et al. (1982) Platelet function and fibrinolytic activity following distance running. Scand J Haematol 29:425–430.

19. Yilmaz MB, Saricam E, Biyikoglu SF, Guray Y, Guray U, et al. (2004) Mean platelet volume and exercise stress test. J Thromb Thrombolysis 17:115–120.

20. Li N, He S, Blombäck M, Hjemdahl P (2007) Platelet activity, coagulation, and fibrinolysis during exercise in healthy males: effects of thrombin inhibition by argatroban and enoxaparin. Arterioscler Thromb Vasc Biol 27:407–413.

21. Whittaker JP, Linden MD, Coffey VG (2013) Effect of aerobic interval training and caffeine on blood platelet function. Med Sci Sports Exerc 45:342–350.

22. Kahan T, Schwieler JH, Wallén H, Nussberger J, Hjemdahl P (2013) Platelet activation during exercise is not attenuated by inhibition of the renin angiotensin system: the role of physical activity. J Hypertens 31:2103–2104.

23. Bakovic D, Pivac N, Eterovic D, Breskovic T, Zubin P, et al. (2013) The effects of low-dose epinephrine infusion on spleen size, central and hepatic circulation and circulating platelets. Clin Physiol Funct Imaging 33:30–37.

24. Hilberg T, Menzel K, Gläser D, Zimmermann S, Gabriel HH (2008) Exercise intensity: platelet function and platelet-leukocyte conjugate formation in untrained subjects. Thromb Res 122:77–84.

25. Otto JM, Montgomery HE, Richards T (2013) Haemoglobin concentration and mass as determinants of exercise performance and of surgical outcome. Extrem Physiol Med 2:33.

26. Cho HC, Kim J, Kim S, Son YH, Lee N, et al. (2012) The concentrations of serum, plasma and platelet BDNF are all increased by treadmill VO$_2$max performance in healthy college men. Neurosci Lett 519:78–83.

27. Guthikonda S, Alviar CL, Vaduganathan M, Arikan M, Tellez A, et al. (2008) Role of reticulated platelets and platelet size heterogeneity on platelet activity after dual antiplatelet therapy with aspirin and clopidogrel in patients with stable coronary artery disease. J Am Coll Cardiol 52:743–749.

28. Mangalpally KK, Siqueiros-Garcia A, Vaduganathan M, Dong JF, Kleiman NS, et al. (2010) Platelet activation patterns in platelet size sub-populations: differential responses to aspirin in vitro. J Thromb Thrombolysis 30:251–262.

29. Colkesen Y, Muderrisoglu H (2012) The role of mean platelet volume in predicting thrombotic events. Clin Chem Lab Med 50:631–634.

30. Mei-Dan O, Lippi G, Sánchez M, Andia I, Maffulli N (2010) Autologous platelet-rich plasma: a revolution in soft tissue sports injury management? Phys Sportsmed 38:127–135.

31. Mishra A, Harmon K, Woodall J, Vieira A (2012) Sports medicine applications of platelet rich plasma. Curr Pharm Biotechnol 13:1185–1195.

32. World Anti-Doping Agency. The 2014 Prohibited List. International Standard. Available at: http://list.wada-ama.org/. Accessed: 16 August 2014.

33. Wasterlain AS, Braun HJ, Harris AH, Kim HJ, Dragoo JL (2013) The systemic effects of platelet-rich plasma injection. Am J Sports Med 41:186–193.

34. Kasuya N, Kishi Y, Sakita SY, Numano F, Isobe M (2002) Acute vigorous exercise primes enhanced NO release in human platelets. Atherosclerosis 161:225–232.

35. Jones AM (2013) Dietary nitrate supplementation and exercise performance. Sports Med 44 Suppl 1:S35–45.

36. Kuffler DP (2013) Platelet-rich plasma and the elimination of neuropathic pain. Mol Neurobiol 48:315–332.

37. Kennedy G, Norris G, Spence V, McLaren M, Belch JJ (2006) Is chronic fatigue syndrome associated with platelet activation? Blood Coagul Fibrinolysis 17:89–92.

38. Gardner MJ, Demetrakopoulos D, Klepchick PR, Mooar PA (2007) The efficacy of autologous platelet gel in pain control and blood loss in total knee arthroplasty. An analysis of the haemoglobin, narcotic requirement and range of motion. Int Orthop 31:309–313.

39. Everts PA, Devilee RJ, Brown Mahoney C, van Erp A, Oosterbos CJ, et al. (2008) Exogenous application of platelet-leukocyte gel during open subacromial decompression contributes to improved patient outcome. A prospective randomized double-blind study. Eur Surg Res 40:203–210.

40. Fanning J, Murrain L, Flora R, Hutchings T, Johnson JM, et al. (2007) Phase I/II prospective trial of autologous platelet tissue graft in gynecologic surgery. J Minim Invasive Gynecol 14:633–637.

41. Raeissadat SA, Sedighipour L, Rayegani SM, Bahrami MH, Bayat M, et al. (2014) Effect of Platelet-Rich Plasma (PRP) versus Autologous Whole Blood on Pain and Function Improvement in Tennis Elbow: A Randomized Clinical Trial. Pain Res Treat 2014:191525.

42. Andia I, Latorre PM, Gomez MC, Burgos-Alonso N, Abate M, et al. (2014) Platelet-rich plasma in the conservative treatment of painful tendinopathy: a systematic review and meta-analysis of controlled studies. Br Med Bull 110:99–115.

43. Hamid MS, Yusof A, Mohamed Ali MR (2014) Platelet-rich plasma (PRP) for acute muscle injury: a systematic review. PLoS One 9:e90538.

18

The Pro-Resolving Lipid Mediator Maresin 1 (MaR1) Attenuates Inflammatory Signaling Pathways in Vascular Smooth Muscle and Endothelial Cells

Anuran Chatterjee*, Anjali Sharma, Mian Chen, Robert Toy, Giorgio Mottola, Michael S. Conte

Cardiovascular Research Institute (CVRI) and Department of Surgery, University of California San Francisco, San Francisco, California

Abstract

Objective: Inflammation and its resolution are central to vascular injury and repair. Maresins comprise a new family of bioactive lipid mediators synthesized from docosahexaenoic acid, an ω-3 polyunsaturated fatty acid. They have been found to exert anti-inflammatory and pro-resolving responses in macrophages, neutrophils and bronchial epithelial cells and impart beneficial actions in murine models of peritonitis and colitis. We investigated the impact of maresin-1 (MaR1) on tumor necrosis factor alpha (TNF-α) induced inflammatory responses in human vascular endothelial (EC) and smooth muscle cells (VSMC).

Methods: Primary cultures of human saphenous vein EC and VSMC were employed. We tested the naturally occurring MaR1 as modulator of TNF-α effects, with examination of monocyte adhesion, oxidant stress, and intracellular inflammatory signaling pathways.

Results: MaR1 attenuated TNF-α induced monocyte adhesion and reactive oxygen species (ROS) generation in both EC and VSMC, associated with down-regulated expression (cell surface) of the adhesion molecule E-selectin (in EC) and NADPH-oxidases (NOX4, NOX1, NOX2). MaR1 attenuated TNF-α induced release of pro-inflammatory mediators by EC and VSMC. MaR1 caused an attenuation of TNF-α induced NF-κB activation in both cell types associated with inhibition of I-κ Kinase (IKK) phosphorylation, IκB-α degradation and nuclear translocation of the NF- κB p65 subunit. MaR1 also caused a time-dependent increase in intracellular cyclic AMP (cAMP) in both naive and TNF-α stimulated VSMC and EC.

Conclusions: MaR1 has broad anti-inflammatory actions on EC and VSMC, which may be partly mediated through up-regulation of cAMP and down-regulation of the transcription factor NF-κB. The results suggest that the pro-resolving lipid mediator MaR1 exerts homeostatic actions on vascular cells that counteract pro-inflammatory signals. These findings may have direct relevance for acute and chronic states of vascular inflammation.

Editor: Anthony Peter Sampson, University of Southampton School of Medicine, United Kingdom

Funding: Funding was provided by American Heart Association- Scientist Development Grant (13SDG16940069) to AC, National Institutes of Health- National Heart Lung and Blood Institute (HL119508) to MSC. The funders had no role in study design, data collection and analysis, decision to publish, or preparation of the manuscript.

Competing Interests: The authors would also like to declare no competing interests related to the funding agency "American Heart Association."

* Email: anuran.chatterjee@ucsf.edu

Introduction

Acute inflammatory responses are associated with vascular endothelial (EC) and smooth muscle cell (VSMC) activation and transmigration of leukocytes across blood vessels, resulting in vascular leak and edema at the site of infection or injury. Counter-regulatory mechanisms such as production of anti-inflammatory cytokines and negative feedback loops of pro-inflammatory signals blunt the inflammatory response and assist in the attainment of homeostasis. It has further become apparent that distinct bioactive mediators regulate the "resolution phase" of inflammation. Employing an unbiased lipidomics approach using liquid chromatography mass spectrometry (LC/MS-MS), novel ω3-polyun-saturated fatty acid derived lipids were discovered in mouse peritoneal inflammatory exudates, giving rise to the discovery of a new genus of "specialized pro-resolving mediators (SPM)" [1]. Docosahexaenoic acid (DHA) and eicosapentaenoic acid (EPA) present in blood and edema were found to serve as precursor ω3-PUFA for SPMs, which include protectin D1, D-series (Resolvin-D1, D2, D3, D4, D5) and E-series resolvins (Resolvin-E1, E2). Maresins (**Ma**crophage mediators in **res**olving **in**flammation) are a newly discovered class of lipid mediators synthesized by macrophages in the presence of DHA [2]. Maresin1 (MaR1) is biochemically synthesized from 14-lipoxygenation of DHA by human macrophage 12-lipoxygenase (hm12-LOX) that produces 14-hydroperoxy-docosahexaenoic acid (14-HpDHA which in turn produces an epoxide intermediate 13S, 14S-epoxide that is hydrolyzed to bioactive MaR1. The complete stereochemistry of MaR1 is established and shown to be 7R, 14S-dihydroxy- docosa-4Z,8E,10E,12Z,16Z,19Z-hexaenoic acid [3].

The profile of biological activity of SPMs is an area of considerable interest in the field of inflammation [4]. Resolvins are extensively investigated both *in vitro* and *in vivo* in models of inflammatory diseases, and were found to induce "pro-resolution" activities through cessation of neutrophil infiltration, enhancement of macrophage efferocytosis (removal of dead cells from the inflammatory milieu), and showed dose-dependent actions on attenuation of organ injury, inflammatory signaling and mortality [5]. The mechanisms through which resolvins exert their biological actions involve down-regulation of NF-κB and AP-1 activity and are thought to be mediated via G-protein coupled receptors (GPCRs) [6,7]. Along these lines, maresins also enhance macrophage phagocytosis of apoptotic neutrophils, limit neutrophil infiltration (in a mouse model of zymosan induced peritonitis) and reduce neuropathic pain in mice by blocking transient receptor potential V1 (TRPV1) currents in dorsal root ganglion neurons [3]. In a recent study, MaR1 was shown to exert a protective effect on human bronchial epithelial cells exposed to organic dust by attenuating cytokine production and PKCα and PKCε activation [8]. In a murine model of colitis, MaR1 dose-dependently reduced colon injury, blocked expression of inflammatory mediators and reduced NF-κB activation in the colon [9]. Interestingly, it was also shown that higher levels of MaR1 were associated with an increase in M2 macrophages (associated with homeostasis of inflammation) versus M1-macrophages (pro-inflammatory subtype), thereby signifying a homeostatic and pro-resolution function of MaR1 [10].

Inflammation and its resolution are central to the processes of vascular injury and repair, which are directly relevant to clinical problems such as failure of angioplasty, stenting, and vascular grafts in patients with advanced atherosclerotic disease. In recent studies, we characterized the anti-inflammatory and pro-resolving activities of resolvin-D1 (RvD1) in human VSMC and in a rabbit model of vascular injury induced by balloon angioplasty [7]. In the present study, we sought to investigate the biological activity of MaR1 in vascular cells, and to define a potential role for MaR1 as a therapeutic target in vascular healing.

Materials and Methods

Reagents, cells and treatment protocol

Human greater saphenous veins discarded at the time of coronary or peripheral bypass grafting operations at The University of California- San Francisco (approved by the Institutional Review Board; UCSF Committee on Human Research- Number: 10-03395; the committee waived the need for informed consent) were used to prepare primary cell cultures of EC and VSMC, as described previously [11]. VSMC were maintained in Dulbecco's Modified Eagle's Medium (DMEM; low glucose; HyClone, Logan, UT) containing 10% FBS (Life Technologies, Grand Island, NY) penicillin/streptomycin/amphotericin B (Lonza 1760) and used between passages 2 and 5. EC (passage 2 to 7) were maintained in Media 199 with Earle's Balanced Salt Solution (Hyclone, Logan, UT) supplemented with 10% FBS, penicillin/streptomycin/amphotericin B (Lonza 1760), ECGS (BD Cat no. 356006) and heparin (17.5 U/ml). U937 monocytes were maintained in RPMI-1640 Medium (Hyclone Laboratories, Logan, UT) supplemented with antibiotics (Lonza 1760) and 10% FBS, 1% Glutamine, 1% Sodium Pyruvate and 1.2% HEPES. MaR1 (7R, 14S-dihydroxy-4Z,8E,10E,12Z,

16Z,19Z-docosahexaenoic acid) and resolvin-D1 (7S, 8R, 17S-trihydroxy-4Z,9E,11E,13Z,15E,19Z-docosahexaenoic acid) were obtained from Cayman Chemicals ((Ann Arbor, MI). In most experiments (except where indicated) we utilized a pre-treatment protocol where cells were exposed to MaR1 at indicated doses for 30 min prior to the addition of TNF-α.

Monocyte adhesion assay

VSMC and EC, grown to 100% confluency in black 96-clear bottom plates were utilized in a static monocyte adhesion assay as described previously [12]. In brief, VSMC and EC were pre-treated with MaR1 for 30 min and activated with TNF-α for 4 hr. U937 monocytes were labeled with calcein-AM (Life Technologies, Carlsbad, CA) for 30 min at 37°C in PBS and were washed once and resuspended in PBS at a concentration of 1 million cells/ml. Labeled monocytes (0.2 million/well) were added to EC or VSMC after 4 hr of TNF-α incubation and allowed to incubate for 20 min at 37°C and 5%CO$_2$. In separate experiments (Fig S1B), only the monocytes were incubated with MaR1 at various nM concentrations along with calcein-AM for 30 min at 37°C and after one wash with PBS, were placed on top of TNF-α activated VSMC (0.2 million/well). Unbound monocytes were washed off with cold PBS and fluorescence measurements (excitation 494 nm, emission 517 nm) of bound monocytes were made with a plate reader (SpectraMax M2e Molecular Devices, Sunnyvale, CA). To visualize adhesion response in EC (Fig 1 A, B, C) cells were grown in 24 well plates to 100% confluency and after performing the adhesion assay (same protocol as above), cells were washed twice with ice-cold PBS, fixed with methanol for 10 min and were visualized under a microscope with 10× objective.

Measurement of reactive oxygen species (ROS)

For measurement of ROS in VSMC, we used the cell-permeable reagent "dihydroethidium" (DHE) as an indicator of superoxide, which binds to superoxide anions and is rapidly oxidized to ethidium bromide, which then binds to DNA and stains the nucleus red. VSMC were seeded in 8-well chamber slides (EMS, Hatfield, PA) at the concentration of 15000 cells per chamber and were treated with MaR1 the next day in serum free media for 30 min, followed by 4 hr of TNF-α (10 ng/ml). DHE was added at a final concentration of 3 μM per well and incubated for 30 min at 37°C and 5%CO$_2$, protected from light. VSMC were then washed 3 times in warm PBS (in dark) and mounted with "Vectashield" mounting medium with DAPI nuclear counter-stain (Vector Laboratories, Burlingame, CA). Fluorescence was detected in a fluorescence microscope, allowing the detection of DHE at excitation/emission wavelength of 488 nm/590 nm. Multiple images (random) were taken from each treatment group (wells) and the mean nucleus-DHE fluorescence per nucleus area was calculated from all images of each well (group) using Image J software (NIH).

TNF-α is known to induce an apoptotic effect in EC and the release of cytochrome c from mitochondria into the cytoplasm is known to give a false positive signal for DHE, interfering with superoxide detection in EC [13]. Therefore in EC, we used CellRox Deep Red reagent (Life Technologies, Carlsbad, CA) as an indicator of ROS (mainly O$_2^{\cdot-}$ and OH$^{\cdot}$ radicals). The cell-permeant dye is non-fluorescent in reduced state and binds preferentially to superoxide and hydroxyl radicals emitting a fluorescent signal with absorption/emission maxima at 644 nm/665 nm. Endothelial cells were seeded in human fibronectin coated 96-well black plates at a density of 50000 cells/well and were assayed the next day for ROS. The treatment protocols were similar to VSMC but the TNF-α dose was 1 ng/ml and we

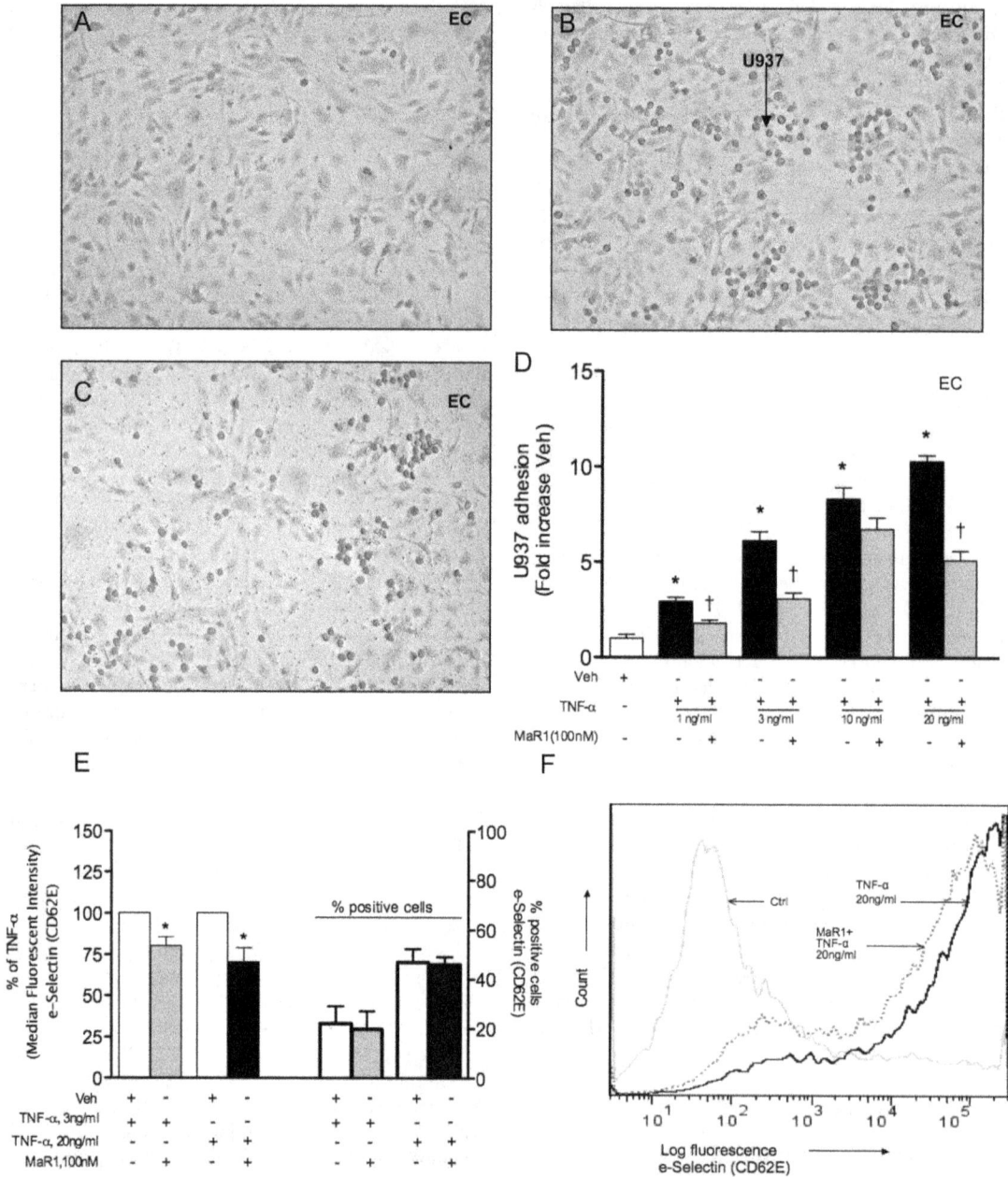

Figure 1. MaR1 attenuates TNF-α induced monocyte adhesion. (A, B, C) Endothelial cells grown in 24-well plates were treated with vehicle (A, B) or 100 nM MaR1 (C) for 30 min, followed by TNF-α at 1 ng/ml (B, C) for 4 hr and adhesion of labeled U937 monocytes were visualized under a microscope. (D) EC were grown in 96-well plates and adhesion of labeled U937 monocytes (4 hr post TNF-α) were quantified using a fluorescence plate reader. Treatment protocol of MaR1 was same as (Fig 1A, B, C). N≥4. N = each well of a 96-well plate. ANOVA (oneway) with Dunnett's posthoc test (p = 0.003). *:p≤0.05 compared to vehicle control, †: p≤0.05 compared to TNF-α alone (t-test). (E) EC grown in 12-well plates were treated with vehicle or 100 nM MaR1 as (Fig 1A, B, C) and after 4 hr of TNF-α, analyzed for cell surface E-selectin expression by flow cytometry. N≥5. N = each well of 12-well plate. *:p≤0.05 compared to TNF-α alone (t-test). Error bar = SEM. (F) Representative histogram of (E) for TNF-α at 20 ng/ml.

analyzed ROS production 2 hours post TNF-α. This was based on a preliminary time-course study in EC that showed a peak in the CellRox signal at 2 hr post TNF-α (data not shown).

Western blotting

VSMC and EC were lysed in CellLytic M buffer (Sigma, Cat no. C2978) and were saved in −80°C after three pulses of low watt sonication on ice. The lysates were centrifuged at 21000 g for 20 min and the supernatants (whole cell lysates) were run on Mini-

Protean TGX gels (Biorad, Hercules, CA), transferred on PVDF membranes and probed with appropriate primary antibodies. Sources of primary antibodies are as follows: NOX4 (Cat no. ab109225) from Abcam Inc (Cambridge, MA); NOX2 (Cat no. 20782), NOX1 (Cat no. SC5821) and IκB-α (Cat no. SC371) from Santa Cruz biotechnology (Dallas, TX); iNOS (PA-1036) from Thermo Scientific-Pierce (Rockford, IL); Phospho IKK α/β (Ser 176/180, Cat no. 2694) and IKK (Cat no. 2684) from Cell Signaling Inc (Danvers, MA). We used streptavidin bound Q-dot

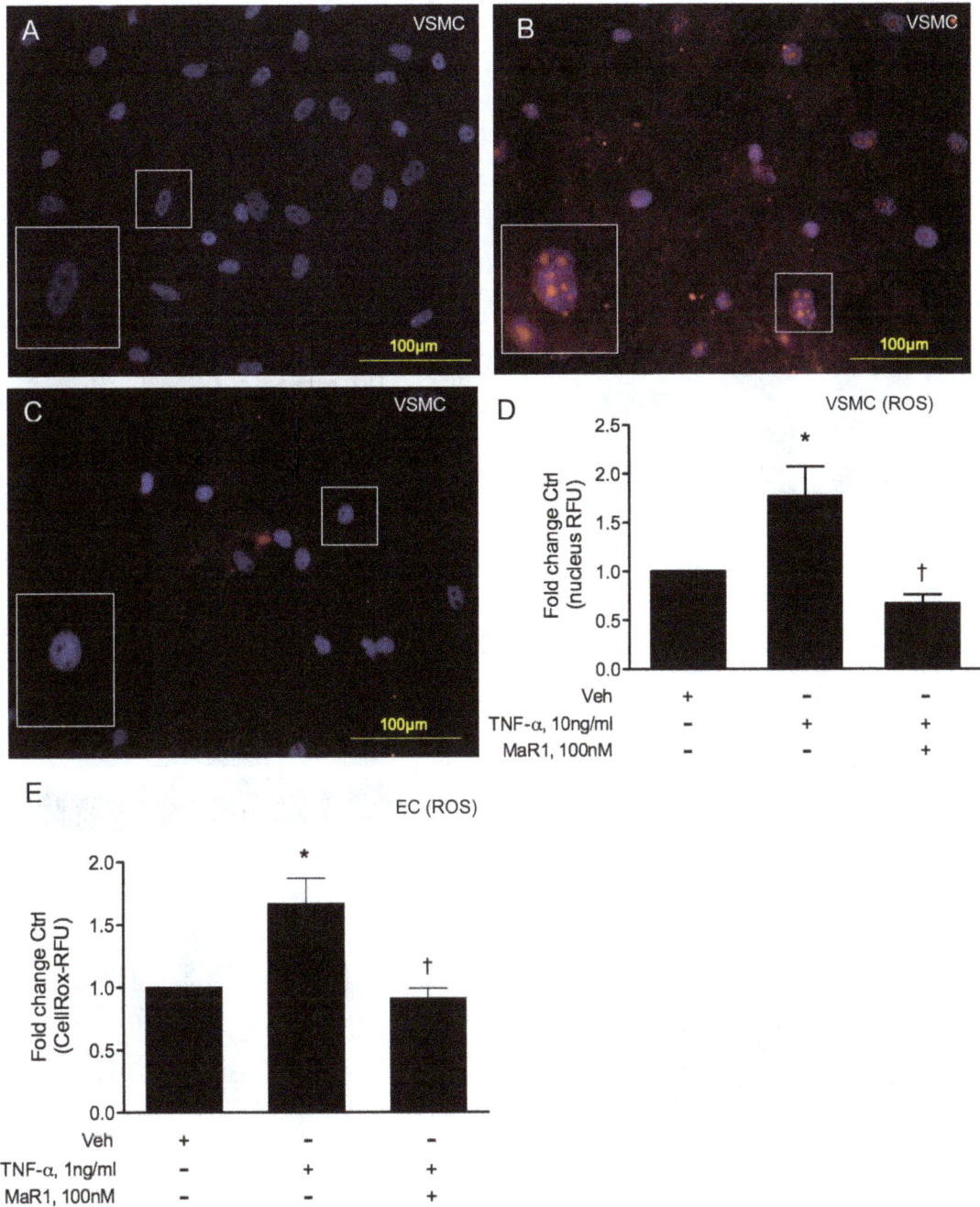

Figure 2. MaR1 attenuates TNF-α induced ROS production in vascular smooth muscle and endothelial cells. (A–C) Representative images of dihydroethidium/DHE stained (red) vascular smooth muscle cells counterstained with DAPI (nucleus). VSMC were grown in 8-well chamber slides and received vehicle (A, B) or 100 nM of MaR1 (C) for 30 min, followed by TNF-α, 10 ng/ml for 4 hr (B, C). (D) Quantitative analysis of mean DHE intensity (nucleus RFU/area of nucleus) of vascular smooth muscle cells, N≥3 per group. N = each well of an 8-well chamber slide. (E) EC grown in 96-well plates, received 100 nM of MaR1, 30 min prior to TNF-α and ROS production was measured 2 hr post TNF-α, using a ROS specific dye CellRox Deep Red reagent, N≥3 per group. N = each well of a 96-well plate. *:p≤0.05 compared to vehicle control, †: p≤0.05 compared to TNF-α alone (t-test). Error bar = SEM.

nano crystals (Life Technologies, Carlsbad, CA) for detection of the proteins bound to biotinylated secondary antibodies. For iNOS, we used HRP labeled secondary antibodies (Santa Cruz Biotechnology, Cat no. SC2030) and detected bands using Western Bright Quantum HRP substrate (Advansta, Menlo Park, CA).

Array for analysis of secreted cytokines

Protein expression analysis of inflammatory cytokines were performed using "human antibody inflammation arrays" (Raybiotech, Norcross, GA, Cat no. AAH-INF-3) according to the manufacturer's protocol. Briefly, EC and VSMC were grown to confluency in 6-well plates and were serum starved for 24 hrs, followed by MaR1 treatment (30 min) and TNF-α for 18 hrs.

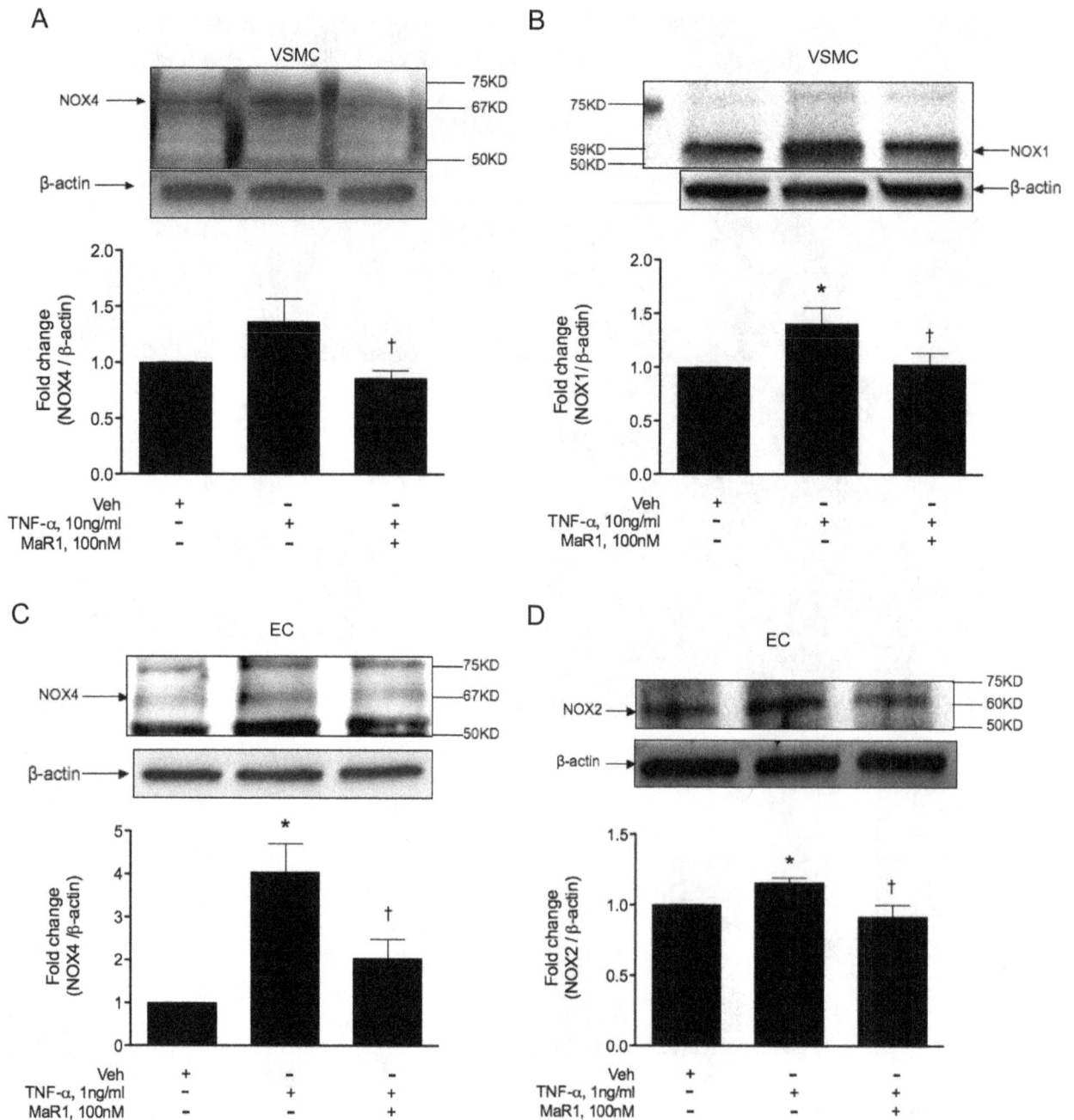

Figure 3. MaR1 attenuates TNF-α induced expression of NADPH-oxidases. VSMC (A, B) and EC (C, D) were treated with 100 nM of MaR1 for 30 min, followed by TNF-α for 6 hr. After TNF-α treatment, cells were lysed and probed for NOX-4, NOX-1 and NOX-2. (A) N = 14 per group, (B) N = 17 per group, (C) N ≥ 7 per group, (D) N = 3 per group. *:p≤0.05 compared to vehicle control, †: p≤0.05 compared to TNF-α alone (t-test). N = each well of a 6-well plate. Error bar = SEM.

Conditioned cell culture media was saved at −80°C for antibody microarray analysis. Data was normalized to protein content per well. Densitometric analysis was performed using Biorad Chemidoc Software (Image Lab 4.0.1).

Immunofluorescence for p65 localization

Cells were seeded on 8-well chamber slides (EMS, Hatfield, PA) and after treatment, were briefly rinsed in PBS and fixed with 2% paraformaldehyde for 20 min at room temperature, followed by permeabilization in ice-cold acetone (10 min at −20°C) and 1% Triton-X100 (20 min at room temperature). Cells were incubated

in a humidified chamber overnight with anti-p65 antibody (Santa Cruz Biotechnology, Dallas, TX, Cat no. SC-372) at 4°C, followed by ALEXA-Fluor 488 tagged secondary antibody (Life Technologies, Carlsbad, CA) and were visualized under a fluorescence microscope. Quantitation of fluorescent signals in nucleus and cytoplasm were performed using GIMP 2.8 software (www.gimp.org).

cAMP assay

Cyclic AMP assay was performed using an ELISA kit (Enzo Life Sciences Inc, Farmingdale, NY, Cat no. ADI-900-066). Confluent

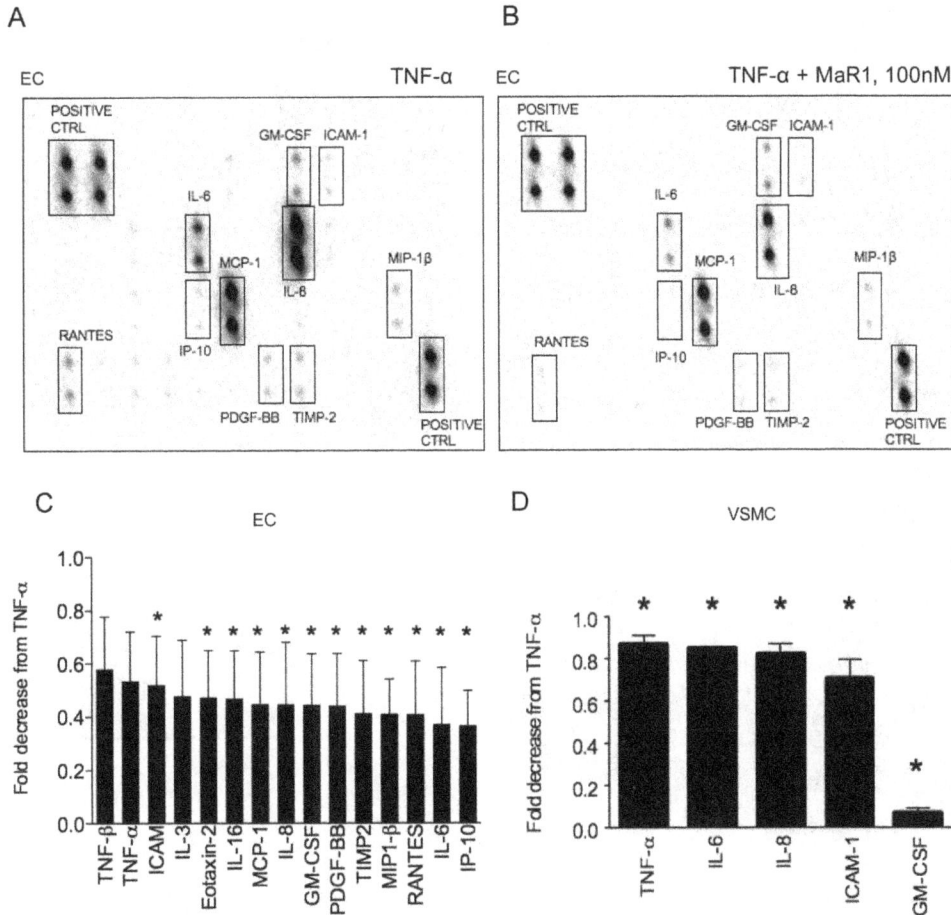

Figure 4. MaR1 attenuates TNF-α induced inflammatory pathways. EC were treated with 100 nM MaR1 for 30 min followed by 18 hr of TNF-α (1 ng/ml), after which the conditioned medium was analyzed for the presence of 40 different inflammatory mediators using antibody arrays. (A, B) Representative images of three independent experiments done on EC. (C) After densitometric analysis of individual spots (in duplicate) normalized to protein content (cell lysates), inflammatory mediators that were down-regulated significantly in TNF-α+ MaR1 (t-test: p≤0.05), compared to TNF-α alone are shown in the bar-graph, N = 3. (D) Graphical representation of down-regulated inflammatory proteins found in the media from VSMC that underwent same treatment protocol as (Fig 4 A–C) but with TNF-α at 10 ng/ml. N = 3. *:p≤0.05 compared to TNF-α alone (t-test). N = each well of a 6-well plate. Error bar = SEM.

VSMC and EC were grown in 24-well plates and following treatment, cells were lysed in 0.1 N HCl with 1% TritonX-100 and subsequently cAMP was acetylated and assayed following manufacturer's instructions. Values were calculated from a standard curve generated from acetylated-cAMP supplied by the manufacturer.

Flow cytometry

Endothelial cells grown to 90% confluency in 12-well plates were used for flow cytometry analysis of E-selectin following a previously published protocol [14]. Since cell surface antigens are sensitive to trypsin we first stained the cells with E-selectin antibody, followed by trypsin digestion. After treatment protocol, EC in each well were washed twice with warm PBS and blocked for 10 min with mouse IgG1 in PBS (with 0.5% FBS) in an orbital shaker followed by APC-conjugated mouse-antihuman E-selectin (clone 68-5H11, BD Pharmingen, Cat# 551144) for 30 min in the dark at room temperature. EC were trypsinized briefly with trypsin/EDTA (0.05% Trypsin, Hyclone, Cat # SH30236.01) for 4 min, washed, resuspended in PBS (with 0.5% FBS) and analyzed in BD FACSVerse flow cytometer. Median fluorescence intensity (MFI) and percentage APC positive cells were analyzed by FlowJo software.

Reporter assay

The NF-κB luciferase reporter plasmid (pGL4.32[luc2P/NF-κB-RE/Hygro] Vector) and renilla luciferase reporter plasmid (pGL4.74[h-Rluc/TK] vector) were purchased from Promega corporation (Madison, WI). The NF-κB plasmid contains 5 repeats of NF-κB response element that drives transcription of the luciferase reporter gene luc2P (*Photinus pyralis*). The renilla pRL-TK Vector was used as an internal control reporter vector and contains the herpes simplex virus thymidine kinase (HSV-TK) promoter to provide low to moderate levels of Renilla luciferase expression in co-transfected mammalian cells. VSMC were seeded in 96-well plates at 70% confluency and were co-transfected with 75 ng of DNA (both vectors) in serum and antibiotic-free DMEM media for 1 day, followed by MaR1 or vehicle pre-treatment of 30 min and TNF-α (10 ng/ml) for 6 hr. Cells were then lysed and induced NF-κB reporter activity was corrected for the constitutive renilla luciferase expression using a Dual Luciferase Kit (Promega, WI, Cat no. E1910) and a Glomax-20/20 luminometer. Results

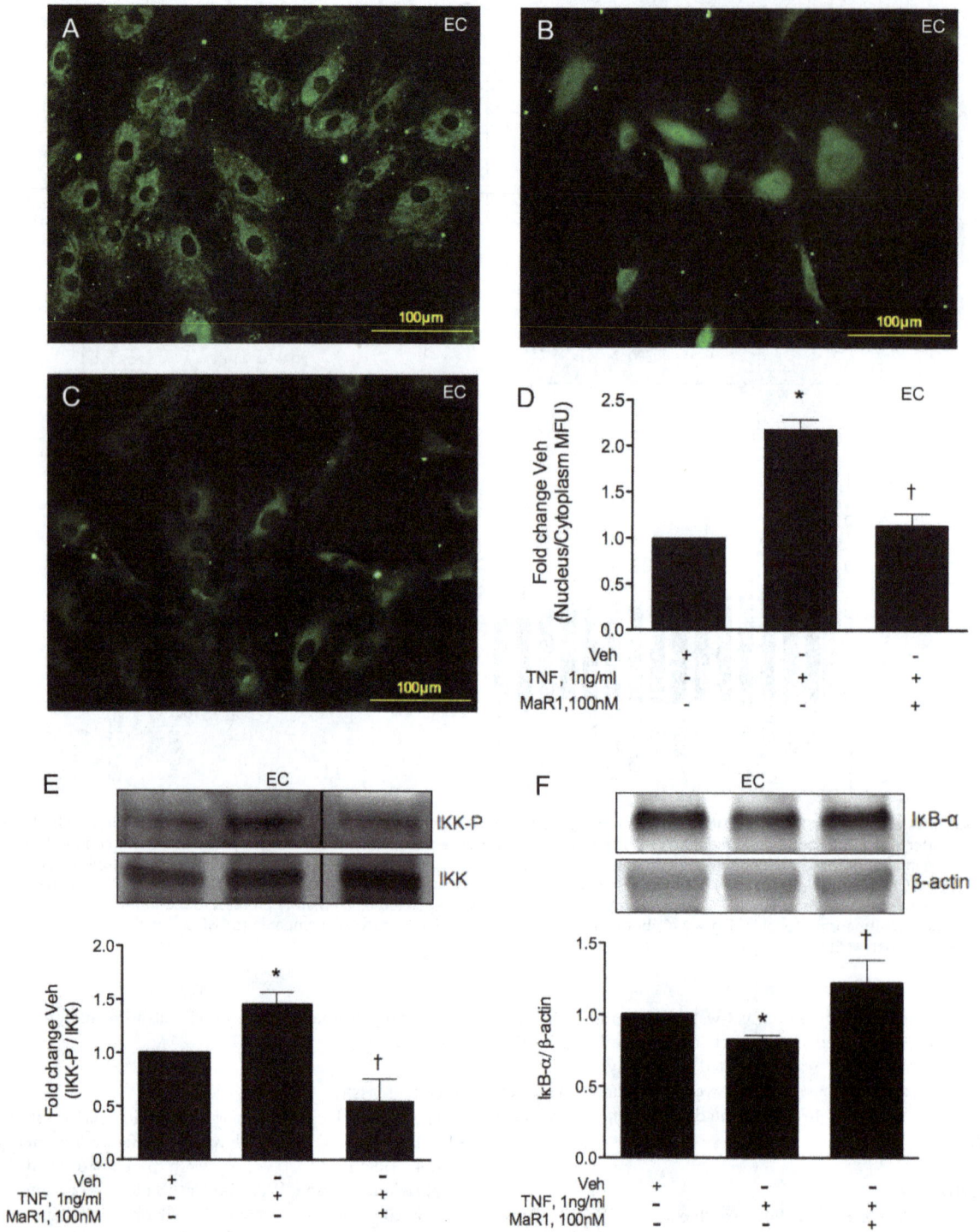

Figure 5. MaR1 attenuates TNF-α induced NF-κB activation in endothelial cells. (A–C) Representative images of nuclear translocation of p65 NF-κB subunit in EC treated with vehicle (A), vehicle + TNF-α, 2 hr (B), 100 nM of MaR1 (30 min) + TNF-α, 2 hr (C). (D) Quantitative analysis of p65 translocation (ratio of nuclear to cytoplasmic fluorescence) in EC. N≥3 where N = each well of an 8-well chamber slide. (E) Endothelial whole cell extracts were analyzed for phospho- and total-IKK, 15 min post TNF-α addition that received 100 nM MaR1, 30 min prior to TNF-α. N = 3 where N = one 10 cm plate. *:p≤0.05 compared to vehicle control, †: p≤0.05 compared to TNF-α alone (t-test). (F) EC received vehicle or 100 nM MaR1 for 30 min and TNF-α for 1 hr, after which they were lysed and probed for IκB-α. *:p≤0.05 compared to vehicle control, †: p≤0.05 compared to TNF-α alone (t-test) Error bar = SEM.

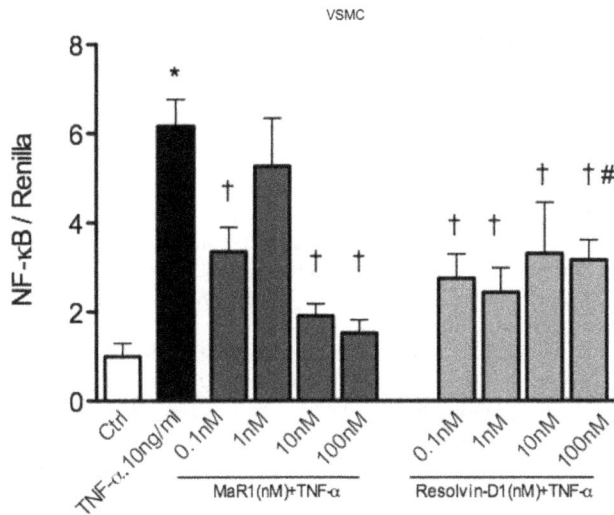

Figure 6. MaR1 and Resolvin-D1 attenuates TNF-α induced NF-κB reporter activity in vascular smooth muscle cells. VSMC transfected with firefly luciferase (NF-κB) and renilla luciferase vectors were treated with MaR1 and resolvin-D1, followed by TNF-α for 6 hr and were analyzed for firefly and renilla luciferase activity. Net NF-κB activity is shown as a ratio of firefly luciferase activity normalized to renilla luciferase for transfection efficiency. N≥6 per group. *:p≤0.05 compared to vehicle control, †: p≤0.05 compared to TNF-α alone (One way ANOVA with Dunnett's post hoc test). #: p = 0.01 (t-test) compared to MaR1, 100 nM +TNF-α. N = each well of a 96-well plate. Error bar = SEM.

were subtracted from background reading obtained from a non-transfected control.

Results

MaR1 attenuates TNF-α –induced monocyte adhesion to vascular cells

Exposure of vascular cells to pro-inflammatory mediators like TNF-α results in an increase in the adhesion of leukocytes through receptor-ligand interactions (e.g. integrins). TNF-α (1–20 ng/ml) induced a 2.9–10.3 fold increase in U937 adhesion to EC (Fig 1 D) and a 1.7–2.4 fold increase in U937 adhesion to VSMC (Fig S1A). Pre-incubation of EC and VSMC with MaR1 (100 nM) resulted in a significant attenuation of the TNF-α induced adhesion response. This decrease in adhesion was not due to cell death as measured by cytotoxicity (MTT) assays in both cell types (data not shown). We also observed (data not shown) inhibition of monocyte adhesion with MaR1 at 10 nM with TNF-α at 10 ng/ml(VSMC) and 1 ng/ml(EC). In a different experiment, we pre-treated only the monocytes with MaR1 (0.1–100 nM) and exposed them to TNF-α activated VSMC to examine direct effects of MaR1 on monocytes. We observed a dose-dependent attenuation of U937 adhesion to activated VSMC, with a maximum inhibition of 46% with 100 nM MaR1 (Fig S1B).

In order to investigate the mechanisms associated with this inhibition of cell-cell adhesion, we examined cell surface VCAM-1 and ICAM-1 in both cell types, and E-selectin expression in EC following TNF exposure (Fig 1E, F). We did not identify a significant reduction in cell surface VCAM-1 and ICAM-1 expression by MaR1 (10–100 nM, data not shown), however we observed a significant, modest decrease (20–30%) in endothelial E-selectin expression (Fig 1E) by MaR1 (100 nM).

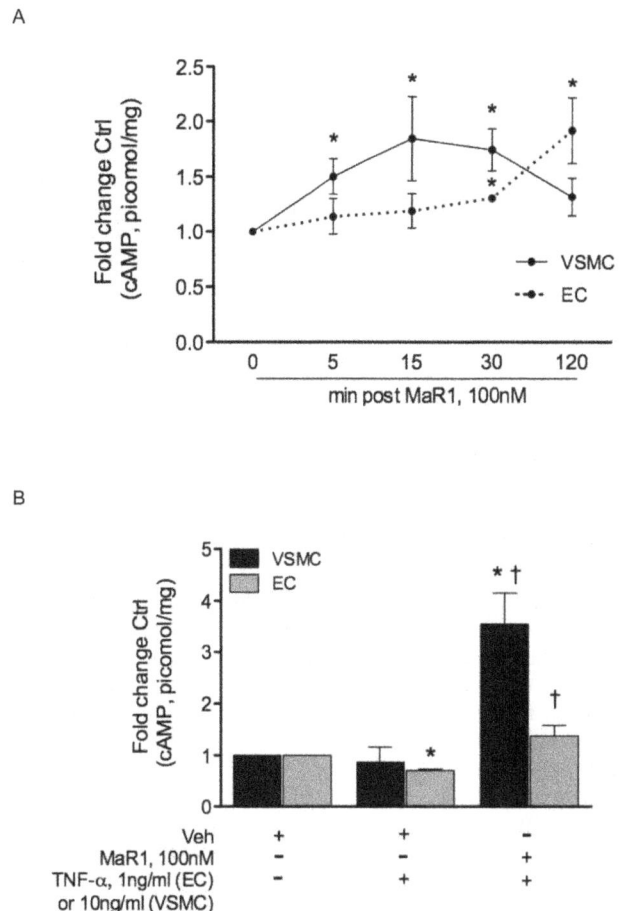

Figure 7. MaR1 increases cAMP levels in vascular smooth muscle and endothelial cells. (A) VSMC and EC were seeded to confluency in 24-well plates and were treated with 100 nM MaR1 for the indicated time-points and cAMP levels were determined and normalized to mg protein. N = 3 per time-point (B) VSMC and EC were treated with vehicle or MaR1 (100 nM) for 30 min, followed by TNF-α (10 ng/ml for VSMC, 1 ng/ml for EC) for 120 min and assayed for cAMP. N = 4. *:p≤0.05 compared to vehicle control (0 min) (t-test); †: p≤0.05 compared to TNF-α + vehicle (t-test). N = each well of a 24-well plate. Error bar = SEM.

MaR1 abrogates TNF-α induced oxidative stress and NOX expression in vascular cells

We selected the dosage of TNF-α at 1 ng/ml for EC and 10 ng/ml for VSMC for all subsequent experiments, as these doses gave optimum induction of the experimental parameters studied.

TNF-α binds to its receptor TNFR-I in VSMC and EC and results in ROS production in a time and dose-dependent manner. A family of ROS producing enzymes, classified as NADPH-oxidases (NOX) form the major source of TNF-α induced ROS [15,16,17]. We investigated the extent of ROS production under TNF-α exposure and analyzed expression of the major ROS producing NOX isoform, NOX-4 (in both VSMC and EC), NOX-1 (VSMC) and NOX-2 (EC). TNF-α (4 hr treatment) caused a significant increase in dihydroethidium (DHE) fluorescence in the nuclei of VSMC (1.77 fold Ctrl, ±0.30 SEM), indicating formation of fluorescent ethidium bromide-DNA adducts (Fig 2B, D). MaR1 treatment at 100 nM caused a significant decrease in DHE fluorescence below baseline values

(0.67 fold Ctrl, ±0.09 SEM, p = 0.001) in VSMC and significantly decreased ROS generation (0.91 fold ctrl ±0.08 SEM) in EC.

We investigated expression of NADPH-oxidases (NOX) in order to see if the reduced ROS generation was related to altered NOX expression. In VSMC, NOX4 showed up as a clearly defined band at 67 KD (isoform NOX4B) as found by others [18] whereas in EC there were a few non-specific bands in addition to the predicted 67KD weight. In this study, we have quantified this predominant NOX4 isoform (NOX4B) in both cell type. We found TNF-α to up-regulate NOX4 in VSMC (p = 0.08) 4 hr post TNF-α addition (Fig 3A), whereas MaR1 (100 nM) caused a significant attenuation of NOX-4 expression (p = 0.02 compared to TNF-α alone). In EC, MaR1 (100 nM) showed similar inhibitory effect on NOX4 expression (p = 0.042), 6 hr post TNF-α addition (Fig 3C). In VSMC, there was a significant attenuation in NOX-1 levels by 100 nM MaR1 (Fig 3B, p = 0.048) and in EC, MaR1 almost completely abolished NOX-2 expression (Fig 3D, p = 0.046).

MaR1 attenuates TNF-α induced pro-inflammatory pathways

TNF-α augments endothelial pro-inflammatory gene transcription and subsequently the release of cytokines in the extracellular milieu that amplify local inflammation in a paracrine fashion [19,20]. We looked at the effect of MaR1 on the levels of these secreted inflammatory mediators using an antibody-based membrane array. Out of the 40 proteins we studied using the human inflammation array-3 (refer: http://www.raybiotech.com/c-series-human-inflammation-array-3-8.html), we found many to be significantly down-regulated (~50%–60%), 18 hr post TNF-α (1 ng/ml) by MaR1 (100 nM) in EC (Fig 4C). In VSMC, MaR1 (100 nM) caused a modest but significant decrease in several mediators (Fig 4D) with the strongest inhibitory effect seen in GM-CSF levels (Fig 4D). Additionally, in endothelial cells, we observed a dramatic attenuation of expression of inducible nitric oxide synthase (iNOS) by MaR1 (Fig S2).

TNF-α signaling is known to involve the coordinated activity of multiple transcription factors in endothelial and smooth muscle cells (e.g. NF-κB, AP-1), resulting in enhanced transcription of a spectrum of inflammatory mediators [21]. The NF-κB family of transcription factors (p65/p50 heterodimer being the most abundant type) are involved with activation of various pro-inflammatory genes in response to TNF-α [22]. Binding of TNF-α to its receptor TNFR-I results in activation of a series of down-stream signaling intermediates that phosphorylate I-kappa kinases (IKK) which in turn phosphorylates I-kappa α and results in its proteosomal degradation, releasing p65 from the I-kappa α/p65-p50 complex and its translocation into the nucleus [23]. We examined these key steps in VSMC and EC exposed to TNF-α with or without MaR1 preteatment at 100 nM. In both EC (Fig 5) and VSMC (Fig S3), MaR1 significantly reduced p65 nuclear translocation in response to TNF-α (Fig 5C, D; Fig S3 C, D). In endothelial cells, TNF-α enhanced IKK-phospho levels to 1.45 fold control and MaR1 decreased the phosphorylation to 0.55 fold control levels (Fig 5E). In smooth muscle cells TNF-α caused a 31% increase in IKK-p whereas MaR1 brought down IKK-phospho levels below control levels (Fig S3E). As shown in Fig 5F and Fig S3F, there was a significant inhibition of IκB-α degradation in both cell types by MaR1(100 nM). Finally, we looked at the net extent of NF-κB activation over a longer time-period (6 hrs) in VSMC, utilizing a luciferase based reporter assay (Fig 6). We tested MaR1 and the pro-resolving mediator resolvin-D1 at four different doses in order to compare dose-dependent effects of these two distinct lipid mediators. Our results show a significant inhibition of NF-κB activation by both MaR1 and Resolvin-D1, however at 100 nM, MaR1 was slightly more effective that resolvin-D1 (Fig 6).

MaR1 stimulates cAMP production in naive and TNF-α activated VSMC and EC

Since cyclic-AMP modulates inflammatory signals in a wide variety of cells, and is involved with promoting an anti-inflammatory [24] and anti-oxidant effect in vascular cells [25], we determined the effects of MaR1 on intracellular cAMP levels in both naive and TNF-α activated VSMC and EC. There was a time-dependent increase in intracellular cAMP levels in both cell types by MaR1, where vascular smooth muscle cells showed enhanced elevation of cAMP in comparison to endothelial cells in early time-points (Fig 7A). There was a 50%, 84% and 75% increase in cAMP in VSMC, 5 min, 15 min and 30 min post addition of MaR1 and a modest 30% increase in cAMP levels in EC, 30 min post MaR1 treatment. We investigated cAMP levels, 2 hr post TNF-α in both cell types (Fig 7B) where VSMC/EC received 100 nM MaR1 or vehicle for 30 min followed by TNF-α for 2 hrs. We found that in both cell types MaR1 significantly elevated cAMP levels in TNF-α treated cells. In VSMC, cAMP levels were 3.5 fold (±0.60 SEM) higher in MaR1 treated group versus vehicle control group, compared to 0.87 fold (±0.28 SEM) in TNF-α alone group (Fig 7B). In EC, TNF-α exposure led to reduced cAMP levels to 0.70 fold control (±0.02 SEM, p≤0.05) whereas MaR1 pre-treatment caused an increase in cAMP levels of 1.37 fold (±0.20 SEM) control (Fig 7B).

Discussion

Acute vascular injury (e.g. resulting from angioplasty, stents, bypass grafting etc.) involves endothelial and smooth muscle cell activation resulting in adhesion and sequestration of monocytes and neutrophils and subsequent tissue injury to the vessel wall. The inflammation that succeeds the vascular injury induces a phenotypic switch in VSMC that results in their proliferation and migration to the *tunica intima*, resulting in development of intimal hyperplasia. Therefore, modulation of the inflammatory response forms one of the pre-eminent therapeutic strategies to attenuate the severity of vascular injury. The findings reported in this study have clinical relevance to a broad range of vascular diseases e.g. atherosclerosis, vascular injury associated restenosis, diabetes and peripheral vascular disease among many others as most of them have persistent vascular inflammation as an important contributor in the pathogenesis of the disease. Since the discovery of pro-resolving lipid mediators by Serhan et al. [1] in an acute murine model of peritonitis, there has been an exponential growth in the number of investigations on DHA and EPA derived SPMs, especially in relation to inflammatory diseases. Resolvin-E1 is under active investigation in clinical trials for dry eye, asthma and other diseases (Source: www.clinicaltrials.gov). Compared to other SPMs, relatively little is known about the biological activity of the macrophage synesized lipid mediator MaR1. Moreover, its effects on endothelial and smooth muscle cells have not been characterized. Since Maresins and D-series resolvins share the same precursor (DHA), and we have previously shown that D-series resolvins exert potent anti-inflammatory and homeostatic effects in vascular cells [7,26] we hypothesized MaR1 to possess similar properties.

We have observed an anti-adhesive effect of MaR1 on both cell types. When MaR1 was incubated with monocytes alone, we also saw an inhibition of the adhesive effect, which might imply that MaR1 interferes with monocyte function. Flow-cytometry based analyses showed that MaR1 causes a 20–30% reduction in cell surface E-selectin expression, which is involved with "rolling" phenomenon of monocytes that precedes firm adhesion. Surprisingly, we did not see any significant inhibition of cell surface expression of VCAM-1 and ICAM-1 in EC and VSMC by MaR1. Investigations are underway in our lab in order to better characterize the mechanisms of reduced adhesion in the presence of MaR1, looking at multiple pathways that may affect monocyte interactions to EC and VSMC.

TNF-α causes generation of reactive oxygen species in endothelial and smooth muscle cells primarily through activation of NADPH-oxidase 4 (NOX-4). Other cell-specific isoforms of NOX, like NOX-1 (in VSMC) and NOX-2 (in EC) are also involved with TNF-α-induced ROS generation but to a much lesser extent compared to NOX-4 [17,27]. Two recent studies show RvD1 [28] and RvE1 [29] to reduce ROS production in macrophages, however to our knowledge, no study has examined the effects of MaR1 on ROS generation in EC or VSMC. Our results show MaR1 to attenuate ROS production, associated with reduced NOX protein expression in both cell types. As ROS is known to play a potentially detrimental role in inflammation, the observed beneficial effects of MaR1 could be partially linked to attenuation of the ROS response. Additional studies involving mRNA and protein expression of components of NOX-4 enzyme complex (e.g. p22 phox), NOX-4 enzyme activity, and characterization of ROS species (hydrogen peroxide, superoxide etc.) are under way to further elucidate mechanisms of ROS attenuation.

TNF-α activates multiple pro-inflammatory transcription factors in EC and VSMC that result in gene transcription and release of the mediators (e.g. cytokines and chemokines) in the extracellular milieu, that act in a paracrine and autocrine fashion to modulate the inflammatory responses. We investigated the effects of MaR1 on extracellular release of 40 different inflammatory mediators in TNF-α activated EC and VSMC 18 hr post TNF-α, and found MaR1 to attenuate a number of the mediators including chemokines and chemoattractants like Interferon gamma induced protein-10 (IP-10), MCP-1, RANTES, MIP-1β, IL-8, Eotaxin-2, IL-16 and cytokines such as GM-CSF and IL-3 which are involved with proliferation and maturation of cells of myeloid lineage. Interestingly, MaR1 also attenuated PDGF-BB release from endothelial cells, an important regulator of VSMC proliferation and migration. MaR1 has been shown *in vivo* to block NF-κB activation in colonic tissues in a murine colitis model [9], however MaR1 was found to have no inhibitory effect on NF-κB activation in human bronchial epithelial cells [8]. Our results show a strong inhibitory effect of MaR1 on NF-κB activation in both cell types, involving several key steps involved with NF-κB activation including phosphorylation of IKK and IκB-α degradation.

RvD1 and RvE1 receptors have been identified, and their actions are known to be mediated through GPCRs in a pertussis toxin sensitive fashion, indicating involvement of Go/Gi type GPCRs [7,30,31,32,33]. MaR1 receptors are still unknown, however a recent report showed partial inhibition of the effects of MaR1 in dorsal root ganglion neurons, in the presence of pertussis toxin, suggestive of a decrease in cAMP mediating MaR1's effects in neurons [3]. In this study, we report MaR1 to elevate intracellular cAMP levels in naive smooth muscle and endothelial cells. A recent study also showed time-dependent elevation of cAMP and PKA activity by resolvin-D1 in mouse RAW 264.7 macrophages [28]. Moreover, we found that MaR1 led to increased cAMP levels in TNF-α treated cells. Cyclic-AMP has been shown to impart anti-inflammatory actions on cytokine activated human endothelial cells and vascular smooth muscle

cells, by blocking NF-κB activation [34,35] and reducing adhesion molecule expression [24,36,37,38], and therefore forms an important line of investigation related to MaR1's anti-inflammatory actions on vascular cells.

Increased levels of 14-HpDHA have been found in subcutaneous fat surrounding foot wounds in patients with peripheral vascular disease (PVD), suggesting activation of resolution pathways involving MaR1 in PVD [39]. In another study, bacterial lipopolysaccharide was found to enhance the synthesis of 14-HpDHA and MaR1 in human Caco-2 epithelial cells and foam macrophages [40]. These observations highlight the importance of MaR1 in activating "anti-inflammatory" and "resolution" signaling pathways in the inflammatory zone or region and underscores its importance in turning "ON" pro-resolution pathways in these inflammatory diseases. In summary, in the present study we report MaR1 to impart a strong anti-inflammatory phenotype in human vascular smooth muscle cells and endothelial cells, associated with reduced monocyte adhesion and TNF-α induced production of ROS and inflammatory mediators. At the molecular level, we found MaR1 to reduce NOX expression and inhibit NF-κB activation and increase intracellular cAMP levels in both cell types. Hence, we conclude that MaR1 has potent anti-inflammatory actions in vascular cells of human origin and modulates signaling pathways under basal and TNFα-stimulated conditions. These findings suggest a therapeutic potential for maresins and their emergence as a novel family of DHA-derived SPMs to treat vascular inflammatory diseases.

Supporting Information

Figure S1 MaR1 attenuates TNF-α induced monocyte (U937) adhesion in VSMC. (A) U937 monocyte adhesion in TNF-α activated VSMC that received 30 min pre-treatment of vehicle or MaR1(100 nM). (B) U937 monocyte adhesion on TNF-α activated (10 ng/ml) VSMC where only the monocytes were pre-treated with MaR1 (0.1–100 nM) for 30 min. N≥4 per group. ANOVA (oneway) with Dunnett's posthoc test (Fig S1A: p = 0.007, Fig S1B:p = 0.003). *:p≤0.05 compared to vehicle control, †: p≤0.05 compared to TNF-α alone. N = each well of a 96-well plate. Error bar = SEM.

Figure S2 MaR1 attenuates TNF-α induced iNOS expression in endothelial cells. Confluent EC grown in 6-well plates were treated with vehicle or TNF-α (1 ng/ml) for 6 hrs with/without 30 min pretreatment with 100 nM MaR1. Whole cell lysates were probed with iNOS and beta-actin. N = 3.*:p≤ 0.05 compared to vehicle control, †: p≤0.05 compared to TNF-α alone (t-test). N = each well of a 6-well plate. Error bar = SEM.

Figure S3 Effect of MaR1 on TNF-α induced NF-κB activation in VSMC. VSMC were treated with vehicle (A, B) or 100 nM MaR1 (C) for 30 min followed by TNF-α (10 ng/ml, B, C) for 2 hr. (A–C) Representative images of VSMC showing nuclear translocation of p65 (in green) (D) Quantitative analysis of A, B, C. N≥3. N = each chamber of an 8-well chamber slide. (E, F) VSMC whole cell extracts were analyzed for phospho- and total-IKK (15 min post TNF-α) and IκB-α (1 hr post TNF-α). (E) N = 3. N = each10 cm plate and (F) N = 5. N = each well of a 6-well plate. Graph represents densitometric analyses of western blots. *:p≤0.05 compared to vehicle control, †: p≤0.05 compared to TNF-α alone. Error bar = SEM.

Author Contributions

Conceived and designed the experiments: AC MSC. Performed the experiments: AC AS RT MC GM. Analyzed the data: AC AS MC GM. Contributed reagents/materials/analysis tools: AC RT MC. Wrote the paper: AC MSC.

References

1. Serhan CN, Clish CB, Brannon J, Colgan SP, Chiang N, et al. (2000) Novel functional sets of lipid-derived mediators with antiinflammatory actions generated from omega-3 fatty acids via cyclooxygenase 2-nonsteroidal antiinflammatory drugs and transcellular processing. J Exp Med 192: 1197–1204.
2. Serhan CN, Yang R, Martinod K, Kasuga K, Pillai PS, et al. (2009) Maresins: novel macrophage mediators with potent antiinflammatory and proresolving actions. J Exp Med 206: 15–23.
3. Serhan CN, Dalli J, Karamnov S, Choi A, Park CK, et al. (2012) Macrophage proresolving mediator maresin 1 stimulates tissue regeneration and controls pain. Faseb J 26: 1755–1765.
4. Serhan CN (2014) Pro-resolving lipid mediators are leads for resolution physiology. Nature 510: 92–101.
5. Fredman G, Serhan CN (2011) Specialized proresolving mediator targets for RvE1 and RvD1 in peripheral blood and mechanisms of resolution. Biochem J 437: 185–197.
6. Lee CH (2012) Resolvins as new fascinating drug candidates for inflammatory diseases. Arch Pharm Res 35: 3–7.
7. Miyahara T, Runge S, Chatterjee A, Chen M, Mottola G, et al. (2013) D-series resolvin attenuates vascular smooth muscle cell activation and neointimal hyperplasia following vascular injury. Faseb J 27: 2220–2232.
8. Nordgren TM, Heires AJ, Wyatt TA, Poole JA, Levan TD, et al. (2013) Maresin-1 reduces the pro-inflammatory response of bronchial epithelial cells to organic dust. Respir Res 14: 51.
9. Marcon R, Bento AF, Dutra RC, Bicca MA, Leite DF, et al. (2013) Maresin 1, a proresolving lipid mediator derived from omega-3 polyunsaturated fatty acids, exerts protective actions in murine models of colitis. J Immunol 191: 4288–4298.
10. Dalli J, Serhan CN (2012) Specific lipid mediator signatures of human phagocytes: microparticles stimulate macrophage efferocytosis and pro-resolving mediators. Blood 120: e60–72.
11. Wang GJ, Sui XX, Simosa HF, Jain MK, Altieri DC, et al. (2005) Regulation of vein graft hyperplasia by survivin, an inhibitor of apoptosis protein. Arterioscler Thromb Vasc Biol 25: 2081–2087.
12. Patricia MK, Kim JA, Harper CM, Shih PT, Berliner JA, et al. (1999) Lipoxygenase products increase monocyte adhesion to human aortic endothelial cells. Arterioscler Thromb Vasc Biol 19: 2615–2622.
13. Benov L, Sztejnberg L, Fridovich I (1998) Critical evaluation of the use of hydroethidine as a measure of superoxide anion radical. Free Radic Biol Med 25: 826–831.
14. Grabner R, Till U, Heller R (2000) Flow cytometric determination of E-selectin, vascular cell adhesion molecule-1, and intercellular cell adhesion molecule-1 in formaldehyde-fixed endothelial cell monolayers. Cytometry 40: 238–244.
15. De Keulenaer GW, Alexander RW, Ushio-Fukai M, Ishizaka N, Griendling KK (1998) Tumour necrosis factor alpha activates a p22phox-based NADH oxidase in vascular smooth muscle. Biochem J 329 (Pt 3): 653–657.
16. Lee IT, Luo SF, Lee CW, Wang SW, Lin CC, et al. (2009) Overexpression of HO-1 protects against TNF-alpha-mediated airway inflammation by downregulation of TNFR1-dependent oxidative stress. Am J Pathol 175: 519–532.
17. Moe KT, Aulia S, Jiang F, Chua YL, Koh TH, et al. (2006) Differential upregulation of Nox homologues of NADPH oxidase by tumor necrosis factor-alpha in human aortic smooth muscle and embryonic kidney cells. J Cell Mol Med 10: 231–239.
18. Goyal P, Weissmann N, Rose F, Grimminger F, Schafers HJ, et al. (2005) Identification of novel Nox4 splice variants with impact on ROS levels in A549 cells. Biochem Biophys Res Commun 329: 32–39.
19. Sana TR, Janatpour MJ, Sathe M, McEvoy LM, McClanahan TK (2005) Microarray analysis of primary endothelial cells challenged with different inflammatory and immune cytokines. Cytokine 29: 256–269.
20. Zhao B, Stavchansky SA, Bowden RA, Bowman PD (2003) Effect of interleukin-1beta and tumor necrosis factor-alpha on gene expression in human endothelial cells. Am J Physiol Cell Physiol 284: C1577–1583.
21. Bandman O, Coleman RT, Loring JF, Seilhamer JJ, Cocks BG (2002) Complexity of inflammatory responses in endothelial cells and vascular smooth muscle cells determined by microarray analysis. Ann N Y Acad Sci 975: 77–90.
22. Napetschnig J, Wu H (2013) Molecular basis of NF-kappaB signaling. Annu Rev Biophys 42: 443–468.
23. DiDonato JA, Hayakawa M, Rothwarf DM, Zandi E, Karin M (1997) A cytokine-responsive IkappaB kinase that activates the transcription factor NF-kappaB. Nature 388: 548–554.
24. Sands WA, Palmer TM (2005) Inhibition of pro-inflammatory cytokine receptor signalling by cAMP in vascular endothelial cells. Biochem Soc Trans 33: 1126–1128.
25. Gusan S, Anand-Srivastava MB (2013) cAMP attenuates the enhanced expression of Gi proteins and hyperproliferation of vascular smooth muscle cells from SHR: role of ROS and ROS-mediated signaling. Am J Physiol Cell Physiol 304: C1198–1209.
26. Ho KJ, Spite M, Owens CD, Lancero H, Kroemer AH, et al. (2010) Aspirin-triggered lipoxin and resolvin E1 modulate vascular smooth muscle phenotype and correlate with peripheral atherosclerosis. Am J Pathol 177: 2116–2123.
27. Van Buul JD, Fernandez-Borja M, Anthony EC, Hordijk PL (2005) Expression and localization of NOX2 and NOX4 in primary human endothelial cells. Antioxid Redox Signal 7: 308–317.
28. Lee HN, Surh YJ (2013) Resolvin D1-mediated NOX2 inactivation rescues macrophages undertaking efferocytosis from oxidative stress-induced apoptosis. Biochem Pharmacol 86: 759–769.
29. Takamiya R, Fukunaga K, Arita M, Miyata J, Seki H, et al. (2012) Resolvin E1 maintains macrophage function under cigarette smoke-induced oxidative stress. FEBS Open Bio 2: 328–333.
30. Krishnamoorthy S, Recchiuti A, Chiang N, Yacoubian S, Lee CH, et al. (2010) Resolvin D1 binds human phagocytes with evidence for proresolving receptors. Proc Natl Acad Sci U S A 107: 1660–1665.
31. Martin N, Ruddick A, Arthur GK, Wan H, Woodman L, et al. (2012) Primary human airway epithelial cell-dependent inhibition of human lung mast cell degranulation. PLoS One 7: e43545.
32. Mizwicki MT, Liu G, Fiala M, Magpantay L, Sayre J, et al. (2013) 1alpha, 25-dihydroxyvitamin D3 and resolvin D1 retune the balance between amyloid-beta phagocytosis and inflammation in Alzheimer's disease patients. J Alzheimers Dis 34: 155–170.
33. Arita M, Ohira T, Sun YP, Elangovan S, Chiang N, et al. (2007) Resolvin E1 selectively interacts with leukotriene B4 receptor BLT1 and ChemR23 to regulate inflammation. J Immunol 178: 3912–3917.
34. Ollivier V, Parry GC, Cobb RR, de Prost D, Mackman N (1996) Elevated cyclic AMP inhibits NF-kappaB-mediated transcription in human monocytic cells and endothelial cells. J Biol Chem 271: 20828–20835.
35. Oldenburger A, Roscioni SS, Jansen E, Menzen MH, Halayko AJ, et al. (2012) Anti-inflammatory role of the cAMP effectors Epac and PKA: implications in chronic obstructive pulmonary disease. PLoS One 7: e31574.
36. Pober JS, Slowik MR, De Luca LG, Ritchie AJ (1993) Elevated cyclic AMP inhibits endothelial cell synthesis and expression of TNF-induced endothelial leukocyte adhesion molecule-1, and vascular cell adhesion molecule-1, but not intercellular cell adhesion molecule-1. J Immunol 150: 5114–5123.
37. Ghersa P, Hooft van Huijsduijnen R, Whelan J, Cambet Y, Pescini R, et al. (1994) Inhibition of E-selectin gene transcription through a cAMP-dependent protein kinase pathway. J Biol Chem 269: 29129–29137.
38. Panettieri RA, Jr., Lazaar AL, Pure E, Albelda SM (1995) Activation of cAMP-dependent pathways in human airway smooth muscle cells inhibits TNF-alpha-induced ICAM-1 and VCAM-1 expression and T lymphocyte adhesion. J Immunol 154: 2358–2365.
39. Claria J, Nguyen BT, Madenci AL, Ozaki CK, Serhan CN (2013) Diversity of lipid mediators in human adipose tissue depots. Am J Physiol Cell Physiol 304: C1141–1149.
40. Le Faouder P, Baillif V, Spreadbury I, Motta JP, Rousset P, et al. (2013) LC-MS/MS method for rapid and concomitant quantification of pro-inflammatory and pro-resolving polyunsaturated fatty acid metabolites. J Chromatogr B Analyt Technol Biomed Life Sci 932: 123–133.

19

Uptake and Presentation of Myelin Basic Protein by Normal Human B Cells

Marie Klinge Brimnes[1], Bjarke Endel Hansen[1,2], Leif Kofoed Nielsen[3,4], Morten Hanefeld Dziegiel[4], Claus Henrik Nielsen[1]*

1 Institute for Inflammation Research, Department of Infectious Diseases and Rheumatology, section 7521, Copenhagen University Hospital Rigshospitalet, Copenhagen, Denmark, 2 Immudex, Copenhagen, Denmark, 3 Department of Technology, Faculty of Health and Technology, Metropolitan University College, Copenhagen, Denmark, 4 Blood Bank, KI2034, Department of Clinical Immunology, Copenhagen University Hospital Rigshospitalet, Copenhagen, Denmark

Abstract

B cells may play both pathogenic and protective roles in T-cell mediated autoimmune diseases such as multiple sclerosis (MS). These functions relate to the ability of B cells to bind and present antigens. Under serum-free conditions we observed that 3–4% of circulating B cells from healthy donors were capable of binding the MS-associated self-antigen myelin basic protein (MBP) and of presenting the immunodominant peptide MBP85-99, as determined by staining with the mAb MK16 recognising the peptide presented by HLA-DR15-positive cells. In the presence of serum, however, the majority of B cells bound MBP in a complement-dependent manner, and almost half of the B cells became engaged in presentation of MBP85-99. Even though complement receptor 1 (CR1, CD35) and CR2 (CD21) both contributed to binding of MBP to B cells, only CR2 was important for the subsequent presentation of MBP85-99. A high proportion of MBP85-99 presenting B cells expressed CD27, and showed increased expression of CD86 compared to non-presenting B cells. MBP-pulsed B cells induced a low frequency of IL-10-producing CD4+ T cells in 3 out of 6 donors, indicating an immunoregulatory role of B cells presenting MBP-derived peptides. The mechanisms described here refute the general assumption that B-cell presentation of self-antigens requires uptake via specific B-cell receptors, and may be important for maintenance of tolerance as well as for driving T-cell responses in autoimmune diseases.

Editor: Thomas Forsthuber, University of Texas at San Antonio, United States of America

Funding: MKB received funding from The Danish Multiple Sclerosis Society, grant number 959531218. The funder had no role in study design, data collection and analysis, decision to publish, or preparation of the manuscript.

Competing Interests: The authors declare that affiliation to Immudex, along with any other relevant declarations relating to employment, consultancy, patents, products in development or marketed products, etc., does not have any competing interests.

* Email: claus.henrik.nielsen@rh.regionh.dk

Introduction

In addition to producing antibodies, B cells are highly efficient antigen-presenting cells (APCs) and produce a variety of cytokines [1]. B cells are capable of taking up small amounts of their cognate antigen and presenting it to T cells [2]. Complement receptors (CRs) may contribute to antigen uptake by B cells, either by cross linking CR2 and the B-cell receptor (BCR), or as a BCR-independent internalisation receptor [3,4]. In contrast to antigen-specific BCRs, CRs recognise antigens coated with fragments of complement component 3 (C3) or in the context of complement-coated immune complexes [4–11]. CR2-mediated antigen uptake by B cells bypasses the need for antigen specificity, and increases the proportion of B cells engaging in antigen-presentation [12]. We have previously shown that CR2 contributes to B-cell binding of the self-antigen thyroglobulin, which is capable of forming immune complexes with naturally occurring or disease-associated autoantibodies [12,13]. It is not known, however, whether CR2-dependent uptake is sufficient for presentation of self-antigens to occur. Depending on the circumstances, this could either potentiate immune responses or mediate T-cell tolerance.

Recently, much research has focused on a subset of B cells with immunoregulatory potential, known as regulatory B cells (Bregs) [14–17]. These B cells assist in maintaining peripheral tolerance by secreting immunoregulatory cytokines [15,17]. The phenotypic definition of Bregs is still controversial because production of the immunomodulating cytokine interleukin-10 (IL-10) is their only hallmark [14]. Moreover, several studies have demonstrated crosstalk between Bregs and regulatory T cells (Tregs) [18–20] and, apart from IL-10 production [20], especially the expression of CD80 and CD86 seems important in this interaction [18,20]. Activated B cells derived from MS patients show decreased IL-10 production [21]. Usually, polyclonal stimuli such as toll-like receptor ligands are used to stimulate human B cells to produce IL-10 (for review see [22]), but the self-antigen thyroglobulin also induces IL-10 production by approximately 1% of normal B cells [23].

Propathogenic B cells are involved in the maintenance of autoimmune diseases, as demonstrated by the beneficial effect of the B cell-depleting antibody rituximab in a number of autoimmune diseases [24]. These include relapsing-remitting multiple sclerosis (MS) [25,26], an inflammatory, demyelinating disease of the central nervous system (CNS) characterised by an immunological attack on the myelin sheath in the CNS orchestrated by autoreactive CD4+ T cells [27]. MS is associated with the human histocompatibility leukocyte antigen (HLA)-DR15 haplotype [28], indicating that major histocompatibility complex class II-restricted presentation of CNS-derived antigens is important in the disease process. Reduced relapse rates in the first 24 weeks of B-cell depletion without a significant influence on total antibody level [25] suggest that the pathogenic role of B cells is associated with antigen-presentation [29] and secretion of pro-inflammatory cytokines [30], rather than with antibody production. B-cell numbers are elevated in the CNS in the majority of MS patients [31].

B-cell antigen presentation is usually studied by indirect measurement of the resulting T-cell response [5,6,10,12,32]. Using CD4+ T-cell activation as read-out, we and others have previously examined the ability of B cells to present self-antigens such as thyroglobulin [23] and aggrecan [33]. However, antigen presentation that leads to downregulation of T-cell responses is difficult to assess in this manner, and information about the proportion and phenotype of the B cells presenting the antigen is usually missing. Here we examine directly the B-cell uptake and presentation of the self-antigen myelin basic protein (MBP), a self-antigen considered to be involved in the pathogenesis of MS [27], exploiting the recognition of the immunodominant peptide MBP85-99 presented on HLA-DR15 by mAb MK16 [28]. We also aimed to determine the role of complement receptors in the process, and to characterise the phenotypic profile of the B cells that most efficiently present MBP85-99.

Materials and Methods

Cells and serum

Peripheral blood mononuclear cells (PBMCs) and serum were isolated from healthy blood donors attending the Blood Bank at Copenhagen University Hospital Rigshospitalet in tubes containing heparin or no anti-coagulant (BD Bioscience, San Jose, CA). Buffy coats or heparin blood derived from 6 HLA-DR15-positive donors were used for experiments analysing the presentation of MBP peptide. Another 25 healthy blood donors with unknown HLA-tissue type were used for i) assessing the role of complement inactivation and blockade of CR1/CR2/FcRs on surface binding of MBP, ii) verifying classical complement activation in the presence of serum and iii) in co-culture studies of B cells and T cells. The donors were anonymous to the investigators, and thus no local Ethical Committee approval was required according to Danish legislation. Gradient centrifugation over LymphoPrep (Axis-Shield, Oslo, Norway) was used to isolate PBMCs. The cells were washed twice in phosphate buffered saline (GIBCO, Invitrogen, Carlsbad, CA, USA) and were resuspended in Roswell Park Memorial Institute (RPMI) 1640 medium containing HEPES (Biological Industries Israel Beit-Haemek Ltd, Kibbutz Beit-Haemek, Israel), L-glutamine (GIBCO) and gentamicin (GIBCO). Cells were either used directly in MBP surface-binding experiments or stored in liquid nitrogen before use in MBP peptide-presentation experiments. PBMCs were labelled with 5-carboxy-2′,7′-dichlorofluorescein diacetate succinimidyl ester (CFSE) at 0.25 μM in RPMI 1640 for 10 min at 37°C. CD19+ B cells and CD3+ T cells were purified from freshly purified PBMCs using the Human B cell Enrichment Kit or CFSE-labelled PBMCs using the Human CD3 Selection Kit (StemCell Technologies Inc, Vancouver, Canada).

Unless otherwise stated, serum from blood group AB donors (Lonza, Basel, Switzerland) was used as the source of normal human serum (NHS).

Antigens

Whole human MBP was purchased from HyTest Ltd. (Turku, Finland) and was used either unconjugated or conjugated with biotin using the LYNX rapid conjugation kit (AbD serotec, Kidlington, UK), according to the manufacturer's instructions. Tetanus toxoid (Statens Serum Institut, Copenhagen, Denmark) and thyroglobulin (Biogenesis Ltd., Poole, England) were used as control antigens.

Antibodies

The monoclonal antibody MK16 that recognizes MBP85-99 in the context of HLA-DRB1*1501 [28] was used as probe for antigen presentation. MK16 was originally obtained by phage display technology [28] in the Fab format, and was subsequently modified into a murine IgG1 antibody expressed in Chinese hamster ovary (CHO) cells [34]. The MK16 IgG1 antibody (referred to in the following as MK16) was affinity-purified by protein A from the supernatant of the MK16-expressing CHO cells grown in HAMS F-12 media (GIBCO) supplemented with 10% fetal calf serum (FCS; Biological Industries) and 0.8 mg/ml geneticin (Invitrogen, Carlsbad, CA, USA). Murine anti-human CR1 IgG1 antibody (mAb3D9) was kindly donated by Dr John O'Shea (Frederick Cancer Research and Development Center, Frederick, MD, USA), and polyclonal sheep anti-human CR2 was purchased from R&D Systems (Minneapolis, MN, USA). Mouse antibody against human glycophorin A (GP-A, CD235a) was purchased from Beckman Coulter (Brea, CA, USA). FITC-anti-human C3 (recognising C3, C3b and iC3b) and biotin-anti-human C1q for detection of C3 and C1q deposit on B cells was purchased from LifeSpan BioSciences, Inc, Seattle, WA, USA and Abcam, Cambridge, MA, USA respectively.

For flow cytometric characterisation of B-cell and T-cell subsets, the following fluorochrome-conjugated monoclonal antibodies were used: FITC-anti-human CD3, PE-Cy7-anti-human CD4, PerCP-anti-human CD14, APC-anti-human CD19, FITC-anti-human CD19, PE-anti-human CD27, APC-anti-human CD86 and PE-Cy7-anti-human CD80 (all from BD Biosciences, San José, CA, USA).

Proliferation assay in co-cultures of B cells and T cells

250,000 CFSE-labelled CD3+ T cells were mixed with 100,000 CD19+ B cells plus 30 μg/ml MBP. Cells were cultured in RPMI 1640 in round-bottomed 96-well plates containing 30% (v/v) NHS for 7 days at 37°C and 5% CO_2. As positive controls, 250,000 CFSE-labelled CD3+ T cells were added to wells coated with anti-CD3 (OKT3) at a concentration of 0.5 μg/ml (eBioscience, San Diego, CA, USA). At day 7, cells were stained for expression of CD4, and proliferation was measured by flow cytometry on a FACS Calibur cytometer (BD Biosciences). Background proliferation was assessed in cultures without added MBP.

IL-10 and TNF-alpha secretion assay

500,000 CD3+ T cells were mixed with 100,000 CD19+ B cells ±30 μg/ml MBP. Cells were cultured in RPMI 1640 in flat-bottomed 96-well plates containing 30% (v/v) autologous serum for 18 h at 37°C under 5% CO_2. As positive control, cells were cultured with staphylococcal enterotoxin B (SEB) at a concentration of 1 μg/ml. Cultures containing only T cells were used as negative controls. Production of IL-10 and TNF-alpha were measured using MACS cytokine secretion assay for IL-10 and TNF-alpha according to the manufacturer's instructions (Miltenyi Biotec, Bergisch Gladbach, Germany). Samples containing only detection antibodies were included as controls and these values were subtracted from all other samples. B-cell preparations contained 97.7±0.47% B cells, 1.5±0.43% T cells, and 0.68±0.15% monocytes, while T-cell preparations contained 98.9±0.40% T cells, 0.92%±0.38 B cells, and 0.15±0.05% monocytes. For each sample, between 100,000 and 150,000 CD4+ T cells were recorded using a FACS Canto flow cytometer (BD Biosciences).

Assessment of MBP deposition on B cells

0.3×10^6 PBMCs from healthy donors were incubated for 30 min at 37°C under 5% CO_2 in LGM-3 media (Lonza, Walkersville, MD, USA) with 30 µg/ml biotinylated MBP either in the absence of serum, or in the presence of 30% (v/v) autologous serum, 30% (v/v) heat-treated (30 min at 56°C) autologous serum, or 30% (v/v) autologous serum containing 50 mM EDTA or sodium polyanethole sulfonate (SPS) at a concentration of 0.2 mg/ml or 2 mg/ml respectively (Sigma, St Louis, MO). Cells were washed twice in PBS/2% FCS and then incubated with 0.6 µg/ml streptavidin-PE and APC-anti-human CD19 for 30 min at 4°C. Binding of MBP to B cells was measured as mean fluorescence intensity (MFI) values on the total CD19+ population. Cells were analyzed by flow cytometry using a FACS Calibur cytometer (BD Biosciences). To stain for dead cells, 7-actinomycin D (7-AAD) (BD Biosciences) was added to samples before acquisition.

Assessment of MBP presentation

Aliquots of MK16 were conjugated with biotin using the LYNX rapid conjugation kit (AbD serotec, Kidlington, UK), according to the manufacturer's instructions, or with fluorescein isothiocyanate (FITC; Sigma-Aldrich GmbH, USA) to an FITC:protein ratio of 6:1.

0.5×10^6 HLA-DR15+ PBMCs were incubated for 18 h at 37°C under 5% CO_2 in media containing 30% v/v AB serum plus 30 µg/ml of whole MBP. In some experiments thyroglobulin and tetanus toxoid were included as controls at a final concentration of 30 µg/ml. Next, the cells were incubated with IgG for intravenous use (IVIg; CSL Behring, Bern, Switzerland) at a concentration of 6 mg/ml and 2% mouse serum (Statens Serum Institut, Copenhagen, Denmark) to block unspecific binding. Subsequently, MK16 was incubated at a concentration of 50 ng/ml for 30 min at 4°C in 2% FCS; antibodies against cell-surface markers were included in the same step. Following two washes, streptavidin-PE (BD Biosciences) was incubated with the samples for 30 min at 4°C in experiments using biotinylated MK16. Finally, cells were analysed on a FACS Canto flow cytometer (BD Biosciences). To exclude dead cells, 7-AAD was added to samples before acquisition.

Assessment of complement deposition on B cells

0.3×10^6 PBMCs were incubated for 5 or 15 min at 37°C in LGM-3 media ±30 µg/ml of MBP and ±30% v/v autologous serum. Afterwards the tubes were kept on ice, and cells were stained with FITC-anti-human C3, biotin-anti-human C1q, and PE-Cy7-anti-human CD19 followed by a second stain by streptavidin-PE. To exclude dead cells, 7-AAD was added to samples before acquisition. Cells were analysed on a FACS Canto flow cytometer (BD Biosciences).

Inhibition of B-cell binding and presentation of MBP by CR1 and CR2 blockade

To inhibit uptake and presentation of MBP by B cells, 0.3×10^6 PBMCs and 1×10^6 PBMCs respectively were incubated for 30 min at room temperature with monoclonal anti-CR1 (clone 3D9), polyclonal anti-CR2 antibodies, or a combination of the two, each at a final concentration of 10 µg/ml. As negative control, an irrelevant antibody, anti-human glycophorin (GP)-A (CD235a) was used at a concentration of 10 µg/ml. In experiments analysing presentation of MBP, cells were incubated for 1.5 h or 4 h at 37°C with 30 µg/ml MBP in media containing 30% v/v NHS. Excess MBP was washed away, and cells were incubated for 18 h at 37°C in media containing 30% v/v NHS. Otherwise, the experiments were carried out as described above. Background MFI values from samples incubated without MBP were subtracted from all values.

Statistics

Data was analysed using FACS Diva (BD Biosciences) or FlowJo v.X, (TreeStar, Inc, Ashland, OR, USA).

Student's paired t-test was used. Kolmogorov-Smirnovs test was used to test for normality. P-values<0.05 were considered statistically significant.

Results

Binding of MBP to normal B cells

We assessed the binding of MBP to B cells in cultures of normal PBMCs. In the absence of serum, little binding occurred: only 2.5±1.5% (mean±SEM) of the cells stained positive for MBP binding (Figs. 1A and B). By contrast, addition of autologous serum to the medium resulted in a shift of the entire B-cell population towards higher MBP binding. Under these conditions, 65.4±8.2% of the cells had MFI values above the negative control (no addition of MBP).

In view of previous findings that complement promotes the uptake of antigens by B cells [6,9,10,12], we examined the effect of heating serum to 56°C, which is known to inactivate heat-labile factors of the complement system [35]. Moreover, we also added EDTA or sodium polyanethole sulphonate (SPS) as a different means of preventing complement activation [36,37]. As shown in Fig. 1C, heat treatment of serum lowered the binding of MBP to B cells by 61.3% on average, while EDTA reduced the binding by 86.1%. SPS reduced the binding of MBP to B cells by 71.6% at a concentration of 0.2 mg/ml and 81.9% at 2.0 mg/ml. Taken together, these data strongly imply that complement enhances the binding of MBP to B cells. Accordingly, we observed that C3-fragments and C1q co-deposited with MBP on the B-cell surface (Figs. 2A and B).

Antibody-mediated blockade of either CR1 or CR2 markedly lowered the binding of MBP to the B cells, while simultaneous blockade of both receptors virtually abrogated MBP binding (Figs. 2C and D). On the contrary, blockade of FcγRIIa,b,c (CD32) known to be expressed by B cells, did not affect the binding of MBP to the B cells (Fig. S1).

Presentation of the MBP85-99 peptide by normal HLA-DR15+ B cells after culture with whole MBP protein

To study antigen presentation by B cells, isolated PBMCs from HLA-DR15-positive donors were incubated with whole MBP. Subsequently, the mAb MK16 was used as probe for presentation of the immunodominant MBP peptide MBP85-99 [28] (Figs. 3A and B). As shown in Fig. 3B, only 3.7±2.4% CD19+ B cells

A

B

C

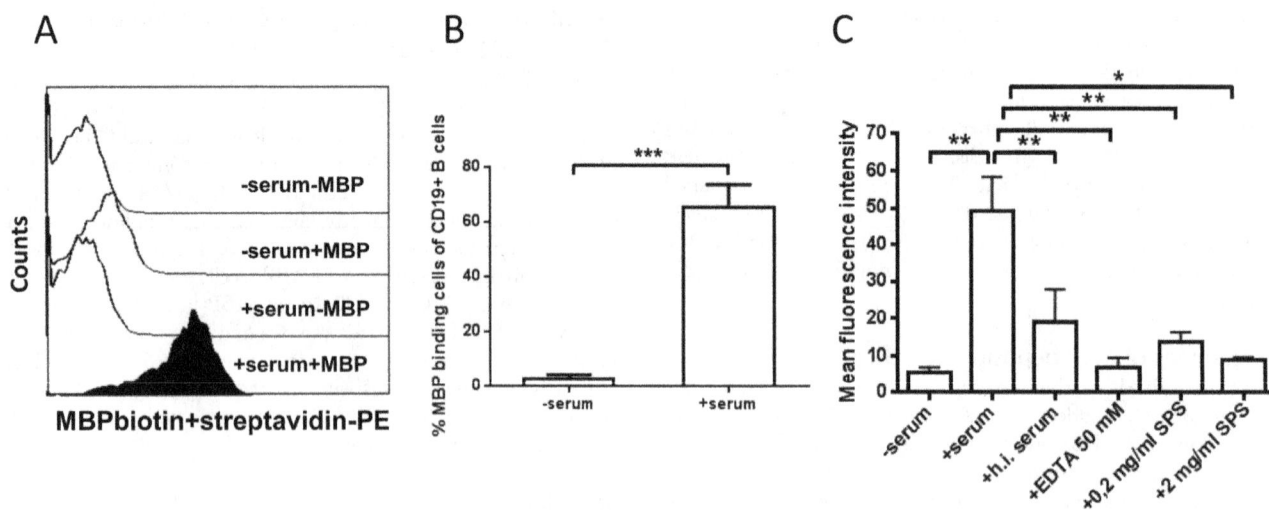

Figure 1. Serum complement promotes the binding of MBP to normal B cells. PBMCs from healthy donors were incubated for 30 min with or without 30 µg/ml biotinylated MBP in medium containing normal serum (30% v/v), or in pure medium. (A) Histogram plot depicting MFI values of MBP binding to B cells in one representative healthy donor. B) The binding of MBP to B cells from 7 healthy donors is shown, expressed as percentage MBP-positive B cells. C) Before addition to the culture media, serum was treated in one of three ways: heat-inactivated (h.i.) by heating to 56°C for 30 min, or supplemented with EDTA or sodium polyanethole sulphonate (SPS) in different concentrations. The resulting MFI values from 5–7 healthy donors are shown. Bars and error bars represent means and SEM *p<0.05 **p<0.01 and ***p<0.001.

presented MBP peptides in the absence of serum. In the presence of serum, however, 42.2±9.4% of the B-cell population presented MBP85-99. Binding of the MK16 antibody to B cells from DR15-negative donors was also examined to validate the antibody's specificity (Fig. 3C). As expected, MK16 did not bind to MBP-stimulated B cells from DR15-negative subjects, nor to B cells incubated with a different self-antigen, human thyroglobulin, or tetanus toxoid, a foreign recall antigen.

Influence of serum concentration and complement activity on B-cell presentation of MBP85-99

Little B-cell presentation of MBP85-99 was observed after incubation of PBMCs with MBP in medium containing only 0.1% of serum (Fig. 4A). At serum concentrations above 3%, however, the peptide was efficiently presented. To examine if complement was the serum factor responsible for enhancing the presentation of MBP85-99, in analogy to its role in binding of MBP by B cells, SPS was used as complement inhibitor and, indeed, dose-dependently reduced the presentation of MBP85-99 (Fig. 4B).

The presence of polyclonal anti-CR2 antibodies during incubation of PBMCs with MBP for 1.5 or 4 h markedly lowered the presentation of MBP85-99 by B cells (Fig. 4C). By contrast, co-incubation with anti-CR1 mAb had no effect (Fig. 4C).

Phenotypic characterisation of MBP85-99-presenting B cells

To characterise the phenotype of B cells presenting MBP85-99 (Fig. 5A), we co-stained B cells for the expression of the surface markers CD19, CD27, CD5, CD1d, CD24, and IgM.

The most outstanding finding was that a high proportion (around 50%) of B cells presenting MBP85-99 (MK16 positive cells) expressed CD27, which is considered a memory B-cell marker [38], compared to only 20% of the MK16 negative B cells, as shown in Fig. 5B.

Notably, MBP85-99-presenting B cells were not enriched with any of the markers CD5, CD1d, or CD24, which have all been associated with Bregs [20,23,39], nor with IgM (Fig. S2). CD86

and CD80 were found to be constitutively expressed by B cells, and their expression was independent on addition of MBP (Figs. 5C and D). Interestingly, however, B cells presenting MBP85-99 showed increased expression of CD86 compared to MBP85-99 negative B cells (Fig. 5C). We did not observe a corresponding increase in the expression of CD80 (Fig. 5D).

In agreement with their lack of phenotypic Breg markers, B cells presenting MBP85-99 with high efficiency did not produce IL-10 or IL-6 when stimulated with MBP alone (Fig. S3).

Low frequency of IL-10 secreting MBP specific CD4+ T cells in co-cultures of T cells and B cells

In co-cultures of purified CD3+ T cells and purified CD19+ B cells pulsed with MBP, no T-cell proliferation was induced, whereas anti-CD3 stimulated T cells proliferated as expected (data not shown). We did, however, observe a low frequency of IL-10 producing CD4+ T cells in co-cultures of B cells and T cells from three out of six donors, suggesting B cells presenting MBP peptides in some cases drive an immunoregulatory T-cell response (Figs. 6A and C). MBP-pulsed B cells did not induce T-cell production of TNF-alpha in any of the donors tested (Figs. 6B and D).

Discussion

While the ability of B cells to take up and present foreign antigens has been investigated intensively (for review see [40]), little is known about the capacity of human B cells to take up and present self-antigens and thereby modulate CD4+ T-cell activation. In this study we dissect the uptake and presentation of the self-antigen MBP by B cells.

We observed that 2.5±1.5% of normal B cells were capable of binding MBP when suspended in serum-free medium. We previously showed that a similar proportion of B cells bound a different self-antigen, human thyroglobulin, under similar conditions [12]. It is likely that the B-cell subsets in question bear

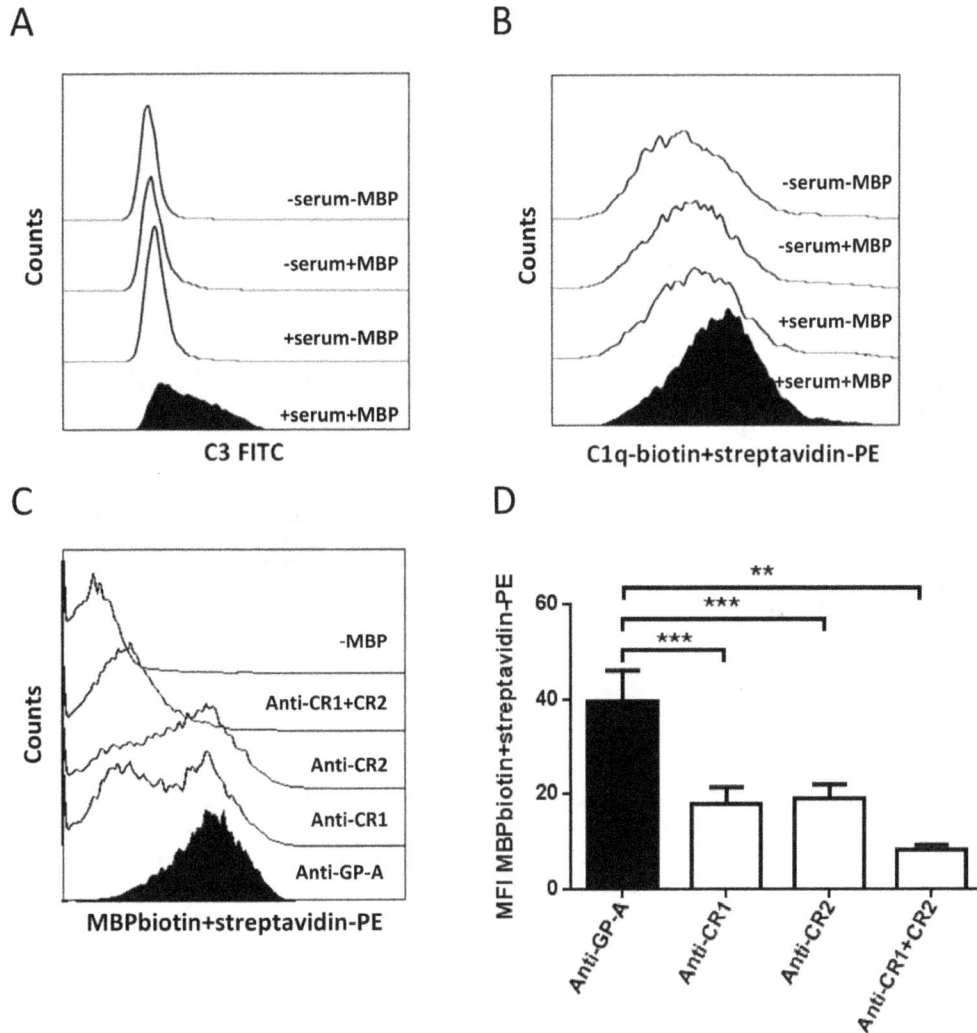

Figure 2. C1q and C3 co-deposit with MBP on B cells, which take up MBP via CR1 and CR2. PBMCs from healthy donors were incubated with or without 30 µg/ml MBP in medium containing normal autologous serum (30% v/v), or in pure medium. The resulting deposition of C3 and C1q on B cells was measured by flow cytometry after 5 min incubation (N = 3). Representative histogram plots show A) C3-deposition, and B) C1q-deposition on B cells. C) The binding of MBP was assessed using biotinylated MBP as probe and subsequent staining with streptavidin-PE. Blockade of CR1 or CR2 was achieved by pre-incubation of PBMCs with mAb3D9 and polyclonal sheep anti-human CR2 respectively. Monoclonal anti-glycophorin (GP)-A was used as negative control. D) Mean fluorescence intensity (MFI) values of 5–6 experiments are shown; background values (of samples with no MBP added) have been subtracted. Bars and error bars represent means and SEM. **p<0.01, ***p<0.001.

polyreactive B-cell receptors reactive with a variety of self-and non-self-antigens [41].

In the presence of 30% (v/v) serum, the majority of B cells bound MBP. We show here that B-cell uptake of MBP is dependent on active complement and functional complement receptors. Thus, the binding of MBP was markedly reduced by: i) heat inactivation of serum complement; ii) EDTA-mediated chelation of calcium and magnesium, essential for complement activation; iii) inactivation of complement by SPS [37]; and iv) blockade of CR1 or CR2. Accordingly, we observed that C1q and C3 co-deposited with MBP on B cells. Taken together with the finding that NHS contains antibodies capable of binding MBP [42,43], this suggests that MBP is incorporated into immune complexes that activate complement via the classic pathway of activation, facilitating the uptake of MBP by B cells as previously shown for exogenous antigens [4–6,9–12,32] and thyroglobulin [12]. We did not detect any lowered binding of MBP when

blocking CD32a, b, c indicating that FcγRs do not participate in this process.

When examining the presentation of MBP85-99 peptides after culturing of B cells with whole MBP we found that 3.7±2.4% of B cells presented MBP85-99 in the absence of serum, and that approximately half of the B cells presented the peptide when the serum concentration exceeded 3% (v/v). Thus, a surprisingly high proportion of B cells became engaged in antigen-presentation when serum was present. Inhibition of complement by SPS and antibody-mediated blockade of CR2 abrogated presentation, while anti-CR1 antibody did not inhibit presentation, even though it significantly reduced binding of MBP to B cells. CR2 thus seems to be the important receptor for antigen internalisation by B cells in our system, supporting prior observations [4,44]. Using a monoclonal antibody recognising the 46–61 determinant from hen egg lysozymes presented on mouse MHC class II molecule I-A^k one study has previously demonstrated presentation of peptides

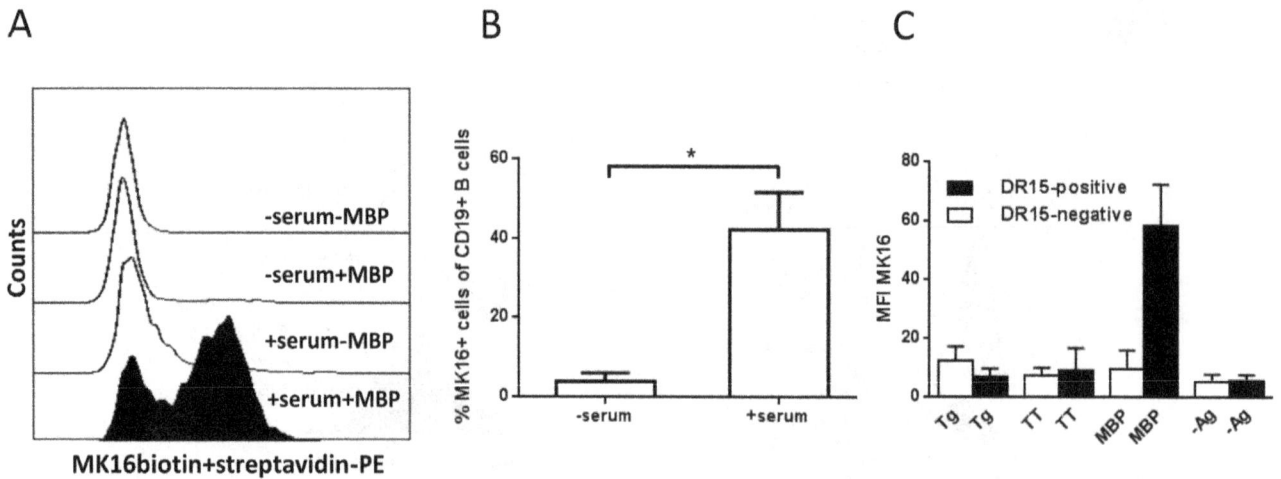

Figure 3. Presentation of MBP85-99 by HLA-DR15+ B cells. PBMCs from HLA-DR15+ individuals were incubated with MBP (whole protein) in the presence or absence of normal serum (30% v/v) for 18 h. Biotinylated mAb MK16 and streptavidin-PE were used as markers of MBP85-99 presentation. A) Representative histogram plot of 5 healthy donors showing binding of MK16 to live (7AAD-negative) B cells in the absence or presence of serum and MPB. B) The percentages of MK16-positive live B cells in 5 healthy HLA-DR15+ donors are shown; background values (no MBP added) have been subtracted. C) MK16 staining of B cells incubated with 30 μg/ml thyroglobulin (Tg), tetanus toxoid (TT), myelin basic protein (MBP) or no antigen (-Ag) in 4 healthy HLA-DR15+ donors (black bars) and 4 healthy HLA-DR15/16 negative donors (white bars). Means and SEM are shown. *p<0.05.

by bulk non-specific B cells after administration of soluble protein [45], supporting our findings. The fact that bulk B cells can engage in antigen presentation may have important implications for maintenance of tolerance by Bregs [17], as well as for B-cell-driven pathogenic processes in MS, where pathogenic T cells are believed to be activated outside the blood-brain barrier [46]. Our data suggest that B cells, irrespective of specificity, may take up and present MBP via CR2 in lymph nodes and spleen, or take up MBP outside lymphoid tissue and migrate to secondary lymphoid organs

to present MBP-derived peptides to T cells. Transitional B cells may take up MBP outside the blood-brain barrier and, as described by Lee-Chang et al. [31,47], cross the barrier by virtue of α4 and β1 integrin expression. The majority of MS patients show elevated numbers of B cells in the CNS [31]; B cells have been demonstrated in a subset of cortical lesions in patients with early-stage MS [48], and some patients have ectopic B-cell follicles containing T cells, B cells and plasma cells in the cerebral meninges [49,50]. Complement-activating immune complexes

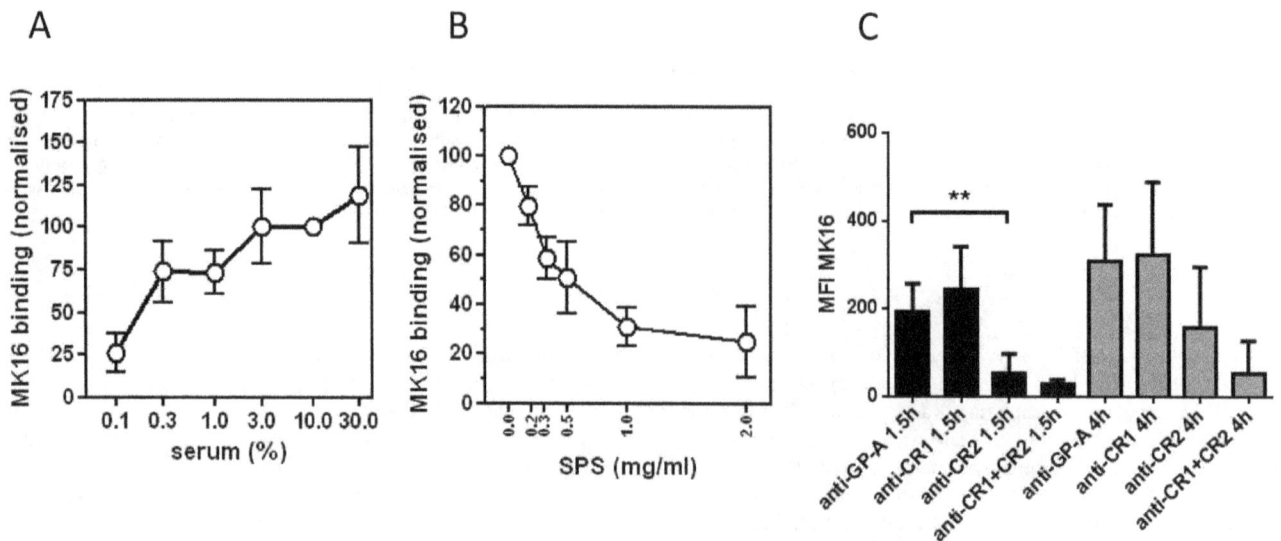

Figure 4. Influence of complement on the presentation of MBP85-99 by DR15+ B cells. PBMCs from healthy HLA-DR15+ donors were incubated for 18 h with MBP in media containing normal serum. Cells were stained with FITC anti-CD19 and biotinylated MK16, followed by streptavidin-PE. (A) The binding of MK16 at different serum concentrations is shown as mean fluorescence (MFI) values normalised to that of 10% serum, (N=4). B) Before addition of serum (30% v/v), different concentrations of the complement inhibitory compound sodium polyanethole sulphonate (SPS) were added. MFI values are shown, normalised to samples without SPS, (N=6). (C) The PBMCs were pre-incubated with the anti-CR1 mAb3D9 or polyclonal sheep anti-human CR2, or both, before addition of serum (30% v/v) and MBP. Anti-glycophorin (GP)-A was used as negative control. Data are shown as means±SEM, (N=4-6). **p<0.01.

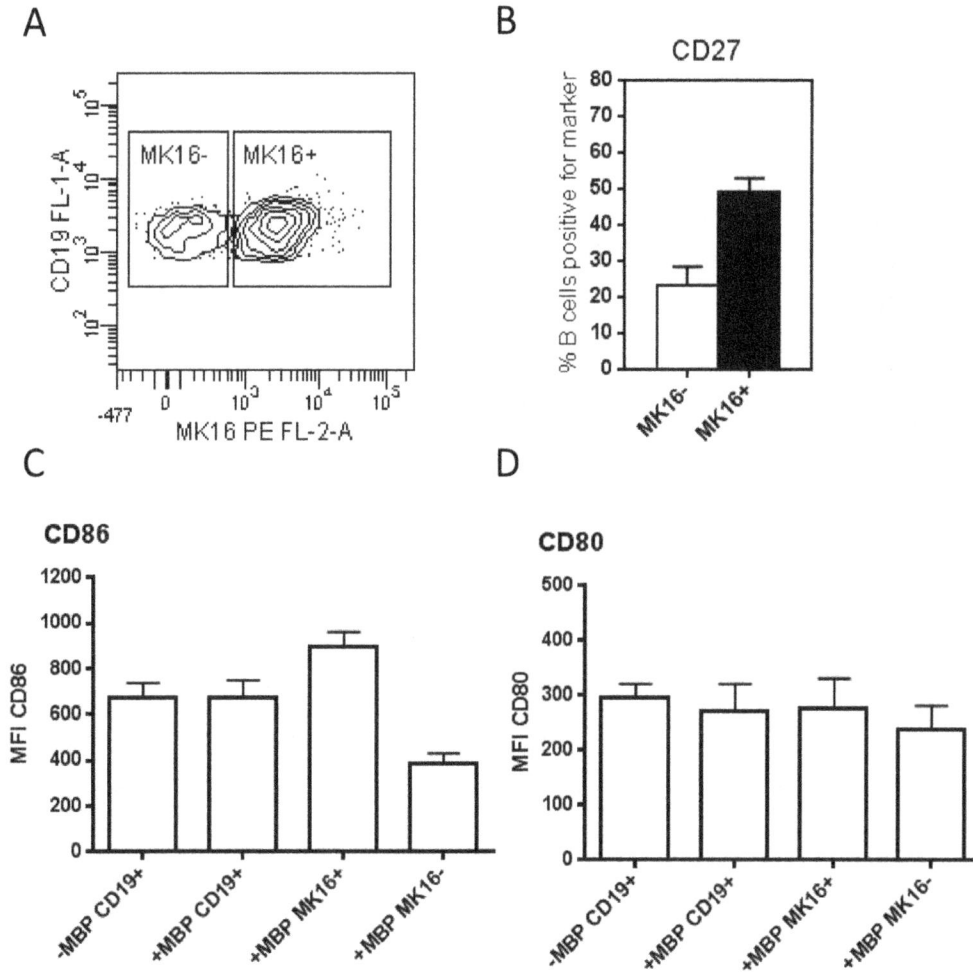

Figure 5. Phenotype of MBP85-99-presenting B cells. PBMCs from healthy HLA-DR15+ donors were incubated with MBP (30 µg/ml) in RPMI containing 30% (v/v) normal serum for 18 h. The presentation of MBP85-99 by CD19+ B cells was assessed using biotinylated MK16 and streptavidin-PE. A) Representative dot plot showing a subset of B cells that present MBP58-99 (MK16+) and a subset that do not (MK16−). Expression of various surface markers was evaluated in these subsets. B) The percentages of MK16+ (black bar) or MK16− (white bar) B cells expressing CD27 are shown (N = 4). B-cell expression of the co-stimulatory molecules C) CD86 and D) CD80 is shown as mean fluorescence intensity (MFI) values (N = 5). 7-AAD was used to exclude dead cells. Data are shown as means and SEM.

may also form intrathecally, when anti-MBP antibodies are present in cerebrospinal fluid, as is the case in children at least [42], and immunopathological evidence of complement activation has been demonstrated in plaques [51]. It is possible that higher quantities and affinities of anti-MBP antibodies in patients, as compared to healthy controls, may lead to formation of immune-complexes with stronger pro-inflammatory potential than those involved in this study.

We were not able to identify subsets with particular pro- or anti-inflammatory potential among MBP85-99-presenting B cells, neither in terms of production of IL-10 or IL-6, nor in terms of expression of CD24, CD1d, CD5 or IgM, which have been associated with Bregs [20,23,39]. Approximately half of the B cells presenting MBP85-99 expressed CD27, which has been associated with a Breg phenotype [52,53]. However, it is usually considered a memory B-cell marker [38], hence the significance of this observation is not clear. We did not investigate if the expression of CR1 and CR2 on MBP85-99-presenting B cells was similar to that of B cells not engaged in presentation of the peptide. Others have shown that CD27+ memory B cells have been shown to

express higher levels of CR1, but not CR2, than CD27- naïve B cells [54]. Moreover, we observed significantly upregulated expression of CD86 on MBP85-99-presenting B cells. Increased expression of co-stimulatory molecules has usually been associated with an immune activating phenotype of APCs [55], but recently expression of B7 (CD80/CD86) on murine B cells was shown to be central to regulation of CD4+CD25^{high} Tregs in experimental autoimmune encephalomyelitis [18]. Accumulating data also support a role for B cells in the generation of human Tregs [56]. Concordantly, B cells pulsed with MBP induced low frequencies of IL-10-producing CD4+ T cells in half of the co-cultures tested in this study, while MBP induced no TNF-alpha-producing CD4+ T cells. This is to be expected if B cells are involved in the silencing of potentially self-reactive T cells in healthy humans, as indicated by animal experiments [15,17].

In conclusion, our study demonstrates that B cells, irrespective of specificity, can become engaged in the presentation of the MS-relevant auto-antigen MBP in a complement-dependent manner. While CR1 and CR2 cooperate in the binding of MBP, engagement of CR2 is crucial for subsequent presentation of the

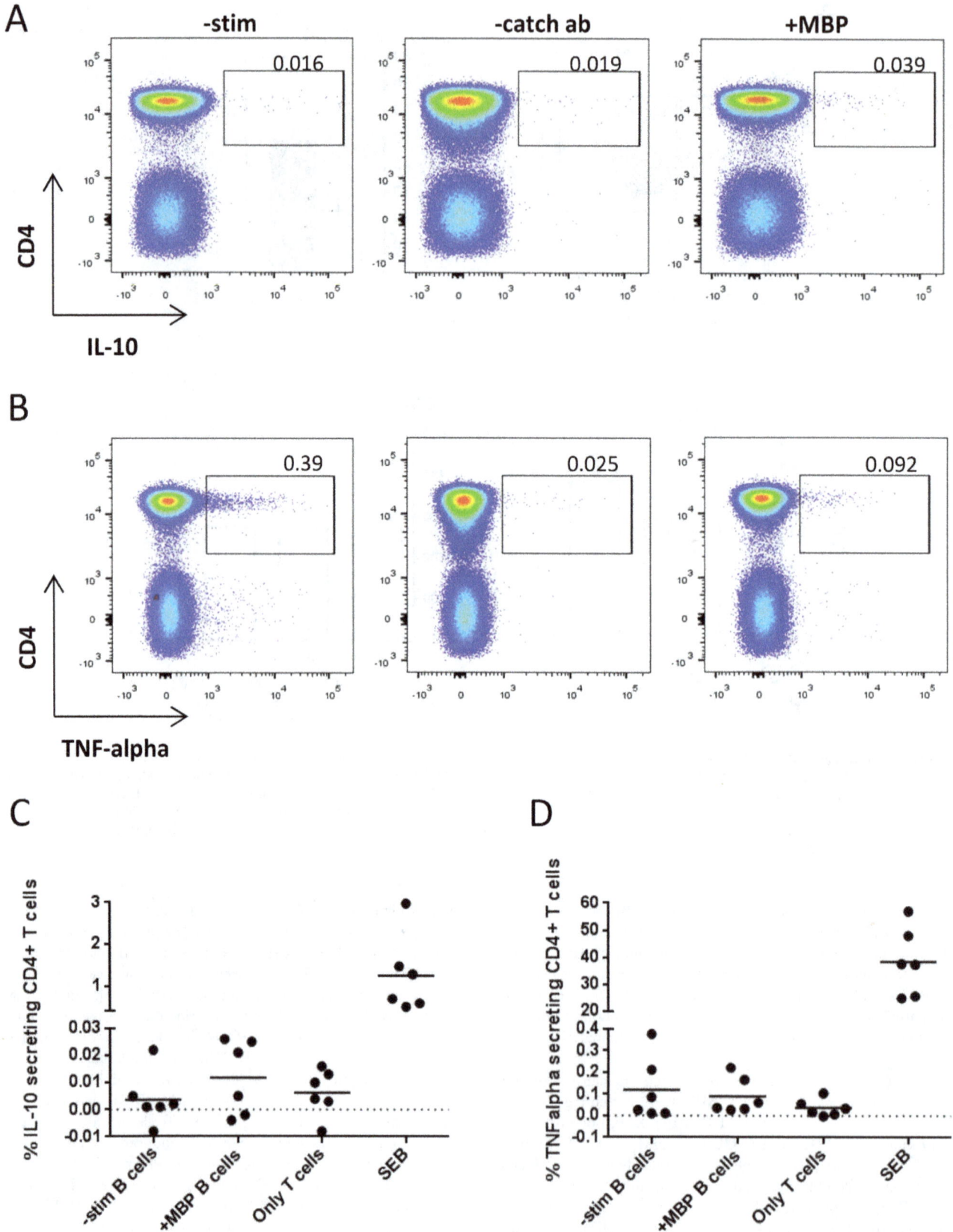

Figure 6. IL-10 and TNF-alpha secretion by MBP specific CD4+ T cells in co-cultures of T cells and B cells. 500,000 CD3+ T cells were cultured with 100,000 CD19+ B cells ±30 µg/ml MBP for 18 h and the resulting IL-10 and TNF-alpha production in CD4+ T cells were measured. Shown is representative dot plots of (A) IL-10 and (B) TNF-alpha production in CD4+ T cells and individual values of the proportion of CD4+ T cells producing (C) IL-10 or (D) TNF-alpha (N = 6). Cultures stimulated by staphylococcal enterotoxin B (SEB) were used as positive controls and cultures

containing only T cells were used as negative controls. Samples containing only detection antibodies (-catch ab) were included to correct background staining of the assay and these values were subtracted from all other samples.

immunodominant peptide MBP85-99. Increased expression of CD86 on normal B cells presenting MBP in the presence of NHS indicates a role of these cells in maintenance of tolerance, but different qualities of T cells, B cells and immune complexes in MS may associate the mechanisms described in this study with the pathogenesis of MS.

Supporting Information

Figure S1   Contribution of Fcγ-receptors to the binding of MBP to B cells. PBMCs from three healthy donors were incubated for 30 min. with monoclonal antibodies against FcγRI (anti-CD64, clone10.1), FcγRII (anti-CD32a,b,c, clone AT10) or FcγRIII (anti-CD16, clone 3G8), of which FcγRIIa, -b, and –c are present on mature human B cells, in medium containing 30% (v/v) normal serum. Subsequently, MBP-biotin (30 μg/ml) was added, followed by streptavidin-PE. An antibody against glycophorin-A (anti-GP-A) was used as an additional negative control, and a combination of anti-CR1 antibody (3D9) and polyclonal antibodies against CR2 were included as positive controls for inhibition. The binding of MBP-biotin/streptavidin-PE was assessed by flow cytometry. The resulting mean fluorescence intensity (MFI) values are shown as mean±SEM.

Figure S2   Phenotype of MBP85-99-presenting B cells. PBMCs from four healthy HLA-DR15+ donors were incubated with MBP (30 μg/ml) in RPMI medium containing 30% (v/v) normal serum. The presentation of MBP85-99 by CD19+ B cells was assessed by flow cytometry using FITC-conjugated MK16 antibody (A) or biotinylated MK16+streptavidin-PE (C–D).

Shown is the percentage of MK16- and MK16+ B cells expressing CD5 (A), CD24 (B), CD1d (C), or IgM (D) among B cells. MFI values are shown as mean±SEM.

Figure S3   Cytokine secretion by MBP85-99 presenting B cells. PBMCs from four healthy HLA-DR15+ donors were incubated for 18 hours with or without MBP (30 μg/ml) in RPMI medium containing 30% (v/v) normal serum. Cells were stained with PerCP anti-human CD19, biotinylated MK16+PE-streptavidin, APC-anti-human IL-10, FITC anti-human IL-6 and life/dead cell discriminator LIVE/DEAD Fixable Near-IR. A) Representative dot plot showing IL-10 and IL-6 secretion by MBP85-99 presenting, live B cells. B) The percentages of IL-10 producing or C) IL-6 producing, live B cells are shown as means and SEM. As positive control, a combination of MBP, phorbol myristate acetate and ionomycin (PMAiono) was used as stimulating agent.

Acknowledgments

We thank Winnie Hansen for expert technical assistance and Alistair Reeves for editing the manuscript.

Author Contributions

Conceived and designed the experiments: MKB BEH CHN. Performed the experiments: MKB BEH. Analyzed the data: MKB BEH CHN. Contributed reagents/materials/analysis tools: LKN MHD. Wrote the paper: MKB CHN.

References

1. Pistoia V (1997) Production of cytokines by human B cells in health and disease. Immunol Today 18: 343–350.
2. Lanzavecchia A (1985) Antigen-specific interaction between T and B cells. Nature 314: 537–539.
3. Carroll MC (1998) The role of complement and complement receptors in induction and regulation of immunity. Annu Rev Immunol 16: 545–568.
4. Barrault DV, Knight AM (2004) Distinct sequences in the cytoplasmic domain of complement receptor 2 are involved in antigen internalization and presentation. J Immunol 172: 3509–3517.
5. Arvieux J, Yssel H, Colomb MG (1988) Antigen-bound C3b and C4b enhance antigen-presenting cell function in activation of human T-cell clones. Immunology 65: 229–235.
6. Boackle SA, Morris MA, Holers VM, Karp DR (1998) Complement opsonization is required for presentation of immune complexes by resting peripheral blood B cells. J Immunol 161: 6537–6543.
7. Nielsen CH, Matthiesen SH, Lyng I, Leslie RG (1997) The role of complement receptor type 1 (CR1, CD35) in determining the cellular distribution of opsonized immune complexes between whole blood cells: kinetic analysis of the buffering capacity of erythrocytes. Immunology 90: 129–137.
8. Nielsen CH, Svehag SE, Marquart HV, Leslie RG (1994) Interactions of opsonized immune complexes with whole blood cells: binding to erythrocytes restricts complex uptake by leucocyte populations. Scand J Immunol 40: 228–236.
9. Thornton BP, Vetvicka V, Ross GD (1996) Function of C3 in a humoral response: iC3b/C3dg bound to an immune complex generated with natural antibody and a primary antigen promotes antigen uptake and the expression of co-stimulatory molecules by all B cells, but only stimulates immunoglobulin synthesis by antigen-specific B cells. Clin Exp Immunol 104: 531–537.
10. Thornton BP, Vetvicka V, Ross GD (1994) Natural antibody and complement-mediated antigen processing and presentation by B lymphocytes. J Immunol 152: 1727–1737.
11. Villiers MB, Villiers CL, Jacquier-Sarlin MR, Gabert FM, Journet AM, et al. (1996) Covalent binding of C3b to tetanus toxin: influence on uptake/ internalization of antigen by antigen-specific and non-specific B cells. Immunology 89: 348–355.
12. Nielsen CH, Leslie RG, Jepsen BS, Kazatchkine MD, Kaveri SV, et al. (2001) Natural autoantibodies and complement promote the uptake of a self antigen, human thyroglobulin, by B cells and the proliferation of thyroglobulin-reactive CD4(+) T cells in healthy individuals. Eur J Immunol 31: 2660–2668.
13. Nielsen CH, Hegedus L, Leslie RG (2004) Autoantibodies in autoimmune thyroid disease promote immune complex formation with self antigens and increase B cell and CD4+ T cell proliferation in response to self antigens. Eur J Immunol 34: 263–272.
14. Mauri C, Bosma A (2012) Immune regulatory function of B cells. Annu Rev Immunol 30: 221–241.
15. Mauri C, Gray D, Mushtaq N, Londei M (2003) Prevention of arthritis by interleukin 10-producing B cells. J Exp Med 197: 489–501.
16. O'Garra A, Howard M (1992) IL-10 production by CD5 B cells. Ann N Y Acad Sci 651: 182–199.
17. Fillatreau S, Sweenie CH, McGeachy MJ, Gray D, Anderton SM (2002) B cells regulate autoimmunity by provision of IL-10. Nat Immunol 3: 944–950.
18. Mann MK, Maresz K, Shriver LP, Tan Y, Dittel BN (2007) B cell regulation of CD4+CD25+ T regulatory cells and IL-10 via B7 is essential for recovery from experimental autoimmune encephalomyelitis. J Immunol 178: 3447–3456.
19. Carter NA, Vasconcellos R, Rosser EC, Tulone C, Munoz-Suano A, et al. (2011) Mice lacking endogenous IL-10-producing regulatory B cells develop exacerbated disease and present with an increased frequency of Th1/Th17 but a decrease in regulatory T cells. J Immunol 186: 5569–5579.
20. Blair PA, Norena LY, Flores-Borja F, Rawlings DJ, Isenberg DA, et al. (2010) CD19(+)CD24(hi)CD38(hi) B cells exhibit regulatory capacity in healthy individuals but are functionally impaired in systemic Lupus Erythematosus patients. Immunity 32: 129–140.
21. Duddy M, Niino M, Adatia F, Hebert S, Freedman M, et al. (2007) Distinct effector cytokine profiles of memory and naive human B cell subsets and implication in multiple sclerosis. J Immunol 178: 6092–6099.
22. Fillatreau S, Gray D, Anderton SM (2008) Not always the bad guys: B cells as regulators of autoimmune pathology. Nat Rev Immunol 8: 391–397.
23. Langkjaer A, Kristensen B, Hansen BE, Schultz H, Hegedus L, et al.(2012) B-cell exposure to self-antigen induces IL-10 producing B cells as well as IL-6- and TNF-alpha-producing B-cell subsets in healthy humans. Clin Immunol 145: 1–10.

24. Nielsen CH, El FD, Hasselbalch HC, Bendtzen K, Hegedus L (2007) B-cell depletion with rituximab in the treatment of autoimmune diseases. Graves' ophthalmopathy the latest addition to an expanding family. Expert Opin Biol Ther 7: 1061–1078.

25. Hauser SL, Waubant E, Arnold DL, Vollmer T, Antel J, et al. (2008) B-cell depletion with rituximab in relapsing-remitting multiple sclerosis. N Engl J Med 358: 676–688.

26. Bar-Or A, Calabresi PA, Arnold D, Markowitz C, Shafer S, et al. (2008) Rituximab in relapsing-remitting multiple sclerosis: a 72-week, open-label, phase I trial. Ann Neurol 63: 395–400.

27. Sospedra M, Martin R (2005) Immunology of multiple sclerosis. Annu Rev Immunol 23: 683–747.

28. Krogsgaard M, Wucherpfennig KW, Cannella B, Hansen BE, Svejgaard A, et al. (2000) Visualization of myelin basic protein (MBP) T cell epitopes in multiple sclerosis lesions using a monoclonal antibody specific for the human histocompatibility leukocyte antigen (HLA)-DR2-MBP 85-99 complex. J Exp Med 191: 1395–1412.

29. Weber MS, Prod'homme T, Patarroyo JC, Molnarfi N, Karnezis T, et al. (2010) B-cell activation influences T-cell polarization and outcome of anti-CD20 B-cell depletion in central nervous system autoimmunity. Ann Neurol 68: 369–383.

30. Barr TA, Shen P, Brown S, Lampropoulou V, Roch T, et al. (2012) B cell depletion therapy ameliorates autoimmune disease through ablation of IL-6-producing B cells. J Exp Med 209: 1001–1010.

31. Cepok S, Rosche B, Grummel V, Vogel F, Zhou D, et al. (2005) Short-lived plasma blasts are the main B cell effector subset during the course of multiple sclerosis. Brain 128: 1667–1676.

32. Jacquier-Sarlin MR, Gabert FM, Villiers MB, Colomb MG (1995) Modulation of antigen processing and presentation by covalently linked complement C3b fragment. Immunology 84: 164–170.

33. Ciechomska M, Wilson CL, Floudas A, Hui W, Rowan AD, et al. (2014) Antigen-specific B lymphocytes acquire proteoglycan aggrecan from cartilage extracellular matrix resulting in antigen presentation and CD4+ T-cell activation. Immunology 141: 70–78.

34. Jensen LB, Riise E, Nielsen LK, Dziegiel M, Fugger L, et al. (2004) Efficient purification of unique antibodies using peptide affinity-matrix columns. J Immunol Methods 284: 45–54.

35. Johnson AH, Mowbray JF, Porter KA (1975) Detection of circulating immune complexes in pathological human sera. Lancet 1: 762–765.

36. Nielsen CH, Pedersen ML, Marquart HV, Prodinger WM, Leslie RG (2002) The role of complement receptors type 1 (CR1, CD35) and 2 (CR2, CD21) in promoting C3 fragment deposition and membrane attack complex formation on normal peripheral human B cells. Eur J Immunol 32: 1359–1367.

37. Palarasah Y, Skjoedt MO, Vitved L, Andersen TE, Skjoedt K, et al. (2010) Sodium polyanethole sulfonate as an inhibitor of activation of complement function in blood culture systems. J Clin Microbiol 48: 908–914.

38. Agematsu K, Hokibara S, Nagumo H, Komiyama A (2000) CD27: a memory B-cell marker. Immunol Today 21: 204–206.

39. Yanaba K, Bouaziz JD, Haas KM, Poe JC, Fujimoto M, et al. (2008) A regulatory B cell subset with a unique CD1dhiCD5+ phenotype controls T cell-dependent inflammatory responses. Immunity 28: 639–650.

40. Lanzavecchia A (1990) Receptor-mediated antigen uptake and its effect on antigen presentation to class II-restricted T lymphocytes. Annu Rev Immunol 8: 773–793.

41. Nakamura M, Burastero SE, Ueki Y, Larrick JW, Notkins AL, et al. (1988) Probing the normal and autoimmune B cell repertoire with Epstein-Barr virus. Frequency of B cells producing monoreactive high affinity autoantibodies in patients with Hashimoto's disease and systemic lupus erythematosus. J Immunol 141: 4165–4172.

42. O'Connor KC, Lopez-Amaya C, Gagne D, Lovato L, Moore-Odom NH, et al. (2010) Anti-myelin antibodies modulate clinical expression of childhood multiple sclerosis. J Neuroimmunol 223: 92–99.

43. O'Connor KC, Chitnis T, Griffin DE, Piyasirisilp S, Bar-Or A, et al. (2003) Myelin basic protein-reactive autoantibodies in the serum and cerebrospinal fluid of multiple sclerosis patients are characterized by low-affinity interactions. J Neuroimmunol 136: 140–148.

44. Boackle SA, Holers VM, Karp DR (1997) CD21 augments antigen presentation in immune individuals. Eur J Immunol 27: 122–129.

45. Zhong G, Reis e Sousa, Germain RN (1997) Antigen-unspecific B cells and lymphoid dendritic cells both show extensive surface expression of processed antigen-major histocompatibility complex class II complexes after soluble protein exposure in vivo or in vitro. J Exp Med 186: 673–682.

46. Goverman J (2009) Autoimmune T cell responses in the central nervous system. Nat Rev Immunol 9: 393–407.

47. Lee-Chang C, Top I, Zephir H, Dubucquoi S, Trauet J, et al. (2011) Primed status of transitional B cells associated with their presence in the cerebrospinal fluid in early phases of multiple sclerosis. Clin Immunol 139: 12–20.

48. Lucchinetti CF, Popescu BF, Bunyan RF, Moll NM, Roemer SF, et al et al. (2011) Inflammatory cortical demyelination in early multiple sclerosis. N Engl J Med 365: 2188–2197.

49. Magliozzi R, Howell O, Vora A, Serafini B, Nicholas R, et al. (2007) Meningeal B-cell follicles in secondary progressive multiple sclerosis associate with early onset of disease and severe cortical pathology. Brain 130: 1089–1104.

50. Serafini B, Rosicarelli B, Magliozzi R, Stigliano E, Aloisi F (2004) Detection of ectopic B-cell follicles with germinal centers in the meninges of patients with secondary progressive multiple sclerosis. Brain Pathol 14: 164–174.

51. Lucchinetti C, Bruck W, Parisi J, Scheithauer B, Rodriguez M, et al. (2000) Heterogeneity of multiple sclerosis lesions: implications for the pathogenesis of demyelination. Ann Neurol 47: 707–717.

52. Iwata Y, Matsushita T, Horikawa M, Dilillo DJ, Yanaba K, et al. (2011) Characterization of a rare IL-10-competent B-cell subset in humans that parallels mouse regulatory B10 cells. Blood 117: 530–541.

53. Bouaziz JD, Calbo S, Maho-Vaillant M, Saussine A, Bagot M, et al. (2010) IL-10 produced by activated human B cells regulates CD4(+) T-cell activation in vitro. Eur J Immunol 40: 2686–2691.

54. Isaak A, Gergely P, Jr., Szekeres Z, Prechl J, Poor G, et al. (2008) Physiological up-regulation of inhibitory receptors Fc gamma RII and CR1 on memory B cells is lacking in SLE patients. Int Immunol 20: 185–192.

55. Lenschow DJ, Walunas TL, Bluestone JA (1996) CD28/B7 system of T cell costimulation. Annu Rev Immunol 14: 233–258.

56. Lund FE, Randall TD (2010) Effector and regulatory B cells: modulators of CD4+ T cell immunity. Nat Rev Immunol 10: 236–247.

Permissions

All chapters in this book were first published in PLOS ONE, by The Public Library of Science; hereby published with permission under the Creative Commons Attribution License or equivalent. Every chapter published in this book has been scrutinized by our experts. Their significance has been extensively debated. The topics covered herein carry significant findings which will fuel the growth of the discipline. They may even be implemented as practical applications or may be referred to as a beginning point for another development.

The contributors of this book come from diverse backgrounds, making this book a truly international effort. This book will bring forth new frontiers with its revolutionizing research information and detailed analysis of the nascent developments around the world.

We would like to thank all the contributing authors for lending their expertise to make the book truly unique. They have played a crucial role in the development of this book. Without their invaluable contributions this book wouldn't have been possible. They have made vital efforts to compile up to date information on the varied aspects of this subject to make this book a valuable addition to the collection of many professionals and students.

This book was conceptualized with the vision of imparting up-to-date information and advanced data in this field. To ensure the same, a matchless editorial board was set up. Every individual on the board went through rigorous rounds of assessment to prove their worth. After which they invested a large part of their time researching and compiling the most relevant data for our readers.

The editorial board has been involved in producing this book since its inception. They have spent rigorous hours researching and exploring the diverse topics which have resulted in the successful publishing of this book. They have passed on their knowledge of decades through this book. To expedite this challenging task, the publisher supported the team at every step. A small team of assistant editors was also appointed to further simplify the editing procedure and attain best results for the readers.

Apart from the editorial board, the designing team has also invested a significant amount of their time in understanding the subject and creating the most relevant covers. They scrutinized every image to scout for the most suitable representation of the subject and create an appropriate cover for the book.

The publishing team has been an ardent support to the editorial, designing and production team. Their endless efforts to recruit the best for this project, has resulted in the accomplishment of this book. They are a veteran in the field of academics and their pool of knowledge is as vast as their experience in printing. Their expertise and guidance has proved useful at every step. Their uncompromising quality standards have made this book an exceptional effort. Their encouragement from time to time has been an inspiration for everyone.

The publisher and the editorial board hope that this book will prove to be a valuable piece of knowledge for researchers, students, practitioners and scholars across the globe.

List of Contributors

Chen Yu, Qing-Zhong Li and Hong-Juans Li
School of Pharmacy, Binzhou Medical University, Yantai, Shandong, China

Dong Qi
Department of Nephrology, Yantai Yu-Huang-Ding/Qingdao University Hospital, Yantai, Shandong, China

Wei Lian
Yantai Yan-Tai-Shan Hospital, Yantai, Shandong, China

Hua-Ying Fan
School of Pharmacy, Yantai University, Yantai, Shandong, China

Jörg U.Hammel and Michael Nickel
Institut fu¨ r Spezielle Zoologie und Evolutionsbiologie mit Phyletischem Museum, Friedrich-Schiller-Universita¨t Jena, Erbertstr. 1, 07743, Jena, Germany

Sujit V. Janardhan and Reinhard Marks
Department of Pathology, The University of Chicago, Chicago, Illinois, United States of America

Thomas F. Gajewski
Department of Pathology, The University of Chicago, Chicago, Illinois, United States of America
Department of Medicine, The University of Chicago, Chicago, Illinois, United States of America

Jacques Robert, Leon Grayfer, Eva-Stina Edholm, Brian Ward and Francisco De Jesú s Andino
Department of Microbiology and Immunology, University of Rochester Medical Center, Rochester, United States of America

Ste´phanie Madec
Laboratoire Universitaire de Biodiversite´ et Ecologie Microbienne (EA3882), SFR48 ScInBios, Universite´ de Bretagne Occidentale (UBO), UEB, ESIAB, Technopoˆ le Brest Iroise, 29280, Plouzane´ , France

Vianney Pichereau, Fabienne Guèrard, Mathieu Paillard, Jean-Louis Nicolas and Christine Paillard
Laboratoire des Sciences de l'Environnement Marin, UMR 6539 UBO/CNRS/IRD/Ifremer, Universitè de Bretagne Occidentale (UBO), Institut Universitaire Europèen de la Mer, Technopô le Brest Iroise, 29280, Plouzanè , France

Annick Jacq
Institut de Ge´ne´tique et de Microbiologie, UMR8621, CNRS-Universite´ Paris-Sud, 91405, Orsay, France

Claire Boisset
Centre de Recherche sur les macromole´cules ve´ge´tales, CERMAV-CNRS, BP53, 38041 Grenoble, France

Michelle J. Hansen, Sheau Pyng J. Chan, Shenna Y. Langenbach, Lovisa F. Dousha, Jessica E. Jones, Selcuk Yatmaz, Huei Jiunn Seow, Ross Vlahos, Gary P. Anderson and Steven Bozinovski
Lung Health Research Centre, Department of Pharmacology and Therapeutics, The University of Melbourne, Victoria, Australia

Peng Dong, Siya Zhang, Menghua Cai, Ning Kang, YuHu, Lianxian Cui and Wei He
Department of Immunology, Institute of Basic Medical Sciences, Chinese Academy of Medical Sciences and School of Basic Medicine, Peking Union Medical College, State Key Laboratory of Medical Molecular Biology, Beijing, China

Jianmin Zhang
Department of Immunology, Institute of Basic Medical Sciences, Chinese Academy of Medical Sciences and School of Basic Medicine, Peking Union Medical College, State Key Laboratory of Medical Molecular Biology, Beijing, China
Neuroregeneration and Stem Cell Programs, Institute for Cell Engineering, Department of Neurology, Johns Hopkins University School of Medicine, Baltimore, MD, United States of America

Nathalie Delesque-Touchard, Caroline Pendaries, Cécile Volle-Challier, Laurence Millet, Véronique Salel, Caroline Hervé , Anne-Marie Pflieger, Jean-Marc Herbert, Pierre Savi, Franc͵oise Bono
Early to Candidate (E2C), Sanofi, Toulouse, France

Laurence Berthou-Soulie and Catherine Prades
SCP Biologics, Sanofi, Vitry-Sur-Seine, France

Tania Sorg
Department of Scientific Operations PhenoPro, Mouse Clinical Institute (MCI), Strasbourg, France

Taehoon Lee
Department of Allergy and Clinical Immunology, Asan Medical Center, University of Ulsan College of Medicine, Seoul, Korea
Department of Internal Medicine, Ulsan University Hospital, University of Ulsan College of Medicine, Ulsan, Korea

Jinhee Kim
National Evidence-based Healthcare Collaborating Agency, Seoul, Korea
Department of Nursing, College of Medicine, Chosun University, Gwangju, Korea

Sujeong Kim
Department of Allergy and Clinical Immunology, Asan Medical Center, University of Ulsan College of Medicine, Seoul, Korea
Department of Internal Medicine, Kyungpook National University School of Medicine, Daegu, Korea

Kyoungjoo Kim, Yuri Kim and Yoon
National Evidence-based Healthcare Collaborating Agency, Seoul, Korea

Yunjin Park
Department of Statistics, Dongguk University, Seoul, Korea

Su Lee, Hyouk-Soo Kwon, You Sook Cho, Hee-Bom Moon and Tae-Bum Kim
Department of Allergy and Clinical Immunology, Asan Medical Center, University of Ulsan College of Medicine, Seoul, Korea

Sae-Hoon Kim and Yoon-Seok Chang
Department of Internal Medicine, Seoul National University College of Medicine, Seoul, Korea

An-Soo Jang
Department of Internal Medicine, Soonchunhyang University Bucheon Hospital, Bucheon, Korea

Jung- Won Park
Department of Internal Medicine, College of Medicine, Yonsei University, Seoul, Korea

Dong-Ho Nahm
Department of Internal Medicine, College of Medicine, Ajou University, Suwon, Korea

Ho-Joo Yoon
Department of Internal Medicine, College of Medicine, Hanyang University, Seoul, Korea

Sang-Heon Cho
Department of Internal Medicine, Seoul National University College of Medicine, Seoul, Korea

Young-Joo Cho
Department of Internal Medicine, College of Medicine, Ewha Womans University, Seoul, Korea

Byoung Whui Choi
Department of Internal Medicine, College of Medicine, Chung-Ang University, Seoul, Korea

Adeliane Castro da Costa
Laboratório de Imunopatologia das Doenc͵as Infecciosas, Instituto de Patologia Tropical e Saúde Pública, Universidade Federal de Goiás, Goiânia, Goiás, Brazil

Abadio de Oliveira Costa-Júnior
Laboratório de Imunopatologia das Doenc͵as Infecciosas, Instituto de Patologia Tropical e Saúde Pública, Universidade Federal de Goiàs, Goiânia, Goiàs, Brazil

Fàbio Muniz de Oliveira
Laboratório de Bacteriologia Molecular, Instituto de Patologia Tropical e Saúde Pública, Universidade Federal de Goiás, Goiânia, Goiàs, Brazil

Sarah Veloso Nogueira
Laboratório de Imunopatologia das Doenc͵as Infecciosas, Instituto de Patologia Tropical e Saúde Pública, Universidade Federal de Goiás, Goiânia, Goiás, Brazil

Joseane Damaceno Rosa
Laboató rio de Imunopatologia das Doenc,as Infecciosas, Instituto de Patologia Tropical e Sau´de Pu´ blica, Universidade Federal de Goia´s, Goiaˆnia, Goia´s, Brazil

Danilo Pires Resende
Laboató rio de Imunopatologia das Doenc,as Infecciosas, Instituto de Patologia Tropical e Saúde Pú blica, Universidade Federal de Goiàs, Goiânia, Goiàs, Brazil

André Kipnis
Laboató rio de Bacteriologia Molecular, Instituto de Patologia Tropical e Saúde Pú blica, Universidade Federal de Goiàs, Goiaˆnia, Goiàs, Brazil

Ana Paula Junqueira-Kipnis
Laboató rio de Imunopatologia das Doenc,as Infecciosas, Instituto de Patologia Tropical e Saúde Pú blica, Universidade Federal de Goiàs, Goiaˆnia, Goiàs, Brazil

Sujin Kang, Taeyun A. Lee, Eun A. Ra, Eunhye Lee, Hyun jin Choi, Sungwook Lee and Boyoun Park
Department of Systems biology, College of Life Science and Biotechnology, Yonsei University, Seoul, South Korea

Romina Soledad Coloccini, Dario Dilernia, Yanina Ghiglione, Gabriela Turk, Andrea Rubio, Horacio Salomo´ n and Marı´a A´ ngeles Pando
Instituto de Investigaciones Biome´dicas en Retrovirus y SIDA (INBIRS), Universidad de Buenos Aires-CONICET, Buenos Aires, Argentina

Natalia Laufer
Instituto de Investigaciones Biomédicas en Retrovirus y SIDA (INBIRS), Universidad de Buenos Aires-CONICET, Buenos Aires, Argentina
Hospital Juan A. Fernandez, Buenos Aires, Argentina

María Eugenia Socías, María Iné s Figueroa, Omar Sued and Pedro Cahn
Hospital Juan A. Fernandez, Buenos Aires, Argentina
Fundación Huésped, Buenos Aires, Argentina

Nathan Dissinger
Center for Retrovirus Research, The Ohio State University, Columbus, Ohio, United States of America

Department of Veterinary Biosciences, The Ohio State University, Columbus, Ohio, United States of America

Nikoloz Shkriabai
Center for Retrovirus Research, The Ohio State University, Columbus, Ohio, United States of America
College of Pharmacy, The Ohio State University, Columbus Ohio, United States of America

Sonja Hess
Proteome Exploration Laboratory, Beckman Institute, California Institute of Technology

Jacob Al-Saleem
Center for Retrovirus Research, The Ohio State University, Columbus, Ohio, United States of America
Department of Veterinary Biosciences, The Ohio State University, Columbus, Ohio, United States of America

Mamuka Kvaratskhelia
Center for Retrovirus Research, The Ohio State University, Columbus, Ohio, United States of America
College of Pharmacy, The Ohio State University, Columbus Ohio, United States of America

Patrick L. Green
Center for Retrovirus Research, The Ohio State University, Columbus, Ohio, United States of America
Department of Veterinary Biosciences, The Ohio State University, Columbus, Ohio, United States of America
Comprehensive Cancer Center and Solove Research Institute, Columbus, Ohio, United States of America
Department of Molecular Virology, Immunology, and Medical Genetics, The Ohio State University, Columbus, Ohio, United States of America
Pasadena, California, United States of America

Orla M. Finucane
Institute of Molecular Medicine, School of Medicine, Trinity Centre for Health Sciences, St. James Hospital, Dublin 8, Ireland
Nutrigenomics Research Group, School of Public Health & Population Science, UCD Conway Institute, University College Dublin, Dublin 4, Ireland

Clare M. Reynolds
Nutrigenomics Research Group, School of Public Health & Population Science, UCD Conway Institute, University College Dublin, Dublin 4, Ireland
Liggins Institute, University of Auckland, Auckland, New Zealand

Fiona C. McGillicuddy
Nutrigenomics Research Group, School of Public Health & Population Science, UCD Conway Institute, University College Dublin, Dublin 4, Ireland

Karen A. Harford
Nutrigenomics Research Group, School of Public Health & Population Science, UCD Conway Institute, University College Dublin, Dublin 4, Ireland

Martine Morrison
Nutrigenomics Research Group, School of Public Health & Population Science, UCD Conway Institute, University College Dublin, Dublin 4, Ireland

John Baugh
School of Medicine and Medical Science, UCD Conway Institute, University College Dublin, Dublin 4, Ireland

Helen M. Roche
Nutrigenomics Research Group, School of Public Health & Population Science, UCD Conway Institute, University College Dublin, Dublin 4, Ireland

Anuran Chatterjee, Anjali Sharma, Mian Chen, Robert Toy, Giorgio Mottola and Michael S. Conte
Cardiovascular Research Institute (CVRI) and Department of Surgery, University of California San Francisco, San Francisco, California

Marie Klinge Brimnes
Institute for Inflammation Research, Department of Infectious Diseases and Rheumatology, section 7521, Copenhagen University Hospital Rigshospitalet, Copenhagen, Denmark

Bjarke Endel Hansen
Institute for Inflammation Research, Department of Infectious Diseases and Rheumatology, section 7521, Copenhagen University Hospital Rigshospitalet, Copenhagen, Denmark
Immudex, Copenhagen, Denmark

Leif Kofoed Nielsen
Department of Technology, Faculty of Health and Technology, Metropolitan University College, Copenhagen, Denmark, Blood Bank, KI2034, Department of Clinical Immunology, Copenhagen University Hospital Rigshospitalet, Copenhagen, Denmark

Morten Hanefeld Dziegiel
Blood Bank, KI2034, Department of Clinical Immunology, Copenhagen University Hospital Rigshospitalet, Copenhagen, Denmark

Claus Henrik Nielsen
Institute for Inflammation Research, Department of Infectious Diseases and Rheumatology, section 7521, Copenhagen University Hospital Rigshospitalet, Copenhagen, Denmark

Index

www.ingramcontent.com/pod-product-compliance
Lightning Source LLC
Chambersburg PA
CBHW082023190326
41458CB00010B/3250